SURGERY

An Illustrated History

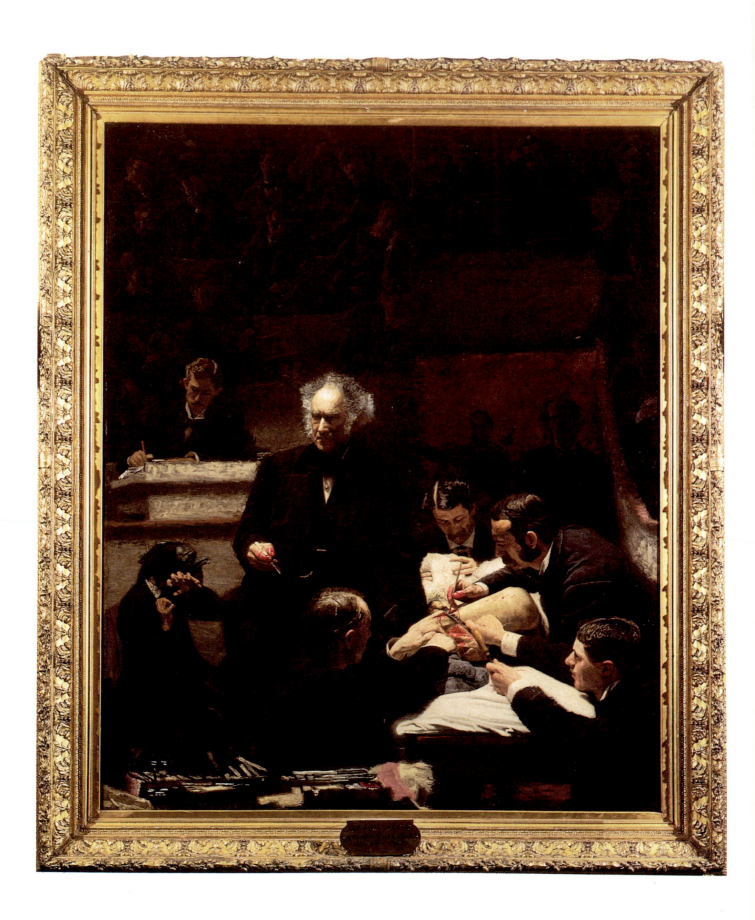

SURGERY
An Illustrated History

IRA M. RUTKOW, M.D., M.P.H., Dr.P.H.
Clinical Associate Professor of Surgery
University of Medicine and Dentistry of New Jersey
Newark, New Jersey

with 368 illustrations, including 102 in full color

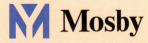
Mosby

St. Louis Baltimore Boston Chicago London Madrid Philadelphia Sydney Toronto

Published by Mosby–Year Book, Inc.
in Collaboration with Norman Publishing.

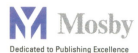

Publisher: George Stamathis
Editor: Susie Baxter
Developmental Editor: Anne Gunter
Project Manager: Patricia Tannian
Production Editor: Ann E. Rogers
Manuscript Editor: Mary McAuley
Designer: Jeanne Wolfgeher
Manufacturing Supervisor: Theresa Fuchs

Front Cover Photo: Courtesy of the University of Pennsylvania School of Medicine, Philadelphia

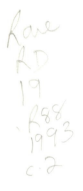

Printed in the United States of America
Composition by Clarinda Company
Printing/binding by Walsworth Publishing Co.

Mosby–Year Book, Inc.
11830 Westline Industrial Drive
St. Louis, Missouri 63146

Library of Congress Cataloging in Publication Data

Rutkow, Ira M.
   Surgery: An illustrated history / Ira M. Rutkow (1948-)
      p.   cm.
   Includes bibliographical references and index.
   ISBN 0-8016-6078-5
   I. Title.
   [DNLM: 1. Surgery—history.   WO 11.1 R977i 1993]
RD19.R88   1993
617'.09—dc20
DNLM/DLC   93-9820
   for Library of Congress   CIP

93 94 95 96 97 / 9 8 7 6 5 4 3 2 1

To my wonderful family:
my wife *Beth,*
our children *Lainie* and *Eric,*
my parents *Bea* and *Al Rutkow.*
They often wonder whether my mind is in
the present or somewhere in the past.

PREFACE

❧

It was a unique honor to be asked to write *Surgery: An Illustrated History*. To understand and set forth the past of one's profession is to better comprehend that discipline's present and anticipate its future. The opportunity to organize such a project was an undertaking that I approached with utmost respect for all my surgical forebears.

Whether the study and understanding of surgical history are important to the maturation and continued education of a surgeon remains a rhetorical question. On the other hand, it is hardly necessary to dwell on the heuristic value that an appreciation of history provides in developing adjunctive humanistic, literary, and philosophical tastes.

Clearly the practice of medicine is a lifelong learning process that should be an enjoyable and rewarding experience. I would argue that for a surgeon the understanding of surgical history will greatly contribute toward making this learning process more pleasurable and provide constant invigoration. To trace the evolution of what one does every day and to appreciate that work from a historical perspective are enviable goals. In reality there is no way to separate today's surgery and our own practice from the experiences of all the surgeons who have preceded us.

It is a magnificent adventure for the budding surgeon to recognize what he or she is currently learning within the context of past and present social, cultural, and economic institutions. The active but perhaps bored practitioner will find that historical studies of his or her profession, dealing, as they must, with all aspects of human culture, afford an excellent outlet for reappreciating previous clinical ideas and concepts. Most important, surgical history provides a ready escape from the mental stagnation, ennui, and enervation that are the consequence of today's drive toward ever-increasing specialization and from parochialism in the professional thought process. To study the past of our profession is fun, illuminating, humbling, and enormously useful. To be engrossed in surgical history is to accept an invitation to learn, a solicitation no surgeon should resist.

It has become evident that the writing of medical history must go beyond the simple understanding of a great doctor's life or the straightforward narration of the development of clinical or surgical techniques. It is no longer adequate to summarize medical history as if it were simply an unrelated series of contributions by individual physicians. There can be little dispute with the modern assumption that medical history involves not only biological content but socioeconomic and political elements as well. The flowering of medicine is a central theme in our human experience.

This modern approach to medical history seeks to place developments in medicine and surgery within the broad sweep of societal changes. However, this new social and medical history must include an appreciation of the basic medical sciences and clinical methods and concepts. Because of the technical intricacies of surgical operations, surgeons have knowledge and experience that place them in a unique position to assess historical facts and direct surgical historical inquiry.

Cognizant of the aforementioned concepts, I organized this book to have three major levels of historical content. The first level is intended to provide an understanding of significant developments in world history that were occurring during a particular surgical era. In this regard, time lines have been provided for the Middle Ages, the Renaissance, and the seventeenth, eighteenth, and nineteenth centuries, at the beginning of Chapters 7, 8, 9, 10, and 11. At a quick glance the reader is able to determine what well-known personalities were alive during a given period in the fields of science and technology, religion and philosophy, literature and theater, music, and the visual arts. In addition, each chapter begins with a short section on political events during particular eras or in particular countries. When such nonmedical historical information is made available, placing surgical history within the context of evolving world history becomes an easier task.

The second level concerns the important process of the professionalization of surgery. For many centuries surgical intervention was looked on disdainfully as little more than a frightening technical exercise that was just one of many therapeutic regimens available within the broad expanse of medicine. At what point was surgery no longer considered a mere physical craft but instead, a true science based on legitimate scientific research corroborated by independent clinical observations? A complex interaction of social, political, economic, and institutional factors contributed to this professionalization of the surgeon and his skills. How did this surgical independence occur? Did it pass from one European country to the next, or was it more of an ongoing process that engulfed all of European medicine at the same time? Did surgeons in the United States go through the same phases of surgical maturation that their European peers experienced?

What of the sharp division between physician and surgeon before the modern era? Physicians were always regarded as a university-educated elite within the confines of medicine. Conversely, surgeons and barber-surgeons were considered uneducated craftsmen. They learned their skills by serving as apprentices to the guild masters. When did these centuries-old arrangements end and surgery assume its own social and hierarchical structure within the whole of medicine? Most important, when did the concept of surgical specialization become an integral part of surgical care?

The third historical level consists of a detailed understanding of the lives of the great surgeons. Although biographies alone do not constitute an adequate medical history, there is an understandable thrill in reading about the surgical experiences of such renowned figures as Vesalius, Paré, Pott, Dupuytren, Lister, Billroth, Halsted, and Kocher. Accordingly, the section on medicine and surgery within each time line contains the names of the surgeons for whom biographical data are presented in that particular chapter. Almost 1000 biographical entries invest the daily lives and professional activities of these individuals with new meaning.

Because the use of eponyms remains widespread in the modern practice of surgery, I have made a deliberate attempt to incorporate as many surgical eponyms as possible into the numerous surgical biographies. To accomplish this I have used information from *Stedman's Medical Dictionary,* Skinner's *The Origin of Medical Terms,* and Kelly's *Encyclopedia of Medical Sources.*

The publication of *Surgery: An Illustrated History* marks the personal culmination of many years of book collecting and historical research both in the United States and in Europe. The actual first writing of the text took place from December 1990 through August 1991. Revision of the manuscript along with selection of illustrations was concluded by June 1992.

Although in writing this text I consulted primary works, most of my sources have been secondary, or the writing of others. Thus I owe a special debt of gratitude to the many physicians and surgeons in the past who researched and authored works on surgical history. I drew inspiration from the excellent tradition established by such renowned surgeon-historians as Bick, Billings, Cope, Fergusson, Gross, Gurlt, Hirschberg, Kelly, Leonardo, Malgaigne, Mumford, Portal, Ravitch, Ricci, Smith, South, Thoms, Trendelenburg, Wangensteen, Whipple, Wright, Zimmerman, and countless others.

Of the many works listed in the bibliography, I have used most heavily the following books for information: Billings's chapter, "The History and Literature of Surgery," in Dennis's *System of Surgery* (1876); Buck's *The Growth of Medicine from the Earliest Times to about 1800* (1917) and *The Dawn of Medicine* (1920); Fisher's discussion of the history of surgery in Ashhurst's *International Encyclopedia of Surgery* (1881); Garrison's *An Introduction to the History of Medicine* (1929); Gelfand's *Professionalizing Modern Medicine* (1980); Haeger's *Illustrated History of Surgery* (1988); Hurwitz and Degenshein's *Milestones in Modern Surgery* (1958); Leonardo's *History of Surgery* (1943) and *Lives of Master Surgeons* (1948); Lyons and Petrucelli's *Medicine: An Illustrated History* (1978); Meade's *Introduction to the History of General Surgery* (1968); Miles's *The Edinburgh School of Surgery before Lister* (1918); Norman's edition of *Morton's Medical Bibliography* (1991); Parker's *The Early History of Surgery in Great Britain* (1920); and Zimmerman and Veith's *Great Ideas in the History of Surgery* (1961). Although the bulk of my work represents not original historical research but, more properly, the collation of past writings on surgical history, I accept responsibility for any factual error or unsubstantiated opinion.

Many individuals are owed a great debt of gratitude for their assistance. Among these are Tom Horrocks, Jean Carr, and Kevin Crawford of the Historical Collections at the Library of the College of Physicians of Philadelphia, and Robin Siegel of CentraState Medical Center in Freehold, New Jersey. I must extend a special thank you to my business partner, Alan Robbins, of The Hernia Center and to our office manager, Susan Disbrow, for allowing me the necessary time to complete this project.

To the Mosby staff go my heartfelt thanks, in particular, to George Stamathis and Terry Van Schaik for aiding me during the conception of this book and to my editor, Susie Baxter, and her developmental assistant, Anne Gunter, for their sage advice. To my production editor Ann Rogers, manuscript editor Mary McAuley, and book designer Jeanne Wolfgeher I am most grateful. To the many other unnamed individuals involved in the production and marketing of this book I also wish to acknowledge my gratitude.

My most sincere thanks are extended to Jeremy Norman for his in-depth review of the manuscript and assistance in determining which illustrations would best serve this work. His expertise in the field of rare medical-book collecting combined with a scholar's understanding of what constitutes masterful medical and surgical history cannot be too strongly stressed. Jeremy's role in authoring most of the legends for the illustrations must also be acknowledged. Finally, to Martha Steele, for her unceasing and always cheerful assistance in obtaining the actual illustrations along with necessary documentation to permit their use, I remain forever grateful.

Ira M. Rutkow
Marlboro, New Jersey

CONTENTS

12
THE TWENTIETH CENTURY   505

BIBLIOGRAPHY   535

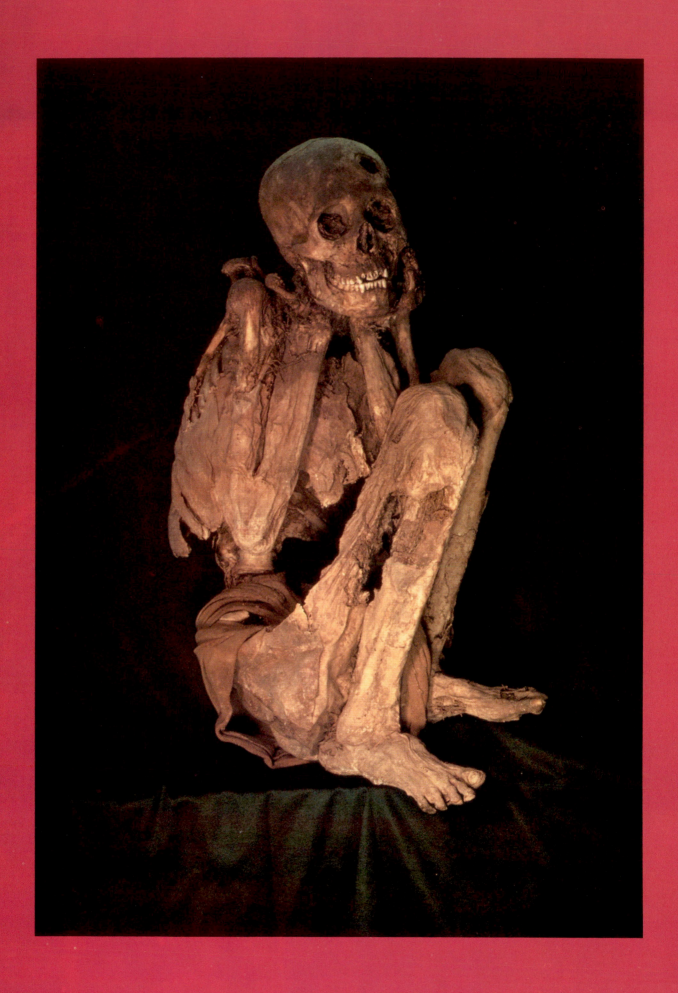

CHAPTER 1

PRESCIENTIFIC AND PRIMITIVE SURGERY

❧

Surgery, derived from the Greek *cheir* (hand) and *ergon* (to work) and the Latin *chirurgia,* is defined as "the treatment of disease, injury, or deformity by manual or instrumental operations, as the removal of diseased parts of tissue by cutting." The word *chirurgeon,* or surgeon, known since the 1300s, was probably introduced during the linguistic period called Middle English (1150-1475).

Although there is no way of knowing when the earliest surgical operations were performed, it is not unreasonable to assume that frequent attempts at "surgery" were completed by our most distant prehistoric ancestors. The attempt to remedy day-to-day external discomforts by means of manual manipulations must have been among the evolutionary efforts of the human species. Presumably the earliest attempts at surgery were mainly devoted to the treatment of injuries and included procedures to alleviate nuisances, such as removing splinters, piercing boils or blisters, treating burns, and excising traumatized tissue.

Unfortunately archeologists who have studied Paleolithic (Old Stone Age, e.g., Cro-Magnon and Neanderthal) humans can tell us little about how these surgical operations were conducted. The practices of numerous present-day nonindustrialized societies in which relatively primitive surgical operations continue to be performed provide indirect information about surgical feats accomplished by early humans. Among these contemporary methods are bloodletting (via scarification, cupping, venesection, or leeching), sex organ and decorative mutilation, hemostasis and counterirritation, treatment of dislocations and fractures, amputations, and trephination.

Trephination remains the earliest example of actual major surgery. That prehistoric humans, using the most rudimentary surgical instruments, were able to bore open a human skull—and that the patient survived—is an incredible medical achievement. When and how skull boring originated are matters of scientific conjecture. However, skulls from the Mesolithic (Middle Stone Age) cultural period have been found to have round depressions suggestive of primitive trephination efforts, which would date initial efforts at trephination at 10,000 to 5000 B.C.

Certainly, since many Neolithic (New Stone Age) trephinated skulls have been found in Western Europe and Asia, it can be stated that trephination was widely used by 3000 to 2000 B.C., when humans were developing polished stone tools and weapons, raising cattle, and laying the basic technological and social foundations of modern civilization.

That trephination was practiced throughout the civilized world has been confirmed in the discovery of more than 10,000 well-preserved mummies from pre-Inca Peru (dating back to 2000 B.C.): more than 6% of these mummies demonstrate evidence of trephination. In many instances the skull defects are multiple, ranging from two to a record of seven in a single patient. They are placed

1. *Facing page,* Peruvian trephination subject, seated. Circa A.D. 400. *(Warren Museum, Harvard Medical School.)*

all over the cranium, including suture lines, and frequently expose large segments of the superior longitudinal sinus. The defects can be quite large, up to 7 by 11 centimeters.

Why would Stone Age humans resort to trephination? There is little archeological evidence to suggest that this practice was used for the treatment of diseases such as osteomyelitis or syphilitic lesions of the cranium: most trephinations were performed on intact skulls with no prior signs of violence. It is more likely that trephinations were carried out for spiritual or magical reasons and used in cases of mental illness, epilepsy, or headache.

That magic and evil spirits can live in one's head is an ancient superstition still with us today. In primitive, prescientific times a hole drilled in the head could have been perceived as a way for these evil spirits to escape, and the weak and infirm may have undergone trephination as a possible means of relieving their disabilities by ridding themselves of evil spirits. It has even been speculated that leaders of a clan could have had round holes prophylactically drilled in their skulls, through which, they presumably believed, evil vapors could continually escape. If they survived this operation and were thought to be free of the evil spirits that plagued their followers, the leaders would have possessed a magical power over their people.

Because of the smooth edges of many trephination defects, it has been estimated that at least 50% of all individuals survived the operation. How, then, was trephination accomplished? A number of different methods have been suggested, all of which, in this preanesthetic era, would have required a stoic patient. The simplest but crudest method would have been simply to scrape a hole in the cranium, using a sharpened rock or shell. A second method would have required a circular cut in the bone with a flint or obsidian knife. Boring a series of holes in a circular or oval pattern and later cutting through the separating partitions to join the holes would have been another possible scheme. Finally, a crude hammer and chisel could have been used to create four grooves in a cross

2. Trephined skulls, showing a variety of shapes and sizes of skull openings. Some of the trephinations were accomplished by boring a series of small holes in a circular pattern. The pattern of crude intersecting grooves around the opening on one skull indicates that the trephination was probably made by a hammer and chisel. *(Mütter Museum, College of Physicians of Philadelphia.)*

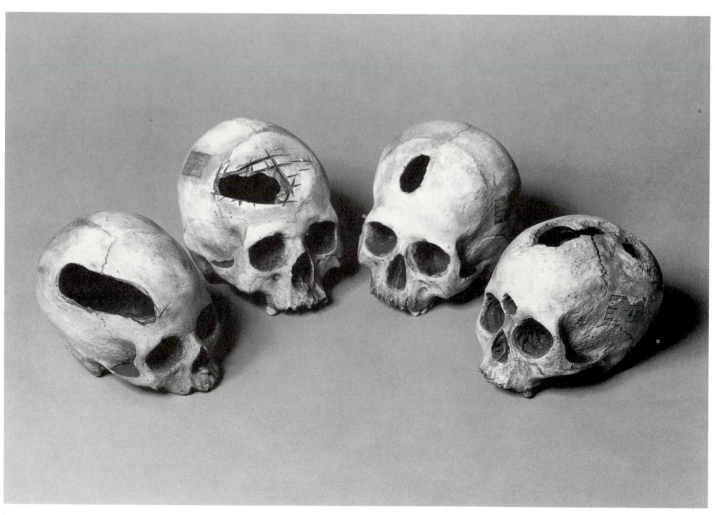

shape so that the square piece of center bone could then be lifted out. This button of bone, also called a rondelle, was frequently worn as an amulet or used in magic or religious ceremonies to ward off evil spirits.

Technical difficulties and ensuing complications certainly must have tested the ingenuity of prehistoric humans. The first stage of incision required an ability to control bleeding. What the prehistoric surgeon used is conjectural, but various possibilities were available, including bandages, hemostatic plants, pressure tamponade, and cautery. At the conclusion of the procedure a number of options had to be considered. Should the opening be covered with a hard substance such as gourd, shell, or bone, or should it be left open? If it were left open, would the individual suffer damage to the brain? Infection is not likely to have been a serious problem, since communities were small and for the most part unpolluted. Was a primitive form of anesthesia available? Much remains unknown, but it is likely that prehistoric surgeons had at their disposal various herbs and plant extracts that would have decreased pain.

Trephination appears to have been conducted for different reasons in different locales. The South American Incas performed trephination primarily for spiritual, magical, and religious reasons. In Europe, trephination appears to have been practiced most frequently in areas where weapons that produced skull fractures were used. Such injuries could have been associated with patient distress or bizarre behavior. For traumatic injuries, it has been estimated, little more than 30 minutes would have been required to complete a trephination. Empirical evidence eventually must have shown the prehistoric surgeon that removal of depressed bone fragments and wounded tissue could possibly restore an individual's health.

Neolithic surgeons probably carried out other surgical operations apart from trephination; however, little archeological evidence of such operations exists. Pictures in prehistoric caves in Europe depict human hands with missing fingers. Whether these represent amputations carried out for sacrificial or propitiatory rites or more mundane matters such as trauma and frostbite remains unknown.

Although surgery has continued to advance in a natural evolutionary course, attitudes and knowledge about the craft of surgery in many cultures in the modern world remain prescientific and primitive. In most instances the surgical authority in primitive cultures resides in a single individual who has absolute authority under a supernatural aegis. The unique surgical methods of these aboriginal tribes provide an ongoing reflection of the accomplishments of prehistoric humans.

The surgical achievements of prehistoric and primitive humans are unquestionably impressive in view of their lack of knowledge of wound healing, anatomy, physiology, and basic instrumentation. Although the performance of trephination or digital amputation for magical or spiritual reasons may be considered spurious, supernatural, and certainly antiscientific, there is little doubt that certain patients were aided by the primitive surgeon's technical skills. A combination of this technical skill, empirical information, and confidence in the surgeon probably brought about successful restoration of health in many cases of trauma and illness.

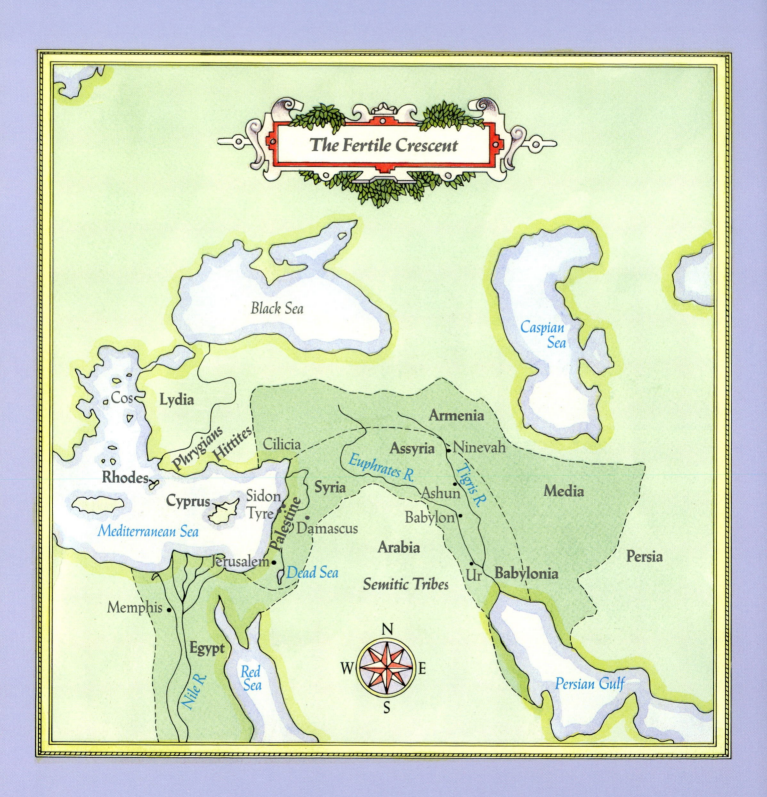

The Fertile Crescent

Black Sea

Caspian Sea

Cos

Lydia

Phrygians

Hittites

Cilicia

Armenia

Assyria

Ninevah

Euphrates R.

Tigris R.

Media

Rhodes

Cyprus

Sidon
Tyre

Palestine

Syria

Ashun

Babylon

Persia

Mediterranean Sea

Damascus

Arabia

Jerusalem

Dead Sea

Semitic Tribes

Ur

Babylonia

Memphis

Egypt

Nile R.

Red
Sea

Persian Gulf

N
W E
S

CHAPTER 2
ANCIENT CIVILIZATIONS

MESOPOTAMIANS

The late Neolithic and early Bronze ages, a period from about 3500 B.C. to 750 B.C. that varied widely in different areas, was characterized by the alloying of copper with tin to produce tools and weapons. During that time a succession of powerful tribes appeared in Southwest Asia. This region between the Tigris and Euphrates rivers, known as Mesopotamia, would become the root area of modern Western civilization. The Fertile Crescent, tilled for wild wheat and barley for more than 10,000 years, attracted nomads from the fringes of the Arabian desert and mountain tribes from the north and east. Here Western civilization's initial attempts were made to develop a system of writing and construct cities.

The most prominent early inhabitants of the region were the Sumerians in their city-state of Sumer, from whom originated the world's oldest written language, cuneiform, probably around 3500 B.C. For almost 2000 years many dynastics flourished at Sumer, but the Sumerians were gradually absorbed into the superior culture of the Semitic Akkadians to the south. With the rise of the great Akkadian ruler Sargon of Agade (circa 2400 B.C.) and his city-state of Akkad, the world's first empire came into existence.

The center of another major civilization in Mesopotamia was Babylon, a sizable city as early as 4000 B.C. Cuneiform inscriptions describe it as an important center during the reign of Sargon. Babylon's population was essentially Amorite, and the most reknowned ruler of the many early Babylonian dynasties was Hammurabi (1958–1916 B.C.). Babylon fell successively to the Assyrians, Chaldeans, and Persians, and to the Greeks under Alexander the Great (356–323 B.C.).

The development of Babylonian medicine and surgery culminated during the age of the Chaldean Empire (625–539 B.C.). The Chaldeans, a late Babylonian people, found their zenith under King Nebuchadnezzar (606–562 B.C.), who conquered Jerusalem, destroyed King Solomon's temple, and forced the Jews into exile.

The culture of ancient Mesopotamia was quite complex. The city-states were ruled by priest-kings, and inequality of social classes was a fundamental principle of Babylonian law. A basic tenet of criminal jurisprudence was retaliation. If a surgeon performed an operation on a patient who died as a result of the procedure or suffered other losses, the physician's own fingers were cut off in retribution.

Medicine was highly respected by the ancient Babylonians. Many of the more than 30,000 excavated cuneiform tablets relate to the healing arts. On one of them is the world's first prescription; another contains the shield of a surgeon, Urlugaledin (circa 2300 B.C.), which displays two knives together with gods and herbs. In most instances diseases were presumed to be caused by evil spirits and

3. *Facing page,* Map of the Fertile Crescent in the Pre-Christian Era. Medicine and surgery were significantly advanced by the ancient Babylonians. *(From Donahue MP: Nursing: the finest art: an illustrated history, St Louis, 1985, Mosby.)*

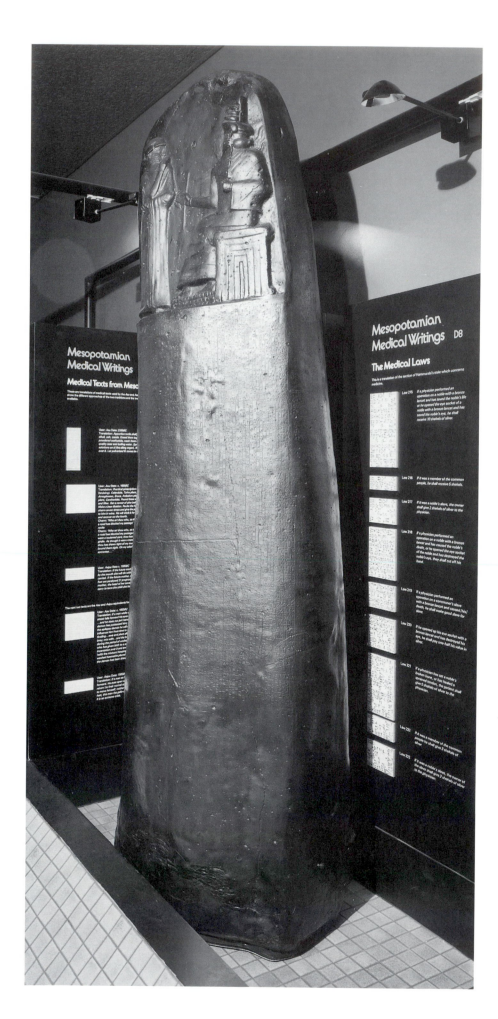

4. This black diorite stele, nearly 8 feet tall, has engraved around it in Assyrian cuneiform symbols the 282 laws of King Hammurabi's Code. Several of the laws concern the practice of surgery. At the top of the stone Hammurabi is shown receiving the laws from the sun god, Shamash. The stone was found broken by a French expedition in 1901. The stone was reassembled, the code translated, and the translation published within a year of discovery. It is now preserved in the Louvre. *(Reproduced by permission of the Trustees of the Science Museum, London; 1053/82.)*

cosmic demons. Consequently cures were obtained with the assistance of astrologers and priests and their surrogates. Even this early in the development of medicine and surgery, society made the distinction between the learned physician who worked with books and theories to prescribe remedies and the usually illiterate but highly practical surgeon who worked with his hands. Perceived as craftsmen or technicians rather than men of learning, surgeons were viewed prejudicially as an inferior caste.

The most important legacy from Assyro-Babylonian medicine is the Code of Hammurabi. Although no specific cuneiform tablets devoted solely to surgery have been found, many of the rules in Hammurabi's code concern the outcome of operations. Thus it can be assumed that surgical therapy was carried out. The first statements regarding surgical instrumentation can be found in the Code of Hammurabi. It would appear that a certain kind of bronze was used in the manufacturing of surgical knives, but no archeological evidence of such tools remains. Guidelines for surgical therapy, as stated in the code, included the following:

> If a physician shall cause on anyone a severe operation wound with a bronze operating-knife and cure him, or if he shall open a tumor (abscess or cavity) with a bronze operating-knife and save the eye, he shall have ten shekels of silver; if it is a slave, his owner shall pay two shekels of silver to the physician.
>
> If a physician shall make a severe wound with the bronze operating-knife and kill him, or shall open a growth with a bronze operating-knife and destroy his eye, his hands shall be cut off.
>
> If a physician shall make a severe wound with a bronze operating-knife on the slave of a freed man and kill him, he shall replace the slave with another slave. If he shall open an abscess (growth, tumor, cavity) with a bronze operating-knife and destroy the eye, he shall pay the half of the value of the slave.
>
> If a physician shall heal a broken bone or cure diseased bowels, he shall receive five shekels of silver; if it is a matter of a freed slave, he shall pay three shekels of silver; but if a slave, then the master of the slave shall give to the physician two shekels of silver.

The 282 provisions of Hammurabi have proven to be the first set of laws governing the practice of medicine and surgery. Despite such extensive regulations, little is known of actual Babylonian surgical techniques. Archeologists have been able to contribute little to current understanding because almost all traces of Babylonian culture and civilization were destroyed by wars.

JEWS

Closely connected in spirit and substance with Assyro-Babylonian and Sumerian-Semitic surgery is the surgery of the ancient Jews. After their Assyrian and Babylonian captivities (722 B.C. and 604 B.C., respectively), the Jews practiced medicine that was closely aligned with the thoughts and beliefs of the great dynasties of Mesopotamia. The Jews continued to believe that diseases were part of divine punishment and that proper treatment for those afflicted was to apply to their priests. Through appropriate prayers and religious ceremonies ailments could be cured. Although in biblical times a class of professional physicians practiced medicine, the priestly caste discouraged the people from seeking advice outside the temples. An obviously antagonistic relationship among the various groups of healers was aggravated by religious beliefs and superstitions, as is evident in the sarcasm invoked in a biblical story regarding King Asa's illness and death:

> And in the thirty and ninth year of his reign Asa was diseased in his feet; his disease was exceeding great; yet in his disease he sought not to the Lord, but to the physicians.
>
> And Asa slept with his fathers, and died in the one and fortieth year of his reign.
> (2 Chronicles 16:12-13.)

Biblical physicians, a group separate from the priests, were known as "rophe." The rophe participated in both medicine and surgery, whereas barbers and other uneducated castes were allowed to engage in the practice of bloodletting and other minor surgical procedures. The doctors who limited themselves entirely to surgical procedures were referred to as "uman."

The principal sources of knowledge concerning ancient Jewish surgery are the Pentateuch (Torah), that is, the Five Books of Moses (Genesis, Exodus, Leviticus, Numbers, and Deuteronomy), and the Talmud. The former contains written laws, whereas the latter consists of those transmitted by oral tradition.

The Five Books were first collected in the time of King Solomon (circa 1000 B.C.), although Moses himself lived six centuries earlier. Around the time of Solomon, the Iron Age—the archeological phase from around 1000 B.C. to the beginning of the Christian Era—was marked by a change in technology that resulted from the discovery of iron smelting. The use of iron, an improvement over the previously employed copper and bronze, would have an important effect on surgical instrumentation.

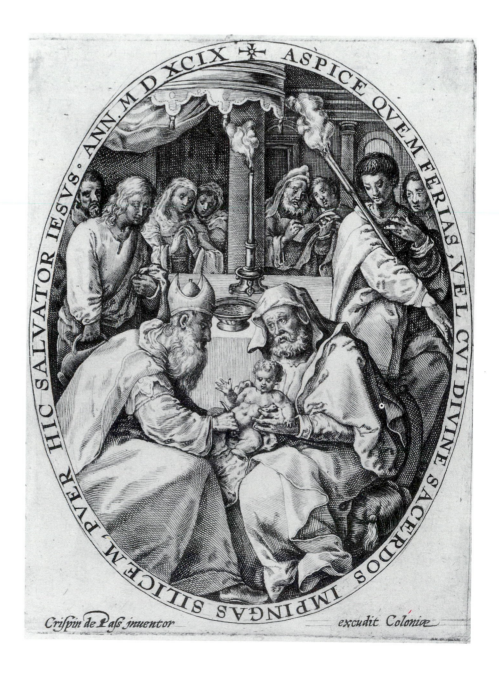

5. Surgery as a ritual and social event: the ceremony of circumcision is depicted in this engraving, dated 1599, by the Dutch artist Crispin de Passe the Elder. *(Charles M. Lea Collection, Philadelphia Museum of Art.)*

The earliest operation described by the Jews was circumcision. According to the Torah, the first religious circumcision, in which a sharp stone was used as a knife, was performed on Abraham (circa 1900 B.C.) when he was 90 years old:

> And God said unto Abraham: "And as for thee, thou shalt keep My covenant, thou and thy seed after thee throughout their generations.
> This is My covenant, which ye shall keep, between Me and you and thy seed after thee: every male among you shall be circumcised.
> And ye shall be circumcised in the flesh of your foreskin; and it shall be a token of a covenant betwixt Me and you.
> And he that is eight days old shall be circumcised among you, every male throughout your generations, he that is born in the house, or bought with money of any foreigner, that is not of thy seed.
> He that is born in thy house, and he that is bought with thy money, must need be circumcised; and My covenant shall be in your flesh for an everlasting covenant.
> And the uncircumcised male who is not circumcised in the flesh of his foreskin, that soul shall be cut off from his people; he hath broken My covenant.
>
> (Genesis 17:9-14.)

Other fleeting references to religious circumcision can be found, especially relative to instrumentation:

> Then Zipporah took a flint and cut off the foreskin of her son . . .
>
> (Exodus 4:25.)

> At that time the Lord said unto Joshua: Make thee knives of flint, and circumcise again the children of Israel the second time.
> And Joshua made him knives of flint, and circumcised the children of Israel at Gibeath-ha-araloth.
>
> (Joshua 5:2-3.)

The earliest known and most blatant use of surgery as an instrument of political and moral revenge is found in the story of Dinah and her brothers, the siblings of Jacob. Dinah was raped by Shechem, a Hivite. Subsequently Shechem fell in love with her and asked his father, Hamor, to secure Dinah as his wife. Hamor spoke with Jacob and his sons, imploring them to allow Dinah to become his daughter-in-law. The father and brothers, knowing the rigors of circumcision and its attendant postoperative pain, responded:

> ". . . We cannot do this thing, to give our sister to one that is uncircumcised; for that were a reproach unto us.
> Only on this condition will we consent unto you: if ye will be as we are, that every male of you be circumcised; then will we give our daughters unto you, and we will take your daughters to us, and we will dwell with you, and we will become one people.
> But if ye will not hearken unto us, to be circumcised; then will we take our daughters, and we will be gone."
> And their words pleased Hamor, and Shechem . . .
> And Hamor and Shechem . . . came unto the gate of their city, and spoke with the men of their city . . .
> Only on this condition will the men consent unto us to dwell with us, to become one people, if every male among us be circumcised, as they are circumcised . . .
> Shall not their cattle and their substance and all their beasts be ours? Only let us consent unto them . . .
> And unto Hamor and unto Shechem . . . all that went out of the gate of his city; and every male was circumcised . . .
> And it came to pass on the third day, when they were in pain, that two of the sons of Jacob . . . took each man his sword, and came upon the city unawares, and slew all the males.
> And they slew Hamor and Shechem his son with the edge of the sword, and took Dinah out of Shechem's house, and went forth.
> The sons of Jacob came upon the slain, and spoiled the city, because they had defiled their sister.
>
> (Genesis 34:14-27.)

Another common operation among Jews in the time of the Old Testament was the earlobe perforation, in which an awl was used as the surgical instrument. Earlobe perforation was performed when a Jewish slave, after serving his master for 6 years, refused his freedom. According to law, the master was required to respond as follows:

> . . . then thou shalt take an awl, and thrust it through his ear and into the door, and he shall be thy bondman for ever . . .
>
> (Deuteronomy 15:17.)

Although specific surgical operations other than circumcision and earlobe perforation are not discussed in the Old Testament, a roller-bandage for fractures is referred to as follows:

> Son of man, I have broken the arm of Pharaoh king of Egypt; and, lo, it hath not been bound up to be healed, to put a roller, that it be bound up and wax strong, that it hold the sword.
>
> (Ezekiel 30:21.)

Wounds were dressed, as in all ancient civilizations, with oil, wine, and balsams prepared as therapeutic ointments:

> . . . But wounds, and bruises, and festering sores: they have not been pressed, neither bound up, neither mollified with oil.
>
> (Isaiah 1:6.)

A rich collection of surgical lore is found in the Talmud. This mass of verbal tradition (Mishna) with interpretations and commentaries (Gemara) began to accumulate after the Babylonian captivity. The information was later codified in the Jerusalem and Babylonian Talmuds (A.D. 370–390 and A.D. 352–427, respectively). The information in these books provides a more definite and detailed characterization of surgical practices than does the half-legendary narrative of the Bible.

The Talmud discusses various surgical procedures, including how to suture wounds and clean traumatized edges, methods for dealing with imperforate anus, how to determine whether bleeding emanates from the uterus or only from the vagina, the advantages of lessening pain during a surgical procedure, reduction of dislocations, amputations and the use of wooden prostheses, attempts to repair defects by replacing or restoring the cranial bones, cesarean section, excision of the spleen, and detailed instructions concerning the use of artificial teeth constructed of hard wood or metal, especially gold. A veterinary surgeon is also mentioned in the Talmud.

EGYPTIANS

The ancient history of Egypt can be divided into a number of major periods. Around 3500 B.C. the two kingdoms of Upper and Lower Egypt were united under King Menes. The subsequent millennium (first through fifth dynasties) has become known as the Old Kingdom. The period of the fourth dynasty is termed the Pyramid Age, and during the reign of Cheops (circa 2900 B.C.) the Great Pyramid was built in Gizeh.

After the Pyramid Age royal authority rapidly declined, primarily because the fabulously wealthy nobles and priests of endowed temples negated any efforts to preserve centralized administration by usurping those very functions. The triumph of the forces of particularism and parochialism marked the Feudal Age (circa 2500–2200 B.C., the sixth through tenth dynasties).

During the eleventh and twelfth dynasties (2200–1800 B.C.) the Middle Kingdom was established with the restoration of royal authority and centralized government. Intefo, the founder of the eleventh dynasty, extended his rule with the city of Thebes as a nucleus. The succeeding dynasty of Amenemhet I completed the task of royal reconstruction in an era that has also been called the "Classical Age" because of its reinvigoration of learning and the prominent place that medicine held.

In about 1800 B.C. Egypt was conquered by the Hyksos, who came from Asia Minor. Their use of cavalry and archers gave them a great tactical advantage, which enabled them to conquer the land of the Nile with comparative ease. They also introduced the horse to Egyptian culture. The Hyksos held sway for nearly 200 years, and many of their gods and customs merged into Egyptian life.

Hyksos domination was finally shattered by Ahmose, founder of the eighteenth dynasty (circa 1580 B.C.), and his immediate successor, Amenhotep I. With the establishment of the New Kingdom (1580–1200 B.C.) Egypt entered one of its most spectacular and brilliant eras. In 1501 B.C. Queen Hatshepsut ascended the throne. The first female ruler of all Egypt, Queen Hatshepsut greatly enhanced the power and influence of her country. Her consort, Thutmose III, became ruler in his own right in 1479 B.C. He extended Egyptian dominance over much of the known world while Babylonia languished under Kassite domination and Assyria was still in its infancy. Among his most lasting monuments is the temple of Karnak.

The reign of Amenhotep III (1412–1376 B.C.) was a period of luxury and prodigious extravagance. He was succeeded by his son, Amenhotep IV, who married Queen Nefertiti. Of the succeeding rulers of the eighteenth dynasty much interest has been centered on Amenhotep IV's son-in-law and successor, Tutankhamen (also, *Tutankhaten*) (circa 1300 B.C.). The discovery in 1922 of his sealed tomb filled with magnificent jewelry, splendid furniture, and other objects of art proved an outstanding contribution to Egyptology.

After Tutankhamen's rule power shifted back to a dynasty of Hyksos derivation. The biblical story of the enslavement of the Jews probably dates from this period. Temporary recovery of the power and prestige of the kingdom came during the nineteenth dynasty in the reign of Ramses II (1300–1233 B.C.), who was the builder of the great temple of Abu Simbel and may have been pharaoh during the Exodus.

As the power of Ramses declined, the vast kingdom began to fall apart. Foreign possessions were irretrievably lost, and internecine strife produced total chaos. Consequently Egypt fell easy prey to the hegemony of Assyria and Persia. Liberation from Persian rule was promptly followed by incorporation into the empire of Alexander the Great. With the division of Alexander's empire in 301 B.C. Egypt came under the rule of a Greco-Egyptian dynasty started by Ptolemy I (367–285 B.C.), who served as King of Egypt. He extended the empire to Cyrene, Crete, and Cyprus and made Egypt a great commercial nation. Autonomy was maintained until the defeat of the forces of Marcus Antonius (83–30 B.C.) and his wife, Cleopatra VII (69–30 B.C.), last of the Ptolemaic leaders, at the battle of Actium (31 B.C.). This defeat firmly established Roman rule in the land of the Nile.

Egyptian Surgery

Most current knowledge of Egyptian surgery is obtained from several ancient papyruses. In addition, hieroglyphics found on Egyptian ruins furnish further information, as do the comments of later Greek and Roman writers. The Egyptians learned quite early to write on papyrus, and it is believed that during the Old Kingdom the first treatises on surgery (circa 2900 B.C.) were being completed. Speculation exists that the author of one such text may have been no less a personage than Imhotep. He was grand vizier, architect, and physician to King Zoser (2980–2900 B.C.). Such was the fame of Imhotep that his status was eventually elevated to that of a god, and he served as one of the principal deities of healing. Imhotep was worshipped for hundreds of years, and his essence was incorporated into the Greek god Asclepios and the Roman counterpart, Aesculapius.

Numerous examples of other Egyptian physicians in the Old Kingdom are known; this suggests the presence of an organization of the medical profession almost 5000 years ago. From the same period, the world's oldest known depiction of a surgical operation, a circumcision, has been found drawn into the doorpost of a royal tomb at Memphis.

The two most renowned surgical papyruses are named for Georg Ebers (1837-1898), a German antiquities professor, and Edwin Smith (1822-1906), an American Egyptologist. The Ebers papyrus is the longest of all known ancient papyruses and has been precisely dated to 1550 B.C. Mainly concerned with the naming of ailments without diagnostic description, the Ebers papyrus is regarded as a compilation of recipes for treatment interspersed with magical spells and religious chants.

According to the Ebers papyrus, every treatment had to be followed by prayers and verbal charms addressed to an appropriate god. Most of this ancient text is devoted to the medicinal treatment of disease; surgical interference was limited to instructions for minor operations. The bites of crocodiles or men were cured by the placement of raw meat. At least two remedies existed for burns, including the application of either "a frog warmed in oil" or "goat dung in yeast that is fermenting." A number of ointments were used in the extraction of splinters, including "male and female semen" and the "skull of the shadfish, cooked in oil." Treatment of wounds included exact methods of applying dressings with bandages of linen soaked in honey and myrrh; removal of the dressings in 4 days was required.

6. The surgical practice of circumcision as both ceremony and ritual seems to have originated for hygienic reasons in Egypt. This carving, circa 2500 B.C., was found in the Sakkara cemetery at Memphis, once the home of Imhotep, the great physician, sage, and architect. The scene suggests that circumcision operations might have been undertaken in a manner of "mass production." This carved relief is the earliest known pictorial representation of a surgical operation. *(Wellcome Institute Library, London.)*

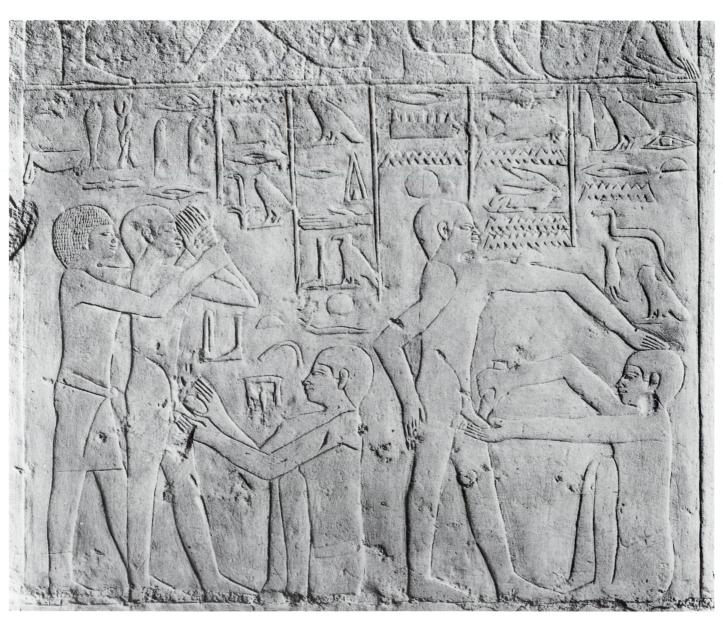

Actual operative surgery often involved the use of a cautery, whereas abscesses and various tumors (i.e., sebaceous cysts, lipomas, and the like) were provided such different treatments as the following:

> When thou comest upon a tumor of the flesh in any part of the body of a person and thou dost find it like skin on his flesh; it is moist; it moves under thy fingers save when thy fingers are held still, then its movement is caused by thy fingers. So shalt thou say: "It is a tumor of the flesh, I will treat the disease since I will try to cure it with fire, as the metal-worker cures."

> When thou findest a purulent swelling with the apex elevated, sharply defined and of a rounded form, then sayest thou, "It is a purulent tumor which is growing in the flesh. I must treat the disease with a knife."

> When thou findest a fatty growth in the neck, and findest it like an abscess of the flesh and soft to the fingers, then sayest thou, "He has a fatty growth on his neck. I will treat the disease with the knife, paying heed to the vessels."

Experience taught practitioners that not all tumors were amenable to incision or excision:

> When thou meetest a large tumor of the God Xensu in any part of the limb of a person, it is loathsome and suffers many pustules to come forth; something arises therein as though wind were in it, causing irritation. The tumor calls with a loud voice to thee: "Is it not like the most loathsome of pustules?" It mottles the skin and makes figures. All the limbs are like those which are affected. Then say thou: "It is a tumor of the God Xensu. Do thou nothing there against."

The most important document in the study of ancient Egyptian surgery has been the Edwin Smith papyrus. It was acquired at Thebes in 1862 but not fully deciphered and translated until 1930. Although its age has been a matter of some controversy, the actual Smith papyrus itself (circa 1600 B.C.) is generally accepted to be at least a generation older than the Ebers papyrus. However, the Smith papyrus is believed to be a copy of another manuscript first written circa 3000 B.C.

The original text (circa 3000 B.C.) of the world's oldest known surgical treatise dates back to the Old Kingdom and appears to have been authored by an individual with an avid interest in surgery. Some centuries later it was copied, presumably by another "surgeon." Fortunately that writer added a series of 69 "glosses," or explanations. These constitute a short dictionary of terms that were distributed throughout the original treatise, which was already so old in 2600 B.C. that many of these terms were no longer used, were totally incomprehensible, and required explanation.

The Smith papyrus was apparently rewritten from the second-generation copy by a scribe who was not a "surgeon." This individual had a beautiful cursive writing style but was unfamiliar with the factual text and made many errors, corrections, and omissions. Unlike other medical papyruses, the Smith text deals strictly with surgical problems. It does not include magical spells or charms, and incantations and prescriptions are kept to a minimum. Unfortunately the work, systematically arranged like a textbook of surgery, remains incomplete. The 48 cases commence with the skull and overlying soft tissue and brain (cases 1 to 10) and proceed downward by way of the nose (cases 11 to 14), face and ears (cases 15 to 27), throat and neck (cases 28 to 33), clavicle (cases 34 and 35), humerus (cases 35 to 38), thorax, sternum, overlying soft tissue, and true ribs (cases 39 to 46), shoulders (case 47), and spinal column (case 48, incomplete). At this point the treatise is discontinued, leaving the document incomplete. The scribe stopped his work in mid-sentence, and why he did so is not explained.

The discussion of each case follows a definite pattern. Each case commences with a "title," usually beginning with the word *instructions*. An identifying designation of the injury is then given, together with indication of the region or organ affected and, sometimes, additional details. This introduction is followed

7. Case Six from the *Edwin Smith Surgical Papyrus,* circa 1600 B.C. Written in hieratic, a cursive version of simplified hieroglyphs, the case describes a gaping wound in the head with compound comminuted fracture of the skull and rupture of the meningeal membranes. This case is the first mention of the brain and its envelope in any medical document. The unknown surgeon describes the wound as "an ailment not to be treated." Edwin Smith purchased the papyrus in Thebes in 1862. It remained at the New York Historical Society until James Breasted of the Oriental Institute of Chicago finally examined it in 1920. Breasted's masterful two-volume translation and commentary on the world's oldest surgical document is a landmark in Egyptology. *(From Breasted J: The Edwin Smith Surgical Papyrus, Chicago, 1930, University of Chicago.)*

by the "examination," which takes the form of a teacher instructing a pupil that the pupil shall do certain specific things. This element of "examination" invites conjecture that perhaps this papyrus is no more than a surgical instruction book. However, indications are that the treatise developed as the product of an effort to record the instructions of a master in the exact words that he used in the process of instruction. Thus the text could be likened more to a series of clinical presentations than to an actual "how to" text. On the basis of the examination, which includes interrogation, inspection, palpation, and the observation of movements performed at the direction of the surgeon, a "diagnosis" is reached and is always introduced by the words "thou shouldst say concerning him. . . ." A description of the ailment is then provided. Included in this section is the "verdict," a statement of the surgeon's decision regarding outcome: "An ailment which I will treat," "An ailment with which I will contend," or "An ailment not to be treated." The first type of ailment is considered curable. For the second, therapy is instituted, although the surgeon has doubts about the curability. With the third verdict the surgeon emphasizes the seriousness of the case, thus relieving himself of personal responsibility in the event of a fatal outcome. He refrains from immediate therapy and restricts himself to watching, waiting, and thorough observation of the patient.

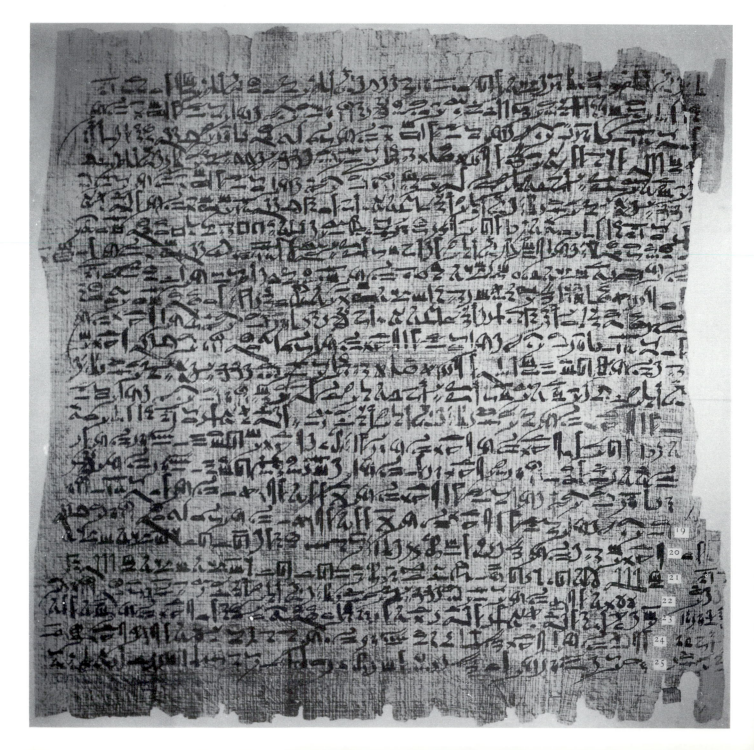

The next-to-last section in each case concerns "treatment," which includes the following choices: (1) exclusively mechanical or surgical treatment, (2) a combination of surgical treatment and use of external medicines, and (3) exclusive use of medicines applied externally. A final section of "glosses" is contained in 29 of the cases as a means of clarifying lost knowledge.

The Smith papyrus provides an exciting glimpse into the state of surgical knowledge in ancient Egypt. The anatomical observations are quite descriptive, and terms are created to designate structures. In the case of a skull injury, the pulse is recorded and a digital exploration of the wound is attempted to ascertain whether there is a depressed fracture of the skull. Feeble pulse and fever are noted in cases of hopeless head injuries.

The ancient commentator carefully explains the concepts of fracture, compound fracture, and compound comminuted fracture, including various techniques for reduction of dislocated bones. Numerous skeletal structures are noted, including the mandible, the temporomandibular joint, clavicles, ribs, and shoulder blades. The coronoid process and condyle of the ramus of the mandible are likened to the claw of a two-toed bird that clasps the temporal bone.

Deafness in fracture of the temporal bone is discussed, as is fever in a knife wound of the pharynx and esophagus. In dislocation of the cervical vertebrae, paralysis of the arms, legs, and sphincters is described; the author even goes so far as to note the occurrence of seminal emission, priapism, and involuntary urination after such an injury. There is an awareness of the relation between the location of a cranial injury and the side of the body involved.

The treatment of wounds seems almost modern. The traumatized skin edges are placed close together, and bandages soaked in a type of glue hold them in position. Fresh meat, perhaps for its hemostyptic value, is the usual dressing for the first day. Subsequently, soothing and protective substances are applied. Applications of both heat and cold are suggested for the appropriate situations.

Most impressively, the ancient Egyptians knew of a cardiac system and were approaching recognition of the circulation of the blood. They were aware that the heart was the center and the pumping force of a system of distributing vessels.

Excerpts from the Smith papyrus follow.

Case 6

[Title]   Instructions concerning a gaping wound in his head, penetrating to the bone, smashing his skull, [and] rending open the brain of his skull.

[Examination]   If thou examinest a man having a gaping wound in his head, penetrating to the bone, smashing his skull, [and] rending open the brain of his skull, thou shouldst palpate his wound. Shouldst thou find that smash which is in his skull [like] those corrugations which form in molten copper, [and] something therein throbbing [and] fluttering under the fingers, like the weak place of an infant's crown before it becomes whole—when it has happened there is no throbbing [and] fluttering under thy fingers until the brain of his [the patient's] skull is rent open—[and] he discharges blood from both his nostrils, [and] he suffers with stiffness in his neck,

[Diagnosis]   Thou shouldst say: "An ailment not to be treated."

[Treatment]   Thou shouldst anoint that wound with grease. Thou shalt not bind it; thou shalt not apply two strips upon it: until thou knowest that he has reached a decisive point.

[Gloss A]   As for: "Smashing his skull, [and] rending open the brain of his skull," [it means] the smash is large, opening to the interior of his skull, [to] the membranes enveloping his brain, so that it breaks open his fluid in the interior of his head.

[Gloss B]   As for: "Those corrugations which form on molten copper:" it means copper which the coppersmith pours off [rejects] before it is forced into the mould, because of something foreign upon it like wrinkles. It is said: "It is like ripples of pus."

Case 25

[Title]   Instructions concerning a dislocation in his mandible.

[Examination]   If thou examinest a man having a dislocation in his mandible, shouldst thou find his mouth open [and] his mouth cannot close for him, thou shouldst put thy thumb [s] upon the ends of the two rami of the mandible in the inside of his mouth, [and] thy two claws [meaning two groups of fingers] under his chin, [and] thou shouldst cause them to fall back so that they rest in their places.

[Diagnosis]   Thou shouldst say concerning him: "One having a dislocation in his mandible. An ailment which I will treat."

[Treatment]   Thou shouldst bind it with ymrw, [and] honey every day until he recovers.

Case 45

[Title]   Instructions concerning bulging tumors on his breast.

[Examination]   If thou examinest a man having bulging tumors on his breast, [and] thou findest that swellings have spread over his breast; if thou puttest thy hand upon his breast upon these tumors, [and] thou findest them very cool, there being no fever at all therein when thy hand touches him; they have no granulation, they form no fluid, they do not generate secretions of fluid, and they are bulging to thy hand,

[Diagnosis]   Thou shouldst say concerning him: "One having bulging tumors. An ailment with which I will contend."

[Treatment]   There is no treatment. If thou findest bulging tumors in any member of a man, thou shalt treat him according to these directions.

[Gloss A]   As for: "Bulging tumors on his breast," it means the existence of swellings on his breast, large, spreading and hard; touching them is like touching a ball of wrappings; the comparison is to a green hemat-fruit, which is hard and cool under thy hand, like touching those swellings which are on his breast.

As becomes apparent when the back side of the Smith papyrus is read, Egyptian surgery was a peculiar blend of superstition, ceremony, and rational thinking. The text is from a much later period than are the surgical cases and contains invocations against pestilential winds, formulas for the rejuvenation of the aged, and other mystical prescriptions. Apparently one of two types of medical doctrine was predominant in Egypt, depending on the dynasty in power. The surgical portion of the Smith papyrus invoked little magic, was largely naturalistic, and provided an uncomplicated guide for the surgeon and his pupil. The later document was supernatural in emphasis: mystical incantations were employed, and the healer is more of a priest than a physician.

Because adherence to tradition was rigorous in Egyptian medicine, little in the way of individual initiative occurred. Medicine and surgery had never been divorced completely from religion, but gradually mystical incantation began to have more influence than any rational treatment plan. As a result, within each historical period the progress of surgery was only slightly advanced. The Ebers papyrus, written after the Smith treatise, demonstrates convincingly the growing power of charms and incantations. Although it contains much in the way of sound medical and surgical advice, the belief in demoniacal possession is clearly evident. Consequently the practice of surgery was slowly engulfed by mystical and religious exorcisms, and Egypt itself eventually sank into relative obscurity. It is ironic that surgery and its various techniques were apparently more advanced and important to Egyptian culture during the earlier Old Kingdom than during the Middle and New Kingdoms.

It must be assumed that an ancient Egyptian surgeon had working knowledge of human anatomy because the practice of mummification was prevalent. Embalmers were skilled in opening the body and removing the viscera, with the exception of the heart and its close appendages. They were also experts in bandaging and often taught surgeons this art. A type of adhesive tape made by impregnating gums, honey, and myrrh into linen strips was used to pull gaping wounds together. The ceremony of embalming was a religious rite, and physicians did not dissect the bodies. Nevertheless, the opening of the body cavities in the preparation of mummies paved the way toward future surgical dissection by decreasing fears and avoidances associated with the study of dead bodies.

Egyptian surgical instruments made of bronze were fashioned for specialized purposes, and several kinds of surgical blades were made of stone, metal and papyrus reed. Excavations from tombs have unearthed forceps, needles, hooks, and scarification instruments.

In the fifth century B.C. the Greek historian Herodotus (484–425 B.C.) wrote as follows about the Egyptian physician:

> Medicine with them is distributed in the following way: every physician is for one disease and not for several, and the whole country is full of physicians of the eyes; others of the head; others of the teeth; others of the belly, and others of obscure diseases.

Specialization was carried to absurd lengths. For instance, around certain pharaohs and their courts virtually every organ or sickness acquired its own specialist. One royal personage had one physician for his right eye and another for his left eye. In the Old Kingdom there was Iry, who was "keeper of the king's rectum," and Hesi-Re, a tooth specialist. Such specialization, however, is not necessarily evidence of an advanced system of medicine, and how the practice of surgery was incorporated into this hierarchy of specialization remains uncertain.

In studying Egyptian surgery, special attention should be paid to circumcision, an ancient operation that appears to have originated in that country. As mentioned earlier, the Jews, who must have learned of circumcision during their Egyptian bondage, eventually made it part of their religious beliefs. The beginnings of this surgical procedure are cloaked in mystery. Apparently circumcision was initiated in Egypt either as a sign of distinction or to increase fertility; only later did it become a religious ceremony. Once a sign of the priesthood, circumcision was later extended to the pharaohs and their families. Thus sanctioned by the king, the practice began to spread as a symbol of distinction to children of nobility and the warrior classes. Eventually the operation lost part of its religious significance, and apparently the practice was enforced for hygienic reasons in all male children in Egypt.

According to Herodotus, Egyptian public hygiene was of a much higher order than Egyptian medicine and surgery. The average Egyptian paid significant attention to cleanliness of body and home. The purgings, vomitings, and enematizing that ancient Egyptians engaged in monthly were symbolic cleansings of sorts, as well as methods of clearing their bodies of dangerous intestinal content. For many reasons, especially because of surgery's dependence on fluctuating societal elements such as religion and royal authority, it is difficult to assign surgery a definitive role within Egyptian culture.

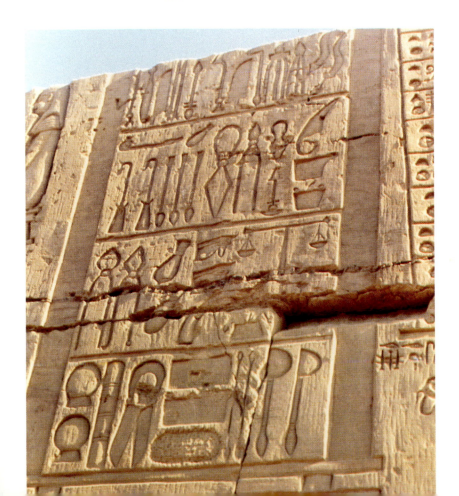

8. Many surgical instruments, including knives and several kinds of forceps, are shown in this carving on the wall of the Ptolemaic temple at Kom Ombo, just north of Aswan. *(From Ring ME: Dentistry: an illustrated history, New York, 1985, Harry N Abrams.)*

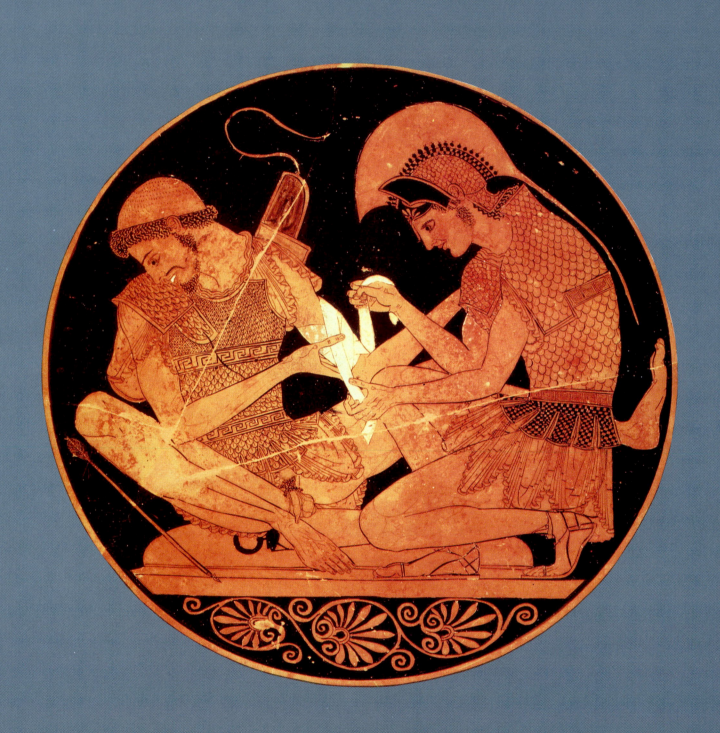

CHAPTER 3

THE CLASSICAL WORLD

❧

GREECE

❧

The ancient Greeks were a composite people whose diverse elements created a self-willed, independent civilization. This overwhelming social heterogeneity, however, prevented the Greeks from ever forming a unified national government. The origins of Greek civilization are found at least as early as 3500 B.C. in the Minoan civilization on Crete. By 1700 B.C. the Minoans had developed a flourishing sea trade with Egypt and had constructed an elaborate palace at Knossos for King Minos. About a century later, Greeks from the mainland captured Knossos, and 400 years after the capture of Knossos a second group of invaders destroyed most of Minoan culture. In later times, the Greeks had only fading memories of the Minoans and many of these were incorporated into Greek mythology. King Minos himself was deemed a son of Zeus and after his own demise became one of the three judges of the dead.

The Greek Bronze Age first developed in Hellas, the mainland of Greece, around 1500 B.C. Late Helladic civilization is often called Mycenaean because Mycenae, in southern Greece, was the largest city. Agamemnon, the king of Mycenae, was the richest and most powerful ruler on the mainland. According to tradition, the Helladic peoples fought against Troy in Asia Minor from 1194 to 1184 B.C. Homer (circa 800 B.C.) wrote of the war in the *Iliad*. If this conflict actually occurred, it was the last vestige of Helladic might, since shortly thereafter waves of migrating tribes submerged Helladic civilization.

By 500 B.C. Cyrus the Great and his Persian empire had become the strongest military power in the world. Among the countries the Persians hoped to conquer was Greece, but in 490 B.C. the outnumbered Greeks threw back the first Persian invasion at the Battle of Marathon. Ten years later the Athenians defeated the Persian fleet at Salamis.

With the end of the Persian Wars Athens became the strongest naval power in Greece and entered its Golden Age (461–431 B.C.): Pericles (490–429 B.C.) came to power in 461 B.C., Herodotus wrote history, Aeschylus (526–456 B.C.) and Sophocles (496–406 B.C.) authored tragedies, Aristophanes (448–380 B.C.) produced comedies, and Hippocrates (460–370 B.C.) founded modern medicine.

From 431 to 404 B.C. the Peloponnesian War was fought, and the Athenian military historian Thucydides (471–400 B.C.) wrote about the conflict. During this period Socrates (470–399 B.C.) taught and Euripides (480–406 B.C.) wrote plays. Sparta eventually defeated Athens and assumed leadership of the Greek city-states. Spartan rule was quite harsh, and in 371 B.C. the Thebans defeated the Spartans at Leuctra and assumed the leadership of Greece.

The Thebans accomplished little more than to allow weakness and political decay to enter Grecian life. Athens continued to hold unquestioned cultural leadership. The great philosophers Plato (427–347 B.C.) and Aristotle (384–322 B.C.) wrote during this period.

9. *Facing page,* Attic bowl (circa 500 B.C.) by the Greek potter Sosias portrays Achilles applying a roller bandage to the arm of his friend Patroclus during the Trojan War (circa 1200 B.C.). Patroclus eventually learned the healing art from Achilles. *(Bildarchiv Preussicher Kulturbesitz, Berlin.)*

As the Greek city-states declined in power, expansionistic Macedonia to the north grew steadily. The Macedonian king, Philip II (382–336 B.C.), extended his power southward and eventually defeated the Greeks at Chaeronea in 338 B.C. Four years later Alexander the Great, son of Philip II, attacked and conquered the Persian empire with an army of Macedonians and Greeks. Alexander was a great admirer of Greek culture, and by spreading Greek traditions and language, he profoundly affected world history. This period is known as the Hellenistic Age.

After Alexander's death in 323 B.C. his Macedonian empire weakened. By 197 B.C. the Romans easily conquered Greece and Macedonia for the first time. Between 146 and 27 B.C. the Romans completed their conquest of the entire Hellenistic world.

Greek Surgery

The initial development of surgery in ancient Greece is difficult to reconstruct because few medical documents survive from before the age of Hippocrates. The oldest sources of knowledge are the Homeric poems, the *Iliad* and the *Odyssey,* which, it is generally agreed, were written between 700 and 800 B.C. but were derived from customs and events that had occurred five or six centuries earlier.

Derived from the Cretan-Mycenaean culture, the *Iliad* presents one of the world's first literary accounts of war injuries. More than 100 passages give realistic descriptions of 147 battle wounds: 106 spearings (80% mortality), 17 sword thrusts (100% mortality), 12 arrow wounds (42% mortality), and 12 slingshot injuries (67% mortality). Apparently the Homeric surgeon could best treat arrow injuries, had difficulty with spearings and slingshot wounds, and was incapable of handling sword trauma.

Two episodes from the *Iliad* demonstrate the capabilities of a Greek military surgeon. King Menelaos, Helen's forsaken husband, is wounded in the abdomen by an arrow. Agamemnon orders a doctor, Makaon, the son of Asclepios, to aid the stricken warrior. Makaon draws out the arrow:

> and when he drew it out, its sharp barbs broke. He loosened the shining belt and the mail-coat under, and last the girdle, bronzed by wondrous smiths. But seeing the wound where the painful arrow entered, he sucked out the blood, then adeptly smoothed on salve which Cheiron once had kindly given his father.

Cheiron was a centaur who had brought up the god Asclepios and served as his mentor in the art of healing. What the salve was remains locked in medical mystery, since no other clues to its contents are given in the *Iliad.*

In another episode the thigh of the warrior Euryplus is wounded by an arrow. His friend Patroclus attends to him:

> The attendant . . . spread the ox hide couch: then as he lay reclined, Patroclus with his dagger, from the thigh cut out the biting shaft; and from the wound with tepid water cleansed the clotted blood; then pounded in his hand, a root applied, astringent, anodyne, which all his pain allayed; the wound was dried, and stanched the blood.

In the *Odyssey,* when Ulysses is gored by a wild boar, pre-Hippocratic surgery invokes the following mixture of rational and irrational elements:

> With bandage firm Ulysses' knee they bound; then, chanting mystic lays, the closing wound of sacred melody confessed the force: the tides of life regained their azure course.

The preceding passages demonstrate the necessity of looking in two directions for the basic features of Homeric surgery. Greek military forces were skilled in the extraction of embedded weapons, the arrest of hemorrhage, and the alleviation of pain. Wounds were washed and picked clean of detritus. Conversely, there was a psychological need for mystic-religious rites, which were important adjuncts to therapies.

The anatomical terms used by Homer relate mainly to the exterior of the body and do not imply any extensive knowledge of visceral anatomy. This lack of knowledge regarding basic anatomy, pathology, and physiology contributed to the continued combination of religious and secular medical practices during the immediate post-Homeric age.

The mythological origin of the art of healing, attributed to the Greek gods, is most evident in the legend of Asclepios. The son of Apollo and the nymph Koronis, Asclepios was raised by the centaur Cheiron. He became such an adept doctor that Hades, god of the underworld, became distraught at the decreasing death rate. Hades complained to Zeus, who found the complaint justified and killed Asclepios with a thunderbolt. Asclepios was then raised to the rank of a healing deity and received divine honors as the Greek god of medicine and surgery. Asclepios's daughter was Hygieia, who became the goddess of health care and provides the etymological origin for the word "hygiene." Another daughter was Panaceion, the protectress of healing plants. The concept of a "panacea" derives from her status as a god.

The cult surrounding Asclepios reached its greatest strength in the fifth and sixth centuries B.C. By that time hundreds of temples of Asclepios were located throughout the Greek empire. Apparently a collection of physicians who were not priests gathered in the vicinity of the temples. Those who gathered belonged to an association or a brotherhood whose members either claimed to be descendants of Asclepios or were admitted to the guild by adoption in an elaborate ceremony. These individuals, known collectively as the "asclepiads," were distinctly different from the priests who ministered in the temple. There is little doubt that the priests also gave medical advice, but apparently it was of a more religious nature. The asclepiads, or lay physicians, kept records that were handed down from father to son and preserved as a valuable family heritage.

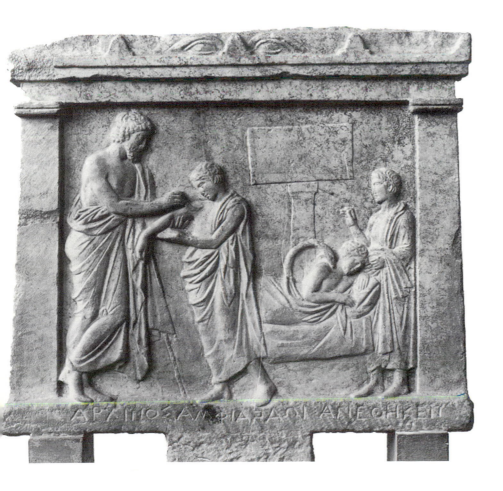

10. The god as surgeon. This votive relief from the Hellenistic period (circa 350 B.C.) depicts the patient, Achinos, with a shoulder ailment, dreaming in healing sleep in the temple of the god Amphiaraos. (National Museum, Athens.)

21

Few written medical or surgical documents from the early temples of Asclepios exist. Clearly the most important ingredient in the effectiveness of the Asclepian temples was the religious faith of supplicants. Their belief in the god of healing, assisted by a mood of relaxation, aided in the overall therapeutic process. The only kinds of active surgical procedures known to have been performed were incisions of abscesses and boils.

Concurrent with the asclepiads was the blossoming of a more scientifically oriented medical philosophy. Two influential thinkers at Miletos, Anaximander and Anaximenes (circa 550 B.C.), began to refute the old doctrine of disease as a mystic imbalance. The former taught that water was the principal element and source of all life; Anaximenes believed it to be air. Other philosopher-scientists were also investigating the human condition. Pythagoras (circa 530 B.C.) considered all surgical procedures to be forbidden, since they might interfere with the soul.

Numerous "schools" of medicine, associations of philosophers, priest-physicians, practitioners, and students, were beginning to develop throughout Greece. The two most important were located at Cnidos and Cos. The Cnidians as early as 700 B.C. appear to have moved away from religiously based medicine and relied more on bedside observation. The "Cnidian Sentences," a collection of medical treatises, are only partially preserved as part of the later writings of Hippocrates. There are archeological hints, not necessarily reliable, that minor surgical procedures were performed by the Cnidians.

On Cos, a small island off the coast of Greece, Hippocrates (460–370 B.C.) was born. His reputation as "the father of modern medicine" is said to rest on three major achievements. He was able to permanently disassociate medicine from the religious mysticism that previously coexisted with it; through his abilities as a teacher he crystallized the existing knowledge of the Cnidian and Coan schools into a systematic science; and, most important, he made physicians understand the high moral inspiration under which they practiced medicine.

Confusion abounds concerning the identity of Hippocrates. He is thought to have come from an asclepiad family, so his profession of medicine would have been preordained. There is little doubt that a clever physician named Hippocrates was an active teacher at the school of Cos and throughout Greece. When Ptolomey I made Alexandria his capital (fourth century B.C.), he ordered that Hippocratic medical writings be collected under a single title. This collection of 72 medical works has become known as the *Corpus Hippocraticum.* Whether a single person authored all of them or, more likely, whether they were derived from a circle of doctors associated with Hippocrates, either during or shortly after his lifetime, remains uncertain. Undoubtedly the works of others were included in the *Corpus,* so when the writings of Hippocrates are discussed, it is reasonable to presume more than one author.

Teachers and medical practitioners at the time of Hippocrates no longer regarded illness solely as a punishment from the gods. The Coan school achieved prognosis by extensively studying the symptoms of disease. Its cornerstone was each patient's individual reaction to illness, and treatment centered on assisting the patient through his or her own symptoms. The Cnidian school concentrated on the disease rather than the patient. Diseases were classified according to specific therapies.

Greek physicians, particularly surgeons of the fourth and fifth century B.C., remained a class of craftsmen. However, their social status must have been somewhat enhanced as a result of changing societal attitudes toward health and cleanliness. Medical training was by apprenticeship, and apparently for a fee the student received instruction, participated in the care of patients, and assisted his mentor in whatever tasks needed to be completed. There were many practitioners, but whether some served strictly as surgeons is difficult to ascertain.

Since general medicine and operative surgery are both part of the *Corpus,* there is little doubt that some Hippocratic physicians utilized many types of treatment. The *Corpus* had been transmitted from one generation to the next in the form of handwritten manuscripts. Shortly after the invention of printing in

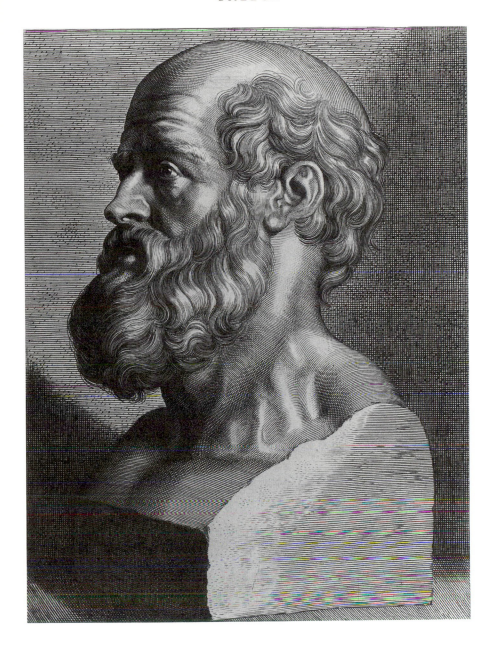

11. Few demonstrably authentic portraits of scientific or medical figures survive from ancient Greece or Rome, and portraits of Hippocrates reflect primarily the artists' imaginations. This engraving by Paul Ponce, after a drawing of a classical bust by Peter Paul Rubens, was published in 1638, probably in Antwerp. It is certainly one of the most artistically significant portraits of Hippocrates. (Jeremy Norman & Co., Inc.)

the second half of the fifteenth century, individual Hippocratic writings appeared as printed books. However, the first complete printed edition of Hippocrates was a Latin text issued in 1525 from Rome under the auspices of Pope Clement VII (1478-1534). In the following year the first Greek edition from the Aldine press in Venice was published. During subsequent centuries numerous translations were published; the first complete English edition was published in the mid-nineteenth century.

The subject matter in the *Corpus* is not arranged in any coherent plan. However, the surgical books, including Wounds and Ulcers, Hemorrhoids, Fistulas, Injuries of the Head, Fractures, Articulations, and Mochlicus (Bones, Their Injuries and Displacements, and Instruments of Reduction), are the most lucid and brilliant sections of the entire work. Scholars believe these to be "genuine" writings of the individual named Hippocrates.

Anatomy, with no systematized presentation, is sketchily treated. This treatment is not surprising, since a thorough knowledge of human structure was not essential to the Hippocratic physician. Instead, general medicine was built on the doctrine of four humors. A proper balance of the humors (warm, dry blood; cold, dry, yellow bile; warm, wet, black bile; and cold, wet mucus) implied a state of good health. Any lack of balance resulted in illness, and treatment was directed toward restoring humoral balance.

Detailed analysis of human anatomy, if any, is found in the three books dealing with the skeletal system. They reflect a wide experience in the management of many types of bony injuries. Reduction was accomplished by traction combined with manual manipulation of the fragments. Bandages were applied initially, while extension was being maintained, but splints were not incorporated until 7 to 11 days had elapsed. Great inventiveness is evident in the various devices used to aid reduction. For a broken humerus with shortening of the extremity, the patient was hung by the axilla over a trapezelike arrangement. The fractured arm was bent at the elbow into a horizontal position, and an assistant supported the wrist. Then a weight was hung in a silken bandage as close to the elbow as possible. With this downward pull, the surgeon could easily manipulate the broken bone ends into contact with each other. A similar configuration was used for treatment of a fractured femur.

The importance of timing in wound treatment is continually emphasized, especially in the early management of wounds. Hippocratic physicians generally favored the "dry" treatment of wounds, with occasional application of wine as a dressing. In a badly contused injury, however, they attempted to promote suppuration by the use of ointments as a means of lessening inflammation and preventing complications. The concept of "laudable pus" can be reliably traced back at least to the time of Hippocrates.

The use of a seton for the cure of fistula-in-ano is described. It was tied gradually tighter until it cut through by pressure necrosis and lay the tract completely open. Cauterization, especially for the relief of hemorrhoids, is mentioned a number of times. Hemorrhage is controlled by both positioning the part and using compression, styptics, tamponade, or mere watching. There is no mention of ligation of vessels. The following Hippocratic observation concerning the efficacy of fire in controlling hemorrhage would be the cause of an

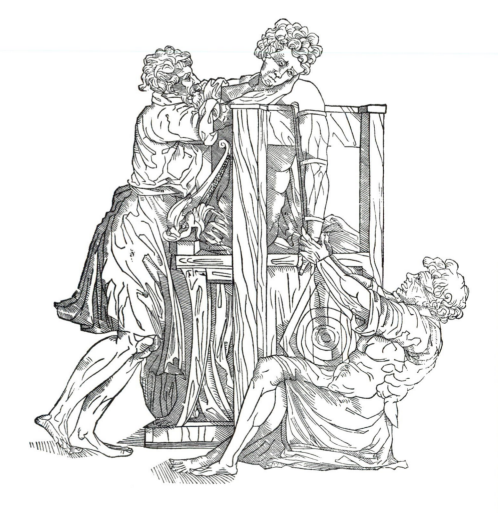

12. Reduction of a dislocation of the shoulder using the ambe of Hippocrates, as depicted in a woodcut probably after a drawing by Francesco Salviati in Guido Guidi, *Chirurgia E Graeco In Latinum Conversae* (Paris, 1544, Gaultier). Although the Greeks could perform only the most elementary surgical procedures, they were relatively advanced in the treatment of fractures and in bandaging. Ancient Greek procedures and bandaging methods, sometimes attributed to Hippocrates, were still actively employed in the sixteenth century, more than 2000 years after their invention. *(Jeremy Norman & Co., Inc.)*

enormous amount of suffering and poor surgical results into the eighteenth century:

> . . . diseases which are not cured by medicines are cured by iron; those which are not cured by iron are cured by fire; those not cured by fire are incurable. . . .

Numerous operative details are discussed, including the operating room, lighting, personnel, instruments, positioning of the patient, and techniques of bandaging and splinting. The treatment of empyema was accomplished by making a small opening in the chest wall and inserting a tube for drainage of the pus. Five types of cranial injuries are recognized: simple fractures or fissures of various kinds or sizes; contusion, without fracture or depression; depressed fractures; fractures of the outer table alone; and contrecoup fractures. Trephination was performed most frequently for depressed fractures. Infections of the scalp and skull and other processes such as erysipelas, bone necrosis, tetanus, and meningitis were all recognized.

Hippocrates does not discuss amputation of limbs through living tissue or with a view to forming a functional stump as a viable surgical alternative. In cases of gangrene resulting from crush injuries or occurring after fractures, when bandages were placed too tightly, it is written that most patients will recover by allowing the gangrenous portion of the extremity to fall off.

Two surgical operations are conspicuous in their absence from the *Corpus:* no mention is made of bladder stone or inguinal hernia. These were among the most common maladies of ancient peoples, but no reasons are given for their not being included in the surgical books.

Excerpts from the *Corpus Hippocraticum* follow:

> The things relating to surgery, are—the patient; the operator; the assistants; the instruments; the light, where and how; how many things, and how; where the body, and the instruments; the time; the manner; the place.
>
> The operator is either sitting or standing, conveniently for himself, for the person operated upon, for the light. There are two kinds of light, the common and the artificial; the common is not at our disposal . . . the part that is operated upon should be opposite the light, and the operator opposite the part operated upon, except in so far as he does not stand in his own light; for in this case the operator will indeed see, but the thing operated upon will not be seen. With regard to himself: when sitting, his feet should be raised to a direct line with his knees, and nearly in contact with one another; the knees a little higher than the groins, and at some distance from one another, for the elbows to rest upon them. The robe, in a neat and orderly manner, is to be thrown over the elbows and shoulders equally and proportionally. . . . When standing, he must make his inspection, resting firmly and equally on both feet; but he must operate while supporting himself upon either leg, and not the one on the same side with the hand which he makes use. . . . The person operated upon should accommodate the operator with regard to the other parts of his body, either standing, sitting, or lying; so as that he may continue to preserve his figure, avoid sinking down, shrinking from, turning away; and may maintain the figure and position of the part operated upon, during the act of presentation, during the operation, and in the subsequent position.
>
> The nails should be neither longer nor shorter than the points of the fingers; and the surgeon should practice with the extremities of the fingers, the index-finger being usually turned to the thumb. . . . It greatly promotes a dexterous use of the fingers when the space between them is large, and when the thumb is opposed to the index. . . . One should practice all sorts of work with either of them, and with both together (for they are both alike) endeavoring to do them well, elegantly, quickly, without trouble, nearly, and promptly.
>
> The instruments, and when and how they should be prepared, will be treated of afterwards; so that they may not impede the work, and that there may be no difficulty in taking hold of them, with the part of the body which operates. . . .
>
> Those about the patient must present the part to be operated upon as may seem proper, and they must hold the rest of the body steady, in silence, and listening to the commands of the operator.

No wounds should be moistened with anything except wine unless the wound is in a joint. Because dryness is more nearly a condition of health, and moisture more nearly allied to disease. . . . It is better to leave a wound unbandaged, unless a poultice is applied. Fresh wounds are less suitable for poultices than old ones, and wounds in the joints. Restriction in the amount of food, and drinking nothing but water are most useful in all wounds, more especially in the recent than those which are old, or for some reason inflamed, or likely to become so; or when danger of necrosis exists, or inflamed wounds about the joints, or where there is danger of convulsions; also in wounds of the abdomen, but most of all in fractures of the skull and femur or any other bone. Standing erect does wounds the most harm. . . . Patients ought neither to walk about, or even be allowed the sitting position. Rest and quiet do the most good . . . When the flesh has been lacerated and contused by the weapon, the wound should be treated in such a way as to produce suppuration as quickly as possible. . . . It is a good plan in fresh wounds, except those in the abdomen, to allow a lot of blood to escape. . . . On account of the escape of blood the parts are drier, and less swollen. . . .

It is a good thing to move the bowels by enema in most wounds, especially in head injuries, and wounds of the abdomen and joints; also when there is danger of gangrene, in sutured wounds, in wounds which corrode, and undermine the tissues, and others which are slow to heal. . . . These in which the wound is surrounded by inflammation do not heal until the inflammation has ceased, nor are wounds likely to heal, in case the surrounding parts are blackened either from softened blood, or blood supplied by an adjoining varicosity and they will not heal at all until you get the surrounding parts into a healthy condition.

In addition to the surgical books, the *Corpus* contains many other general medical works. Among the most interesting are the Aphorisms and, in the first of the ethical books, the Oath of Hippocrates.

The Hippocratic oath is the most impressive early document in medical ethics. Although it has been associated with Hippocrates for more than 2000 years, most scholars agree that it is not part of true Hippocratic teachings. There are too many inconsistencies between the oath and other medical and surgical teachings in the *Corpus* for it to have been part of the Coan or Cnidian schools. The oath is as follows:

I swear by Apollo Physician and Asclepios and Hygieia and Panaceion and all the gods and goddesses, making them my witness, that I will fulfill according to my ability and judgment this oath and this covenant:

To hold him who has taught me this art as equal to my parents and to live my life in partnership with him, and if he is in need of money to give him a share of mine, and to regard his offspring as equal to my brothers in male lineage and to teach them this art—if they desire to learn it—without fee and covenant; to give a share of precepts and oral instruction and all the other learning to my sons and to the sons of him who has instructed me and to pupils who have signed the covenant and have taken an oath according to the medical law, but to no one else.

I will apply dietetic measures for the benefit of the sick according to my ability and judgment; I will keep them from harm and injustice.

I will neither give a deadly drug to anybody if asked for it, not will I make a suggestion to this effect. Similarly I will not give to a woman an abortive remedy. In purity and holiness I will guard my life and my art.

I will not use the knife, not even on sufferers from stone, but will withdraw in favor of such men as are engaged in this work.

Whatever houses I may visit, I will come for the benefit of the sick, remaining free of all intentional injustice, of all mischief, and in particular of sexual relations with both female and male persons, be they free or slaves.

What I may see or hear in the course of the treatment or even outside of the treatment in regard to the life of men, which on no account one must spread abroad, I will keep to myself, holding such things shameful to be spoken about.

If I fulfill this oath and do not violate it, may it be granted to me to enjoy life and art, being honored with fame among all men for all time to come; if I transgress it and swear falsely, may the opposite of all this be my lot.

Contradictions are especially evident in the prohibition against the use of a knife. Since physicians on Cos were actively performing surgical operations, for them to have taken an oath that proscribed surgery seems contradictory. Regardless of the oath's origin, the social status of surgeons is evident: there clearly existed a "class" of men who performed surgical operations to the exclusion of other types of healing. Individuals in this class, it seems, were not held in the same regard as physicians who took the oath.

Hippocratic teachings inculcated that a physician must have a worthy appearance, look healthy, and be well nourished. He should be personally immaculate, wear nice clothing, and possess a high degree of sociability.

Hippocratic physicians were masters at clinical observation, which is nowhere more evident than in the following description of *facies hippocratica:*

> With acute ailments, the patient's face should first be inspected, as to whether it resembles a healthy person's or, even better, that person as he usually looks. The contrary is bad, and worst are the following: a protrusive nose, hollow eyes, sunken temples, cold ears that are drawn in with the lobes turned outward, the forehead's skin rough and tense like parchment, and the whole face greenish or black or blue-gray or leaden.

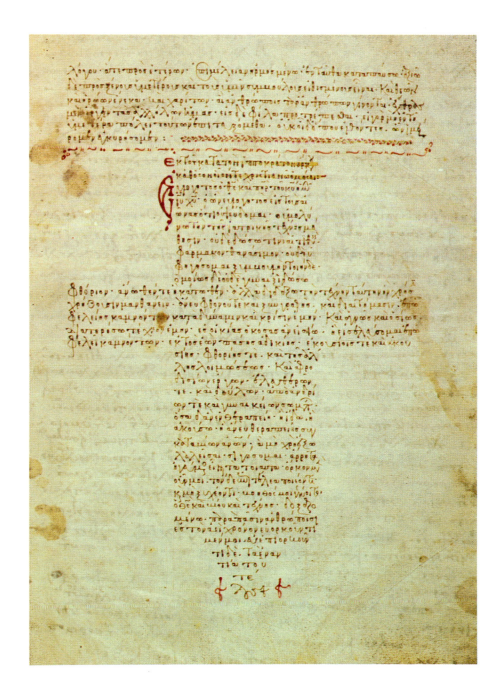

13. The Hippocratic Oath, probably still the greatest brief codification of medical ethics, has remained a standard throughout the evolution of medicine and medical education. In this twelfth-century Byzantine manuscript the oath was written out in the form of a cross, relating it visually to Christian ideas. *(Foto Biblioteca Vaticana)*

Pre-Hippocratic medicine was practiced in a transitional phase between the Bronze and Iron Ages, and this transition was reflected in the metals used to make the surgical armamentarium. Bronze was resistant to corrosion but was not capable of maintaining a good working edge, and iron ultimately proved to be a superior material for knives and other cutting instruments.

At the time of the Trojan War the pre-Hippocratic surgeon would have been expected to have the following in his operating kit: several types of knives, probes or sounds, uterine dilators, bleeding cups, enema syringes, cauterizing irons, raspatories for scraping bone, elevators for depressed fractures, traction or crochet hooks, several forceps, sewing needles, strips of linen, various medications, and some type of hemostatic and anesthetic agents.

The surgeon's instruments would have been replaced by more refined designs during Hippocratic times and still further improved and supplemented by the Romans. The instruments were made of metal and wood; probes, being of lead, tin, or brass, could be bent. Golden wires were used to bind the teeth together in difficult cases of fractured mandibles.

In many respects Hippocratic surgery was no better than that of Egypt and other ancient civilizations. The greatness of Hippocrates lies beyond the mere mechanics of surgical operations or the practice of general medicine. It resides at a simpler level consisting of three principles basic to every physician: observe all, study the patient rather than the disease, and evaluate honestly. Through these principles Hippocrates prepared early practitioners for the scientific foundation of medical practice, and the Hippocratic oath laid the groundwork of medical ethics.

ALEXANDRIA

A major stage in the evolution of surgery resulted from the victories of Alexander the Great and the subjugation of Greece by the Macedonians. With the founding of Alexandria (331 B.C.) in Egypt, Greek science and culture were firmly implanted in that country's ancient civilization. Alexandria became the hub of Mediterranean commerce and the preeminent center for the arts, literature, science, and medicine.

In Alexandria, center of culture, attempts were begun to gather and preserve the knowledge not only of Greece but also of the rest of the world. Scholars were brought from all nations to translate and copy the manuscripts of numerous languages. A museum and library were the focus of this movement, and Aristotle's own private library is said to have served as the nucleus. It is claimed that 700,000 scrolls were eventually housed in the library.

The medical sciences attained new heights, especially in the disciplines of anatomy and surgery, and the achievements of the Alexandrian school were saved for posterity in the later writings of two Roman citizens, Aulus Cornelius Celsus (25 B.C.–A.D. 50) and Galen (A.D. 129–199).

Celsus and Galen recorded that two Alexandrian surgeon-scientists rose in reputation above all others: Herophilos (circa 300 B.C.) and Erasistratos (330–250 B.C.). The former has been called the father of scientific anatomy, and the latter the world's first experimental physiologist.

Herophilos was a pupil of Praxagoras (circa 340 B.C.) and a disciple of the Coan school. Much of modern anatomical nomenclature stems from the Alexandrian school and the influence of Herophilos, who named anatomical structures such as the duodenum and prostate. His main achievements, however, were in the field of neuroanatomy: Herophilos established the brain as the center of awareness and distinguished between motor and sensory nerves.

Erasistratos was a disciple of the Cnidian school and studied under Chrysippus (circa 300 B.C.). Like Herophilos, Erasistratos was concerned with neuroanatomy, but his accurate observations extended to the aortic and pulmonary valves, the chordae tendineae of the heart, the capillary ramifications of the circulatory system, and the common bile duct. Erasistratos also described the functions of the epiglottis.

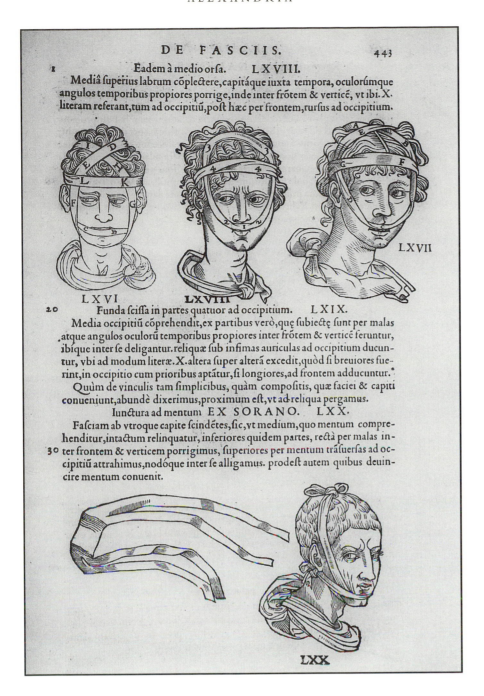

14. Bandaging methods attributed to Hippocrates, from Guido Guidi, *Chirurgia E Graeco In Latinum Conversae* (Paris, 1544, Gaultier). Little advancement had been made in bandaging from the time of ancient Greece to the Renaissance. *(Jeremy Norman & Co., Inc.)*

Both Herophilos and Erasistratos were celebrated for their surgical skills. Herophilos understood much of the actual mechanics of operative surgery but was pragmatic in his use of these techniques. Erasistratos was renowned for his abdominal operations, for his drainage of empyemas, and for the treatment of urethral strictures with an S-shaped catheter.

Perhaps the most important contribution that Herophilos and Erasistratos jointly made was in the systematic dissection of human corpses. For the first time a structured understanding of the human body was being completed. Celsus, in his treatise *De Medicina,* states that actual human vivisections were performed on condemned criminals:

They hold that Herophilos and Erasistratos did this in the best way by far, when they laid open men whilst alive—criminals received out of prison from the kings—and whilst these were still breathing, observed parts which beforehand nature had concealed, their position, color, shape, size, arrangement, hardness, softness, smoothness, relation, processes and depression of each, and whether any part is inserted into or is received into another. For when pain occurs internally, neither is it possible for one to learn what hurts the patient, unless he has acquainted himself with the position of each organ or intestine. . . . Nor is it, as most people say, cruel that in the execution of criminals, and but a few of them, we should seek remedies for innocent people of all future ages. . . .

Erasistratos could not accept humoral pathology; Herophilos firmly believed in it. Their many disciples became more dogmatic and unrealistic in their differing approaches to medicine, studying the texts and following them literally. These students would be embroiled in acrimonious arguments for centuries to come.

By 180 B.C. a so-called philosophy of empiricism had originated in Alexandria, a disciplined reaction against the dogmatic reasoning of the pupils of Herophilos and Erasistratos. The empiricists recognized pure observation of the patient, trial and error, and logical analogies as the cardinal principles of any kind of therapeutic activity. Empiricism moved the fundamental branches of anatomy, physiology, and pathology into the background of medicine. Not surprisingly, the passage of time has made the whole situation somewhat confusing. Nonetheless, it is known that the empiricists performed numerous surgical operations, including lithotomy, herniorrhaphy, and cataract procedures, and devised an apparatus for the reduction of dislocations of the hip.

ROME

Exactly how or when Rome was founded remains uncertain. Tradition states that Romulus and Remus began the city in 753 B.C. A tribe called the Latins are known to have lived on the site of Rome as early as the eighth century B.C. In 509 B.C. the Romans drove out the Etruscans and established Rome as a republic. During the next few centuries the Romans fought a series of wars with neighboring tribes.

In their quest for power the Romans used both military and political methods. To hold conquered territory, the Romans built excellent roads and established frontier forts called colonies. By 264 B.C. Rome had become one of the most powerful nations of the western Mediterranean. Its only neighboring rival was Carthage on the North African coast. Rome and Carthage clashed in a series of struggles called the Punic Wars. In the initial Punic War (264–241 B.C.), the Romans defeated the Carthaginians and Sicily became the first Roman province. Three years later, Rome annexed the islands of Sardinia and Corsica.

The Second Punic War (218–201 B.C.) was initially a series of brilliant victories for the Carthaginian general Hannibal (247–183 B.C.), but the victories never proved entirely decisive and gradually the Romans reconquered their lost territory. Finally, in 201 B.C. Roman armies invaded Africa and defeated Hannibal at Zama.

Although the Romans dominated the whole Mediterranean world, instability and revolution were increasing in Rome. In 60 B.C. Julius Caesar (100–44 B.C.), Pompey (106–48 B.C.), and Marcus Crassus (115–53 B.C.) established three-man rule, called a triumvirate. After gaining decisive military victories in Gaul and Spain, Caesar soon won new territory in Europe. By 54 B.C. he had conquered virtually all barbarian tribes between the Rhine River and the Atlantic Ocean. This Roman achievement laid the Latin foundations of the Middle Ages.

In 49 B.C. Caesar returned to Rome. The Roman Senate feared his new power and ordered him to disband his army before entering Italy. Caesar refused and declared himself sole ruler of Rome. Five years later he was assassinated by Marcus Brutus (85–42 B.C.) and Cassius (?–42 B.C.). Not unexpectedly, the death of Caesar did not restore political stability. Eventually Octavian (63 B.C.–A.D. 14), Caesar's adopted son, gained supremacy after winning the Battle of Actium in 31 B.C.

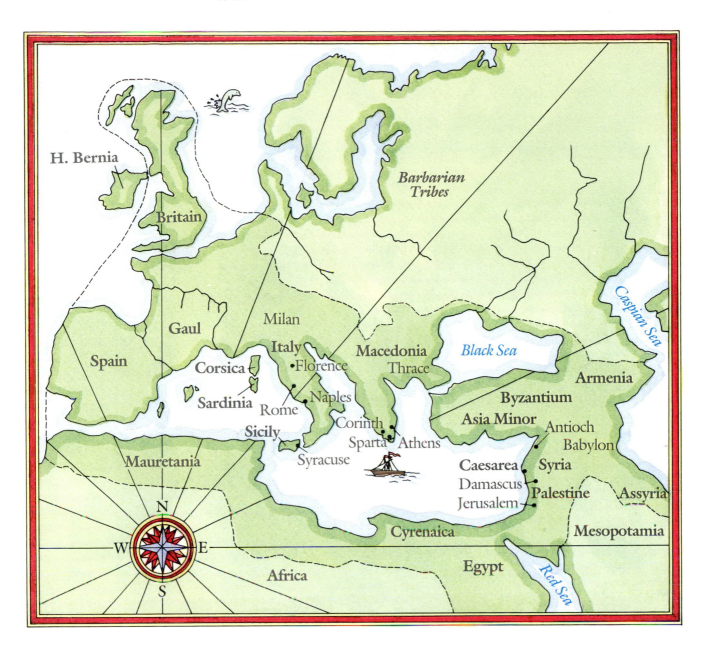

15. Map of the Roman Empire at its greatest extent. *(From Donahue MP: Nursing, the finest art: an illustrated history, St Louis, 1985, Mosby.)*

Four years after the Battle of Actium Octavian took the name of Augustus and became the first emperor of Rome. The reign of Augustus marked the beginning of the Pax Romana, or Roman peace, which lasted for 200 years. No country was strong enough to wage a major war on Rome or pose a serious threat to its borders. Tiberius (42 B.C.–A.D. 37) succeeded Augustus, and during his reign, while Pontius Pilate (dates unknown) was governor of Judea, Jesus Christ was put to death. In A.D. 64 the Emperor Nero (A.D. 37–68) condemned Christians on the charge of setting fire to Rome. In A.D. 70 the Romans crushed a Jewish revolt and destroyed Jerusalem.

Warfare lasting 100 years followed the 200 years of peace. Rome was repeatedly threatened by barbarian tribes in the east and west. The empire had to double the size of its army, which caused continual economic crises. During this time the military put emperors on the throne and removed them at will.

In A.D. 293 Emperor Diocletian (A.D. 245–313) felt that the enormous size of the empire prevented rule by only one man. He divided the empire into eastern and western parts and set up one capital for himself at Nicomedia in Asia Minor.

The arrangement of a divided empire did not last long because a series of struggles commenced among rivals for the throne. After these wars of succession Constantine (A.D. 280–337) became the first Christian emperor of Rome. In A.D. 313 he issued the Edict of Milan, making Christianity legal. In A.D. 330 Constantine created a new capital at Byzantium, later renamed Constantinople.

16. Wounded Roman soldiers receive first aid after combat in this realistic depiction of a battle scene from Trajan's Column. The column, over 100 feet high, was constructed in Rome between A.D. 105 and 114. A flattened-out cast of part of the frieze that runs spirally around the column is shown. If stretched out, the frieze would extend approximately 600 feet. The emperor Trajan ruled from A.D. 98 to 117. His reign saw the last major extensions of the Roman Empire that were gained by the conquest of the Roman frontiers. *(Reproduced by permission of the Trustees of the Science Museum, London.)*

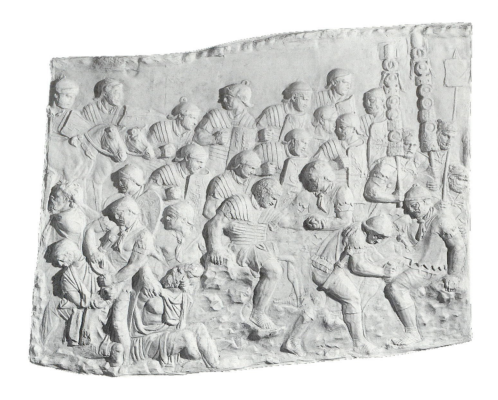

A period of great disorder followed Constantine's death. The only cohesive force within the empire seemed to be the Christian church. The populace was no longer willing to provide enough soldiers to defend the empire and instead hired barbarians as mercenaries. Political and social institutions crumbled, and after Emperor Theodosius (A.D. 346–395) died the two parts of the empire were permanently rent asunder.

The western Roman empire grew steadily weaker. In A.D. 410 the Visigoths captured and sacked Rome, and 50 years later, vandals pillaged and burned Rome. The once mighty city was reduced to waste. The last emperor of Rome was deposed by the barbarian German chief Odoacer (A.D. 434–493) in A.D. 476 Various chieftains and their peoples began to carve up what remained of the empire. Roman rule in the east withstood the crisis and survived until 1453 as the Byzantine empire.

Roman Surgery

Early Roman surgery is poorly understood because little remains in the way of written information. Roman surgery, it is believed, was strongly influenced by Greek medicine and in most aspects reflected the Greek healing traditions. According to Caius Plinius Secundus (Pliny the Elder) (A.D. 23–79), a Roman naturalist and encyclopedist, for at least six centuries before Rome conquered Greece and Macedonia (197 B.C.) his fellow citizens existed without doctors. They apparently relied entirely on medicinal herbs, superstitions, and mystic-religious observances.

In general, upper-class Romans had an aversion to manual work and considered the practice of medicine, especially operative surgery, unworthy of a cultured individual. As itinerant Greek physicians emigrated to Rome, it became only a matter of time before they were accepted into Roman society. The first well-known Greek physician to settle in Rome was Archagathos of Sparta (circa 200 B.C.). Pliny, in his monumental *Historia Naturalis,* recorded that Archagathos was initially well received by the populace. He was considered an outstanding surgeon and was bestowed the title "vulnerarius," or wound healer. It seems that Archagathos later encountered significant operative complications and was repudiated with the name "carnifex," meaning "butcher or executioner."

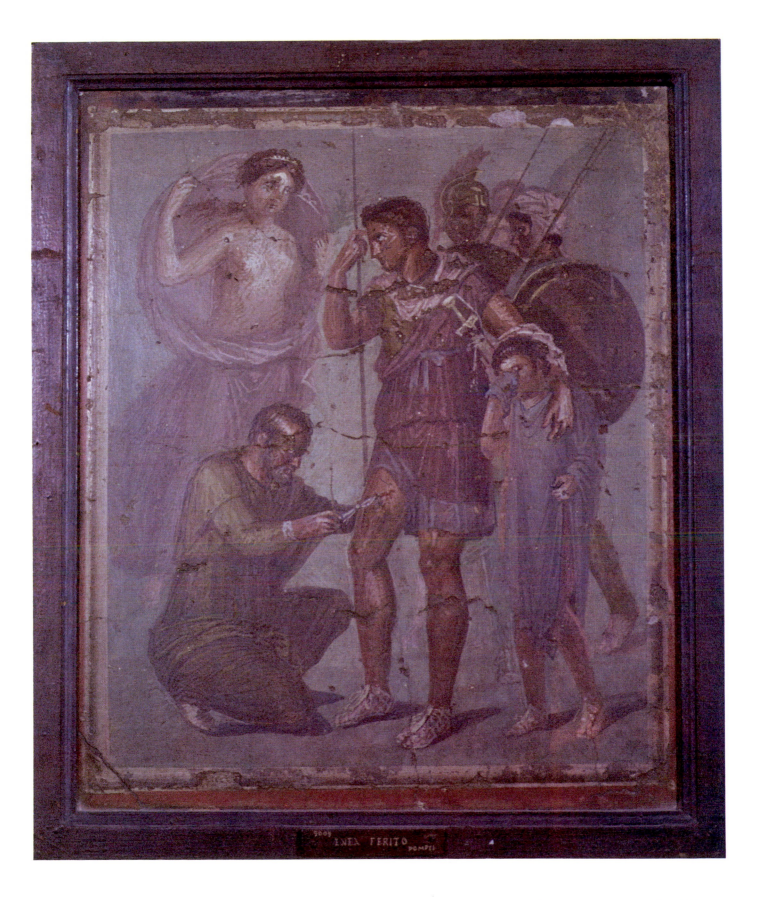

17. In this fresco from Pompeii, which was buried by the eruption of Mount Vesuvius in A.D. 79, Aeneas, the mythical hero of Virgil's (70–19 B.C.) *Aeneid,* is shown being operated on by Japyx before leaving for Troy with his family. *(Museo Nationale, Naples.)*

33

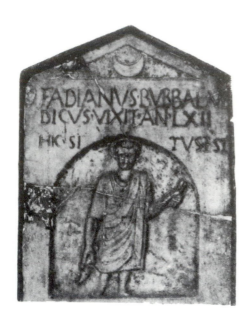

18. Tombstone of a Roman physician, Fadianus Bubbal, from North Africa. He is shown holding a surgical knife. *(Reproduced by permission of the Trustees of the Science Museum, London.)*

Not withstanding an initial Roman contempt for Greek physicians, these Hellenic doctors were eventually called into the best Roman houses and became the leaders in that society's healing traditions. Inevitably the exemplary behavior of Greek doctors and the overall excellence of their medicine and surgery "conquered" their Roman conquerers.

The individual who contributed most to early Roman medicine and surgery was Asclepiades of Bithynia (circa 120–70 B.C.). Although his original writings are lost, his many achievements remain known through references and quotations in the works of Celsus and Galen. Asclepiades practiced surgery and is credited with being the first to propose laryngotomy or tracheotomy. Apparently a man of immense personal charm and eloquence, he was a "society-doctor" who counted among his friends Cicero (106–43 B.C.), Lucius Crassus (140–91 B.C.), Lucretius (96–55 B.C.), and Marcus Antonius.

Asclepiades rejected the medicine of Hippocrates and its reliance on humoral balance. Instead the doctrine of solidism was put forth. He attributed disease to constricted or relaxed conditions of the solid particles (atoms) of the body. The major disciples of Asclepiades, Themison of Laodicia (circa 50 B.C.) and Thessalus of Tralles (circa A.D. 60), exaggerated his beliefs into a formal doctrine of methodism, which became among the most influential of healing systems for centuries afterward.

Thessalus simplified the whole system of medical education and made the claim that medicine and surgery could be learned within 6 months. The latter was said to consist only of the following: foreign bodies, which required removal, fractures and dislocations, tumors or abscesses, which needed excision or incision, and ulcers. As a result of this parochial thought process many uneducated individuals began to study medicine and surgery, which brought the profession into certain disrepute.

Surgery in Rome was practiced almost entirely by Greek physicians, yet the most erudite accounting of it was written by a Roman. Celsus (25 B.C.–A.D. 50) was a nobleman who compiled enormous encyclopedic surveys of various sciences and medical practices for the cultured Roman public. With equal competence he wrote on rhetoric, philosophy, agriculture, military science, and jurisprudence.

Little biographical information is available concerning Celsus. During the Middle Ages his works were lost, but his manuscript on medicine was found in 1433 by Pope Nicholas V (1397-1455). In 1478 *De Medicina* became one of the first medical books to be set into type.

Because Celsus wrote in Latin, not Greek, and because he was not a physician, his works exerted little professional influence during his own time. Even in the handwritten manuscripts of the Middle Ages his name is mentioned only a few times. When first printed during the Renaissance, however, his books on medicine became highly valued for their purity and precision in style and informative value.

De Medicina is the oldest important medical document after the *Corpus Hippocraticum* and provides a cumulative knowledge of medicine and surgery from the time of Hippocrates to the dawn of the Christian era. Of the writings by the 72 medical authors mentioned by Celsus, only the *Corpus* has remained relatively intact. Because of Celsus we have our present knowledge of Greek medicine, Alexandrian surgery, and Roman health practices and we understand many Greek and corresponding Latin medical expressions. As the first important writer on medical history, Celsus established the ultimately high status of Hippocrates, Herophilos, and Erasistratos.

De Medicina consists of eight sections or books; the first four deal with diseases treated by diet and regimen, and the last four describe those amenable to drugs and surgery. Books VII and VIII contain what Celsus considered strictly surgical content, although the last half of Book V and all of Book VI deal with conditions now generally considered surgical. He briefly mentions earlier Greek surgeons, including Meges of Sidon, Tryphon of Gortina, and Euelpistus of Rome.

In the introduction to Book VII Celsus seems to imply that surgery was slowly being accepted as not strictly a handicraft to be practiced by an underclass of citizens:

The third part of the art of medicine is that which cures by the hand. . . . It does not omit medicaments and regulated diets, but does most by hand. The effects of this treatment are more obvious than any other kind; inasmuch as in diseases since luck helps much, and the same things are often salutary, often of no use at all, it may be doubted whether recovery has been due to medicine or a sound body or good luck. . . . But in that part of medicine which cures by hand, it is obvious that all improvement comes chiefly from this, even if it be assisted somewhat in other ways.

The state of Greco-Roman surgery was highly developed, and the breadth of Celsus's work is vast. His observations, when contrasted with the teachings of Hippocrates, evidence considerable progress. Celsus is best remembered for his description of the characteristics of inflammation: redness, swelling, heat, and pain (rubor, tumor, calor, and dolor). *De Medicina* discusses joint dislocations,

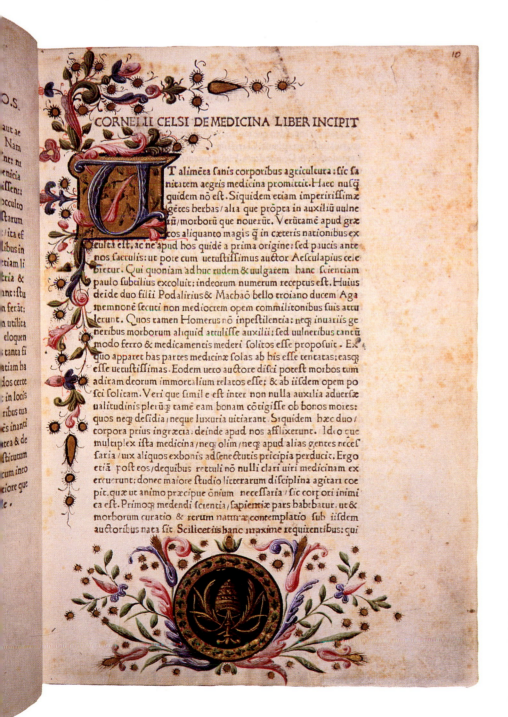

19. The first page of the first printed edition of Celsus's *De Medicina* (Florence, 1478). In this copy the margins and historiated initial have been illuminated in the style of medieval manuscripts. *De Medicina,* the oldest Western medical document after the Hippocratic writings and the first Western history of medicine, also contains authoritative accounts of surgical procedures. It was one of the first medical texts to be printed in the first half-century after Johannes Gutenberg invented printing from movable type in 1455. *(Historical Collections, College of Physicians of Philadelphia.)*

fistulas, traumatic injuries, abscesses, eye, ear, and nose ailments, hernia, varicose veins, urinary tract infections, and fractures. Celsus approaches each therapeutic and surgical maneuver with a thorough understanding, presenting every condition in strict detail. His description of cosmetic surgery includes restoration of the foreskin, apparently because certain Jews in Rome sought to obtain favorable positions and social acceptance by cloaking their origins. Celsus provides a classic description of lateral lithotomy and offers an entire chapter on the proper manner of arresting hemorrhage, including one of the earliest descriptions of ligating and dividing blood vessels. Unlike Hippocrates, Celsus describes inguinal hernia surgery, including detailed anatomical descriptions:

> Now sometimes the inguinal region has to be cut into, sometimes the scrotum. In either case the man for three days before should drink water (only), and for the day before abstain also from food . . . the skin of the groin is rendered tense, the cut is made below the abdominal cavity, where the membranes below are continuous with the abdominal wall. Now the laying open is to be done boldly, until the outer tunic, that of the scrotum itself, is cut through, and the middle tunic reached . . . the index finger of the left hand is introduced, in order that . . . the hernial sac may be freed.
>
> Next the assistant grasping the scrotum with his left hand should stretch it upwards, and draw it away as far as possible from the groin, at first including the testicle itself until the surgeon cuts away with the scalpel all the fine membranes which are above the middle tunic if he is unable to separate it with his finger; the testicle is let go in order that it may slip downwards, and show in the wound and then be pushed out by the surgeon's fingers, and laid along with its two tunics upon the abdominal wall. There whatever is diseased is cut round and away. . . .
>
> The testicle having been thus cleared is to be gently returned through the incision along with the veins and arteries and its cord; and it must be seen that blood does not drop down into the scrotum, or a clot remain anywhere. This will be accomplished if the surgeon takes the precaution of tying the blood vessels; the threads with which the ends of these are tied should hang out of the wound; following upon suppuration they will fall off painlessly. Through the margins of the wound itself two pins are then passed, and over this an agglutinating dressing. . . .

Celsus's writings demonstrate that the surgeon of ancient Rome tried to arrive at an exact diagnosis before undertaking therapy. In so doing, surgeons were beginning to take surgery out of the hands of charlatans. Celsus was demanding in what he considered the ideal surgeon to be:

> A surgeon ought to be in early manhood, or at any rate not much older; have a swift and steady, never-faltering hand, and no less skill in the left hand than the right; have sharp and clear eyesight; appear undistressed, and compassionate inasmuch as he wishes to heal those whom he treats, but does not allow their cries to hurry him more than the circumstances require, or to cut less than is necessary, and permits the patient's groaning to make not the slightest impression on him in anything he does.

Celsus describes many Greco-Roman surgical instruments in detail, although few of the instruments themselves have survived. Roman implements were usually made of copper alloy, often by fine craftsmen. The *armamentarium chirurgicum* was highly specialized. The surgical knife had, as a rule, a blade of steel and a handle of bronze. In most cases the blades were either luted or brazed in permanently. An occasional detachable arrangement would allow for removal and cleaning and provide for the use of several varieties of blades. The ordinary scalpel apparently had a straight, sharp-pointed blade.

According to Celsus, sutures should be of soft thread and not overtwisted. Hippocrates directed that sutures be made of crude flax because the individual strands were stronger than those of finished lint. Neither author mentions catgut, although this substance was known to the Greeks and Romans. Horsehair was used for some manipulative purposes but never for suturing wounds.

Between the times of Celsus and Galen other author-surgeons were prominent in Rome, but their original works for the most part have been lost. The best known was a Greek immigrant in Asia Minor, Soranus of Ephesus (A.D. 98–138). He studied in Alexandria and practiced under the Roman emperor

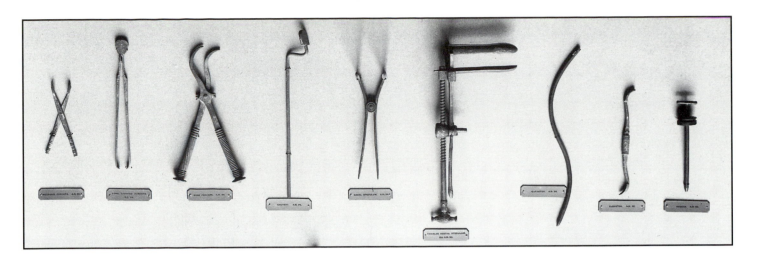

20. Roman surgical instruments used in the second century A.D., from Bingen, Germany, a distant outpost of the far-reaching Roman Empire. *(The Wellcome Institute Library, London.)*

Hadrian (A.D. 76–138). Soranus is considered to have been the leading authority on the gynecology, obstetrics, and pediatrics of Greek and Roman antiquity. Many of his writings were translated from Greek into Latin and incorporated into the works of later authors.

Soranus is credited with introducing the Roman birth stool, which had a crescent-shaped aperture and back and arm supports. Soranus described protection of the perineum and emptying of the bladder with a catheter before delivery and demonstrated an understanding of the menstrual cycle and the various difficulties that can surround labor and delivery, including transverse fetal position. He recognized atresia of the vagina as being congenital or secondary to inflammation. He knew how to tamponade the uterus for hemorrhage and performed a rudimentary hysterectomy for prolapse. Among Soranus's other important works is a treatise on fractures, bandaging, and skull injuries.

Rufus of Ephesus (circa A.D. 100), somewhat older than Soranus, practiced during the reign of Emperor Trajan (A.D. 52–117). Little is known about Rufus other than his celebrated status and his reputation as an outstanding surgeon. His name remained among those most commonly mentioned by medieval physicians. Of 36 works attributed to him, only 12 have survived and sections are missing in many of these.

Rufus's most important achievements were anatomical observations. He correctly described the course of the optic nerves, the crystalline lens, and various membranes of the eye. He recognized the heartbeat as the source of the pulse. His work on anatomical nomenclature is the only pre-Galenic manuscript to list the names of parts of the body in the original Greek. Rufus is particularly remembered for his treatise on hemostasis, which discussed the ligature and the methods of digital compression, styptics, cautery, and torsion.

Heliodorus (circa A.D. 100) practiced surgery in Rome and authored a treatise on surgery, the fragments of which indicate that he must have been a skillful technician. Among his lasting contributions are the ligation and torsion of blood vessels as a method of hemostasis and the use of internal urethrotomy as treatment for stricture. Heliodorus described head injuries, herniorrhaphy that included excision of the sac, and various methods of amputation.

Aretaeus the Cappadocian (A.D. 81–138) apparently practiced surgery in Alexandria, although little biographical information is available. His style of medicine and surgery closely approximated the detailed patient observations of Hippocrates. Most of his works, including at least one volume on surgery, have been lost, but he is substantively quoted in the treatises of later authors. Mentioned in their works are Aretaeus's vivid descriptions of pleurisy, cholera,

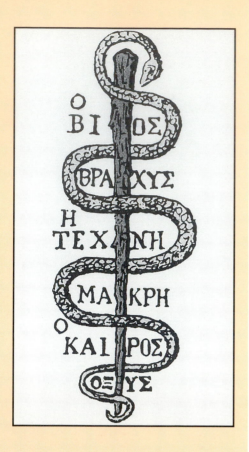

21. The staff of Aesculapius, emblem of medicine: a single serpent coiled around a rough, knotty staff. The Greek inscription is the famous Hippocratic aphorism usually translated, "Life is short, art is long, occasion fleeting . . . ."

diabetes, insanity, ileus, satyrism, and epilepsy. For the latter, surgical therapy consisted of venesection on the dorsum of the hand, application of heat to the head followed by trephining the skull to the diploe, or complete trephination to the level of the meninges with the meninges eventually becoming black and thickened. After formation of a scar the patient was said to be cured.

The regulation of medical and surgical practice in Roman society was at first nonexistent. As centuries passed, however, physicians began to receive exemptions from societal commitments such as taxes and military service. So desirable had the self-proclaimed position of physician become that Emperor Antoninus Pius (A.D. 86–161) had to restrict the privileged exemptions to a limited number and to those who chose to remain in their native regions. Comprehensive laws that regulated training and licensure were finally promulgated during the reign of Emperor Severus Alexander (A.D. ?–235).

Although the practice of surgery and general medicine was leaving behind the era of mysticism and religious incantations, Romans still clung to their belief in Aesculapius. According to legend, the Greek god Asclepios was introduced to Rome (circa 295 B.C.) in the form of a snake sent from the temple of Epidaurus when an epidemic broke out. Roman Aesculapian temples, modeled after their Greek counterparts, were soon to be found throughout the empire. Within a few years the staff of Aesculapius, a single serpent coiled around a rough, knotty staff, became an emblem associated with medicine in Rome. The emblem is said to be significant for medical practice inasmuch as the serpent, because of its long life, annual renewal of skin, and keen sight, is the symbol of healing.

The caduceus preceded the staff of Aesculapius as a symbol of healing. Although reliably traced back to Babylonian times, the caduceus in Greek mythology was the staff of Hermes, an olive branch with garlands and intertwined serpents in coital position symbolizing fecundity. Because Hermes was the messenger of the gods, his staff became the herald's wand and wings were added. The symbol of Hermes was called the *kerykeion*. When translated from Greek to Latin, *Hermes* became *Mercury* and the *kerykeion,* the *caduceus.* This winged staff with two coiled serpents is an ancient symbol, but throughout its early history it actually symbolized commerce and gainful trade. The single-serpent staff of Aesculapius, on the other hand, has always been associated with medicine and the healing arts.

The confusion between these two symbols has persisted for years. It appears that the caduceus was first used inappropriately as a medical emblem in sixteenth-century Switzerland, when it appeared in the crest of a printer of medical books. This mistake has been perpetuated, and confusion still reigns. For instance, the British Royal Army Medical Corps uses as its symbol the staff of Aesculapius and its single serpent. In 1902 the Medical Corps of the United States Army confounded the misidentification by adopting the caduceus, the emblem of Mercury, as its symbol.

The most famous physician of the Greco-Roman period is Galen (A.D. 129–199), of Pergamum, who is considered second only to Hippocrates as the most important physician of all antiquity. His views dominated European medicine for almost 15 centuries, until the time of Andreas Vesalius (1514-1564) and William Harvey (1578-1657).

Unlike Hippocrates, about whom little is known, Galen provided much autobiographical information. His native city of Pergamum was famous for its medical library and Aesculapian temple. Galen's name means "peaceful one," but his writings reveal him to be contentious, argumentative, authoritarian, competitive, and arrogant. Under the stimulus of his father, Galen began the study of medicine when he was 17 years old. After his father's death, Galen continued his education in Smyrna and Corinth and, ultimately, in Alexandria.

In A.D. 158 Galen returned to Pergamum to accept an appointment as chief physician and surgeon to the gladiators. The 5 years that followed provided Galen with unlimited opportunities for the practice of orthopedic, restorative, and traumatic surgery. He again left Pergamum to travel for the first time to Rome, was soon sought out by the nobility, and became quite wealthy. He stopped

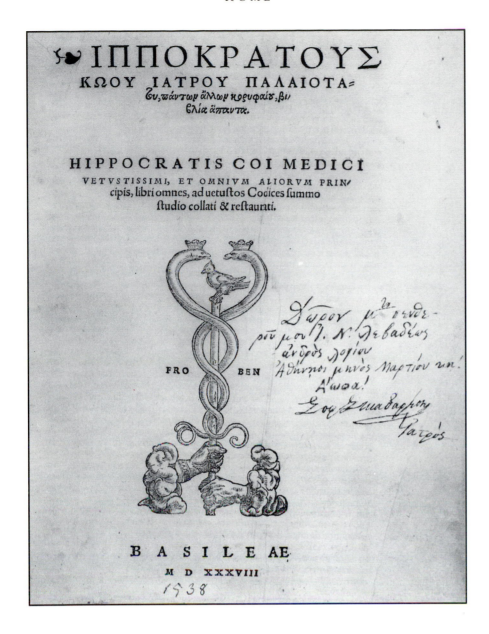

ΙΠΠΟΚΡΑΤΟΥΣ
ΚΩΟΥ ΙΑΤΡΟΥ ΠΑΛΑΙΟΤΑ=
ου, πάντων άλλων κορυφαίε, βι
ελία άπαντα.

HIPPOCRATIS COI MEDICI
VETVSTISSIMI, ET OMNIVM ALIORVM PRIN/
cipis, libri omnes, ad uetustos Codices summo
studio collati & restaurati.

FRO BEN

B A S I L E AE
M D XXXVIII

22. Title page of the Greek edition of Hippocrates' collected works, published by the scholar-printer Johannes Froben of Basel in 1538. Froben's printer's mark, which graced his editions of numerous medical books and other classical texts, incorporated the caduceus, or staff of Hermes, with its intertwined serpents around a staff. This printer's mark may have reflected or possibly originated the confusion between the caduceus and the staff of Aesculapius. (*Jeremy Norman & Co., Inc.*)

performing surgical operations in Rome, but his previous knowledge of surgery formed the basis for his later detailed and outstanding descriptions of surgical treatment.

Galen spent the remainder of his life in Rome, where he became a favorite of the emperor Marcus Aurelius. Because human dissection was not then permitted, Galen conducted public anatomical demonstrations on apes and pigs. Although he repeatedly emphasized the importance of anatomical knowledge for the surgeon, this greatly revered authority drew much human anatomical data from animals rather than humans, which resulted in the perpetuation of countless errors throughout medical literature until the sixteenth century, when the study of anatomy was reformed by Andreas Vesalius and others.

While surrounded by professional success, Galen remained highly suspicious of his fellow physicians. He was uncharitable toward them, and whenever he could, he ridiculed and contradicted their opinions and methods. His self-proclaimed infallibility would have long-lasting negative effects on medical dogma, since scholars of later centuries accepted all that Galen promulgated without subjecting it to further experimentation.

Despite Galen's overbearing personality and ill-formed misconceptions, the breadth and depth of his writings are staggering. Of all the ancient writers Galen wrote the most voluminously, and he was the greatest of the theorists and systematists. His works, a smorgasbord of knowledge, include 9 books on

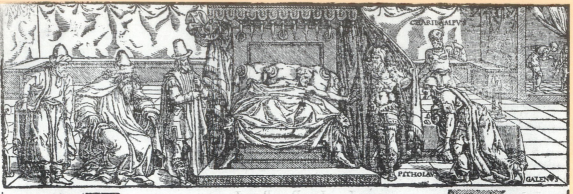

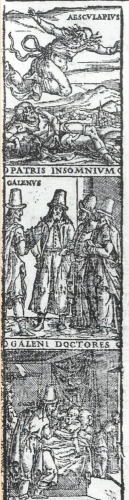

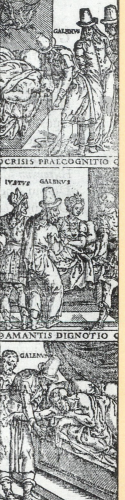

GALENI

LIBRORVM

QVINTA CLASSIS

EAM MEDICINÆ PARTEM,

quæ ad Pharmaciam spectat, exponens; simplicium medicamentorum, substitutorum, purgantium, antido-
torum, componendorum tam per locos, quam
per genera medicamentorum, ponde-
rum denique, ac mensurarum doctrinam comprehendit:

NONA HAC NOSTRA EDITIONE,

non parum ornamenti adepta: locis pluribus quàm alijs superio-
ribus editionibus, ad græcorum librorum fidem emendatis.

Locis etiam Hippocratis in margine indicatis, quos
Galenus sparsim in contextu citat.
Et alijs etiam annotationibus additis.
Librorum numerus proximo folio continetur.

Τὸ Φαρμαχευτιχὸν.

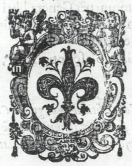

VENETIIS, APVD IVNTAS. MDCXXV.

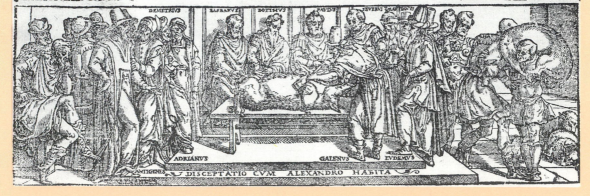

anatomy, 17 on physiology, 6 on pathology, 14 on therapeutics, and 30 on pharmacology and 16 essays on the pulse. It was not until 1525 that the first printed edition of Galen's work was published. This famous five-volume Aldine Greek text was soon followed by Latin editions.

As a clinical observer Galen was unequaled, at least according to his own bragging. Galen was the first contributor to experimental physiology. By means of his animal dissections he described the cranial nerves and the sympathetic nervous system. Experimentation revealed both the importance of the recurrent laryngeal nerve and a rudimentary explanation of the mechanism of respiration. Galen noted paralysis as a result of sectioning various levels of the spinal cord. Among his observations was that urine traveled from the kidney to the bladder via the ureters. He was the first to prove, in opposition to the prevailing views, that arteries contain blood, not air.

Clearly Galen's achievements in pathology, physiology, and general medicine were greater than those in surgery. Although he wrote widely on surgical matters, the writings are diffused throughout his essays and many books and are not summarized in a single volume. Galen also exerted enduring negative influence on surgical technique because he believed in and emphasized that suppuration was an essential element in the healing process of a wound.

Galen was a talented technical surgeon. His operations included the removal of nasal polyps and varicose veins, plastic surgery for cleft lip reconstruction, and intestinal or abdominal wall suture after penetrating injuries of the abdomen. His pragmatism is evident in the following quote:

> All the operations in surgery fall under two heads, separation and approximation. Approximation has to do with the reduction and dressing of fractures, reduction of dislocation of the joints, reductions of prolapsed intestines, uterus, or rectum, sutures of the abdomen and restoration of tissue deficiencies, as in the nose, lips, and ears. Division is concerned with simple incisions, circumcisions, elevations of skin, scalping, excisions of veins, amputation, cauterization, scraping, smoothing, excisions with the saw.

Galen wrote extensively on the use of particular surgical instruments, including scalpels of various sizes, forceps, splints, retractors, and scissors. Most scholars view his treatise on pathological swellings as his foremost contribution to surgery because of its exacting discussion of inflammation and tumors.

In Galen's book on anatomical procedure he forcefully espouses the belief that all surgeons must study anatomy and have an understanding of form and function before undertaking a surgical operation:

> First of all, then, I would ask you to make yourself well-acquainted with the human bones, and not to look on this as a matter of secondary importance. . . . Make it your earnest business, then, not only to learn exactly from the book . . . but to become yourself by the use of your own eyes an eager first-hand observer of human osteology . . . study all the bones, either in the human body or, if possible, in the ape, but preferably in both. Then next we proceed to dissect the muscles. For these two parts (bones and muscles) underlie all the others, like foundation-stones. After these you may learn whatever you like first, whether arteries, veins or nerves. While engaged in the dissection of these you will also learn about the viscera. Next will come a knowledge of the intestines, of fatty tissue, and of glands. . . .
>
> All these observations will be useful to you in surgery as well as in the investigation of functions. For in surgery we are sometimes forced to cut even the muscles themselves, on account of deep-lying abscesses, deposits, or suppurations. And it is most useful to learn the function, so that in case of extensive injuries, where a whole muscle has been cut across, we may know beforehand what function is lost; by forecasting this you will avoid being blamed by censorious individuals (who are in the habit of referring loss of function to the doctor's treatment and not to the original injury).

Why did Galen's writings, among those of all Greco-Roman physicians, exercise such a profound influence for almost 15 centuries?

23. *Facing page,* Title page of the Latin edition of Galen's voluminous medical writings as edited by Fabius Paulinus and published by the Giunta family of Venice in 1625. The success of this edition, which underwent numerous reprints and editorial revisions between 1522 and 1625, reflects Galen's abiding authority and influence on medicine and surgery throughout the sixteenth and early seventeenth centuries. The woodcuts bordering the title page illustrate real and legendary events in Galen's life. Figures are shown in costumes that are a curious blend of sixteenth-century European fashions and those of ancient Rome. At the foot of the page Galen is shown demonstrating anatomy on a pig to his patron, Flavius Boethius. Galen never dissected a human cadaver, and the enduring power of his influence certainly did nothing to encourage human dissection. *(The Library, History/Special Collections, University of California, San Francisco.)*

Galen was a dogmatic, pedantic, and didactic personality. He made certain that his treatises provided answers to questions, even when his knowledge was inadequate. Among his spurious concepts were (1) that the blood obtained "natural spirits" in the liver, with "vital spirits" in the left ventricle being changed into "animal spirits" in the brain, (2) that blood passes from the right to the left ventricle via imaginary invisible pores, and (3) that suppuration is necessary as an essential part of the healing process. Because of his pugnacious personality, Galen never even acquired any true disciples. Nonetheless, because the Middle Ages was a scientifically and culturally unsettled era, there was a need for certainty and authority in medicine. Galen's answers provided the Christian church and lay leaders with their desire for an absolute truth. Reverence for Galen after his death exceeded the reverence he had received during his lifetime. The influence cannot be overestimated of later writers such as Oribasius (A.D. 325–403), Aetius of Amida (A.D. 502–575), Alexander of Tralles (A.D. 525–605), Paul of Aegina (A.D. 625–690), and Rhazes (A.D. 850–923), who propagated Galen's thinking and used his name as the essence of prior medical progress. For all these reasons Galen's contributions to medical science were glorified for 15 centuries.

The evolution of surgery in the classical world concludes with two surgeons whose exploits were described in the works of later authors. Antyllus (second century A.D.) was an outstanding surgeon of whom little is known. Most of his works have been lost, but careful descriptions left by Oribasius, Paul of Aegina,

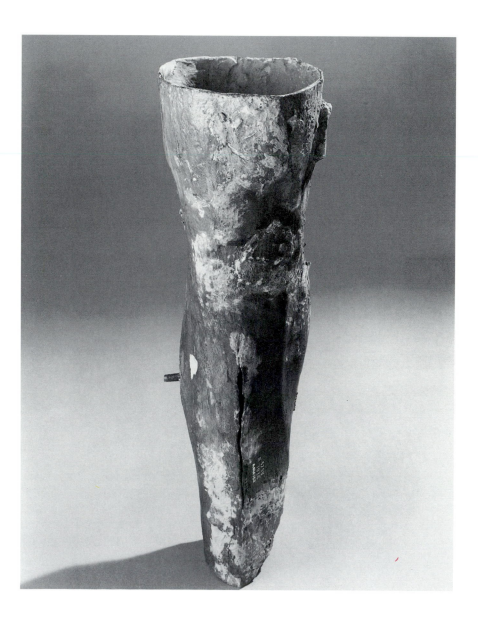

24. Plaster casting of a bronze original of a Roman artificial leg that was formerly in the Royal College of Surgeons, London, but was destroyed in World War II. This artificial leg was designed to replace only the lower part of the extremity. *(Reproduced by permission of the Trustees of the Science Museum, London. Inventory A646752.)*

and Rhazes demonstrated that Antyllus accomplished much in advancing Greco-Roman surgery. He did not belong to any particular philosophical school but tended to rely heavily on self-imposed experience. He is known to have operated on cataracts, performed tracheostomies, excised necrotic bone, and cured hydrocephalus by incising the involved area.

Antyllus, acknowledged as the first vascular surgeon, properly differentiated aneurysms and their causes. Most important, as described in the following passage, he introduced "Antyllus's method" (ligature of the artery above and below an aneurysm, followed by incision into and emptying of the sac):

> There are two kinds of aneurysm. In the first the artery has undergone a local dilatation; in the second the artery has been ruptured. The aneurysms which are due to dilation are longer than the others. The aneurysms by rupture are more rounded. To refuse to treat any aneurysm, as the ancient surgeons advised, is unwise; but it is also dangerous to operate upon all of them. We should refuse, therefore, to treat aneurysms which are situated in the axilla, in the groin, and in the neck, by reason of the volume of the vessels and the impossibility and danger of isolating and tying them. We should not touch an aneurysm of large volume even when it is situated in some other part of the body. We operate in the following manner upon those which are situated upon the extremities and the head: If the aneurysm be by dilatation, make a straight incision through the skin in the direction of the length of the vessel, and, drawing open by the aid of hooks the lips of the wound, divide with precautions the membranes which cover the artery. With blunt hooks we isolate the vein from the artery, and lay bare on all sides the dilated part of this last vessel. After having introduced beneath the artery a probe, we raise the tumor and pass along the probe a needle armed with a double thread in such a manner that this thread finds itself placed beneath the artery; cut the threads near the extremity of the needle, so that there will be two threads having four ends; seizing, then, the two ends of one of these threads, we bring it gently toward one of the two extremities of the aneurysm, tying it carefully; in like manner also we bring the other thread toward the opposite extremity, and in this place tie the artery. Thus the whole aneurysm is between two ligatures. We open then the middle of the tumor by a small incision; in this manner all which it contains will be evacuated, and there will be no danger of hemorrhage. . . .
>
> If the aneurysm owes its origin to the rupture of the artery, we isolate with the fingers as much of the tumor as we can, including the skin, after which we pass underneath the isolated part the needle with the double thread and proceed as before; after which the tumor may be opened at its summit and the superfluous portion of the skin cut away.

Leonides of Alexandria (circa second century A.D.) lived in Rome and is known only through the fragments of his works found in the writings of later authors. He improved many operative methods, including amputation and flap preparation. Leonides especially described incision and drainage of a peritonsillar abscess in adults and children and treatment of breast cancer by amputation involving cautery.

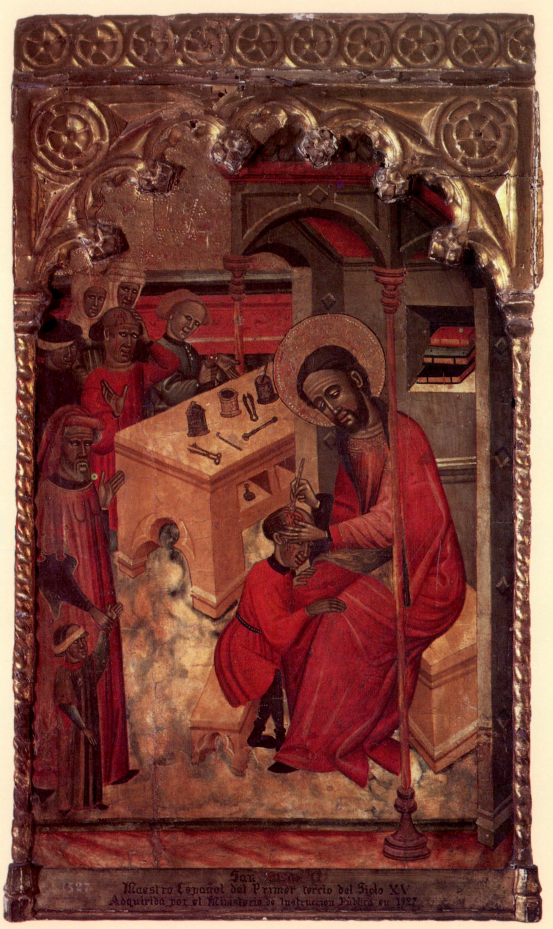

San Lucas (?)
Maestro Español del Primer tercio del Siglo XV
Adquirida por el Ministerio de Instrucción Pública en 1927

CHAPTER 4
THE BYZANTINE EMPIRE

The western Roman empire lasted 500 years; the eastern, or Byzantine, empire would continue for more than 1000 years (A.D. 395–1453). This latter empire served Europe as a defending barrier against barbarian tribes and other invaders such as the Arabs and Turks. The Byzantine period was characterized by the dominance of the Christian church and the preservation of ancient Greek and Roman culture. It served as a connecting link between ancient and modern European culture.

Emperor Constantine, regarded as the founder of the Byzantine empire, transferred the capital of the Roman empire from Rome to Byzantium, later named Constantinople. Under Justinian I (A.D. 483–565) the eastern empire flourished, especially after the codification of Roman law (Justinian Code). Justinian's aggressive military leadership resulted in the regaining of much of the lost territory of the earlier western Roman empire. He especially controlled the Persians, who were situated on his eastern borders.

When Justinian I died, his many conquests and new building projects proved costly. The empire was left bankrupt and the populace angered at his prodigal rule. Successors were left to defend the empire against one invasion after another. By the seventh century a new enemy, the Muslims, won a series of territorial and sea victories. Among the far-flung conquests of the Muslims were the lands of Palestine and Syria (A.D. 636) and Egypt (A.D. 640). The Muslims besieged Constantinople between A.D. 673 and 678 and in A.D. 717 but were defeated both times.

In the ninth and tenth centuries the Byzantine armies again drove the Muslims back on several fronts. During this period Constantinople became a city of extraordinary wealth and luxury. By the late 1000s the Seljuk Turks appeared as another enemy of the Byzantine empire and eventually overran part of Asia Minor. To defend the empire, Christians living in western Europe were called upon to thwart the Turks.

Christian soldiers, also known as the Crusaders, were just as eager to seize the lands of the Byzantine empire as the Turks had been. In A.D. 1204 Constantinople fell to the Venetians, and what was left of the empire was divided into many small states. Soon the Ottoman Turks invaded Asia Minor, and the Serbians advanced into the Balkans. By the end of the fourteenth century all that remained of the Byzantine empire was the immediate area around Constantinople. In A.D. 1453, the city finally fell to the Turks and was renamed Istanbul, and the last of the Byzantine emperors was killed in battle.

Byzantine Surgery

Surgery evolved little during the Byzantine millennium. Virtually all knowledge was inherited from past Greco-Roman traditions via translations of ancient writings. Most of these translations were made in the many Christian monasteries

25. *Facing page,* Luke the Evangelist, patron saint of physicians, operating on a child with a brain tumor. Other sick patients, as well as surgical instruments, medicinal jars, and books, are shown in this fanciful fifteenth-century painting by an artist who shows little evidence of ever having witnessed an actual surgical procedure.

45

26. Reduction of a dislocated mandible, as shown in the oldest extant illustrated surgical manuscript. This is an eleventh-century Byzantine copy of a ninth-century Greek codex, *Commentaries of Apollonios of Chition on the Peri arthron of Hippocrates. (Codice Laurenziana LXXIV, 7 sec IX, Biblioteca Laurenziana, Florence.)*

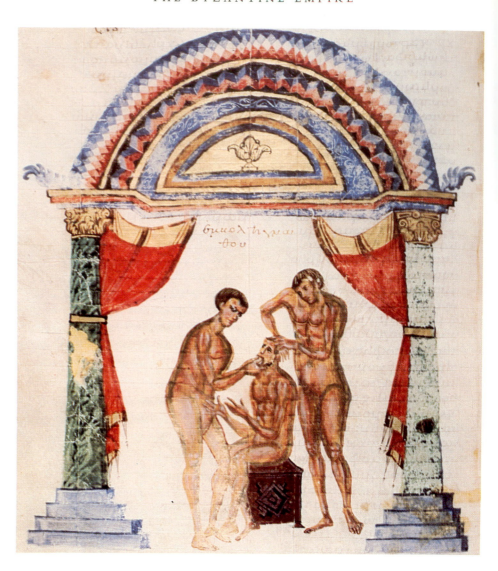

that became seats of science and culture. This compilation of ancient lore has proven to be the most important contribution of Byzantine medicine to European medicine.

Most of what we know of the history of surgery in the Byzantine era, as well as a considerable portion of our knowledge of earlier Greek and Roman surgeons and physicians, is preserved in the encyclopedic writings of Oribasius, Aetius of Amida, Alexander of Tralles, and Paul of Aegina. All these men were physicians of immense learning, and from the firsthand nature of some detailed descriptions of operative techniques we may assume that some of these writers were also accomplished surgeons.

Oribasius (A.D. 325–403) was the first great Byzantine compiler of Greek medical scholarship. A native of Pergamum, he was appointed physician-in-ordinary to Julian the Apostate (A.D. 331–363) and followed him to Gaul. After Julian was named emperor, Oribasius was appointed quaestor at Constantinople.

Oribasius, not considered an original thinker, copied many of the most famous Greek and Roman authorities word for word. He was circumspect in ensuring that appropriate credit was given to any author he abstracted and that the words of the authors were properly quoted. Among the surgeons whose writings he preserved for posterity are Archigenes, Heliodorus, and Antyllus. Oribasius was particularly careful to praise Galen; this praise proved an important force behind Galen's position of influence throughout the Middle Ages.

Oribasius's great *Synagoge,* or *Encyclopedia of Medicine,* was printed for the first time in Venice in 1554. His output was immense: he compiled a digest of medicine, hygiene, therapeutics, and surgery from the time of Hippocrates to his own time in 70 volumes. In addition, Oribasius authored a synopsis of his work

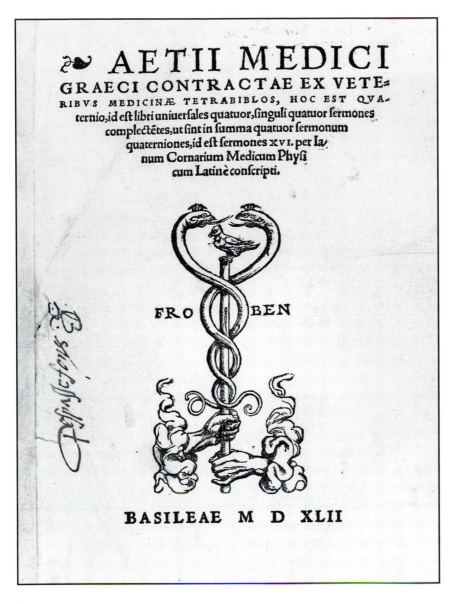

AETII MEDICI GRAECI CONTRACTAE EX VETE=
RIBVS MEDICINÆ TETRABIBLOS, HOC EST QVA=
ternio, id est libri uniuersales quatuor, singuli quatuor sermones
complectetes, ut sint in summa quatuor sermonum
quaterniones, id est sermones XVI. per Ia=
num Cornarium Medicum Physi
cum Latinè conscripti.

FRO BEN

BASILEAE M D XLII

27. Latin translation (Basel: Johannes Froben, 1542) of the *Tetrabiblion (Four Books)* of Aetius of Amida (A.D. 502–575). Aside from his own original surgical work on the treatment of aneurysm by ligation of the brachial artery above the sac, Aetius's writings are valuable for preserving the texts of numerous medical authors who wrote before and during his time, whose work might otherwise have perished. *(Jeremy Norman & Co., Inc.)*

because of its overall unwieldiness. Only 17 volumes of the *Synagoge* have survived. His selections on surgery form the most complete technical treatise that was passed down from generation to generation. Within the volumes is the first treatise exclusively devoted to the treatment of fractures by mechanical means. Oribasius described a screw traction set attached to a narrow wooden bed and devised elaborate multiple-pulley systems. Oribasius elucidated all the symptoms that occur after sectioning of the spinal cord at varying levels, as first described in the experiments of Galen.

Aetius of Amida (A.D. 502–575) studied in Alexandria and was appointed royal physician to Emperor Justinian I and lord high chamberlain at the court of Byzantium. Some speculation exists that Aetius might have been Christian because many of his surgical and medical treatments were accompanied by incantations invoking the name of God. For instance, in explaining how to remove a fishbone from the throat, Aetius advised the surgeon to state the following:

As Jesus Christ drew Lazarus from the grave, and Jonah out of the whale, thus Blasius, the martyr and servant of God, commands 'bone come up or go down.'

Aetius's emphasis on Greek surgical writings was stronger than that of most other Byzantine encyclopedists. His extensive compilation, usually called the *Tetrabiblion,* first printed in 1534, collected surgical thoughts of Rufus of Ephesus, Antyllus, Leonides, Soranus, and Philumenus. In many respects the *Tetrabiblion* supplements what remains of the writings of Oribasius, since it contains copies of some of the sections of the *Synagogue* that had been lost.

The entire *Tetrabiblion* consists of four volumes of four books each. Aetius described many interesting medical conditions including diphtheria, goiter, hydrophobia, ileus, headaches, pleurisy, pneumonia, epilepsy, and elephantiasis. His account of diseases of the eye, ear, nose, throat, and teeth is among the most detailed found in antiquity.

The surgical writings are quite varied. To Aetius is due credit for the first written description of ligation of the brachial artery above the sac for aneurysm:

> An aneurysm located in the bend of the elbow is treated thus. First we carefully trace the artery leading to it, from armpit to elbow, along the inside of the upper arm. Then we make an incision on the inside of the arm, three or four finger-breadths below the armpit, where the artery is felt most easily. We gradually expose the blood vessel and, when it can be lifted free with a hook, we tie it off with two firm ligatures and divide it between them. We fill the wound with incense and lint dressing, then apply a bandage. Next we open the aneurysm itself and no longer need fear bleeding. We remove the blood clots present, and seek the artery which brought the blood. Once found, it is lifted free with the hook, and tied as before. By again filling the wound with incense, we stimulate good suppuration.

As vivid as Aetius's descriptions of surgical operations were (e.g., tonsillectomy, urethrotomy, and hemorrhoidectomy), whether he actually performed any himself remains dubious. He provided practical surgical advice and a rational treatment plan. However, the influence of religion can still be found in many of his charms. In the chapters on obstetrics and gynecology are comments on conception, pregnancy, labor, and lactation. Aetius suggested devices for providing a clean operative field and keeping a patient calm during uterine surgery. Any female patient was to be pitied in this preanesthetic era, since she was placed on the operating table with her knees bent, thighs against the stomach, and legs as wide apart as possible; a rope was tied around one ankle, passed round the knee on the same side, round the back of the neck down to the knee on the other side, and finally to that ankle.

Aetius's most practical suggestion concerned the use of a vaginal speculum for internal inspection. A supposed connection between hypertrophy of the clitoris and heightened sexual instincts was discussed, and clitorectomy was described. He also treated other pathological conditions of the female genitalia, as well as varicose veins and breast cancer. Of the latter he quotes Leonides:

> The cautery is used at first in order to prevent bleeding, but also because it helps to destroy the remains of diseased tissues. When the burning is deep, prognosis is much better. Even in cases where indurated tumors of the breast occur that might be removed without danger of bleeding, it is better to use cautery freely, though the amputation of such a portion down to the healthy parts may suffice.

Alexander of Tralles (525-605) was the youngest of five brothers, all of whom became well known. One of his brothers was the architect of the mosque of St. Sophia in Istanbul. Alexander received his initial medical training from his father and became a skilled physician and an independent scientist with outstanding powers of observation. He was the only Byzantine compiler who demonstrated any special originality. Known as a follower of Galen, Alexander traveled extensively throughout Italy, Gaul, Spain, Greece, and Africa before finally settling in Rome. There he acquired great fame and authored a comprehensive work on medicine in 12 books. His *Practica* was first printed in 1504 and contained various descriptions of diseases and prescriptions that seem to be his own.

The most noteworthy of Alexander's own observations are those concerning worms and vermifuges, which make him the first known parasitologist. He was among the earliest to recommend the use of rhubarb in medicine and was a pioneer in the use of colchicum for gout. Alexander deduced that epilepsy was associated with the brain and that edema, ascites, and splenomegaly could be detected by palpation. Much in his writings concerns pulmonary problems, including tuberculosis and pleurisy. In contrast to other Byzantine writers, Alexander did not emphasize surgical therapy and seems to have been interested in more general medical problems.

As rational and original as Alexander might have been, his writings are heavily imbued with blatantly nonscientific magical and capricious cures. For instance, his use of amulets and incantations included the absurd advice to take a live dung beetle, wrap it in a red rag, and place it on the patient's neck; henbane or hyoscyamus could be administered effectively only if held between the left thumb and index finger when the moon was in a certain position in the sky. For intermittent fever Alexander recommended carrying an olive on which were written mystical but meaningless syllables.

Paul of Aegina (625–690) is considered the last of the Greek eclectics to have dominated the medical culture of the Byzantine period. He studied in Alexandria and practiced there until its conquest by Arab invaders in 641. Little else is known about Paul except that he was greatly admired by his colleagues, especially for his surgical skills. He intended his books to be a compendium of Greek and Roman medicine and succeeded in achieving his purpose.

28. First printing in the original Greek of the *Seven Books* of Paul of Aegina, as issued from the famous Aldine Press of Venice in 1528. The sixth book contains the most complete system of surgery that has been preserved from ancient times. *(Jeremy Norman & Co., Inc.)*

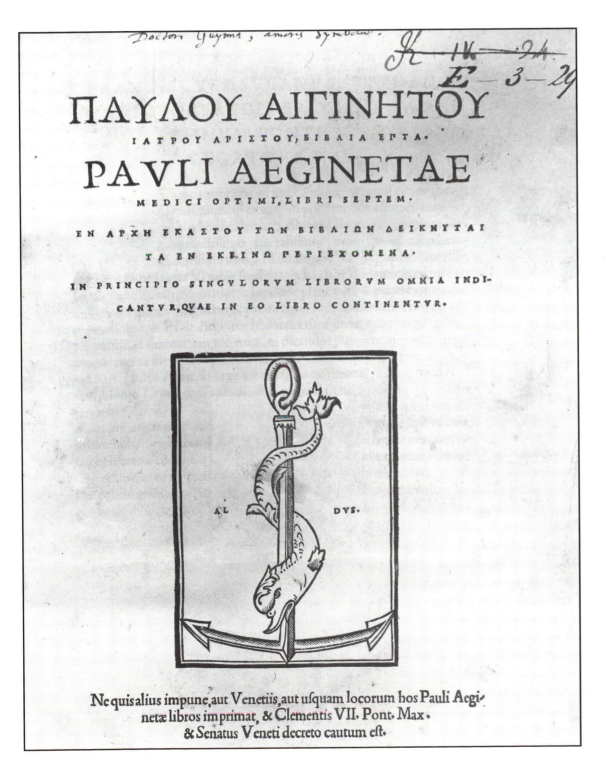

Certain comments by Paul betray the extent to which seventh century medicine had stagnated. He frankly admitted that the authors he wrote about had said all that could be said on a wide variety of subjects and that he functioned as little more than a scribe. The *Seven Books* of Paul first appeared in print in their original Greek text from the famous Aldine Press in Venice in 1528. They form a detailed, carefully selected, concisely expressed compendium and abridgment of the medical literature of his day. Paul related that his main source of information was the works of Oribasius and did not admit to much in the way of personal originality:

It is not because the more ancient writers had omitted anything in the art that I have composed this work, but in order to give a continuous course of instruction; for, on the contrary, everything is handled by them properly and without any omissions, whereas the modern have not only in the first place neglected the study of them, but have also blamed them for prolixity . . .

To remember all the rules of the healing art and all the particular substances connected with it is exceedingly difficult, if not altogether impossible. On this account I have compiled this brief collection from the work of the ancients, and have set down little of my own, except a few things which I have seen and tried in the practice of the art . . .

For being conversant with the most distinguished writers in the profession, and in particular with Oribasius, who, in one work, has given a select view of everything relating to health, I have collected what was best in them, and have endeavored, if possible, not to pass by one distemper. For the work of Oribasius, comprehending seventy books, contains indeed an exposition of the whole art, but is not easily procured by people at large on account of its bulk . . .

Paul succeeded well in his claims, especially concerning surgery. His work was particularly thorough; his writing style was concise and lucid. Because of the systematic organization of his books, large portions of them were incorporated into the texts of the principal Arabic authors. Paul's sixth book, dealing entirely with surgery, was taken over almost word for word by Albucasis of Cordoba (1013-1106), the most famous Arabic surgeon. Thus nearly the entire body of Greek and Roman surgical knowledge was transmitted to Islamic culture through Paul's writings. Later, when the writings of Albucasis were translated from the Arabic back into Latin during the Middle Ages and the Renaissance, large sections of Paul's works were incorporated into the writings of medieval surgeons such as Guy de Chauliac, forming part of the basis of early European surgery.

Paul gave original descriptions of lithotomy, trephination, tonsillectomy, paracentesis, and amputation of the breast but stopped short of describing incision of the chest for empyema. He provided extensive coverage of ophthalmological and military surgery, especially the need for naval physicians. He also provided the first clear description of lead poisoning.

In discussing herniorrhaphy, Paul recommended removal of the testicle, a technique that was perpetuated by the Arabs and continued to be in vogue with European surgeons throughout the sixteenth century.

In Paul's description of a radical operation for hernia, the intestinal or fatty contents were to be pushed back into the abdomen. A large needle with double thread made of 10 strands was then placed through the middle of the incision, incorporating the end of the peritoneum, and tied firmly in cross sutures. The skin was reapproximated with a second ligature, and a wick was placed in the lower end of the incision to provide drainage.

Certain regressive trends that dominated surgical therapy throughout the Middle Ages were being incorporated into Paul's writings. The cauterizing iron was rapidly becoming a most popular surgical instrument, wounds were being treated by the open method involving forced suppuration, and bleeding and cupping were paramount in virtually all therapy.

Paul was evidently quite skillful in military and trauma surgery. His discussions on penetrating wounds and the methods of extracting arrows and other weapons from the human body indicated an extensive personal experience. He used the ligature to arrest traumatic hemorrhage:

> But if the weapon had lodged in any of the larger vessels, such as the internal jugulars or carotids, and the large arteries in the armpits or groins, and if the extraction threaten a great hemorrhage, they are first to be secured with ligatures on both sides, and then the extraction is to be made.

Paul provided the following description of the method of opening the trachea, with indications for this operation:

> The most famous surgeons have also described this operation. Antyllus, therefore, says, 'In cases of cynanche we entirely disapprove of this operation, because the incision is utterly unavailing when all the arteries and the lungs are affected; but in inflammation about the mouth and palate, and in cases of indurated tonsils which obstruct the mouth of the windpipe as the trachea is unaffected, it will be proper to have recourse to pharyngotomy, in order to avoid the risk of suffocation. When, therefore, we engage in the operation we slit open a part of the arteria aspera below the top of the windpipe, about the third or fourth ring. For this is a convenient situation, as being free of flesh, and because the vessels are placed at a distance from the part which is divided. Wherefore, bending the patient's head backwards, so as to bring the windpipe better into view, we are to make a transverse incision between two of the rings, so as that it may not be the cartilage which is divided, but the membrane connecting the cartilages. If one be more timid in operating, one may first stretch the skin with a hook and divide it, and then, removing the vessels aside, if they come in the way, make the incision.' These are the words of Antyllus. We judge that the windpipe has been opened from the air rushing through it with a whizzing noise, and from the voice being lost. After the urgency of the suffocation has passed over, we pare the lips of the incision so as to make them raw surfaces again, and then have recourse to sutures, but sew the skin only, without the cartilage. Then we use the applications proper for bloody or fresh wounds, but if it does not unite we must treat it with incarnants.

As important as Paul's work was in the craft of surgery, he proved to be the last of the great Byzantine encyclopedists, and little evolution in the history of surgery would occur during the next 1000 years.

يا غلنمش ينمق اود سين تاكمحي دشه اندن ضكره مرهله معالجه ايد سين تاكم اوكله

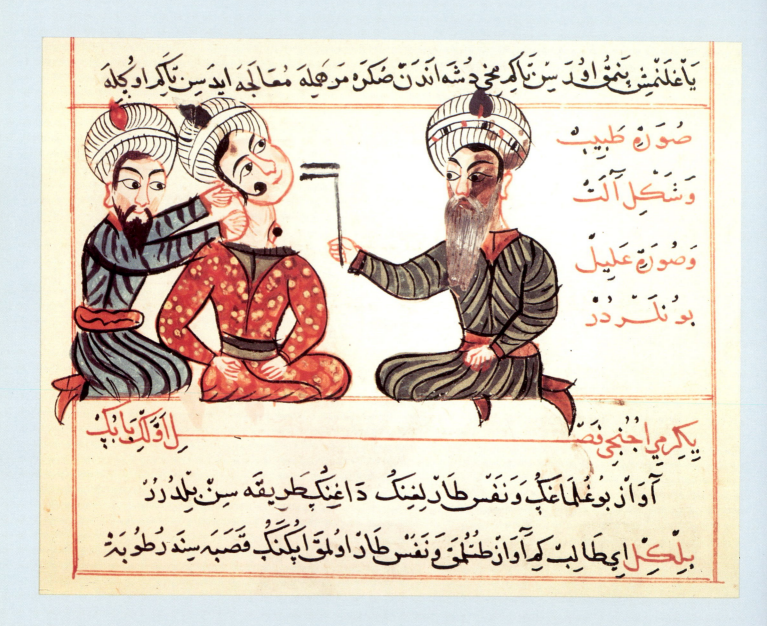

صورة طبيب
وشكل آلت
وصورة عليل
بونلردُرْ

يكرمي اجنبي نص ر اولاعايانك

آواز بوغلماغنك ونفس طارلنك داعنك طريقه سين يلدُرُ د

بلكل اي طالب كه آواز طشلمى ونفس طار اولمق ايكنك قصبه سنده رطوبه

CHAPTER 5

ISLAMIC AND JEWISH SURGERY

uhammad (A.D. 570–632) preached in Mecca (now in Saudi Arabia), but the nobility of that city plotted to assassinate him. On July 16, 622, he fled to Medina and gathered a core of followers. This trip, the Hegira, marked the beginning of the Islamic calendar. Eight years later Muhammad and his followers returned to Mecca, occupied the city, and destroyed all the idols in the pagan temple. Muhammad was acknowledged as a prophet, and Mecca and Medina became the sacred cities of Islam.

Muhammad's teachings soon spread throughout large sections of the civilized world. After Muhammad's death Abu Bakr (573-634) was elected the first caliph, or Muslim ruler. He and his successors encouraged a jihad, or holy war, against the infidels. Within a hundred years they had conquered Syria and Egypt; they went west along the North African coast, crossed the Strait of Gibraltar, and took Spain. They were not stopped until they were well into France; in the east they pushed as far as the Indus River.

The rapid spread of Islamic teachings and culture threatened much of Christian Europe and resulted in numerous wars between Christians and Muslims. The best known of these were the Crusades, undertaken by the Christians from the end of the eleventh century to the conclusion of the thirteenth to recover Palestine.

With the destruction of the library in Alexandria (640), the main repository for all knowledge of the ancient world, the Arabs became the inheritors and preservers of the medicine and science of the Greeks. However, Gundeshapur in Persia would prove more important to the Muhammadan physicians than Alexandria as a cultural center.

Nestorius (?-451), the patriarch of Constantinople, had taught a heretical doctrine concerning Mary and was banished by the general council of the Church. He and his followers were driven into the desert and ultimately to Mesopotamia. Because of religious and social ostracism, the Nestorian heretics were forced to study medicine for their own survival. At Edessa this group gained control of the city's two large hospitals and established a seat of Greek learning in medicine and surgery. The Nestorians inevitably came into conflict with the orthodox bishop of Cyprus, who expelled them from their new home in 489. They fled to Gundeshapur and brought with them the knowledge and scientific zeal they had cultivated at their former medical institution.

A new, soon-to-be-famous school that would become the true starting point of Islamic medicine and surgery was established at Gundeshapur. Greek medicine was cultivated in this city for two centuries, until the Arabs conquered the Middle East, including Persia and Syria, in the seventh century, thus coming into contact with the Nestorians and their Greek medical culture. Greek works in the possession of the Nestorians, already translated into Syrian, were translated into Arabic. During the next two centuries a colossal academic endeavor

29. *Facing page,* Cauterization of swollen lymph nodes of the right side of the neck in a patient with scrofula. From the Sharaf-ad-din ibn Ali manuscript written in 1465. *(Phot. Bibliothèque Nationale, Paris, MS Suppl turc 693, vol 1, fol 29, verso.)*

to translate all the Greek writings into Arabic took place. Consequently, with few exceptions no practical improvements other than translations were made and surgery stagnated.

During the first five centuries of the modern era no advances in medicine and surgery were made in the Christian Roman empire, primarily because of the many physical and spiritual losses of Greek and Roman writings that were the basis of Western civilization. These losses resulted from barbarian invasions of the west, recurrent disasters and pestilence, and the vigorous anti–Greco-Roman feeling of the Christian church. Although the early Christian monks and theologians did study medicine, it was a profession based on rigid beliefs: faith had won out over scientific advances as the most important factor in the healing process.

Early Christian doctrine was vehemently opposed to human vivisection, so the study of anatomy and any consequent advances in surgery were stifled. Eventually the Church decreed that surgery could no longer be practiced by monks and their Christian attendants, leaving the practice of surgery to the uneducated. It eventually fell to itinerant charlatans, sycophants, and ultimately the "barber surgeon."

During these early centuries the Arabic schools were essentially the only seats of active medical learning in the West. Since their instruction was derived from ancient Greek and Roman authorities, teaching continued with a Hellenic foundation. Their medical and surgical masters remained Hippocrates, Celsus, and Galen. Islamic respect for education and learning caused the Arabic conquerors to become the bridge between Greco-Roman knowledge and Latin Europe. Through many centuries of translations, studies, and reinvigoration of Greek and Roman thought the world of Islam reassembled a precious treasure on which the intellectual growth of the West depended. This Arabic period endured up to the close of the fourteenth century.

Although the medical authors of the Islamic period are called "Arabic" because of the language they used, the society was, in fact, polyglot. Many of the authors were Persian- or Spanish-born, some Christian, and a large number Jewish. Because they resided in Muslim-dominated countries, their writings were in Arabic.

Jewish translators occupied a special place in the bridging of Arabic and Latin knowledge. The Muslims were quite tolerant of their subjects' religions and cultures. Realizing that many of the conquered peoples were more advanced in the arts and sciences, the Muslims permitted scholars of all races and religions to pursue their academic studies. Certain Jews, particularly in Muslim-occupied Spain, were especially learned in Arabic, Latin, Hebrew, and other languages. The so-called translators from the Arabic, who made the anonymous Latin translations of Arabic medical and scientific works that were printed during the second half of the fifteenth century and thus profoundly influenced the development of European thought, were chiefly Sephardic Jews.

The main Islamic dynastic caliphates were (1) the eastern, consisting of both Persian Bagdad (the Abbasids, 750-1258) and Cairo (the Fatimids, 909-1171) and (2) the Spanish west, most notably at Cordoba (the Umayyads, 756-1031). Little is known concerning the organization of medicine as a profession in the Arabic countries from the fourth to sixth centuries. However, the rise of the caliphate in Bagdad led to its becoming the earliest dominant center of Arabic medicine and surgery.

The eastern caliphate included such liberal-minded rulers as Al-Mansur (712-775) and Harun al-Rashid (764-809), caliph of the *Tales of the Arabian Nights*. At one time there were said to be 860 licensed physicians and numerous hospitals and schools in Bagdad. The most renowned of the early Arabic physicians was the Nestorian Hunayn ibn Ishaq (808-873), also known as Johannitius. He received his initial education in Gundeshapur under the Christian Arabic translator Johannes Mesue the Elder (777-837), also called Janus Damascenus.

Johannitius was the leading Arabic translator-physician in Bagdad. Under his forceful guidance a board of translators and a council of censors were created.

The latter ensured that no doctor went without necessary education and training. Johannitius studied Hippocrates, Galen, Oribasius, and Paul of Aegina. He also wrote the oldest known Arabic treatise on ophthalmological diseases.

Within the eastern caliphate the greatest physicians were three Persians—Rhazes, Haly Abbas (930-994), and Avicenna (980-1037)—and a Jew, Isaac Judaeus (855-935). A generation after Johannitius came Abu Bakr Muhammad ibn Zakariya al-Razi, known in the Latin world as Rhazes (854-925). He was born near Teheran and did not begin to study medicine until he was over 30 years old. Rhazes eventually became the caliph's personal physician and director of the largest hospital in Bagdad. He is credited with writing 273 manuscripts, most of which are now lost. The clarity of his writings did much to bring Greek medicine, especially Hippocrates and Galen, to the Arabic world. His *Al-Hawi,* or *Continens,* is one of the greatest encyclopedias of ancient medicine. First printed in Latin in 1486, it remains physically the largest and heaviest of the medical books printed before 1501.

Rhazes's fame rests with his descriptions of disease. He provided the first authentic account of smallpox and measles. His ninth book was revised by Vesalius and remained the preeminent source of therapeutic knowledge until long after the Renaissance. Rhazes was known to perform surgical operations, although technical matters did not seem to concern him. His seventh book is on surgery and is taken from Hippocrates, Paul of Aegina, Oribasius, and Aetius of Amida.

Rhazes was a pioneer in the use of animal gut for sutures, and he introduced a number of new remedies such as mercurial ointment. He described an operation for lacrimal fistula and cautioned against injuring the anterior branch of the ophthalmic nerve. It is known that Rhazes excised necrotic bone and wrote authoritatively on resection and removal of the whole tibia, the humerus, the radius, and the ulna. He extensively treated sciatica and spinal curvature and provided many details about bladder catheters. Considered an expert on gonorrhea, he was the first to consistently use urethral injections for its treatment. Rhazes was also the earliest medical writer to devote an entire treatise to diseases of children.

Ali ibn al-Abbas al Majusi (930-994), known in western Europe as Haly Abbas, was born at Ahwaz in southwestern Persia. He considered Rhazes's works to be so overly detailed and diffuse that they were of little practical value. During his residence in Bagdad as a court physician, Haly Abbas authored his *Al-maleki,* or *Liber Regius,* also known as the *Royal Book.* This orderly encyclopedia of medicine and surgery was the leading medical treatise for 100 years, before being displaced by the works of Avicenna. Haly Abbas's sections on anatomy were especially influential in the school at Salerno.

The nineteenth tract of Haly Abbas contains 110 chapters devoted to surgery. Like many books of antiquity, it was originally introduced to western Europe by Constantinus Africanus (1020-1087) under his own name. In the nineteenth tract Haly Abbas advised the excision of goiters. For hydrocele he recommended that the tumor be opened and its tunics dissected out. He provided a description of abdominal paracentesis, three fingers' breadth inferior to the umbilicus, for generalized anasarca. The operative treatment of imperforate anus consisted of the insertion of a sponge or lead tube through the incised membrane to prevent reunion. Haly Abbas's pragmatism as a surgeon is evident in his treatment of brachial artery wounds secondary to careless venesection from the median basilic vein. If cautery is unable to stop the hemorrhage, he advised, the artery should be exposed, carefully isolated, tied in two places, above and below the wound, and then divided between them.

The eastern Arabic work that proved most useful for future physicians was Avicenna's *Canon.* Abu-Ali al-Husayn ibn-adallah ibn-Sina, also known as Avicenna (980-1037), was born at Afshena in Persia, and his influence on Islam and Christendom equaled Galen's. It is said that he was a child prodigy and received his medical education from Nestorians in Bagdad. Eventually Avicenna was made physician-in-chief of the largest hospital in Bagdad. He died in the prime of his life from what has been described as a hedonistic life-style.

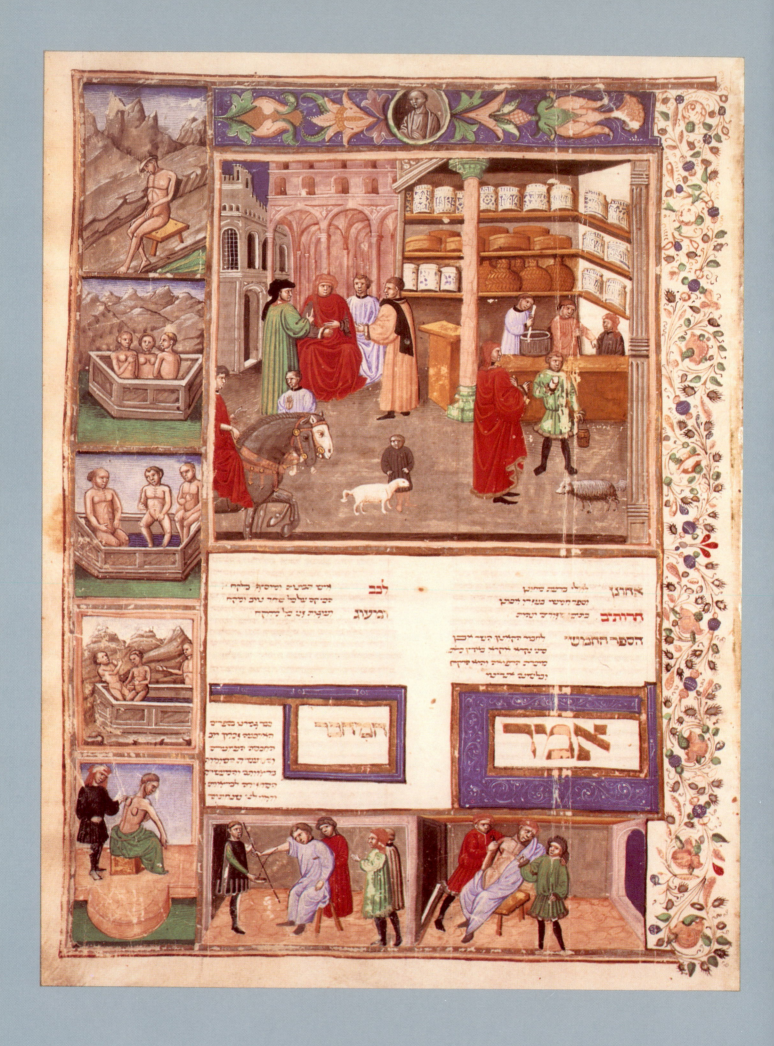

The most renowned of his approximately 100 works is the *Canon*. It dominated the medical schools of Asia and Europe for almost six centuries. The text accompanied the Crusaders on their journeys and accomplished for the Muslims what Galen had done for the Romans. The first complete edition of the *Canon* was printed at Milan in 1473.

The gigantic tome of Avicenna was written in a meticulous style and served as a complete exposition of Galenism. Untold numbers of translators, teachers, students, and practitioners based their medical ideas and procedures on discussions in the *Canon*. On the whole, the influence of this work on medieval medicine was quite negative. Because the *Canon* seemed to confirm doctrine, so compatible with church dogma, that reasoning was more important than proper observation in the overall treatment of patients, it supported the medieval point of view and had little influence on the development of a more modern scientific attitude.

Avicenna regarded surgery and surgeons as little more than a necessary evil. He set back the progress of surgery by suggesting the doctrine that operative surgery was an inferior and separate branch of general medicine. The cauterizing iron was almost the sole treatment that he advised for surgical illnesses. He had a natural aversion to the surgeon's scalpel. Because of Avicenna, therefore, medicine and surgery became truly separate and remained so for many centuries. This attitude paved the way for western Europeans to long consider surgeons of a lower caste than the doctors of internal or general medicine.

Avicenna was an experienced physician and described the etiology of epilepsy and diabetes with glucosuria. He is said to have been the first to discuss the preparation and properties of sulfuric acid and alcohol. Breast cancer was treated by cauterization, to eradicate remnants of the disease and to control hemorrhage. Among Avicenna's surgical recommendations was that broken bones be refractured and reset when they healed with gross deformities. He described tracheotomy and advised that twisted hairs or hog bristles be used instead of silk or hemp as ligatures. Injuries of nerves were described, but actual reapproximation via suturing was not mentioned. One of the most important sections of the *Canon* dealt with the treatment of mandibular fracture. Avicenna emphasized the importance of ascertaining whether proper reduction had occurred; ascertainment could best be accomplished by observing whether the teeth were brought into proper occlusion.

Another prominent medical figure of the eastern caliphate was the Jewish physician Isaac Judaeus (855–935). He was born in Egypt and practiced mainly as an ophthalmologist. He authored a treatise on uroscopy and a work on dietetics. Among his most important contributions was a book of aphorisms in Hebrew.

The western caliphate attained its highest prosperity in the city of Cordoba, where in the eighth century a university with a library said to contain 225,000 volumes was established. At least 50 hospitals were started during the Umayyad dynasty. The leading medical authorities in the western caliphate were the surgeon Albucasis (936–1013), the clinician Avenzoar (1091–1162), and the physician-philosophers Averroes (1126–1198) and Moses Maimonides (1135–1204). Abul Qasim, known as Albucasis, is a prominent figure in the history of surgery. He was born in the Andalusian town of Zahra, near Cordoba. Little other precise biographical information is available. No contemporary evidence exists to confirm the many stories that were later told about him.

What is most evident about Albucasis is the long-lasting effect that his writings had on the course of surgery. He authored the *Altasrif*, or *Collection*, some 30 manuscripts on various phases of medicine. Three of these documents represent the first rational, systematic, and illustrated treatment of the subject of surgery. The *Altasrif* became the leading authority on surgery in the Middle Ages and formed the foundation on which much of European surgery was later fashioned.

Like most of the other handwritten manuscripts of the period, the *Altasrif* is a repetition, with modifications, of the texts of the late Alexandrians, particularly

30. *Facing page,* Manuscript page, written and illuminated in Italy during the first half of the fifteenth century, of Avicenna's *Canon of Medicine* translated into Hebrew. During the Middle Ages Jews living in Spain under Moorish rule were responsible for translating many important Arabic texts into Latin and were known as the "Translators from the Arabic." Much more unusual was the translation of an Arabic medical work into Hebrew. This exquisite illuminated manuscript was possibly prepared for a wealthy Jewish physician living in Bologna, a center of medical and scientific learning in fifteenth-century Italy. It could also have been prepared for a monastic library because members of Catholic religious orders frequently read Hebrew but not Arabic. The images in the outer margin depict bathing for hygienic purposes. Communal bathing for health reasons was common in the Middle Ages; frequently it resulted in the conveyance of venereal disease. *Clockwise to the lower margin,* A physician examines tumors on the back of his patient, and a barber-surgeon bleeds a patient and then operates on the same patient. The center scene depicts a pharmacy with its large medicinal jars. Outside the shop a group of physicians are consulting. *(Codex 2197, fol 492a-38b, Biblioteca Universitaria, Bologna.)*

of Paul of Aegina. Albucasis's declared purpose was to revive the surgical sciences as taught by the ancients. His careful descriptions, pragmatic advice, and personal observations reveal a cautious, ethical, and conscientious practical surgeon. Unlike other Arabic author-physicians, Albucasis described many operative procedures that did not appear in other contemporary manuscripts. The most interesting feature of the text is the large number of illustrations of surgical instruments, which served to clarify many of the operative techniques.

The *Altasrif* had minimal importance in the Arabic world. Although Albucasis was a celebrated physician and surgeon, his surgical writings were never appreciated during his lifetime. Muhammadans in Spain did not approve of surgery, and his appreciation of surgery with a strong emphasis on anatomy was in complete contradiction to accepted practices. As a consequence, among the Arabs his fame was promptly overtaken by Avicenna's. Albucasis stands alone, however, as the only Arab to write a distinct, separate treatise on surgery.

Because Albucasis's work was translated into Latin within a century of his death, it served as the basis for the earliest Italian and French surgical writings. Its concise operative descriptions, systematized approach to surgery, and masterful illustrations were inducements for its use by the Europeans. The first of his three surgical books was devoted to the use of the cautery and caustics. Albucasis described more than 50 surgical conditions and their operative treatment, especially with the cautery. The second book referred to operations for which cutting instruments were necessary and discussed lithotomy, lithotrity, amputa-

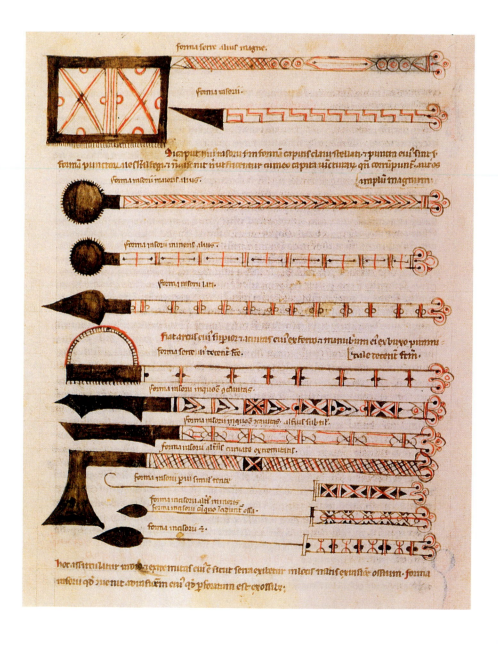

31. Surgical saws and scalpels, from a thirteenth-century Latin translation of Albucasis's *Altasrif,* the first logical, complete, illustrated treatise on surgery and surgical instruments. Abul Qasim, a Moor, was born near Cordoba, Spain. His work remained the standard authority until it was superseded by the surgery of William of Saliceto. *(Phot. Bibliothèque Nationale, Paris, Mss, Lat 7127 [f 38].)*

tions for gangrene, and treatment of wounds. The third book was devoted to fractures, sprains, and dislocations, including spinal fracture with paralysis.

Albucasis is credited with having been the first medical author to write about deformities of the mouth and dental arches. He is the first surgeon to have employed the visual method of teaching by the use of carefully drawn illustrations. Among the many things Albucasis discussed, the following deserve special attention: a tonsil guillotine, a concealed knife and its use in opening abscesses, a trocar for paracentesis, the possibility that Albucasis or his contemporaries invented the true scissors, the use of animal gut as suture material, a rudimentary description of thrombophlebitis migrans, a specially constructed table for extending limbs to reduce dislocation or displaced fractures, and a formula for a kind of plaster cast. Albucasis described ligation of arteries for arterial wounds and aneurysms, excision of scrofulous tumors of the neck, tracheostomy, and intercostal puncture for empyema. He wrote, as follows, the first scientific account of hemophilia:

> I have found men in a certain village who told me that whenever they suffered a severe wound, it bled till they were dead, and they added that when a child rubbed his gums they began to bleed, and went on bleeding till he died. Another also having had a vein opened by a phlebotomist bled to death; and they said that, in general, most of them died thus. I have never seen such a thing save in this village; nor do I find it noticed in ancient writers. I know not the cause of it, but as for the cure, I suppose a cautery should be applied at once; but I have never tried it and the whole thing is marvellous to me.

The efforts of Albucasis to improve the quality of surgical care and, most important, to teach young surgeons according to high ethical and moral standards is quite evident. He writes as follows:

> I thought it well to complete . . . for you . . . this treatise which concerns surgical operating. For the skilled practitioner of operative surgery is totally lacking in our land and time; so that the knowledge of it is on the point of being blotted out and it remains lost; and there is nothing left of it except a few traces in the books of the Ancients; where, however, it has been so corrupted by the hands of scribes, and subjected to error and confusion, that its meaning has become obscured and its value diminished. Therefore I decided to revive this art by expounding, elucidating, and epitomizing it in this treatise . . . Now this is the reason why there is no skilful operator in our day; the art of medicine is long and it is necessary for its exponent, before he exercises it, to be trained in anatomy . . . For he who is not skilled in . . . anatomy . . . is bound to fall into error that is destructive of life . . .
>
> Wherefore you must know . . . that operative surgery is divided into two parts, namely, where operation is associated with the health of the patient, and, on the other hand, where it is for the most part fraught with danger . . . Show, then, caution and care for yourselves and gentleness and perseverance for your patients. Take the best road that leads to health and a happy outcome . . .

Albucasis's legacy to his successors regarding the cautering iron, as follows, is evident in his chapter on treatment of hernia:

> When a rupture occurs in the groin, and part of the intestine and omentum comes down into the scrotum . . . forbid the patient to take food for one day and have him use laxatives to empty the bowel. Then let him lie on his back . . . and bid him hold his breath till the intestine or omentum comes out; then put it back with your finger. Then, below the hernia over the pubic bone, mark a semicircle whose extremities point upward. Then heat a cautery . . . when it is white hot and emits sparks then return the intestine or omentum into his abdominal cavity, and have an assistant put his hand over the place to prevent the exit of the intestine . . . Then apply the cautery to the mark . . . and hold it till it reaches the bone . . . You must take the greatest care that the intestine does not come out while you are cauterizing, lest you burn it and it result in death or grave injury . . . You must understand that if you do not bring the cauterization down to the bone your operation will not be successful . . . dress the site of the cauterization till it heals . . . The patient should lie on his back for forty days so that the wound may cicatrize.

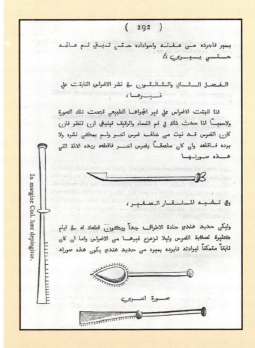

32. The first printing in Arabic of Albucasis's *Altasrif* appeared in this edition by the London pharmacist and Arabist, John Channing. It was issued in 1778 from the Clarendon Press in Oxford in a small edition appropriate for such a specialized work of scholarship. *(Jeremy Norman & Co., Inc.)*

Avenzoar (1091-1162), clinician in the western caliphate, was born in Seville, the son of a Jewish physician. He rejected many teachings of the ancient Greeks, particularly of Galen. His writings, known as *Teisir,* or *Rectification,* were translated into Hebrew in 1280 and eventually printed in Latin (1490). Avenzoar described the itch-mite, serous pericarditis, mediastinal abscess, pharyngeal paralysis, and otitis media. His reports on the total extirpation of the uterus and tracheotomy suggest that he may actually have practiced surgery. Among his many innovative techniques were the use of a rudimentary stomach tube and feeding via the rectum. Avenzoar's description of the treatment of fractures demonstrates that he must have obtained an unusually precise background in anatomy. Although he recommended reliance on one's personal experiences rather than traditional dogma, superstition and mystical beliefs were still invoked for some treatments. For instance, the allegedly curative value of a bezoar is credited to the teachings of Avenzoar.

Averroes (1126-1198) was the best-known pupil of Avenzoar. Primarily a philosopher, Averroes attempted to found a system of medicine based on Aristotle's theories (384-322 B.C.). Although Averroes contributed little to the evolution of surgery, he exerted a profound influence on later Jewish physicians. His pantheistic views were spread throughout Europe by Jewish intellectuals after their expulsion from Spain.

Although great advances in surgery were not made during the Islamic period, other aspects of medicine were quite innovative. General health care, specifically the hospital system, under Islam was superior to that of European society. Although Christian hospitals existed in Europe, they were few, rudimentary, and greatly inferior to those in the Arabic world. One of the eastern caliphs had established a hospital in Damascus as early as 707. However, the finest of all such institutions was the Al-Mansur in Cairo. Founded in 1283, it was a gigantic building with separate departments for patients with different diseases. Al-Mansur contained a dietary kitchen, an outpatient clinic, an orphanage, a chapel, a vast library, and huge lecture halls. Convalescents had separate sections within the hospital complex. Both male and female nurses were employed. On discharge patients received five gold pieces each to support themselves until they could return to work.

Closely connected with Islamic medical culture was the influence of the Jews on European medicine. After the Romans destroyed the homeland of the Jews in Palestine, they settled in colonies in all parts of the Roman empire. Living in the diaspora, or exile, the Jews in Europe suffered hundreds of years of persecution and discrimination. When Christians became dominant in Europe, intolerant leaders persecuted the Jews for rejecting Christianity. In Spain, however, which the Islamic Moors ruled from the eighth to the early fifteenth century, the Jews were treated with respect and an acknowledged religious tolerance, as previously mentioned. Not until the late 1400s did the leaders of the Inquisition began to persecute and prosecute the Jews in Spain. In 1492, King Ferdinand (1452-1516) and Queen Isabella (1451-1504) expelled all Jews from Spain.

Under Arabic domination Jewish physicians were prominent figures at the courts of the caliphs. Fluent in Arabic and Persian, as well as Hebrew and other languages, they were greatly esteemed for their learning, despite their different religious beliefs. Arab tolerance did not extend to Christian physicians, who were generally not learned in Arab culture. Christian authorities also respected learned Jewish physicians, and later, when discrimination against the Jews was pervasive in medieval Europe, the Jewish physicians and surgeons continued to be greatly esteemed.

With the rise of the Christian monks and their monasteries, the priests became the dominant medical practitioners and all progress or improvement in the practice of surgery was nearly at an end. Most of the monks read nothing but simple formularies and relied on relics, exorcisms, and prayers. Greco-Roman and Alexandrian medical teachings were essentially forgotten. Since the Crusades were directed against the Muslims of the East, the Jews in Latin Europe had an opportunity to develop their medical education. Because Jews were the

33. *Facing page,* Medieval illuminated manuscript from southern France of the zodiac man, showing which signs influence each part of the body. This information was used by the physician or surgeon as a guide in determining when operations or treatment would be effective. What is most unusual about this painting, aside from the text in Hebrew, is that the zodiac man is shown circumcised, strongly suggesting that the painting is by a Jewish artist. *(Phot. Bibliothèque Nationale, Paris, Mss Or, Hébreu 1181, f 265.)*

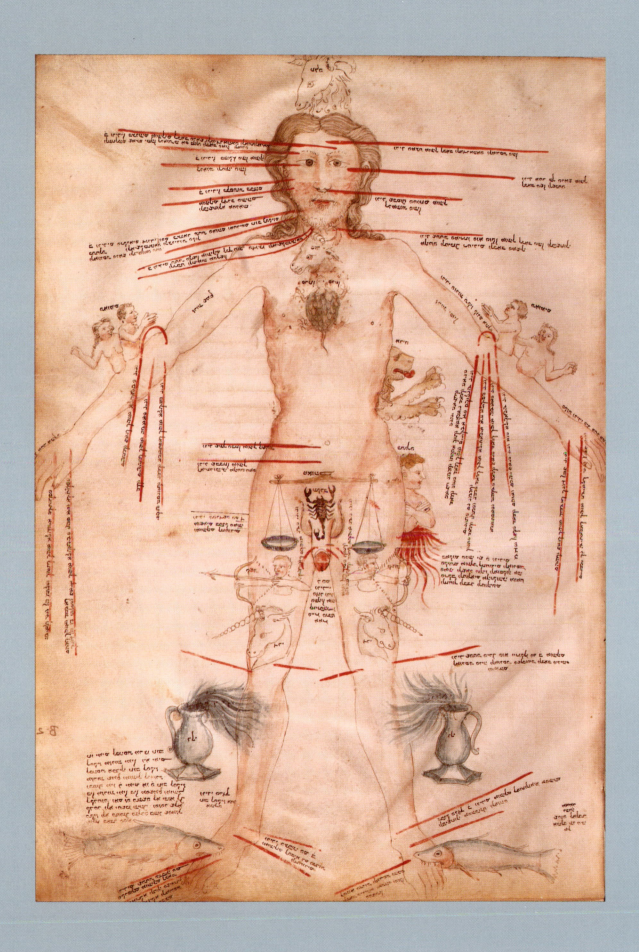

translators of the ancient Greek medical tracts, not unexpectedly the kings and nobility resorted to Jewish physicians. During the tenth and eleventh centuries the Jews were the most important authors and students of medical and surgical topics in Latin Europe. Although general discrimination continued and Jews were forbidden to enter certain cities and regions, to acquire a Jewish physician was tantamount to having an unlawful but important luxury.

The most prominent of Jewish physicians in Arabic medicine was Rabbi Moses ben Maimon (1135-1204), called Moses Maimonides. Born in Cordoba, he served as court physician to the sultan Saladin. Although a proponent of ancient Galenic doctrine, Maimonides practiced pragmatic therapeutics. He authored numerous medical treatises, and translations of his writings from the original Arabic into Hebrew and Latin were read throughout Christian Europe. Perhaps his most memorable writing is the *Oath* or *Prayer of Maimonides,* which provided certain precepts for the practice of medicine:

> In thine eternal providence thou hast chosen me to watch over the life and health of thy creatures. I am now about to apply myself to the duties of my profession. Support me, Almighty God, in these great labors that they may benefit mankind for without thy help not even the least thing will succeed.
>
> Inspire me with love for my art and for thy creatures. Do not allow thirst for profit, ambition for renown and admiration, to interfere with my profession, for these are the enemies of truth and of love for mankind and they can lead astray in the great task of attending to the welfare of thy creatures. Preserve the strength of my body and of my soul that they ever be ready to cheerfully help and support rich and poor, good and bad, enemy as well as friend. In the sufferer let me see only the human being . . . May no strange thoughts divert my attention at the bedside of the sick, or disturb my mind in its silent labors . . .
>
> Grant that my patients have confidence in me and my art and follow my directions and my counsel . . . Should those who are wiser than I wish to improve and instruct me, let my soul gratefully follow their guidance; for vast is the extent of our art . . .
>
> Imbue my soul with gentleness and calmness when older colleagues proud of their age, wish to displace me or to scorn me or disdainfully to teach me . . . For they are old and old age is not master of the passions. I also hope to attain old age upon this earth, before thee, Almighty God!
>
> Let me be contented in everything except in the great science of my profession. Never allow the thought to arise in me that I have attained to sufficient knowledge, but vouchsafe to me the strength, the leisure and the ambition ever to extend my knowledge . . .
>
> Almighty God! Thou hast chosen me in thy mercy to watch over the life and death of thy creatures. I now apply myself to my profession. Support me in this great task so that it may benefit mankind, for without thy help not even the least thing will succeed.

Among Maimonides's medical writings the most voluminous is the *Medical Aphorisms.* Composed of 1500 succinct maxims based mainly on Greek medical writings, the *Medical Aphorisms* contains 25 chapters, each dealing with a different area of medicine. Included are numerous references to surgical topics such as bloodletting, gynecology, and minor operations.

In his *Treatise on Hemorrhoids* Maimonides stated that he disapproved of bloodletting or surgery for hemorrhoids except in severe cases. In general, he regarded operative excision with skepticism because surgery does not remove the underlying causes that produced the hemorrhoids in the first place:

> There was a youth . . . in whom the affliction of hemorrhoids occurred at the mouth of the rectum . . . Because this illness recurred many times, he considered having them extirpated in order to uproot this malady from its source so that it not return again. I informed him of the danger inherent in this, in that it is not clear if these hemorrhoids are of the variety which should be excised or not, since there are people in whom they have once been surgically extirpated and in whom other hemorrhoids develop. This is because the causes which gave rise to the original ones remained and, therefore, new ones develop.

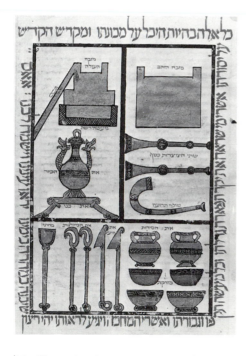

34. Illustration in a manuscript Hebrew bible written and illuminated in Perpignan, France, by the scribe Salomon, son of Raphael, in 1299. Along with sacrificial vessels, circumcision knives are shown in the lower left corner. *(Phot. Bibliothèque Nationale, Paris, Mss Hébreu No 7.)*

Prologus.

℄ Incipiunt aphorismi excellentissimi Raby Moyses se
cundum doctrinam Galieni medicorum principis.

i   N nomie dei pii et misericordis cum quo adiuuo me
Ait Moyses filius teruli dei israeliticus cordubésis
multas cópilatóes cópilauere multi sapientu uia apho
rismoru in diuersis speciebus scientiaru et p ceteris
scientiis hac uia indiget scientia metaphisice que licet
non sit difficilts quo ad intellectu: sicut sunt multe sciétie phisi
ce. nec quo ad cognitóem subiectoru sicut sunt alique scientie
ydiomatu pfectoru: est tamé difficillima quo ad multa que mei
dicum oportet scire et in méoria semp habere. nec tamé omnia
sed solum spéalia que i indiuiduis proxima sunt. ad omniu eni
cóprehensioné sicut probatu est iam nó attingit sciétia alicuius
He autè cópilatónes uia aphoristica cópilate sunt facilis cogni
tóis et retentóis sine dubio. et ad sciendum et retinédum matei
rias necessarias suu adiuuát addiscenté. Et ob hanc câm ypoi
crates precipuus medicoru cópilauit suu libru diuulgatum de
aphorismis. Et multi etiá alii medicoru cópilauerut post eum te
nentes eius uestigia aphorismos ut sunt aphorismi Rasis diuul
gati et aphorismi Susi. et aphorismi Iohannis Mesue Damai
sceni et alioru. et est manifestum cuilibet prouidentu prouisioi
ne máifesta qp quicuq3 cópilator cópilauerit aphorismos in scié
tia aliqua non cópilauit eos uelut sufficiétes ad cóprehendendu
omnes artis radices: sed velut valde vtiles et sufficiétes pre cete
ris cópilatóibus ad cóphendendum materias multas et diuersas
necnó et ad eas in memoria retinédum. Et in summa cópilator
quicunque cópilauit aphorismos nó potuit p ipsos omnia que
sunt necessaria sue scientie. Non ypocras in aphorismis suis
nec ebbussay alfarabii in omnibus hiis que cópilauit uia aphoi
rismoru nec alii qui minores illis fuere. Hec yero premisi ad
excusationé horu aphorismoru quos protuli in psenti libro eos
cóformás. nec dico me compilasse sed elegisse: quia collegi eos
ex verbis Galieni de óibus libris suis et ex eius verbis que dii
xit p viam cóplexionis in expositóe libroru ypocratis. Nec co
arcto me in huiusmodi aphorismis sicut feci in libro qui brei
a.i.

35. First edition, published in Venice in 1489, of the *Aphorisms* of Moses ben Maimon, generally known as Maimonides. This collection of 1500 aphorisms, derived from Galen's works and originally written by Maimonides in Arabic, is Maimonides's most popular medical work. The medical writings of Maimonides, the most famous medieval Jewish physician, philosopher, and theologian, influenced not only Jewish and Muslim physicians but also such surgeons as Henry de Mondeville and Guy de Chauliac. (*Jeremy Norman & Co., Inc.*)

By A.D. 427, the Jewish community in Babylonia had completed the compilation of the Gemara, which with the Mishnah made up the Talmud. However, numerous oral and written comments on the credence of its thoughts continued to be made for centuries, and Maimonides is considered among the most important of these commentators of the Middle Ages. Although the Talmud is primarily a law book, it must be assumed that Maimonides incorporated Jewish religious law into his medical writings and practices.

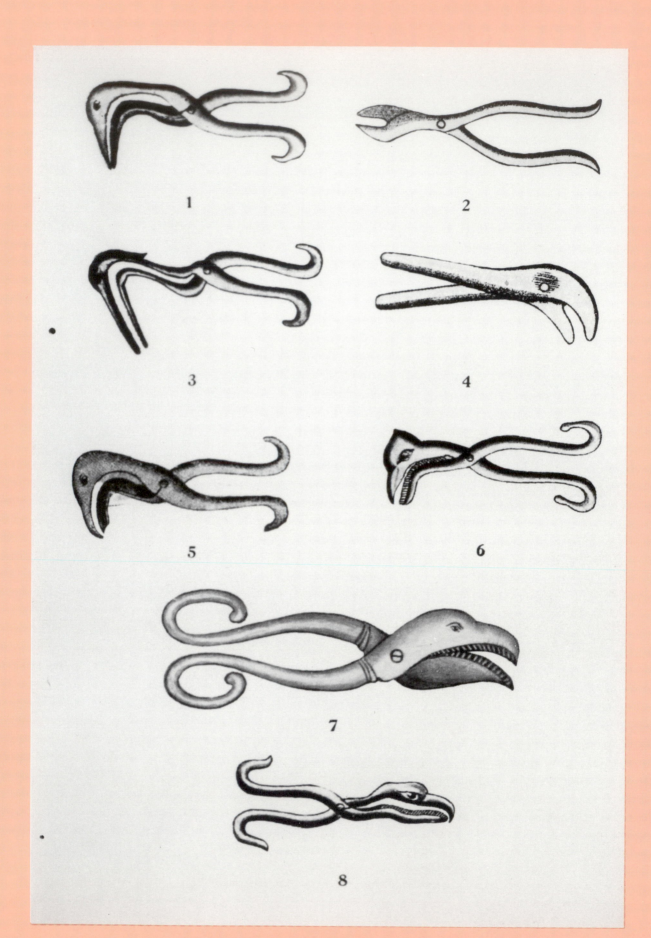

CHAPTER 6
THE FAR EAST

∽

INDIA

The earliest history of India for which archeological evidence exists was centered in Mohenjo-Daro in the Indus River valley. The inhabitants of this area flourished from approximately 2500 B.C. to 1500 B.C. During that time they developed a number of unique public health features such as sanitation systems with both sewers and communal baths. No information is available regarding any surgical operations that might have been performed.

About 1500 B.C. wandering hordes known as Aryans came from the northwest plains of Central Asia, invaded the Indus River valley, and drove the earlier inhabitants into the Indian subcontinent. The influence of the Aryans gradually extended over all of India. The Aryans perfected the Sanskrit language and a method of writing it. They propagated a caste system and brought with them the basis for much of the subsequent religious and cultural development in India. Although the Aryans helped bring Hinduism to India, the religious teacher Gautama Siddhartha (563–483 B.C.), known as the Buddha, was to have an even greater individual impact.

Dated history in India commences in about 500 B.C., when the Persian army of Darius I (558–486 B.C.) seized the northwest region of the country. In 326 B.C. Alexander the Great gained the same area. After the departure of the Macedonian invaders, most of India was governed by the Maurya empire. Its greatest ruler was Asoka (272–232 B.C.), who through military might was able to unify all but the southern tip of the country. He was eventually converted from the Hinduism of his ancestors to Buddhism and established it as the state religion.

After the death of Asoka India was invaded over time by Scythians, Arabs, Greeks, and Bactrians. Eventually another native Indian dynasty, the Gupta, was installed. The Gupta period (A.D. 320 to the end of the fourth century A.D.) is known as the Golden Age of the Sanskrit Renaissance. A great civilization flourished, and India was a center of learning, especially in the field of medicine.

Hinduism is one of the world's oldest living religions, a fusion of the ancient beliefs brought by the Aryans with the religious and cultural traditions of the Indus River valley civilization. The earliest documents concerning Indian medicine are found in the *Vedas,* or books of knowledge, the oldest and most sacred written works of the Hindu religion.

The *Vedas* were initially compiled in Sanskrit between 3000 B.C. and 1000 B.C. During this era, termed the Vedic period, the *Rig Veda, Sama Veda, Yajur Veda,* and *Atharva Veda* were composed. Ayur Veda, or knowledge of life, was the name given to the art of healing. The Hindus believed the *Vedas* emanated from a divine source.

36. *Facing page,* Hindu surgical forceps as described by Sushruta. The eight forceps pictured are known as *Svastika Yantra,* or Cruciform Instruments, since the two parts of an open forceps resemble a cross. The forceps are named after their bird-shaped heads, with Nos. 1 and 2 called the Crow forceps, Nos. 3 and 4 the Heron, No. 5 the Osprey, No. 6 the Blue Jay, No. 7 the Eagle, and No. 8 the Hawk. Hindu surgical instruments were classified as either blunt or sharp, and the heads of the blunt instruments such as forceps were designed to resemble the faces of ferocious beasts, deer, or birds. *(G Mukhopatdhyaya: The Surgical Instruments of the Hindus, vol 2, Calcutta, 1914, plate 13.)*

Ancient Indian healing, called Ayurvedic medicine, was considered a sacred knowledge passed on by the gods. It was based on a vast literature that included the *Vedas,* later commentaries, and a body of allied medical writings from various contributors. The two most renowned authors are Charaka (uncertain, from 600 B.C. to A.D. 200) and Sushruta (uncertain, from 800 B.C. to 600 B.C.).

The earliest Indian medical writings did not include any surgical subjects. As in contemporaneous civilizations, most healers were drawn from upper society. The members of the upper caste (Brahmin) avoided any contact with wounds, injuries, or dead bodies. Consequently, surgical practitioners tended to be members of the lower castes (Kshatriyas or Vaishyas). These individuals were usually illiterate, and most of their knowledge was passed on by oral tradition as opposed to writing. Surgical therapy did not become an accepted branch of Ayurvedic medicine until after the first century A.D. Because ancient Indian healing depended heavily on invocations to the gods, incantations, and magic spells, the growth of scientific medicine and surgery did not occur until approximately 1000 B.C., when the period of rational medicine commenced. Atreya, mentor to Charaka, and Sushruta were considered the founders of rational medicine and surgery, respectively.

The *Charaka Samhita* is acclaimed as the finest medical document of the rational age, and the *Sushruta Samhita* is assigned similar status for the surgical sciences. Scholarly research has been unable to accurately date either of these Indian medical classics. Whether Charaka and Sushruta were actually historical personages or simply legendary figures to whom these collective works were attributed remains uncertain.

It is difficult to discuss ancient Indian medicine without mentioning the influence of ancient Greek ideas. Much scholarly controversy surrounds the question of any influence that occurred between the two cultures. Who borrowed from whom is impossible to clearly determine. However, it is known that the two civilizations first came into contact with one another through the march of Alexander and that contact continued unbroken through the reigns of the Romans and Byzantines. Thus it is fair to say that some ideas from Greek medicine were absorbed by Hindus and some drugs and surgical techniques used by Western physicians were of Indian origin.

After the Muslim conquest of India during the Middle Ages, Indian medicine came under Islamic influence. Not unexpectedly, therefore, Charaka's fame spread to Arabia, and he was extensively quoted by Avicenna and Rhazes. The *Charaka Samhita* was more accurate in its description of illness than was Sushruta's work. The *Charaka Samhita* was arranged in the form of dialogues between master and pupil and was divided into eight books. These eight treatises were eventually translated into Arabic.

Charaka wrote extensively about hospital systems. Included in the many details were location, equipment, food supply, personnel, and entertainment for the patients. Because the Islamic period of medical history saw the flowering of the world's first great hospitals, there is some evidence that this direction was initially received from Charaka's writings.

With the *Sushruta Samhita* the development of ancient Indian surgery reached its climax. Little in the way of written progress was made over subsequent centuries. Sushruta's work was translated into Arabic around A.D. 800. Rhazes often quoted Sushruta as one of the foremost authorities on surgery. An individual needed an excellent medical background to understand the *Sushruta Samhita.* It was divided into six parts and covered all branches of medicine, including hygiene, midwifery, ophthalmology, toxicology, psychosomatic ailments, and materia medica. That Sushruta considered surgery of primary importance in all branches of medicine is evident in his writing:

> All hold this branch to be the most important of all the other branches of the Ayurveda, inasmuch as instantaneous actions can be produced with the help of such appliances as surgical operations, external applications of alkalis, cauterizations, etc., and secondly inasmuch as it contains all that can be found in the other branches of the

sciences of medicine as well, with the superior advantage of producing instantaneous effects by means of surgical instruments and appliances. Hence it is the highest in value of all the medical branches. It is eternal and a source of infinite piety, imparts fame and opens the gates of Heaven to its votaries, prolongs the duration of human existence on earth, and helps men in successfully fulfilling their missions, and earning a decent competence, in life.

Only the union of medicine and surgery constitutes the complete doctor. The doctor who lacks knowledge of one of these branches is like a bird with only one wing.

Sushruta took particular care in selecting an individual who wished to study medicine and surgery. According to him, such an individual:

. . . should be . . . one of the three twice-born castes such as, the Brahmin, the Kshatriya, and the Vaishya, and who should be of tender years, born of a good family, possessed of a desire to learn, strength, energy of action, contentment, character, self-control, a good retentive memory, intellect, courage, purity of mind and body, and a simple and clear comprehension, command a clear insight into the things studied, and should be found to have been further graced with the necessary qualifications of thin lips, thin teeth and thin tongue, and possessed of a straight nose, large, honest intelligent eyes, with a benign contour of the mouth, and a contented frame of mind, being pleasant in his speech and dealings, and usually painstaking in his efforts.

The newly accepted disciple was expected to study for at least 6 years. Before commencement of his training he took a solemn oath, which can be compared to that of Hippocrates or Maimonides:

Thou shalt renounce lust, anger, greed, ignorance, vanity, egotistic feelings, envy, harshness, niggardliness, falsehood, idleness, nay all acts that soil the good name of a man. In proper season thou shalt pare thy nails and clip thy hair and put on the sacred cloth, dyed brownish yellow, live the life of a truthful, self-controlled anchorite and be obedient and respectful towards thy preceptor. In sleep, in rest, or while moving about—while at meals or in study, and in all acts thou shalt be guided by my directions. Thou shalt do what is pleasant and beneficial to me, otherwise thou shalt incur sin and all thy study and knowledge shall fail to bear their wished for fruit, and thou shalt gain no fame. If I, on the other hand, treat thee unjustly even with thy perfect obedience and in full conformity to the terms agreed upon, may I incur equal sin with thee, and may all my knowledge prove futile, and never have any scope of work or display. Thou shalt help with thy professional skill and knowledge, the Brahmin, thy elders, preceptors and friends, the indigent, the honest, the anchorites, the helpless and those who shall come to thee from a distance, or those who shall live closely by, as well as thy relations and kinsmen . . . and thou shalt give them medicine (without charging for it any remuneration whatever), and God will bless thee for that. Thou shalt not treat medicinally a professional hunter, a fowler, a habitual sinner, or him who has been degraded in life; and even by so doing thou shalt acquire friends, fame, piety, wealth and all wished for objects in life and thy knowledge shall gain publicity.

Sushruta's fairly accurate description of the human body is significant in view of Hinduism's major tenet regarding treatment of the dead. According to the code of Manu, an ancient canon of ethics, the dead body was considered sacred and dissection strictly prohibited. Only the bodies of children less than 2 years of age and of animals were to be used for study.

Although surgery was considered the foremost medical science, the use of operative procedures was reserved as a last recourse in the therapeutic armamentarium. Thus Sushruta was well versed in numerous other branches of medicine, especially pharmacology.

The *Sushruta Samhita* provided minute details regarding preoperative and postoperative care, diet, techniques, indications, contraindications, and complications. Surgical procedures were classified into eight types: excision, incision, scarification, puncture, probing, extraction, drainage or evacuation, and suturing. The actual training of a surgeon and the techniques used were described in detail:

The art of making specific forms of incision should be taught by making cuts in the body of a Pushpaphala gourd, Alavu, watermelon, cucumber, or Ervaruka. The art of making cuts either in the upward or downward direction should be similarly taught. The art of making excisions should be practically demonstrated by making openings in the body of a full water-bag, or in the bladder of a dead animal, or in the side of a leather pouch full of slime or water. The art of scraping should be instructed on a piece of skin on which the hair has been allowed to remain. The art of venesection should be taught on the vein of a dead animal, or with the help of a lotus stem. The art of probing and stuffing should be taught on worm eaten wood, or on the reed of a bamboo, or on the mouth of a dried Alavu. The art of extracting should be taught by withdrawing seeds from the kernel of a Vimbi, Vilva or jack fruit, as well as by extracting teeth from the jaws of a dead animal. The act of secreting or evacuating should be taught on the surface of a Shalmali plank covered over with a coat of bee's wax, and suturing on pieces of cloth, skin or hide. Similarly the art of bandaging or ligaturing should be practically learned by tying bandages around the specific limbs and members of a full-sized doll made of stuffed linen. The art of tying up a severed ear-lobe should be practically demonstrated on a soft severed muscle or on flesh, or with the stem of a lotus lily. The art of cauterizing, or applying alkaline preparations should be demonstrated on a piece of soft flesh; and lastly the art of inserting syringes and injecting enemas into the region of the bladder or into an ulcerated channel, should be taught by asking the pupil to insert a tube into a lateral fissure of a pitcher, full of water, or into the mouth of a gourd.

In probably the earliest description of attempts at antisepsis the fumigation of an operating room with fumes of mustard, butter, and salt was described. An undefined level of anesthesia was obtained via alcoholic intoxication. The soporific effects of henbane and Indian hemp were also used.

Sushruta provided a detailed list of at least 125 surgical instruments. They were classified into sharp and blunt varieties and included forceps, pincers, tubes, hooks, catheters, and sounds. The measurements of each instruments were specified, and Sushruta stressed that they be made of pure iron.

It is evident in reading the *Sushruta Samhita* that the practice of surgery had reached masterful levels in ancient India. Fourteen types of dressings were listed. Splints were fashioned from bamboo, tree branches, and bark. Sutures were created from fibers of Indian hemp, the hair of horses, strips of leather, and cotton. Among the various operations described were those for laparotomy and intestinal repair, intestinal obstruction, vesical lithotomy, herniorrhaphy, and harelip. Both cesarean section and various amputations were part of a surgeon's caseload.

The Indian surgeons were skillful at treating cataracts. Couching, or the displacing of the opacifying lens of the eye down and away from the line of vision, was first described as follows:

The doctor chooses a bright morning and sits on a bench at knee height. Opposite is the patient who, after washing and eating, sits tied to the ground. The doctor palpates the impurity in the eye, then the patient stares at his nose while an assistant holds his head firmly. The surgeon holds a lancet with index finger, long finger and thumb, then draws it toward the pupil's edge, half a fingerwidth from the back and one-fourth fingerwidth from the outer eye corner, and next he draws it upward. He cuts in the left eye with his right hand, and in the right with his left. If he has cut properly, a sound is heard, and a drop of water comes out.

Among the preeminent surgical operations pioneered by ancient Indians were those of plastic and reconstructive surgery. The custom of piercing an earlobe and then enlarging the opening to hold an amulet that protected against evil powers was quite common. This procedure often led to rips through the earlobe, or if infection was present, the whole ear could be deformed. The *Samhita* contains 15 methods for repairing such damage, many of which are essentially the same as in modern plastic surgery.

Sushruta is commonly perceived as the originator of reconstructive rhinoplasty. Since cutting off the nose was an official punishment for various transgressions, especially for adultery, the ancient Indian surgeon had ample opportunity to develop techniques for nasal reconstruction. Sushruta's description of the technique is quite extraordinary:

> Now I shall deal with the process of affixing an artificial nose. . . First the leaf of a creeper, long and broad enough to fully cover the whole of the severed or clipped off part, should be gathered; and a patch of living flesh, equal in dimension to the preceding leaf, should be sliced off (from down upward) from the region of the cheek (or forehead) and, after scarifying it with a knife, swiftly adhered to the severed nose. Then the cool-headed physician should steadily tie it up with a bandage decent to look at and perfectly suited to the end for which it has been employed.
>
> The physician should make sure that the adhesion of the severed parts has been fully effected and then insert two small pipes into the nostrils to facilitate respiration, and to prevent the adhesioned flesh from hanging down. After that, the adhesioned part should be dusted with . . . powders . . . and the nose should be enveloped in . . . cotton and several times sprinkled over with the refined oil of pure sesamum. . .
>
> Adhesion should be deemed complete after the incidental ulcer had been perfectly healed up, while the nose should be again scarified and bandaged in the case of a semi or partial adhesion. The adhesioned nose should be tried to be elongated where it would fall short of its natural and previous length, or it should be surgically restored to its natural size in the case of the abnormal growth of its newly formed flesh.

Clearly surgery in India reached admirable heights during the era of Sushruta. As in other comparable ancient civilizations, there was a struggle for surgeons and surgery to mature as a profession. With the rise of the Buddhist period (600 B.C. to A.D. 600) and a consequent religious authoritarianism, dogma, and mysticism, a stagnation of the surgical progress and a lack of further advances became apparent.

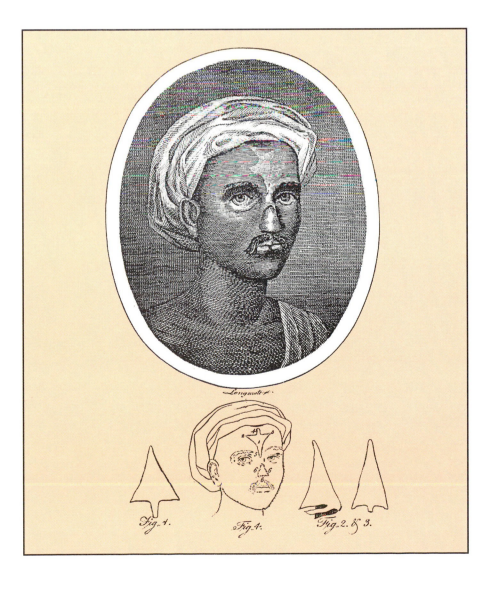

37. To punish adulterers by cutting off their noses was a common practice in ancient India. To remedy this cruel punishment, the Hindus invented rhinoplasty. Sushruta describes the Hindu method of reconstruction of the nose by means of a forehead flap. In 1794 a brief article appeared in *The Gentleman's Magazine,* published in London, describing the Hindu operation; the article was accompanied by this engraving of the patient, Cowasjee, with a restored nose and details of the stages of the operation. The article, signed only with the initials *B.L.,* came to the attention of the English surgeon Joseph Constantine Carpue (1764-1846), who promoted the Hindu method and reestablished rhinoplasty in the West. *(The Gentleman's Magazine, vol 64, 1794, p 891; Jeremy Norman & Co., Inc.)*

CHINA

Surgery in ancient China did not evolve to the monumental heights found in contemporaneous civilizations. Since Confucian tenets concerning the sacredness of the human body and those forbidding human anatomical studies were paramount in Chinese society, any flourishing of surgery as a profession that might have been possible did not occur. As late as the nineteenth century, anatomy was still being taught by means of diagrams and artificial models rather than dissection.

The first Chinese dynasty was the Hsia, which began around 3000 B.C. This empire was followed by the Shang dynasty, which ruled until about 1000 B.C. The Shang rulers were succeeded by the Chou dynasty, which lasted until 256 B.C. During the Chou empire the great Chinese philosophers Lao-tse (604–531 B.C.) and Confucius (557–479 B.C.) lived. Warring feudal states emerged during the Chou dynasty and fought among themselves until the empire was weakened and overthrown by the Ch'in dynasty. During Ch'in rule the Great Wall of China was first built to keep out the Tartars.

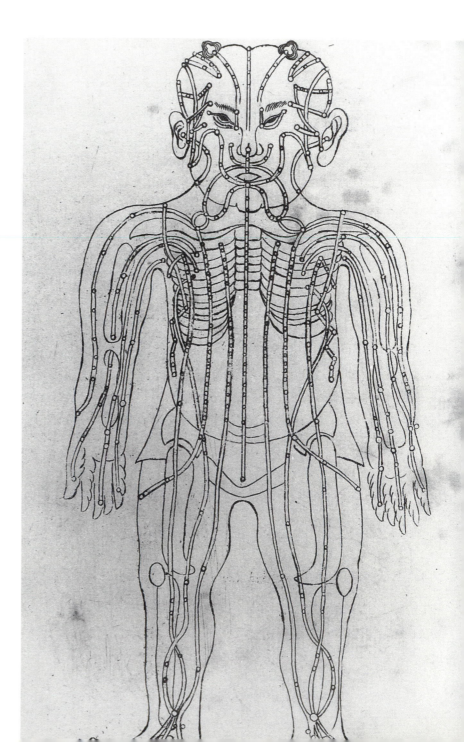

38. These Chinese anatomical and acupuncture charts were the first illustrations of Chinese medical knowledge published in the West. They appeared in the *Specimina Medicinae Sinicae* (Frankfurt, 1682) by Andreas Cleyer, a physician with the Dutch East India Company. Cleyer's 30 plates, chiefly of acupuncture tracts, were taken from Chang Chieh-Pin's *Lei Ching* (1624). *(Jeremy Norman & Co., Inc.)*

As isolated as the Chinese were, they did come into occasional contact with Western and other Eastern cultures. For instance, Buddhism came from India, and occasional contacts were made with the Persian and Islamic civilizations. In the second century B.C. one Chinese official spent more than a decade in Mesopotamia, Syria, and Egypt and brought back aspects of their cultures. The Byzantine culture was introduced into China because the mother of Kublai Khan (A.D. 1216–1294), founder of the Mongol dynasty, was a Nestorian Christian.

In general, Chinese medicine was more concerned with preventive aspects of health care than with active therapeutics. Medicines fascinated the Chinese, who had a rich pharmacopeia. The worse drugs tasted, the more effective they were considered to be. Drugs were classified into five categories: herbs, trees, insects, stones, and grains.

Ancient Chinese medicine was based primarily on classic writings attributed to legendary emperors. The best-known work is that of the Yellow Emperor Huang Ti (2688–2599 B.C.). His *Nei Ching,* or *Canon of Medicine,* was transmitted orally for centuries. Whether it was actually written during Huang Ti's reign or, more likely, later remains historical conjecture. In any case, there is little within this work about surgery.

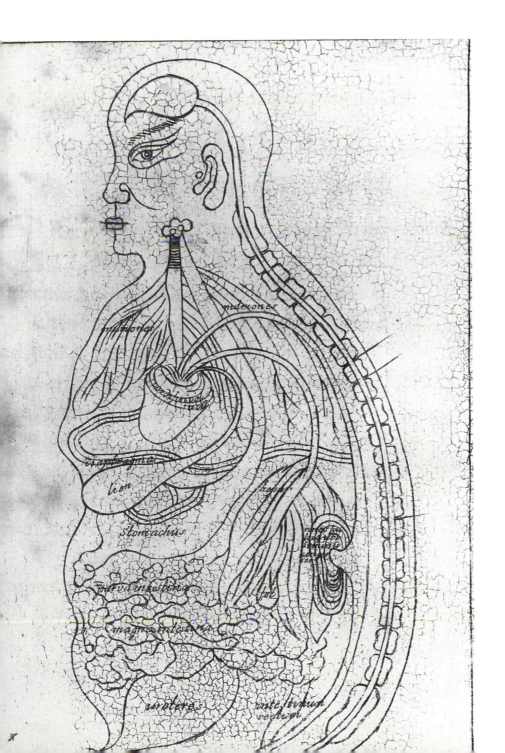

Since Chinese knowledge about human anatomy was limited, it is difficult to imagine how any level of competence in surgery was achieved. However, some surgery was performed, mostly for superficial injuries and in acupuncture and moxibustion. The latter practice is as old as acupuncture, and the same meridians and points on the body are used for placement of the moxa. In moxibustion a powdered plant, usually mugwort, is fashioned into a small mound on the patient's skin and burned, raising a small blister.

The initial references to surgeons can be found in the *Institutions of Chou,* a lengthy compilation of medical works written during the Chou dynasty. The text is restricted to treatment of swellings, ulcers, and wounds. The best known of ancient Chinese surgeons is Hua T'o (circa third or second century B.C.).

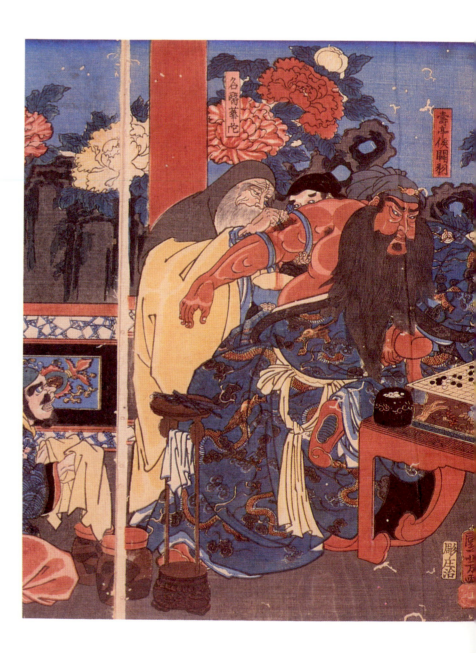

39. Japanese woodblock print of the nineteenth century depicts the Chinese story of the surgeon Hua T'o performing an operation on the arm of General Kuan Kong. Although wounded in the arm by a poisoned arrow, the general played chess until the surgeon arrived. This fearless leader is said to have refused whatever anesthetics were available at that time while the surgeon pulled out the arrow, cleaned the wound, and then sewed up the incision. *(National Library of Medicine, Bethesda, Md.)*

However, all of his writings were destroyed at his death, and few facts about him are known. His exploits became legendary; in fact, he was often worshipped as the deity of surgery. According to legend, his greatest discovery was the use of a potent anesthetic. Supposedly he gave his patients a mixture of hashish and wine or, possibly, a mixture of opium and wine. Hua T'o's surgical accomplishments are said to be numerous, ranging from laparotomy to trephination. His feats were so highly regarded that they were recorded in the later annals of the Wei and Han dynasties. In the Wei dynasty (circa A.D. 225) there is a record of a cesarean section being completed on the wife of a Tartar prince; supposedly both mother and child survived.

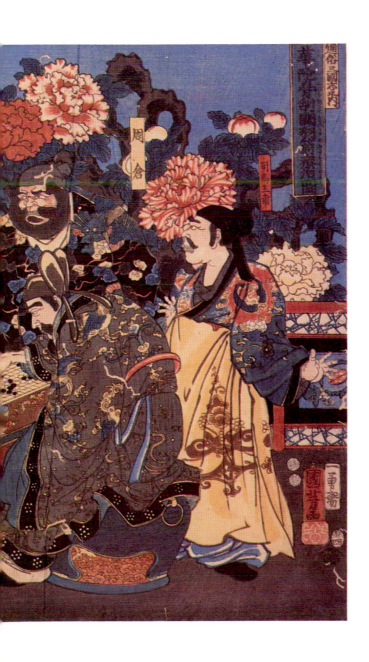

40. Dr. Reifsnyder, a graduate of the Women's Medical College of Philadelphia, performing a successful ovariotomy in Shanghai, as depicted on a Chinese handbill (1885). Western medical knowledge was gradually introduced to China through missionaries and traders, although the influence of a few Westerners on hundreds of millions of individuals in those days of slow communications and traditional thinking could not have been great. In the nineteenth century China remained one of the most male-dominated societies. The traditional practice of foot binding, for example, restricted the roles of women. When Dr. Reifsnyder, a female medical missionary surgeon, performed this operation in Shanghai, the effect must have been sensational. *(Boston Medical Library.)*

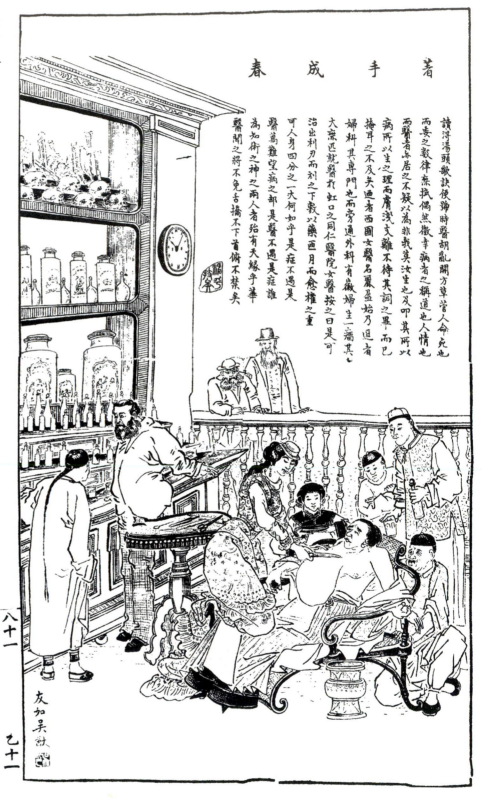

The only widely performed surgical operation was castration. Known since 1000 B.C., castration was important in the Imperial Court because thousands of eunuchs were needed to attend the emperor. More mundanely, castration served as a method of punishment for especially severe crimes. In most cases the procedure was completed after tourniquet-like bandages had been placed around the penis and scrotum. In one swift movement the parts were cut away with a sickle-shaped knife. An astringent powder composed of alum and various resins was applied to the wound, and pressure was exerted until hemorrhage ceased. Then a wooden or metal catheter was introduced into the urethra. The wounds were said to heal in about 3 months, and the death rate was low.

A definite hierarchy of physicians existed in ancient China, including "ulcer doctors." Whether these were a specialized group of individuals who may have been surgeons is unknown. Ancient China also had gynecologists and nose-and-throat experts.

Because of the lack of exact anatomical studies and the preference for bloodless methods, the high standards of surgery achieved by contemporaneous societies were not reached in ancient China. Despite the achievements of Hua T'o and other surgeons, Chinese surgery progressed little after the Tang dynasty (A.D. 619–907) and no books on surgery were written until the mid-nineteenth century.

JAPAN

Japanese aversion toward the performance of surgical operations surpassed that of the Chinese. In the sixth century A.D. Chinese medical practices were introduced into Japan via Korea. By the seventh century A.D. Japanese scholars and physicians were studying in China to gain information and practical experience.

As in China, virtually no ancient Japanese surgical writings are preserved. The surgery of the Heian period (A.D. 784–1186) consisted mainly of minor surgical procedures such as incision of abscesses and cauterization of ulcers. The first monograph on surgery in Japan is believed to have been written in the late ninth century A.D. It was based entirely on Chinese surgical methods and provided little in the way of originality.

41. Trephination. From a nineteenth-century Japanese manuscript by Narabayashi. The tripod instrument is clearly derived from Western examples. (From Nihon igaku no yoake, Tokyo, 1978, Nihon Seron Chōsa Kenkyūjo.)

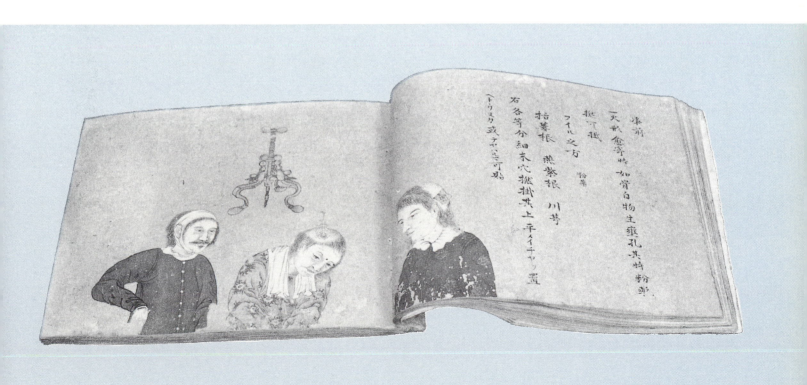

42. Traditional Japanese methods for treating dislocations of the jaw were called "Diving for Pearls." The text describing the "main method" is translated, "Let the patient sit down. The assistant kneels behind him and uses his two hands to hold firmly the two face bones of the patient, with wrists holding the patient's head so that it is immobile. The doctor kneels in front of the patient. He puts his two thumbs into the patient's jaw against the mandible and uses the four fingers on each of his hands to support the bottom of the chin. Then, forcefully, he pushes the mandible toward the throat and at the same time moves it upward. Then the joints will fit together."

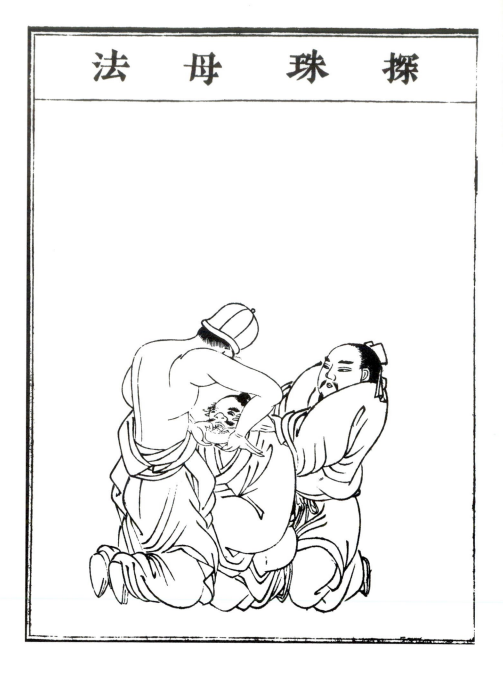

法 毋 珠 探

During the Muromachi period (A.D. 1334–1568) the so-called Kinso-i, or wound surgeons, came into social prominence. This warrior class consisted of wounded soldiers and invalids who, because they were unable to perform any further military duties, studied medicine and assumed the role of military physician to the wounded soldiers. Specific names are lacking, but the exploits of these outstanding trauma surgeons are well known.

Once the religious stigmas attached to caring for the wounded, the bleeding, and the dying were overcome, the Japanese surgeons were able to develop their profession. However, as in China, this development occurred much later than in Western civilizations.

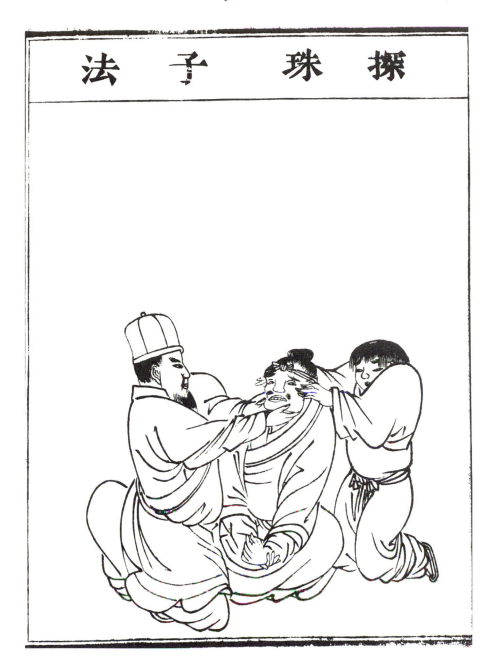

法 子 珠 探

The text describing the "supporting method" is translated, "The assistant does the same as in the main method. The doctor uses his left wrist to hold the patient's right cheek still and uses his four fingers to search for the ends of the teeth bones. Then he forcefully pushes the patient's mandible upward in the same manner as in the main method. The doctor's right hand holds the patient's left cheek firmly so that the patient's head remains immobile." *(Harvard Medical Library.)*

THE MIDDLE AGES

	500	700	900	1100	1300	1500

DAILY LIFE

Plague reduces Europe's population by one half **(542)**

Beds become popular in France and Germany **(750)**

Crossbow **(851)**

Calibrated candles to measure time **(870)**

First recorded appearance of a comet, later called Halley's **(1066)**

Glass windows appear in England **(1180)**

Engagement rings come into fashion **(1200)**

Leprosy imported to Europe by the Crusaders **(1230)**

Coal mined in Newcastle, England **(1233)**

Linen manufactured in England **(1253)**

Glass mirror **(1278)**

The Pied Piper of Hamelin **(1284)**

Spectacles **(1290)**

Bubonic plague, or the Black Death **(1347**

SCIENCE AND TECHNOLOGY

Water wheels for mill drive **(700)**

Vikings sail to Nova Scotia **(1000)**

Bologna University **(1119)**

Marco Polo, Venetian explorer **(1254–1324)**

Apothecaries become popular in Germanic countries **(1300)**

Oriel College, Oxford, and Clare College, Cambridge **(1326)**

Attempts at scientific weather forecasting **(1337)**

RELIGION AND PHILOSOPHY

Incense is introduced into Christian church service **(500)**

Church bells used in France **(550)**

Archepiscopal see of Canterbury **(602)**

Benedictine abbey at Stavelot, Belgium **(652)**

Venerable Bede, English monk and historian **(672–735)**

Easter eggs **(700)**

Charlemagne condemns image worship **(794)**

Jews settle in Germany and develop the Yiddish language **(850)**

Poles converted to Christianity **(966)**

First canonization of saints **(993)**

Westminster Abbey **(1065)**

Thomas Becket, English theologian **(1118–1170)**

Notre Dame, Paris **(1163)**

Francis of Assisi **(1182–1226)**

The Inquisition and torture **(1252)**

Jews expelled from France **(1306)**

The Great Schism, with Popes elected in Rome and Avignon **(1378)**

Printing of the *Constance Mass Book* **(1450)**

LITERATURE AND THEATER

The *Book of Kells,* Latin gospels written in Irish **(760)**

Beowulf **(1000)**

Omar Khayyam, Persian poet **(1027–1123)**

Walther von der Vogelweide, German poet and minnesinger **(1172–1230)**

Wolfram von Eschenbach, German author **(1172–1220)**

The *Nibelungenlied* **(1191)**

Tannhäuser, German poet and minnesinger **(1205–1270)**

Gottfried von Strassburg, German author **(1210–1275?)**

The sonnet in Italian poetry **(1221)**

Dante Alighieri, Italian author **(1265–1321)**

Petrarch, Italian poet **(1304–1374)**

Giovanni Boccaccio, Italian author **(1313–137**

Geoffrey Chaucer, English author **(1340–1400)**

Piers Plowman, a poem in Middle English **(1362)**

The legend of Robin Hood **(1375)**

Ecclesiastical drama flourishes in Ital **(1400)**

THE MIDDLE AGES

	500	700	900	1100	1300	1500

MUSIC

Gregorian church music **(750)**

Schools for church music established in Paris, Cologne, and Metz **(790)**

Polyphonic music **(855)**

Guido d'Arezzo, Italian musical theorist **(995–1050)**

Harp is first noted in Europe **(1050)**

Beginning of troubadour music in France **(1125)**

Philippe de Vitry, French composer **(1290–1361)**

Lute becomes popular in Europe **(1350)**

John Dunstable, English composer **(1369–1453)**

VISUAL ARTS

Crucifix is developed as an ornament **(550)**

Dome of the Rock, Jerusalem **(643)**

Palatine Chapel, Aix-la-Chapelle, France **(796)**

Doge's Palace, Venice **(814)**

St. Mark's Cathedral, Venice **(976)**

Strassburg Cathedral, France **(1015)**

Tower of London **(1078)**

Cathedral of Saint Germain-des-Pres, Paris **(1100)**

The western facade of Chartres Cathedral **(1150)**

Leaning Tower of Pisa **(1174)**

Early Gothic architecture in England **(1200)**

Ciambue, Florentine painter **(1240–1302)**

Giotto, Italian painter **(1266–1337)**

Palace of the Popes, Avignon, France **(1334)**

Lorenzo Ghiberti, Italian sculptor **(1378–1455)**

Donatello, Italian sculptor **(1386–1486)**

Fra Angelico, Italian painter **(1387–1455)**

MEDICINE AND SURGERY

Roger of Salerno, Italian **(late twelfth century)**

Hugh of Lucca, Italian **(1160–1257)**

Roland of Parma, Italian **(mid-thirteenth century)**

Theodoric, Italian **(1205–1296)**

Bruno of Longoburg, Italian **(thirteenth century)**

William of Saliceto, Italian **(1210–1277)**

Jean Pitard, French **(1220–1280)**

Arnald of Villanova, Italian **(1240–1311)**

Lanfranc, Italian **(?–1315)**

Henri de Mondeville, French **(1260–1320)**

Mundinus, Italian **(1275–1326)**

Jean Yperman, Flemish **(1295–1361)**

Guy de Chauliac, French **(1300–1368)**

John of Arderne, English **(1306–1390)**

John of Mirfield, English **(late fourteenth century)**

Peter of Argelata, Italian **(?–1423)**

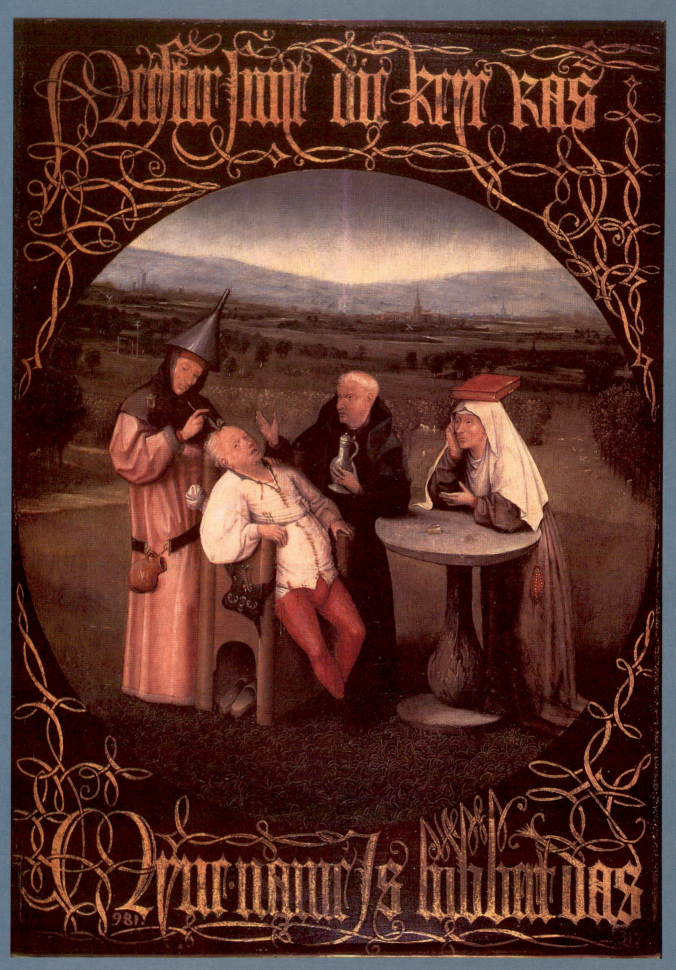

CHAPTER 7
THE MIDDLE AGES

The Middle Ages, or the medieval age, is a period of European history most commonly delineated as beginning with the fall of Rome to the Goths in A.D. 476 and concluding with the fall of Constaninople to the Turks in A.D. 1453. The early Middle Ages, A.D. 476–814, is often referred to as the Dark Ages because it is considered a time of widespread ignorance and lack of social progress.

After the fall of the western Roman empire there was a proliferation of rich and powerful landholders who organized individuals on their estates into small private armies. For the common people the best chance of safety was to hand over their land to the most powerful noble in the district and place themselves under the noble's protection. As this practice grew, western Europe slowly disintegrated into many small, independent units, each under the control of a powerful nobleman, and from these maneuverings feudalism eventually developed.

The greatest political figure of the early Middle Ages was Charlemagne (742-814), who established the Holy Roman Empire and brought the Church into his government. By the end of Charlemagne's reign the conditions for a feudal society were in place; consequently, from the 800s until the end of the Middle Ages feudal government controlled society. Essentially, feudal society comprised three groups: the lords and their knights, the clergy, and the workers, or commoners. Undeniably the one great force that bound all Europeans together was the Church, whose growth and influence were so overwhelming that even powerful kings and nobles often yielded to its dictates.

Trade and commerce grew rapidly during the late Middle Ages, as two new groups, a merchant class and a large number of artisans or craftsmen, emerged. The Crusades brought western Europe into contact with the Near East. As trade expanded and became more profitable, towns became increasingly important. Because the accumulation of wealth became possible, individuals ceased to be bound to the soil, which had been the essence of the economy during the early and middle medieval period. By the end of the late Middle Ages, the Protestant Reformation had disrupted the unity of Christendom and the all-encompassing political and economic power of the Catholic Church was markedly decreased.

The history of medieval medicine is one of Latinization and subsequent Arabization of western Europe and can be divided into the following distinct periods: the rise of Christendom, the papacy, and monasticism (mid-fifth to tenth centuries); the evolution of the School of Salerno (eleventh and twelfth centuries); Byzantine influence (thirteenth century); and the development of scholastic medicine (fourteenth and fifteenth centuries).

While the western Roman empire was disappearing as a political entity, the Catholic Church was becoming the major unifying and cohesive force in Europe. Its strong spiritual appeal, attractive symbolism in Jesus Christ and his apostles, efficient hierarchical organization, and use of the underlying basis of feudalism to protect western European civilization from Islamic invasion could only lead to its eventual domination of medieval life.

43. *Facing page, The Cure of Folly,* by Hieronymus Bosch. Charles de Tolnay, the leading authority, considered this oil painting on wood an early example of Bosch's work. The painting depicts the famous quack operation for removal of stones in the head. The notion that madness is literally caused by objects in the head that are easily removed is perpetuated in the modern slang expression "rocks in the head." In this painting a fat, demented old man is being operated on by a barber-surgeon who is wearing as a head cover the "funnel of wisdom." The nun observing the operation is making the same absurb use of a medical book, which she balances on her head. The round shape of the painting indicates the world. The inscription around the painting may be translated "Master cuts out the stones—My name is Lubbert das [gelded badger]." In the Dutch landscape in the background, to the left of the charlatan's head, a gallows is depicted as a sign of the wickedness of the world. More than a critique of surgical charlatans, the painting alludes to what Bosch perceived as the futility of all worldly healing arts. *(Derechos reservados © Museo del Prado, Madrid.)*

As the clerical organization grew in power, it managed to crush all opposition and doubt about its dogma. Any struggle between collective action and individualism inevitably resulted in the demise of intellectual independence. By the sixth century the gradual passage of science into the hands of the clergy was accomplished. Secular schools of learning were left to wither, and religious zeal and fanatic asceticism became the standard of the day. There was an absolute suppression of experimental science and of the actual verification of self-evident premises. The ultimate result was a return to religious medicine. Illness once again came to be understood as a punishment from God, and treatment was predicated on the denial of the existence of any basis for knowledge or truth.

44. Street scene from a fifteenth-century French illuminated manuscript on politics and court life, *Le Livre du Gouvernement des Princes. Right,* A pharmacy operating under the sign "Bon Hippocras," or "Good Hippocrates." Next to the pharmacy a barber-surgeon plies his trade. *(Phot. Bibliothèque Nationale; Paris, Ms 5062, fol 149 v.)*

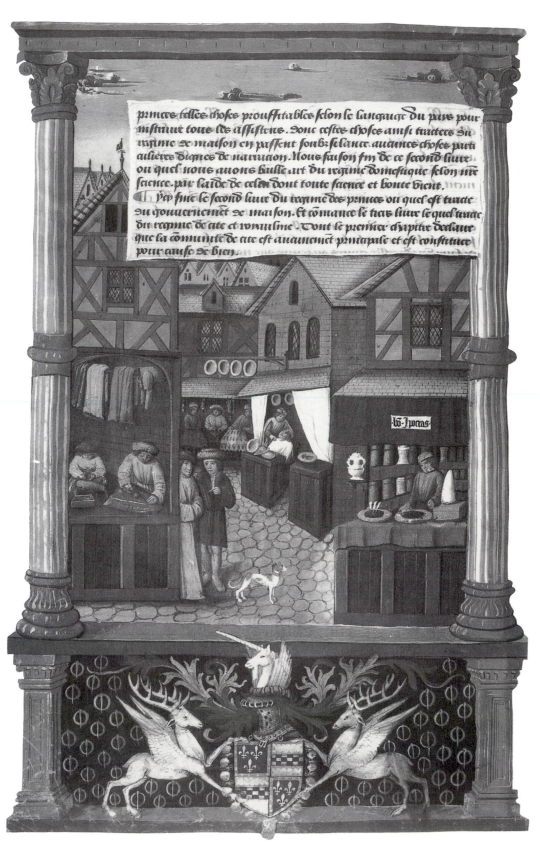

The religious development of monasticism exercised an integrating influence in the early Middle Ages. The essence of monasticism was a withdrawal from worldly society to avoid its wicked and immoral ways. In this way, by forgoing hedonistic urges, an individual could lead a truly righteous life.

The ascetic ideal was first manifested in the early eastern Christian monks who left society to live in squalor and solitude in the desert. Eventually monks began to band together, and by the fourth and fifth centuries sets of monastic rules were being promulgated. The most prominent of these codes was devised by St. Benedict of Nursia (480-543) in his establishment of the monastery of Monte Cassino. By 600, scores of monasteries of the Benedictine type had been founded throughout western Europe.

The monasteries became natural places of congregation for the sick and the weak. The essence of Christian compassion led to new departures in the provision of medical care for these individuals. Out of monastic medicine grew numerous kinds of facilities for the care of the diseased and the oppressed. Among

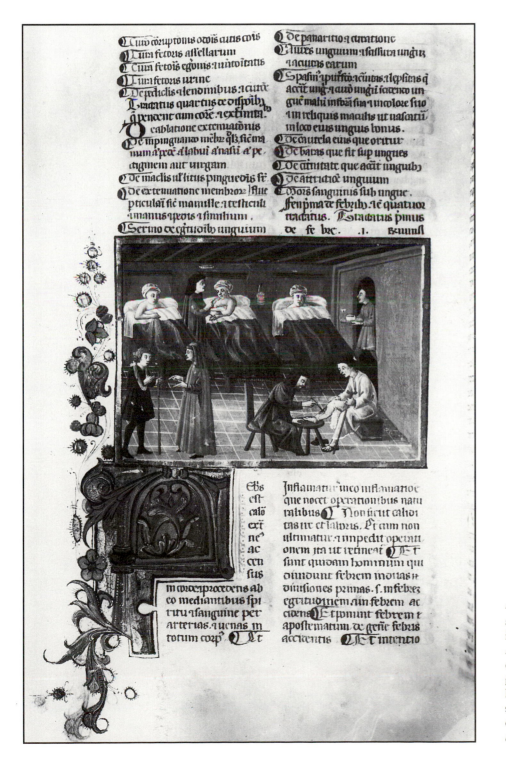

45. A small hospital room with three beds, as depicted in an early fifteenth-century Italian illuminated manuscript of the *Canon* of Avicenna. All the patients and their attendants are wearing hats and seemingly heavy garments, which suggests that the room may have been cold. In the foreground a barber-surgeon is performing some sort of minor operative procedure. *(Biblioteca Laurenziana, Florence, Gaddian, Ms 24, folio 247.)*

the most famous of these early monastic hospitals were those founded by St. Helen, mother of the Roman emperor Constantine in Constantinople (330); a plague hospital built in Edessa by St. Ephraem (circa 350); and one established by St. Basil in Caesarea, capital of Cappadocia (369). Fabiola, a wealthy Roman matron who later became a pupil of St. Jerome, founded the first Christian public hospital in Rome in 394.

Little information is available about the actual care rendered the sick during the Dark Ages. However, an important sixth- and seventh-century offshoot of monastic medicine was the establishment of ascetic houses for women. From these humble beginnings grew the rudimentary structure of nursing. The most famous of these "double monasteries" was founded by St. Radegunde at Poitiers in 559. Nursing care was apparently its chief function; there is no indication that physicians were connected with that monastic community and hospital. Nursing care seems to have been the key to the restoration of health.

The most famous medieval hospitals were the two Hôtels Dieu (God's house) in France. The oldest medieval hospital was initiated in Lyon in 542 and was unique in its freedom from clerical control. The Santo Spirito Hospital in Rome, established in 717 by order of the Pope, was one of the largest (1000 beds) medieval institutions.

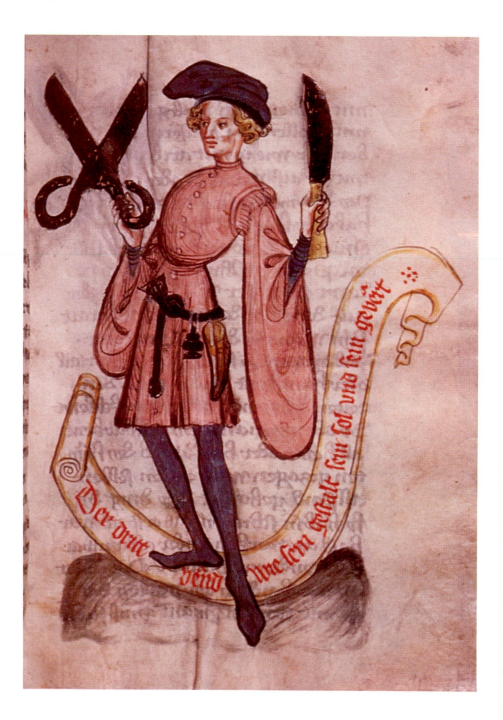

46. Portrait of a medieval barber-surgeon and the tools of his trade, scissors and a knife, in an illuminated manuscript of Jacobus de Cessoli, *Schazabelbuch*, circa 1408. *(By permission of the Houghton Library, Harvard University, Ms Typ 45.)*

Although some innovative changes were made in the delivery of medical care during the Middle Ages, the overall picture was one of stagnation. As barbarian invaders brought down the western Roman empire, the first societal institutions to be dispensed with were those of law and medicine. During the Dark Ages both physician and patient had to increasingly fend for themselves, and the non-clerical physician ultimately ceased to exist.

St. Benedict believed the cure of disease was possible only through prayer and divine intervention; therefore in his monastery the study of medicine was forbidden. His monks continued as "medical practitioners" by resorting solely to relics, prayers, and exhortations to cure the ill. This parochial thinking ensured that all scientific and logical progress in the art of early medieval medicine and surgery would come to an inglorious end. Because the practice of medicine and surgery was under no control whatsoever, virtually anyone who wished to be considered a physician was. Quacks and other uneducated individuals quickly seized upon the practice of surgery.

It is difficult to affix the blame for the stagnation of medical care. The influence of Galen was almost unbelievable; his erroneous views of anatomy and physiology held massive sway over the clerics. The Church looked askance at innovative thinking, which was often termed heresy. If ultimate cure depended on the will of God, how could a surgical operation be worth undertaking?

The classical thinking of earlier civilizations, which viewed surgery as an invaluable adjunct to internal medicine, was completely obfuscated during the early Middle Ages. The clergy carried Galen's belief that surgery was only "a mode of treatment" to the extreme by treating surgeons themselves as lackeys and underlings. Through the influence of the Arabian commentators, there was a genuine belief that it was unclean and unholy to touch another human body with one's hands. More important, the underlying false concept that suppuration via "laudable pus" was essential to the healing of wounds made operative therapy a perilous task. Since all wounds were expected to become "infected," an ultimately poor outcome was ensured.

It must be understood that the medieval surgeon, be he renowned scholar or roving rogue, stood in jeopardy of his life or limb if he operated unsuccessfully on any of the feudal lords. An edict issued from Theodoric (454-526), king of the Ostrogoths, stipulated that any physician whose patient died after an operation should be handed over to the relatives of the patient, who were to do with him as they wished. Consequently the greatest surgeons of the time shrewdly advised their professional brethren to avoid or evade all difficult cases. When an operation was unavoidable, the custom of the day was to require a written guarantee that no harm would befall the surgeon in the event of a fatal outcome.

Although surgery and its practitioners were treated with disdain, some monks themselves continued to perform operative procedures in their monasteries. However, this practice soon came to a definitive conclusion: to ensure that monks would spend all their time on church-related activities and cease their practice of medicine and surgery, the Church began to promulgate a series of edicts to limit all such secular activities.

The first two edicts were issued at Rheims (1125) and Clermont (1130), and the Lateran Council published a third (1139). It was the Council of Tours (1169), however, that first pronounced the infamous edict, *Ecclesia abhorret a sanguine*. By declaring that the shedding of blood was incompatible with a cleric's holy office, the council clearly restricted the educated class from performing any type of surgical practice. In so doing the Church totally abandoned the surgical crafts to the secular arm of medieval society. Thenceforth all surgeons, not only the unskilled, wandering individuals but their competent colleagues as well, were treated as inferior to practitioners of general medicine. The general practice of surgery, including all important operations, was then undertaken by barbers, wandering charlatans, and other, more base peripatetic individuals.

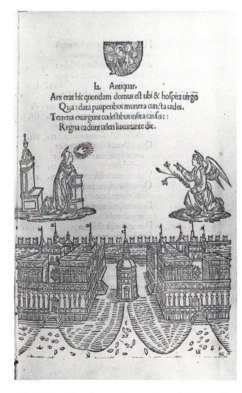

47. Probably the earliest printed illustration of an actual hospital building, the Ospedale Maggiore in Milan, as published in Gilinus's pioneering treatise on hospital history and administration *(Fundatio Hospitalis Magni Mediolani,* 1508). The most important of the early Italian hospitals, the Ospedale Maggiore was founded in the fifteenth century by Francesco Sforza and Maria Visconti. *(Jeremy Norman & Co., Inc.)*

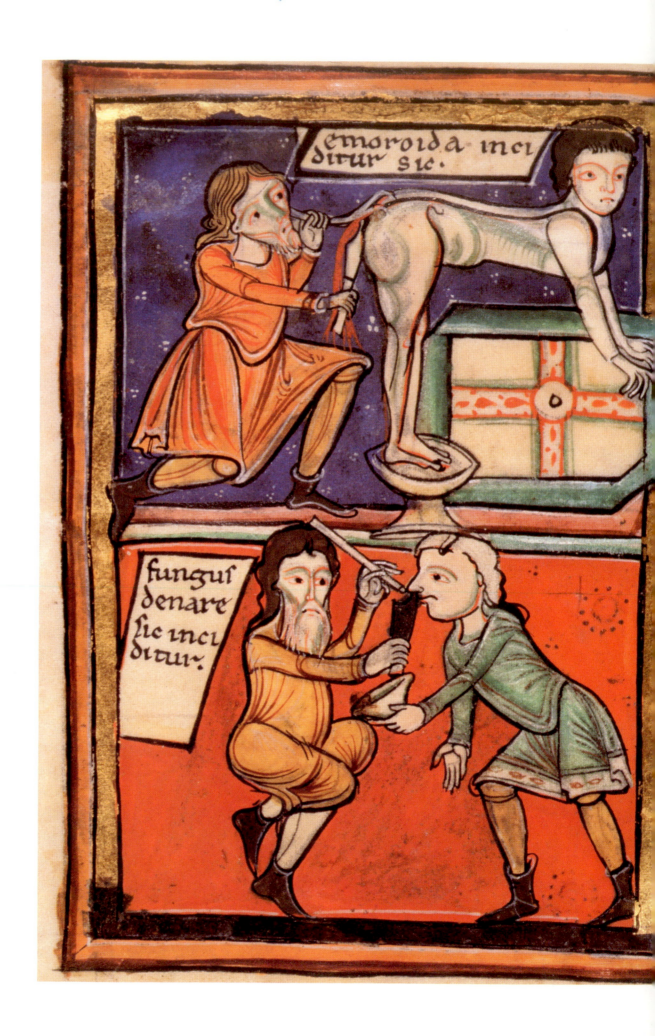

emoroida inci
ditur sie.

fungus
denare
sie inci
ditur.

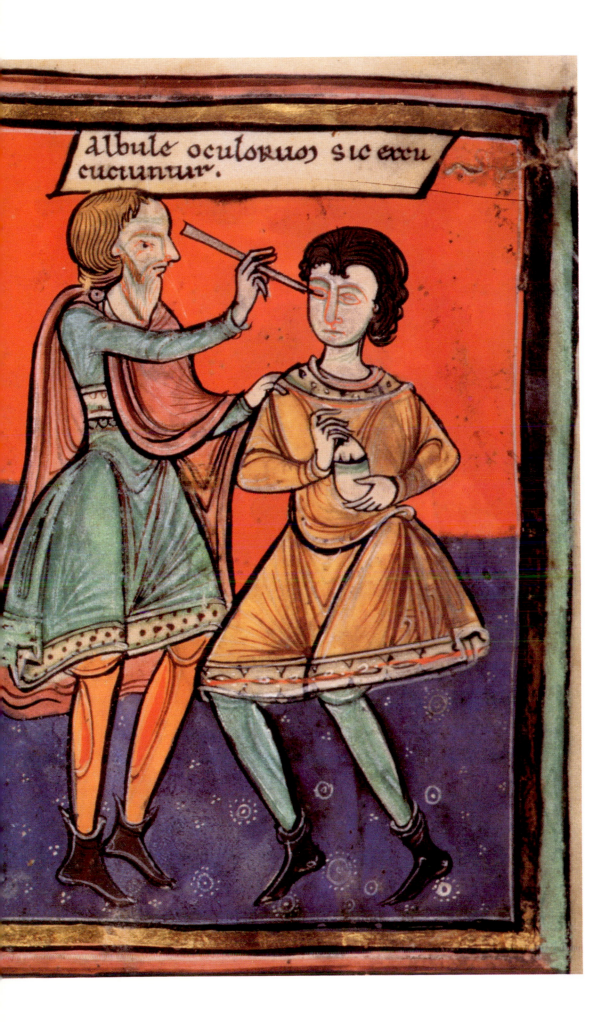

albule oculoruos sic excu
cuciuntur.

48.

48. *Preceding pages,* Operations for hemorrhoids, nasal polyp, and cataract in a manuscript of the late twelfth century. The surgeon excising hemorrhoids uses a clawed separator in his left hand, a knife in his right. The surgeon performing the cataract operation may be using a needle to couch the lens; his patient holds a jar of ointment. *(By permission of the British Library, London, Ms Sloane 1975, f 93.)*

49. *Facing page,* Illustrations from a fourteenth-century manuscript showing, *top left,* preparation of the cautery irons; *top right,* applications for afflictions of the head, treatment of a patient *(lying down)* with an unspecified illness; *bottom left,* treatment of a patient *(standing)* with asthma; and *bottom right,* treatment of hernia. *(The Bodleian Library, Oxford, MS Rawl C328, fol 3v [W945], fol 4r [W3183], fol 5r [W3185], fol 9v [W946].)*

Since monks were forbidden to perform surgical operations, this skill fell mostly to the barbers, who had previously assisted the monks in their surgical therapies and, in particular, had been frequenting monasteries since 1092, when beards were banned. The barbers helped shave the monks and cut their hair in the particular styles of specific religious orders. These barbers soon widened the scope of their professional activities and became specialists. For instance, one operated for hernia, another for bladder calculi, and a third for cataract, the knowledge being handed down from father to son.

By the thirteenth and fourteenth centuries surgical techniques were beginning to mature at the hands of barber-surgeons. These faithful and mostly obscure followers of the craft of surgery, although continuously ostracized by clerical bigots, ensured the ultimate survival of surgery. The principal area of interest in medieval surgical history lies not in changes in general medicine, for those were few, but in the barber-surgeons, who ensured the gradual ascent and development of surgery as a learned profession.

In the study of medieval medicine the most interesting and intriguing area concerns surgical manuscripts. Before the advent of the printing press (mid-fifteenth century), written material was passed from one generation to the next via manuscripts. These tediously handwritten texts, usually found on vellum, a kind of fine parchment prepared from calfskin, lambskin, or kidskin, were reproduced in medieval scriptoriums. The scriptoriums were rooms in a monastery reserved for copying manuscripts, writing, and studying. There the wisdom of past generations was preserved and transmitted.

Although some ancient and many medieval manuscripts have escaped destruction, most have been lost. Thus a philosophical question of history arises: Are the ancient and medieval surgeons and their manuscripts that we know today prominent because they were truly influential during their own times, or do the individual surgeons appear important to us only because their manuscripts managed to survive for so many centuries? There is no historically correct answer to this question, but it must be assumed that once-prominent surgeons whose texts did not survive beyond the Middle Ages have remained unknown.

The resurgence of medical and surgical education in western Europe first occurred at the School of Salerno. Situated near Naples on the Gulf of Paestum, Salerno had long been admired as a place of physical beauty and had served as a health spa during the time of the Roman empire. Although the actual origins of the school remain obscure, the Benedictines were believed to have had a cloister and hospital there in 820. Legend holds that the medical institution was founded by a Jew, Elinus; a Roman, Magister Salernus; a Greek, Pontius; and an Arab, Adala. This apocryphal story certainly may be understood to symbolize the four dominant cultural influences that contributed to the school's eventual success. By the late ninth century the Salernitan school was attracting students from distant locales.

What set the School of Salerno apart from all others was its secular authority. Although the Benedictine monastery of Monte Cassino was nearby, the faculty at Salerno remained remarkably free of clerical control. Perhaps this freedom alone, in view of the Church's promulgations regarding medicine, was responsible for the quality of medicine at Salerno. Ultimately, the School of Salerno became the cradle of modern Western surgery.

The Salernitan masters were the first medieval physicians to cultivate medicine as an independent branch of science. Salernitan surgery became new and innovative; female practitioners served as talented midwives and nurses. By 904 the school was so highly regarded that one of the Salernitan physicians was called to the royal court of France. Eventually, many rulers and members of the clergy sought out the medical and surgical advice of Salernitan faculty.

The most important early medical personage in Salerno was Constantinus Africanus. A native of Carthage, he gained a working knowledge of Greek, Arabic, and Latin during his extensive travels. Constantinus served as the most important link in establishing the spirit of Greco-Roman medicine at Salerno. Through his translations into Latin of ancient Greek medical texts, most often

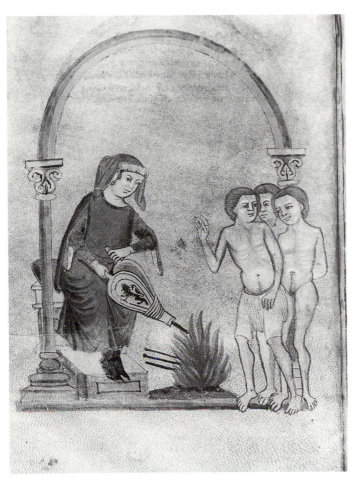

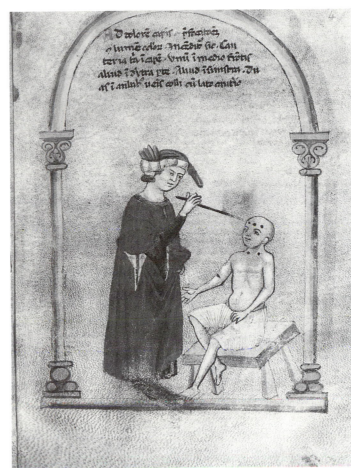

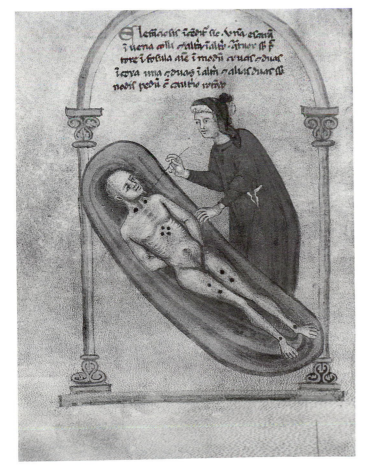

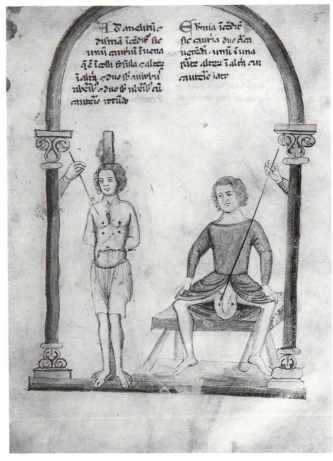

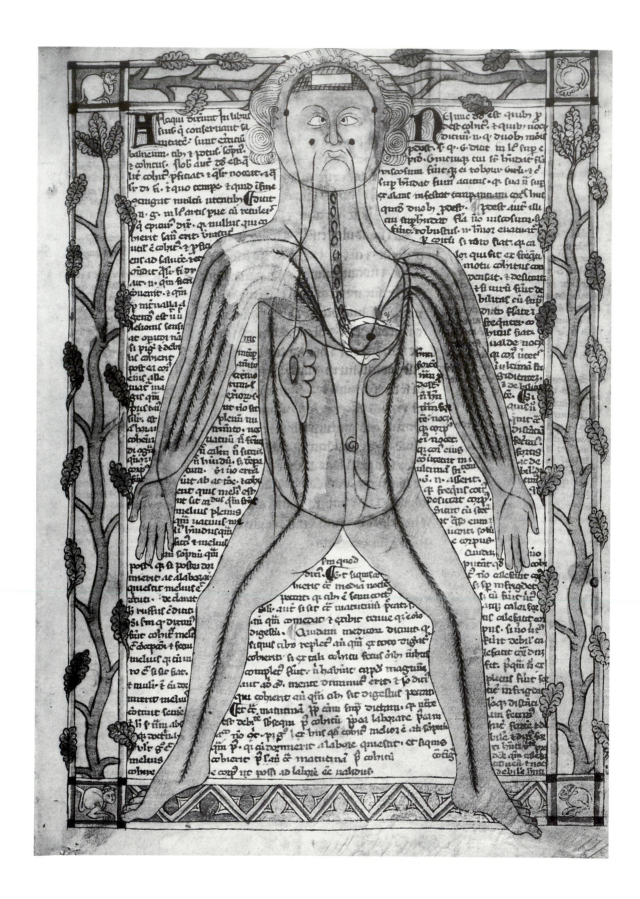

50. Anatomical figure in typical medieval posture illustrating the heart and blood vessels, from a thirteenth-century English manuscript. It is tempting to call this cross-eyed figure an illustration of the circulatory system; however, no concept of the circulation of the blood existed at that time. (*The Bodleian Library, Oxford, MS Ashmole 399, fol 19.*)

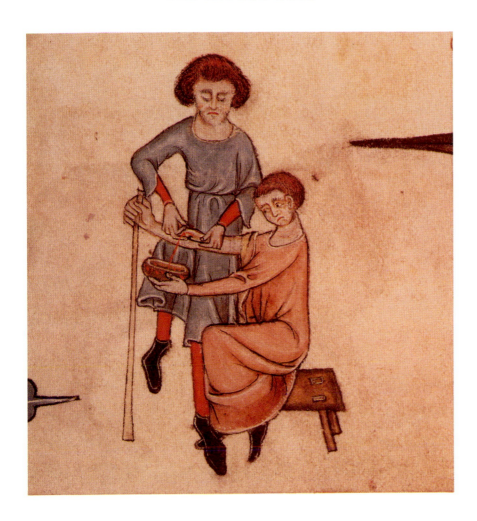

51. A barber-surgeon bleeding a patient, an illustration from the *Luttrell Psalter* (1340). The patient steadies his right arm with a "barber pole" while with his left hand he holds the "bleeding bowl" for the barber. *(By permission of the British Library, London, Add Ms 42130, fol 61.)*

from their Arabic renderings, Salerno became the first European school to make available once again the teachings of the Arabs and thus of the ancients. *Pantegni,* a translation by Constantinus of the royal book *Al-Malaki* by Ali Abba, an Islamic physician and encyclopedist, formed the chief source of early Salernitan surgical knowledge.

Once the educated class learned that the School of Salerno was using the methods of the ancients, the school gained a tremendously favorable reputation. This reputation was quickly enhanced by the country's rulers. King Roger II of Sicily decreed in 1140 that anyone who practiced medicine was required to pass an examination to prove his ability to cure patients and that a permission or license to practice must be obtained. Roger's grandson Frederick II (1194-1250), known as the Great and later to be emperor of the Holy Roman Empire, specified in 1240 that all candidates for medical licensure be publicly examined by Salernitan masters. Most important was Frederick's establishment of examination standards, which ranked surgery as equal to medicine. Frederick provided for two classes of surgeons. Those of the first class were examined by three professors, and the questioning was conducted in Latin. The surgeons of the second class were examined in Italian by only two teachers. The candidates took an oath never to treat internal diseases and could not receive the title of doctor. Frederick also mandated a postgraduate year of study under an experienced physician as a prerequisite for the examination and for a medical license.

The most famous written work of the Salernitan school is the *Regimen Sanitatis Salernitanum,* or *Flos Medicinae,* which was not a surgical text but a popular collection of health rules composed in verse for easy memorization. Believed to have been first composed in the mid-thirteenth century, it was intended to guide the layperson in matters of diet, conservation of health, and prevention of disease. From a basic code of health the *Regimen* gradually evolved into a complete encyclopedia of medicine in verse form. It was translated into almost every

52. Barber-surgeons' volvelle from the fifteenth-century *Guild Book of the Barber-Surgeons of York. Top,* John the Baptist and John the Evangelist, patron saints of the guild. *Bottom,* Cosmas and Damian, the patron saints of surgery. Cosmas holds a urine glass while Damian holds a spatula ready to mix medicine from a compartmentalized box. By setting the indices on the volvelle, the surgeon could determine whether an operation on a particular organ might be auspiciously performed on a certain day. *(By permission of the British Library, London, Egerton MS 2572, f 51.)*

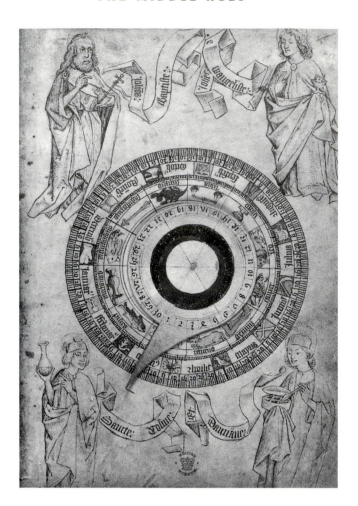

modern language and exists in no fewer than 300 editions. The following is excerpted from one of the verses:

> If thou to health and vigor wouldst attain,
> Shun weighty cares—all anger deem profane,
> From heavy suppers and much wine abstain,
> Nor trivial count it, after pompous fare,
> To rise from the table and to take the air.
> Shun idle, noonday slumber, nor delay,
> The urgent calls of nature to obey.

The first known surgical manuscript from the Salernitan school was written in the middle of the twelfth century by an anonymous author. It has been called the *Bamberg Surgery* because it was found in a library of the principality and bishopric of Bamberg. It was based on the work of Paul of Aegina, on oral tradition, and on Byzantine texts in Latin, including the works of Oribasius and Albucasis. It was never printed in book form and, being the work of multiple authors, was not systematic in scope. The Bamberg manuscript deals with wounds and fractures of the skull, general wounds of the body, surgical lesions of eye and ear, diseases of the skin, fractures and dislocations, hemorrhoids, herniorrhaphy, bloodletting, and cautery. The work is quite pragmatic, especially concerning operative surgery, and includes a number of noteworthy descriptions. Suture of the intestine over a hollow tube and the use of an apparently effective truss to retain inguinal hernia are mentioned. Trephination of the skull for epilepsy and the administration of seaweed for the treatment of goiter are both advised. The use of a "sleep-inducing" or "soporific" sponge is mentioned in a surgical text for the first time. Although such a primitive anesthetic device had been known to earlier civilizations, it had previously been discussed solely in pharmacological texts.

About 20 years after the *Bamberg Surgery* was written, a markedly different type of surgical manuscript appeared at Salerno. Ruggierio Frugardi (circa late twelfth century), usually called Roger of Salerno, authored an original, systematic text called the *Practica Chirurgiae* or the *Surgery of Master Roger*. With topics arranged in sequence from head to lower extremity, it was the preeminent surgical manuscript of the Salernitan school and is the first known independent surgical work in the Western world.

The *Practica* is original in form and content. Although many of the operative techniques can be traced back to Greco-Roman surgery, Roger describes them simply and clearly. He details end-to-end sutures; hemorrhage is controlled with styptics, sutures, or a ligature. Roger states that a nerve with a clean transverse cut, well approximated, will heal better than a nerve with a diagonal cut. Simple and compound fractures are well treated, and mercurial inunction is recommended for treatment of chronic skin diseases. The use of seaweed as treatment for goiter is described in more detail than in the *Bamberg Surgery*. Roger warns against operating for cancer of the uterus or rectum. Like most surgeons of his era, he is well versed in the treatment of wounds and recommends immediate extraction of foreign matter. At that time the belief was still prevalent that wounds could heal properly only by secondary intention, which necessitated the formation of laudable pus. In abdominal injuries with evisceration, Roger recommends that if the intestinal surface has become cold and dry from exposure to the air, the abdomen of an animal be opened and its contents placed over the

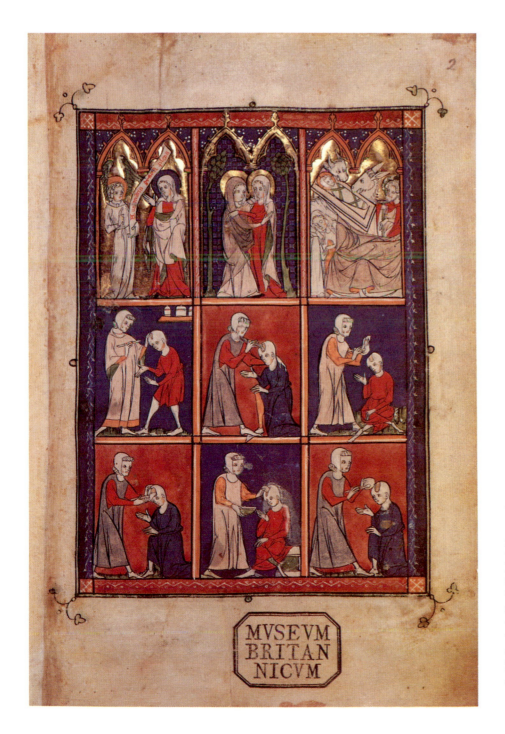

53. Operation for compound fracture of the skull, from what has been called the finest illustrated surgical manuscript of the Middle Ages. Based on the French text of Ruggierio Frugardi (Roger of Salerno) and probably composed near Amiens, the manuscript dates from the first decade of the fourteenth century. The six illustrations of the stages of the operation are remarkable, for that time, for their realism and didactic value. Why the upper three illustrations on the page show incidents in the early life of Christ is unexplained. *(By permission of the British Library, London, Ms. Sloane 1977, f 2.)*

exposed intestine. Once the intestines regained their color and temperature, they could be replaced. Among the most remarkable of his techniques is the repair of injured intestines over a hollow tube:

> If the intestine becomes herniated by any wound of the body and if there is a longitudinal or oblique wound so that the greater part remains uninjured, we are accustomed to treat it as follows: In the first place, if the weather is cold when the intestines are injured, a live animal is cut down the middle and laid upon the intestines and left there until the intestines become warm and regain their natural heat and become softened. In the meanwhile, a cannula is made of elder wood in the shape of the wound of the intestine, but one inch longer than the wound of the intestine and the wound is sewn with a sharp needle and a silk thread. The cannula is placed there in order that the contents of the intestine may pass through it and that the suture of the wound may not make an obstruction. When this has been done the dirt is washed gently from the intestines with a sponge well soaked in warm water. When they have been thoroughly cleaned the intestines are replaced in the abdomen through the wound by which they escaped, and then the patient is placed on a plank and shaken in order that the intestine may slide into their proper position, but if the wound was such that they cannot be replaced, it is made larger and thereafter the wound is left open until you see the intestine stuck together. After suturing the intestine red powder is placed over it. After the wound of the intestine is consolidated the external wound is treated by suture and otherwise as said above.

Roger of Salerno had a number of disciples who continued his teachings and further developed his ideas. The most prominent was Rolando Capelluti, or Roland of Parma (circa mid-thirteenth century), the author of the *Rolandina,* a concise surgical manuscript based on Roger's *Practica.* Roland, however, does not restrict himself entirely to an editorial role. He makes numerous references to Hippocrates, Galen, and Avicenna, who are but vaguely mentioned in the *Practica.* Among the unique reports found in the *Rolandina* is a chest wound with a herniated lung. Roland describes that he was unable to reduce the greatly swollen pulmonary tissue, even after enlarging the wound and attempting to separate the ribs. Consequently, he cut the protruding pulmonary tissue flush with the skin. Roland's work was printed for the first time in a Venetian surgical encyclopedia, *Cyrurgia* (1498).

The works of both Roger of Salerno and his disciple, Roland of Parma, are preserved in the commentary of the "Four Masters of Salerno." Although the identity of these individuals remains uncertain, it is known that they were four Salernitan physicians whose commentary became quite popular and highly successful as a medieval text on surgery. According to the Four Masters, Roger had attributed the decline of surgery to the separation of medicine from the craft of surgery and to the absolute neglect of anatomical studies.

Through the efforts of Roland and the Four Masters the teaching of Roger was widely disseminated and contributed greatly to the tremendous growth of surgery throughout Italy and France. Immediately after the successes of Roger and his surgical disciples, however, the School of Salerno began to disintegrate. Numerous reasons are advanced for this downfall, but primarily it occurred because vigorous university rivals appeared in various parts of Europe. In 1811, a full millennium after the founding of the School of Salerno, the French government under Napoleon I (1769-1821) officially put an end to its existence.

Despite the Church's ban on surgery via its edict abhorring bloodshed, the craft of surgery steadily advanced. Even more surprising, much of this change was accomplished by surgeons from religious orders. The most important of these subsequent advances occurred at the large university in Bologna. Among the early faculty of its medical school was Ugo Borgognoni, commonly called Hugh of Lucca (1160-1257). He served as municipal physician to the city of Bologna, accompanied the Bolognese crusaders in their expedition to Syria and Egypt, and was present at the siege of Damietta in 1219. Hugh was a bold, creative surgeon, but he left no written record of his life or accomplishments. Hugh of Lucca's achievements are known from the writings of his distinguished disciple, Theodoric (Teodorico Borgognoni) (1205-1296), who is thought to have been his son.

Theodoric was a Dominican friar who served as almoner and confessor to Pope Innocent IV (?-1254). Theodoric was named Bishop of Bitonto in 1262 and of Cervia in 1266. While holding clerical office, Theodoric concomitantly practiced surgery. In time his practice became quite extensive and lucrative; Theodoric willed a considerable portion of his estate to charitable causes.

The *Chirurgia* of Theodoric was completed in 1266, and the manuscript was first preserved in printed form in the Venetian surgical collection. In the *Chirurgia* Theodoric described Hugh as an imaginative surgeon. Hugh's greatest contribution concerned the "dry" treatment of wounds. He was said to have insisted on the primary union of injuries. Much to the detriment of surgery's evolution, this belief would not be accepted for many centuries. Hugh's belief, according to the *Chirurgia,* was as follows:

> It is not necessary as Roger and Roland have written, as many of their disciples teach, and as all modern surgeons profess, that pus should be generated in wounds. No error can be greater than this. Such a practice is indeed to hinder nature, to prolong the disease and to prevent the conglutination and consolidation of the wound.

For centuries before Theodoric, growing out of comments of Galen and later distorted by Islamic translations, the doctrine was unshakeable that for any wound to heal properly, suppuration was a necessity. During the medieval era, if suppuration failed to occur, surgeons would probe or pack the injury or dress it with unctuous ointments to promote suppuration. Theodoric's simple but heretical statement places him among the most original and independent surgeons of all time.

Theodoric's *Chirurgia* provides excellent examples of the overall decline of surgery from its previous Greco-Roman sophistication. The influence of Galen, as interpreted by the Islamic translators, was formidable. The doctrine of the humors, for example, was dominant and insinuated itself in all aspects of diagnosis and treatment. Basic surgical precepts were buried in unintelligible jargon. In many respects Theodoric himself did not pursue his own thesis. He sometimes achieved wound reapproximation and healing by bandaging, although suturing remained dominant:

> In whatever part of the body a cut may have occurred, let everything be done in order, according to the rules laid down for wounds in the scalp and face. Indeed, above all else a wound must be made clean. Secondly, having brought the lips of the wound together, they should be replaced accurately in the position which they had in their natural state; if necessary, they should be held there by stitches taken in accordance with the size of the wound. Let the size and depth of the wound determine the closeness and depth of the stitches. For let the physician make no mistake, as has already been said many times, he should be prudent and attentive to every detail. After the suturing has been properly done and the dressings have been carefully arranged, let the wound be bound up skillfully as the position and condition of the part require, that is to say, so that neither the stitches nor the dressings can be disturbed at all. And, just as we have often said before, do not undo the dressing until the third, or fourth, or fifth day if no pain occurs. Afterwards let the dressings be changed every third day unless too much putridity should occur in the wound, in which case it should be changed every day, observing the aforementioned directions. And always, whenever the dressing is changed, by pressing gently upon the wound with a little wine-soaked towel you may express any retained bloody matter. Afterwards let it be bound up according to the aforesaid method and let it be kept thus until the patient has completely recovered. And if proud flesh should become excessive on a wound, as has been said before, put on the green ointment or something similar, for as long as you see that it is necessary.

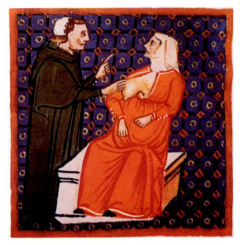

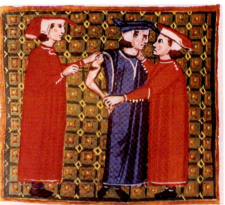

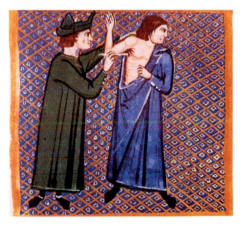

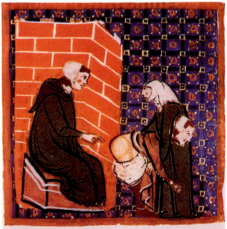

54. Illustrations from a late thirteenth-century illuminated manuscript of the *Chirurgia* of Theodoric Borgognoni. *Top to bottom,* Examination for breast abscess, treatment of an arm wound, probe with an instrument, and rectal examination. *(University Library, Leiden, ms Voss Lat F 3.)*

Theodoric and Hugh are remembered for describing a medieval substitute for general anesthesia. Although the origins of this technique date back to Alexandrian surgery, Theodoric's description of Hugh's soporific sponge is the first detailed account found in a surgical manuscript:

> The composition of a savour to be made by surgeons, according to Master Hugh, is as follows: take of opium, and the juice of unripe mulberry, hyoscyamus, the juice of spurge flax, the juice of leaves of mandragora, juice of ivy, juice of climbing ivy, of lettuce seed, and of the seed of the lapathum which has hard, round berries, and of the shrub hemlock, one ounce of each. Mix these all together in a brazen vessel, and then put into it a new sponge. Boil all together out under the sun during the dog days, until all is consumed and cooked down into the sponge. As often as there is need, you may put this sponge into hot water for an hour, and apply it to the nostrils until the subject for operation falls asleep. Then the surgery may be performed and when it is completed, in order to wake him up, soak another sponge in vinegar and pass it frequently under his nostrils. Likewise the juice of the roots of hay may be put under the nostrils, and the patient will soon be aroused.

Whether this concoction actually relieved pain is unknown. However, Theodoric and Hugh must be commended for their understanding of a need for an anesthetic agent. In the treatment of empyema, of abscesses, of penetrating wounds of the chest, and of both complicated and simple wounds of the skull, these surgeons emphasized the wisdom of using simple measures, of interfering with the parts as little as possible, of abstaining from the use of the probe, and of practicing strict cleanliness. They often soaked their compresses in hot wine before using them, thus attaining a mild antisepsis. Hugh attempted to replace the ends of a fractured rib by manual reduction. Hemorrhage was controlled by cauterization, tamponade, application of a ligature, or complete division of the injured blood vessel. Finally, these surgeons attached great importance to the proper feeding of their patients.

Theodoric's *Chirurgia* is an important milestone in the history of surgery. Despite many shortcomings, including the continued heavy use of cauterization, the treatise demonstrates the beginnings of independence of thought and observation in surgical therapy. Mindful of its obligation to Galen and the Arabists, it contains the first glimmerings of a recovery from the torpid thinking of prior centuries.

Bruno of Longoburg (circa thirteenth century) also advocated the dry or aseptic treatment of wounds. Bruno was a well-known surgeon in southern Italy in whose writings the phrases "healing by first intention" and "healing by second intention" are first found. Bruno's *Chirurgia Magna* was completed in 1252, and many similarities exist between it and the writings of Theodoric. His second major manuscript, the *Chirurgia Parva,* like the *Magna,* contained many extracts from Galen, Avicenna, Hippocrates, and Albucasis, as well as many original observations. Although historical uncertainty makes it difficult to assign definitive credit, Bruno's understanding of wound healing should probably be accorded the same respect accorded the views of Theodoric and Hugh.

A noteworthy contemporary of Hugh and Theodoric, considered the ablest Italian surgeon of the thirteenth century, was Guglielmo Salicetti (1210-1277), known as William of Saliceto. Born in a small village near Piacenza in Lombardy, he obviously had a fine education that included training in both medicine and surgery. In his writings he alluded to extensive experience in military and civilian practice. William was a cleric, as were all those who attended the universities of that era. He was professor at Bologna (circa 1268), later was city physician at Verona, and toward the end of his life composed the renowned *La Ciroxia Vulgarmente Fata.*

William of Saliceto's monumental effort, the *Ciroxia,* was authored primarily for his son Bernardino, who followed in his father's professional path. As a sort of surgical testament, this work was to become one of the most quoted surgical texts during the Renaissance. The *Ciroxia* stands out as a landmark in the history of surgery because it does not separate surgical diagnosis from internal medicine and it includes a remarkable collection of case histories, which William considered the

55. *Facing page,* William of Saliceto lecturing to students, from a Bolognese manuscript of his *Ciroxia (circa 1320). Ciroxia,* written toward the end of the thirteenth century, was one of the most widely quoted surgical texts during the Renaissance. *(Phot. Bibliothèque Nationale, Paris, Mss Lat 14731, f 2.)*

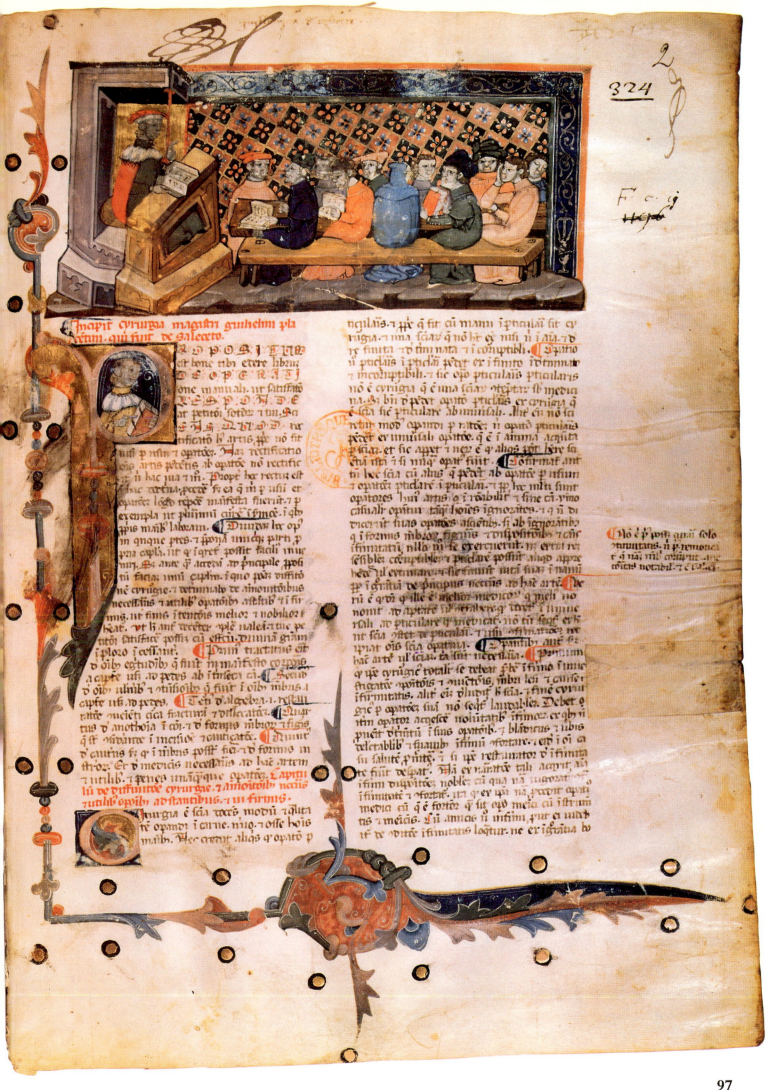

foundation of surgical teaching. Most important, its Book IV contains the first known treatise on regional or surgical anatomy.

William rarely quoted other authors, and most of the observations were original to his own practice. Initially published in Piacenza in 1474, the Italian translation is the first medical book printed in Italian and probably the first work on surgery to be produced from a printing press.

The *Ciroxia* is divided into five books preceded by a short chapter on general methods. Book I is devoted to internal diseases; Book II describes wounds, including those produced by arrows; Book III deals with fractures and dislocation; Book IV contains anatomical descriptions; and Book V encompasses the subject of cauterizing. William shows how to suture divided nerves and diagnose arterial bleeding by the spurting of blood, and he recognizes crepitus as a diagnostic sign of fractures. A careful observer, William describes hydrops as a result of kidney failure and ascribes lesions of the penis to venereal contagion, for which he recommends a prophylactic. Among William's most interesting clinical observations is the rejection of any attempt to remove the testicle as part of a herniorrhaphy. William prefers the knife to a cautering iron but does not comment on Hugh's and Theodoric's "dry" treatment of wounds.

In the introduction to the *Ciroxia* the true personality of William becomes manifest. He provides a detailed description of the approved conduct of the surgeon, the patients, and the assistants. This code of ethics would be repeated by surgeons for many centuries:

> Surgery is a science which teaches the rules and procedures for manual operations on the flesh, nerves and bone of man. One should not believe that such an operation in itself, which is done manually constitutes surgery, in view of the fact that it is one of the special sciences which does not exist but by the action of intelligence . . .
>
> Three things are principally necessary for those who, in this science, operate according to art. The first is that the surgeon should be entirely attentive to the patient in the examination and disposition of the condition of the injured part, thereby to the cause of the ailment, and not commit the least error; for, otherwise, this science is turned to derision, and the surgeon does not at all pursue, by his operation, a result worthy of praise. Those who practice this art should, in addition, acquiesce to the wishes of the patients and conform to them . . . and to comfort the patient by gentle actions, soft words, agreeable and proper, and promise him cure in all cases even though they are hopeless . . . For the mind of the patient feels, from such discourse and promises, a secret influence and a great disposition by which nature acquires vigor and resistance against the disease . . . But it is necessary that the doctor discuss the condition of the illness with the friends or the relatives of the patient . . . so that if the patient should die, one could not say that the doctor has caused the death . . .
>
> Secondly, the patient should neither contradict the physician by his remarks, nor delay the operations by his objections . . . It is suitable, therefore, that the patient accept the words and the actions of the surgeon, at the time that he chooses him to treat his malady . . .
>
> Thirdly, the assistants should bear themselves with kindness toward the patient, they should be agreeable, and they should obey the physicians in everything that seems to relate to the operation.

By the end of the 1200s Italian leadership in surgical education had substantially declined. Among the reasons for this declination was the civil war rampant throughout the country. During the late Middle Ages strong, independent city-states were emerging in Italy. These entities, such as Milan, Genoa, Florence, Pisa, and Venice, became so powerful that they could resist the nobles, even the various emperors, who attempted to bring them under control. Although a prosperous life could have been expected, the lengthy civil wasted the energies and resources of the country.

The Guelphs were a political party that supported the authority of the Pope, and the Ghibellines were an aristrocratic force in opposition. Every city-state was overtaken by internal strife between such groups, and peace occurred only when some powerful family of nobles made itself supreme. Between 1350 and 1500, cities under the rule of such families as the Medicis in Florence were the important centers of learning in Italy.

The principles of the Bologna school were faithfully upheld by William of Saliceto's ablest pupil, Guido Lanfranchi (?-1315), known as Lanfranc of Milan. Little biographical information is available about Lanfranc, except that he was a cleric who received a university degree in medicine. Lanfranc's professional life was devoted almost entirely to the surgical arts; he was said to have enjoyed financial success while practicing in Milan. Although a cleric, he was apparently nonobservant of any vows, since he had several children whom he publicly recognized and one of his sons practiced medicine.

Lanfranc became involved in the squabbles of the Guelphs and Ghibellines in his native city. He took sides against the latter, who to his later misfortune emerged victorious. In 1290 the Visconti banished Lanfranc from his homeland. He sought refuge in Lyon, where he resumed his studies and practice and authored his *Chirurgia Parva*. Professional ambitions caused Lanfranc to resettle in Paris, and in 1295 he arrived in a city that was rapidly becoming the educational and intellectual center of western Europe.

Although his reputation had preceded him, the career of Lanfranc was almost ended prematurely because he was not allowed to obtain a position on the medical faculty at the University of Paris. As might be expected, the university was directly supervised by the French kings and, more important, the Church. The medical faculty for the most part assigned greater status to the practice of medicine than to surgery, and a mandatory supremacy of Christian theology and philosophy over natural science. As early as the twelfth century the medical faculty

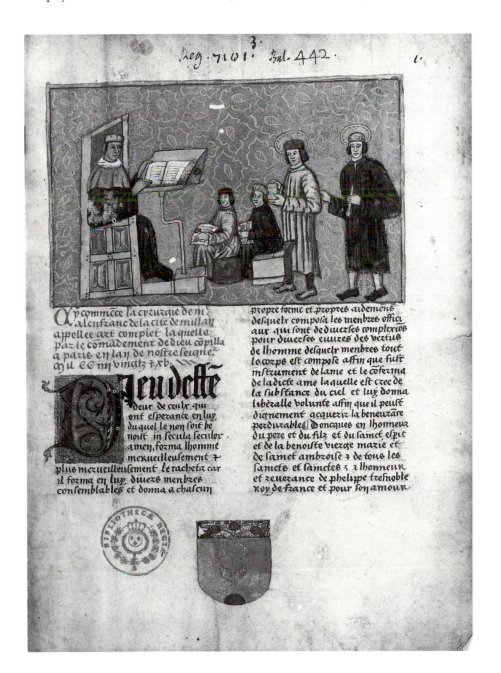

56. Lanfranc of Milan lecturing to two students as seen in a fifteenth-century illuminated manuscript of the French translation of his *Chirurgia*. Behind the two seated students are the much larger figures of Sts. Cosmas and Damian. *(Phot. Bibliothèque Nationale, Paris, Mss, Fr 628, f 1.)*

had excluded all those who wished to work with their hands, so students of medicine had to disavow any intention toward the study of surgery.

Five classes of injuries or diseases were specifically prohibited from being treated: wounds, ulcers, fractures, dislocations, and tumors. Manuscripts on surgery and midwifery began to disappear from the university library. By the splitting asunder of medicine and surgery, the evolution of surgery was forever changed. All university professors were required to be celibate clerics. Therefore Lanfranc became associated instead with a gathering of surgeons called the Confraternity of Sts. Cosmas and Damian.

According to popular tradition, Cosmas and his twin, Damian, were the youngest of five brothers who belonged to a Christian family of some distinction in Persia. They chose the career of traveling physicians and gave their services freely to those in need. During the persecution of the Christians that occurred in the reign of Emperor Diocletian, Cosmas and Damian were tortured and beheaded (circa A.D. 300). They were soon given sainthood for what were regarded as miraculous medical and surgical cures, including the transplantation

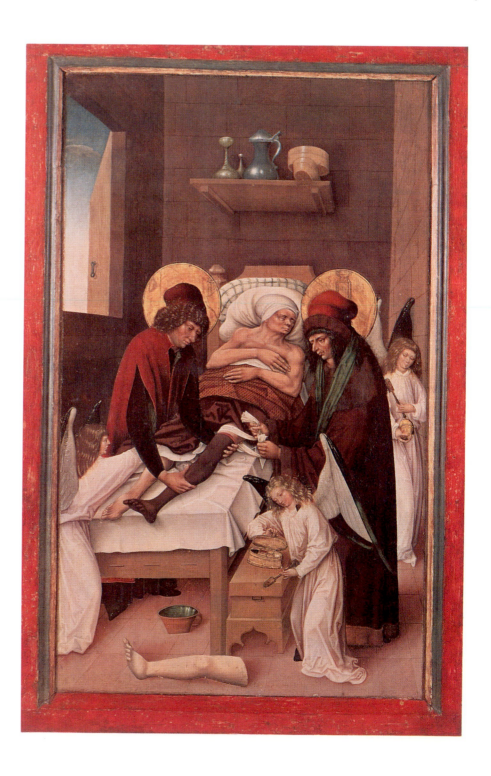

57. The notion of the transplantation of limbs may have had its origin in this legendary exploit of Sts. Cosmas and Damian. In this painting by the Schwäbische Master of the Schnaiter Alter, the saints are shown replacing a Caucasian's amputated leg with one taken from a recently deceased Moor. *(Württembergisches Landesmuseum, Stuttgart.)*

of a leg from a recently deceased Moor to a cancer victim whose leg they had amputated. The Medicis adopted Cosmas and Damian as their particular patron saints, and over the centuries Cosmas and Damian have become recognized as the patron saints of surgery.

The Confraternity of Sts. Cosmas and Damian had been founded by Jean Pitard (1220-1280) in 1255. The educational background of Pitard is unknown, although he might have been of Italian ancestry, having been driven out of his native country by the internecine warfare. Pitard achieved the important post of surgeon to King Louis IX (1214-1270), also known as St. Louis. Pitard's influence with this sovereign would prove important for the future evolution of French and European surgery. Pitard also served as surgeon to Louis's grandson King Philip IV (1268-1314), known as The Fair, who laid the foundation for the French monarchy. No writings from Pitard are known, although it is suspected that he at least compiled a compendium of his surgical work.

By the middle of the 1200s and for centuries afterward, the practice of surgery in France was entirely in the hands of two classes of men, the barbers and the surgeons. As time progressed, the surgeons began to perceive a need for protecting their material interests, which were being increasingly encroached upon by the barbers. This encroachment occurred even though the latter were not allowed by the authorities to include in their professional activities anything beyond haircutting, shaving, cupping, extraction of teeth, application of leeches, incision of boils, and possibly one or two other simple surgical operations.

In 1255, under the leadership of Pitard and with the approval of Louis IX, surgeons gathered themselves into a community of Parisian practitioners. Named after the patron saints of surgery, this confederation was a loosely organized guild containing about 10 "masters." They became affiliated with the newly constructed parish church of Sts. Cosmas and Damian at the corner of rue de la Harpe and rue des Cordeliers, in the academic enclave. Here they met and attempted to assert their common interest and control over the regulation and right of inspection regarding the practice of surgery. In moving to the academic enclave, the probable ulterior goal of this community of surgeons was to obtain scholastic status as part of the true medical faculty at the University of Paris.

Little is known about the early organization of the Confraternity of Sts. Cosmas and Damian. By the beginning of the fourteenth century, however, a guild of Parisian barber-surgeons also was in existence. In general these individuals were not permitted to use a knife, and as a result great jealousy existed between them and the Confraternity. Noting the chaotic state of affairs, Philip IV issued an edict (in 1311) stating that only individuals who underwent an examination administered from a royally authorized source should be allowed to practice surgery in Paris. In this instance the Confraternity assumed the royal order and began academic testing. Those who passed the required examination were entitled to be known as "masters of surgery." By this royal statute the existence and autonomy of the surgeons were officially recognized and reiterated.

Paralleling the surgeons' ambitions to attain university status were the barber-surgeons' aspirations to gain entry into the surgeons' ranks. Unwelcome in the Confraternity, the barber-surgeons obtained from Charles V (1337-1380), also called The Wise, through the intermediary of his personal barber, their own special charter (1372). This charter effectively legalized their professional ambitions and the designation "barber-surgeon." In addition to barbering, the barber-surgeons were now entitled to treat carbuncles, bruises, boils, and any other nonmortal open wounds. Most important, the surgeons of the Confraternity of Sts. Cosmas and Damian were told not to hinder the development of the barber-surgeons. Although the Confraternity attempted to have these prerogatives revoked, they were not able to do so.

Inevitably, over the years the Guild of Parisian Barber-Surgeons and the Confraternity of St. Côme surgeons continually clashed. Suspicions abounded; deprived of teaching and overly sensitive to the haughty manner in which they were treated by the Confraternity, the barber-surgeons approached the university's medical faculty to solicit a merger. The faculty despised both groups of surgeons but had greater disdain for the Confraternity, whose members had always considered themselves the equals of the faculty, but without legitimate academic affiliation. Consequently in 1505 the barber-surgeons signed the first of several contracts with the medical faculty. The barber-surgeons pledged to restrict themselves to the manual aspects of medical and surgical therapy and to treat patients only when a member of the faculty was present or had given prior approval. The barber-surgeons pledged allegiance, honor, and reverence to the faculty and acknowledged the medical physicians as their superiors and mentors. The barber-surgeons agreed to pay annual dues and to have faculty physicians proctor the examinations for prospective master barber-surgeons. The barber-surgeons received from the faculty an agreement to defend the interests of the barber-surgeons' guild, to continue to provide anatomical lessons for its apprentices, and to provide instruction in French instead of Latin.

In 1544 Francis I (1494-1547) honored the Confraternity's request to obtain university privileges. The academic posts included higher social status and pecuniary benefits. These master surgeons were granted the right to wear a "long" university gown, and their community became formally recognized as the "surgeons of the long gown," or the College of St. Côme.

In actuality the College was never a formal part of the faculty of the University of Paris, although the surgeons tried to imitate their academic superiors. Candidates for the surgical degree took examinations and wrote theses in Latin. Imitation was the sincerest form of flattery: even the academic rituals followed by the College closely mimicked those of the university.

For the layperson the distinguishing sign of the barber-surgeons was the shaving dish, made of pewter and hung at the front door of their shops. The surgeons also had a shaving dish, but made of polished brass. Surgeons who were members of the Confraternity were permitted to display at the window a banner bearing the coat of arms of this organization.

At the end of the Middle Ages, therefore, three independent classes of "legitimate" French medical and surgical practitioners existed: the physicians, who were baccalaureates of the faculty of medicine; the surgeons of the Confraternity, or the College of St. Côme; and the Guild of Barber-Surgeons. These ever changing political liaisons continued into the next century. However, the zenith of the College of St. Côme had clearly occurred under the aegis of surgeons like Pitard, Lanfranc, and Henri de Mondeville (1260-1320).

Into the previously described environment Lanfranc settled when he arrived in Paris, where he became one of the founders of modern French surgery. Lanfranc was a man of great erudition and sought to establish surgery as a learned and scientific profession, equal to and an essential part of general medicine. As a member of the Confraternity of Sts. Cosmas and Damian, Lanfranc was a bitter critic of the nonclerical and essentially uneducated barber-surgeons and felt that medicine and surgery should not be split apart:

> Oh, Lord . . . why is there such a great difference between surgeons and physicians? The philosophers have placed the craft in the hands of laymen, for many disdain to work with their hands; and many think it is impossible for one person to know both medicine and surgery. But know this well, that no man can be a good physician who knows no surgery; and conversely, no one can be a good surgeon without knowledge of medicine.

Lanfranc's masterpiece, *Chirurgia Magna,* was completed in 1296. Dedicated to Philip IV, it was first published in Venice in 1490. His works became well known and served as the foundation of French surgical teaching for many years. Lanfranc's ethical advice to the young surgeon is characteristic of his general conservatism:

> Needful it is that a surgeon be of a complexion well proportioned, and that his complexion be tempered . . . . A surgeon must have hands well shaped, long small fingers, and his body not quaking, and all must be of subtle wit, for all things that belong to surgery may not with letters be written. He must study in all the parts of philosophy

and in logic, that he may understand scriptures; in grammar, that he speak agreeably; in art that teaches him to prove his propositions with good reasons; in rhetoric that teaches him to speak seemly. Be he no glutton, nor envious, nor a niggard; be he true, humbly and pleasingly bear he himself to his patients; speak he no ribaldry in the sick man's house. Give he no counsel unless he be asked; speak he not with any woman in folly in the sick man's house; nor chide not with the sick man nor with any of his servants, but courteously speak to the sick man, and in all manner of sickness promise him cure, though thou be despaired of him; but never say the latter to his friends (but) tell them how it stands.

He should shun difficult cures and not intervene in desperate cases. Poor men help he by his might, and of the rich men ask he good reward . . . So learn he physic, that he may with good rules defend his surgery.

Lanfranc's greatest contribution to operative surgery was his description of brain injuries. He was the first to describe concussion of the brain. Depressed fragments and irritation of the dura were his only indications for trephination. Lanfranc recommended percussion of the skull, and if there was no fracture, one heard a sound like an uncracked bell. He also refined the method of tying a waxed string to one of the patient's teeth and holding the string taut. By plucking on it, different tones were produced, which determined whether a skull fracture was present.

Lanfranc carefully distinguished between arterial and venous hemorrhage and cancer and hypertrophy of the breast. Unlike his mentor, William of Saliceto, Lanfranc was a firm believer in the value of cauterization over that of a surgical knife. He was quite conservative in his operative techniques and castigated those who would operate for hernia, cataract, or bladder stones. Among his innovative techniques were intubation of the esophagus and suturing of injured nerves.

A contemporary of Lanfranc who also served as personal surgeon to Philip IV is Henri de Mondeville (1260-1320). Henri, born in Normandy, was the first great French master of surgery. Like his mentor, Theodoric, in Bologna, Henri was a cleric, university educated in medicine, and an ardent devotee of the art of surgery. His major attribute in surgery was his clear understanding of Theodoric's doctrine concerning the primary healing of wounds. Henri was alone among the major surgeons of that era in promulgating this belief and had an almost fanatical enthusiasm expanded by his personal observations in military and civilian surgery.

58. A pharmacy in a fourteenth-century surgeon's office. One assistant cuts herbs in the garden while another, under the doctor's supervision, grinds them in a mortar. From a French illuminated manuscript of the *Chirurgie* of Guy de Chauliac. *(Phot. Bibliothèque Nationale, Paris, Ms 6966, f 154v.)*

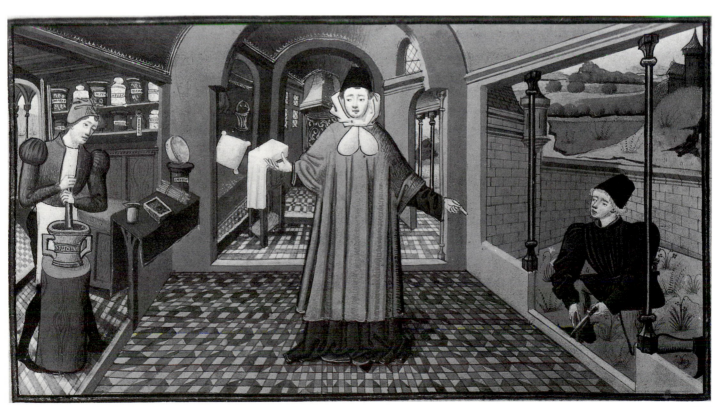

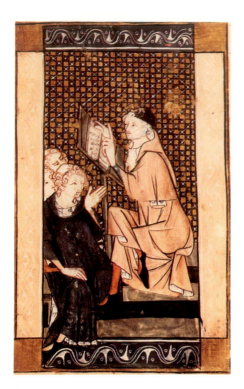

59. Henri de Mondeville lecturing to his students, as seen in a fourteenth-century French illuminated manuscript of his *Chirurgie,* the first surgical textbook by a Frenchman. One of the students appears to be raising his hand to ask a question. Mondeville was the teacher of Guy de Chauliac. *(Phot. Bibliothèque Nationale, Paris, Ms fr 2030.)*

Henri studied at the universities of Montpellier and Paris and apprenticed with Theodoric. On returning to Paris in the 1290s, he was chosen one of the four surgeons to Philip IV. In 1304 Henri delivered a series of anatomical lectures at Montpellier. His many obligations to the royal court caused Henri to set aside his personal interests periodically. Although these services, especially on military expeditions, afforded him the opportunities to acquire great experience in the treatment of wounds, Henri complained bitterly of these interruptions, for which he received little remuneration.

The surgical treatise of Henri de Mondeville was begun in 1306, but his text was never completed because of failing health as a result of asthma and tuberculosis. Not until 1892 was a printed form of the treatise derived and published from several surviving medieval manuscripts. The Church was quite displeased with much of Mondeville's teaching and went to great lengths to suppress any later printing of his work. More important, his contemporaries never gave it the recognition it deserved. Consequently his *Chirurgie* remained in manuscript form and exerted little influence on succeeding generations of French surgeons.

The prominence of Mondeville lies entirely in his early opposition to surgical quackery and empiricism. Henri declared that surgery must belong to all of medicine. He twitted the Church and its hierarchy to explain how its physician-clerks were supposed to learn surgery without being permitted to touch a human body.

Mondeville's text provides a lucid insight into the state of early fourteenth-century surgery. He is quite outspoken about all who surrounded him, including not only his peers but also the rich and the politically powerful:

> It would be in vain for a surgeon today to know all the art, science and operations of surgery if he does not have the art and science of making it pay, since that is his principal intention and a thing is useless if, being intended to arrive at a certain end it does not reach it. Also, it is necessary for the surgeon who wishes to operate, that he has by precaution several valid arguments to accomplish this end. There are, in effect, patients, even rich, who are so miserable, avaricious and stupid as to give nothing, or if they pay, it is a little thing. They believe it satisfactory to the surgeon if they give 12 deniers or 2 sous a day, as if to a mason, a furrier or a cobbler, and do not realize that wealth has no value without health, that there is no poverty that can be compared with sickness . . .
>
> You then, surgeons, if you have operated conscientiously on the rich for a suitable fee, and on the poor for charity, you need not fear fire, rain or wind, you have no need to go into religion, to make pilgrimages, or other acts of the sort, because by your science you have been able to save your souls, live without poverty and die in your homes, live in peace and joy, and exult because your reward is great in the Heavens . . .

The *Chirurgie* was originally intended to appear in five volumes. Mondeville writes in the introduction that he relied principally on Avicenna for anatomy, Theodoric for wounds, and Lanfranc for the treatment of ulcers and other diseases. Volume I deals primarily with anatomy and, because of the Church's decree against human vivisection, provides little of interest. The greatness of Mondeville is found in Volume II. This volume, the longest in the manuscript, concerns the treatment of wounds and ulcers. Here he expresses his solidarity with Theodoric's view that a wound heals more quickly without pus formation. Mondeville opposes the use of ointment on wounds on the grounds that such treatment caused needless suppuration. He advises to simply wash a wound clean and control hemorrhage by styptics, digital compression, acupressure, or torsion of the isolated vessel. Mondeville takes serious objection to any doubters of his therapeutic management.

In the introduction to Volume III, on surgery of the soft tissues other than wounds or ulcers, Mondeville blames the King and the royal court for having taken advantage of his talents as a military physician when he could have been more useful elsewhere:

> On the order of our Lord the King, I have uselessly lost a great deal of time, to my great despair . . . in several of his armies and at his court, hoping that he would pay me what was due me, after which, on further order of the King, renouncing all profit, I have returned to Paris and have lived there, at least for short intervals; I have wished again to take up little by little the work which I have abandoned.

Mondeville was a reformer but knew he would not be able to complete his text. Concerned with his approaching death, he omitted the entire fourth book on fractures and dislocations, to devote his final months to a fifth volume on materia medica. Mondeville was correct in believing that his viewpoints would not influence large portions of the medical community. His greatness was not to be perceived for many centuries.

At the same time that Mondeville's career was coming to an end, the university at Montpellier was beginning to rival the university at Paris as the center of European medical and surgical education. Like Salerno, Montpellier existed on the educational border of the Islamic and Latin worlds. Founded as early as the eighth century, it attained an international reputation because both Jews and Arabs were admitted there. Although 15 universities were established in medieval France, the Church restricted the study of medicine to the faculties in Paris and Montpellier.

Under the influence of Arnald of Villanova (1240-1311) Montpellier achieved its greatest prominence. Arnald wrote one of the best medieval handbooks on the practice of medicine and was especially renowned for his translations of Avicenna. Although Arnald was not generally recognized as a surgeon, there appears to have been no other physician at Montpellier who could be compared to Arnald in professional ability or surgical skills. Arnald's greatest work was the *Parabole,* which contained 345 aphorisms and much original content. He relates that, like all wound surgeons of that era, he did not perform large operations, for fear of "pulsating" hemorrhage. Because of Arnald, many graduates of Montpellier had studied surgery.

The most prominent of these graduates and the individual destined to become the preeminent European surgeon of the late Middle Ages was Guy de Chauliac (1300-1368). A native of France, he received the university training of a cleric, then pursued the study of medicine at Paris and Montpellier and completed a special course in anatomy at Bologna under Niccolo Bertuccio (?-1347). Guy de Chauliac's wide travels and many years of medical education qualified him to be acknowledged as one of the most erudite surgeons of his era.

Guy first began his surgical practice in his native diocese of Mende. Shortly thereafter he was appointed a canon to churches in Rheims (1225) and Lyon (1330). Guy finally settled in Avignon when it was the residency of the Pope and was named private physician and commensal chaplain to Popes Clement VI (?-1352), Innocent VI (?-1362), and Urban V (?-1370). Since Avignon had a magnificent library, Guy had ready access to all the great medical works of past civilizations, especially in their Greek translations. In 1348 an epidemic of the plague occurred in Avignon; among its victims was Laura, love of the poet Petrarch (1304-1374), who was probably cared for by Guy.

Guy de Chauliac's great work is the massive *Inventorium Seu Collectorium Cyrurgie,* first written in 1363. Its initial printed edition, completed in 1478, was the first important medical book published in French *(La Grande Chirurgie).* The work is physically immense and contains more than 3000 quotes from earlier authors. The manuscript must have been quite important in the days before the invention of printing because there remain extant nearly 35 manuscript copies of the *Inventorium.* The printed text went through many editions and translations and served as one of the principal textbooks on surgery for close to two centuries.

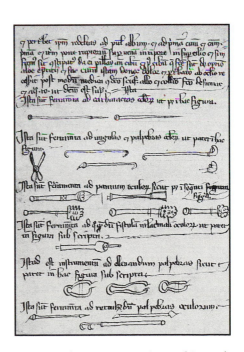

60. Surgical instruments in a thirteenth-century manuscript of the surgical writings of Arnald of Villanova. Arnald's teachings are not generally associated with surgery, but he was considered among the most influential surgeons in the Montpellier school. *(Historical Collections, College of Physicians of Philadelphia.)*

From a reading of his treatise Guy emerges as an independent thinker but more reactionary than Mondeville, particularly in his method of treating wounds. He strongly opposes the theories of Theodoric and believes in healing by the need for suppuration and laudable pus. Guy writes that healing can be accomplished only by the surgeon's interference with salves, plasters, and other invasive meddling, not by letting nature take its course. Guy's attitudes about wound healing, because of his overall influence on the history of surgery, greatly retarded the subsequent evolution of the science.

The *Inventorium* commences with Guy's celebrated "Capitulum singulare." This chapter contains many interesting generalities pertaining to surgery and summarizes the fourteenth-century surgeon's outlook on his profession, thus providing a history of medicine and a discussion of surgery's place in the medieval world:

> Up to the time of Avicenna all writers were both physicians and surgeons, but since that time, either because of the fastidiousness or the excessive occupation of the clerics, surgery has become a separate branch and has fallen into the hands of the mechanics. The sects which have existed in my times among the operators of this art, besides the two general ones of the Logicians and the Empirics, have been five. The first was the school of Roger, Roland and the Four Masters who treated all wounds and abscess alike with cataplasm and poultices, on the ground of the fifth aphorism, "lax things are good, and crude bad." The second was the school of Bruno and Theodoric, which treated all wounds alike with wine, basing their practice exclusively upon the maxim, "the dry is nearest to that which is sound, and the moist to that which is not sound." The third sect was that of William of Saliceto and of Lanfranc,

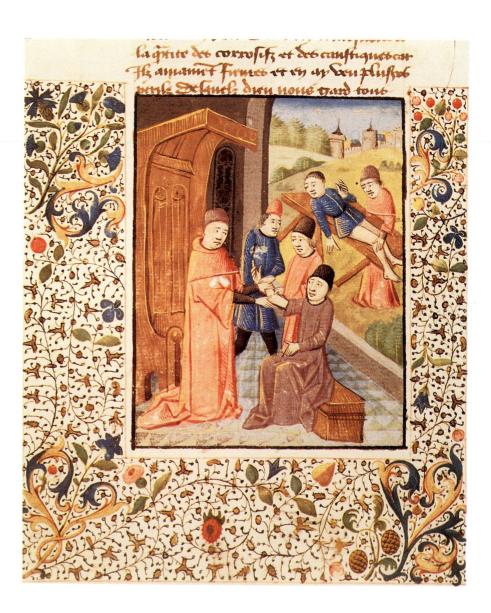

61. Portrait of Guy de Chauliac, with the help of two assistants, reducing a fracture or luxation of the elbow. In the background another patient is being examined for an injured leg. From a fifteenth-century illuminated manuscript of Chauliac, *Inventaire Ou Recueil Chirurgical Ou Medical.* (Phot. Bibliothèque Nationale, Paris, Mss Fr 396, f 80v.)

who wished to pursue the middle course, covering and dressing all wounds with ointments and soft plasters, founding this practice on the fourteenth maxim of the therapeutics, that curation has one sole method, that the treatment shall be gentle and without pain. The fourth sect is composed of all the military men, or German chevaliers and others following the army, who, with conjurations and potions, oil, wool, and cabbage-leaves, dress all wounds, basing their practice on the maxim that God has given his virtue to herbs and stones. The fifth sect is of women and many fools, who refer the sick of all diseases to the saints solely, saying, "God has given me that which pleased Him; God will cure me when it pleases Him to do so; blessed be the name of the Lord. Amen."

The first book of *La Grande Chirurgie* is a topography of the patient, that is, anatomy. Guy considers knowledge of the human body an essential part of a surgeon's education. Since he had taken special instruction in anatomy, it is understandable that he stresses its importance. From the works of Guy and other surgeon-anatomists it becomes evident that the Church's edict against human vivisection was slowly being overlooked while the search for scientific knowledge continued:

> Anatomy is acquired by two means: one is by the teaching from books, which method, though useful, is not always sufficient to explain the things which are not known. . . . The other method is by experience on the dead body. For we practice on the bodies recently dead, that have been decapitated or hanged, at least on the internal organs, the flesh of the muscles, the skin, and of many veins and nerves, especially as to their origin.

Clearly, for that era Guy was a skilled operator. He was among the first to take herniorrhaphy and couching for cataract out of the hands of the itinerant surgeon. Cancer was treated at a relatively early stage with both knife and cautery. Bandages were stiffened by saturating them with egg whites. Guy described in great detail the soporific sponge of Theodoric. His work contains the best summary of medieval dentistry, including the first description of a separate class of individuals (dentatores, i.e., dentists) who operated on teeth. He also provided rules for the care and cleansing of the teeth to prevent decay and advised replacement of lost teeth by other human teeth or by artificial dentures made of bone. Various surgical instruments were described, and the proper contents of a surgeon's case detailed: scissors, speculum, razor, scalpel, needle, and lancet. Guy's inventiveness is obvious in the treatment of fractures and dislocations: he suspended fractures in a sling bandage or by means of weight and pulley.

Guy's methods dominated surgery in France and, to some degree, England for almost 200 years. He provided relatively little that was original, but he achieved distinction in his ability to explain treatments and to place surgery in a proper perspective relative to medicine.

The greatness of thirteenth-century Italian surgery was transferred to France by surgeons like Lanfranc, Mondeville, and Guy, who then disseminated their practical experience, teaching, and writings to numerous pupils. Among the many foreign students attracted to Paris was Jean Yperman (1295-1361), a native of what was then Flanders. He was well educated and became fluent in French and Latin. Like most other university students, Yperman was a cleric but never took holy orders. He moved to Paris and became a student of Lanfranc.

After his apprenticeship Yperman returned to his native land and was appointed attending physician to the Hospital of Belle in a small Flemish town. Within a few years he settled permanently in his native city of Ypres, an area that would achieve infamy during World War I as the first place where the German army used mustard gas, or yperite, as a weapon. For 30 years Yperman maintained a medical and surgical practice in Ypres and became quite famous.

Yperman wrote numerous treatises, but after his death these works became obscured. Not until almost 500 years later was his great work, *La Chirurgie,* first printed. Written in Flemish, the medieval manuscript demonstrates that Yperman was a distinguished surgical authority in the Flemish countries during the late Middle Ages. The manuscript gives splendid accounts of trephination, arrow

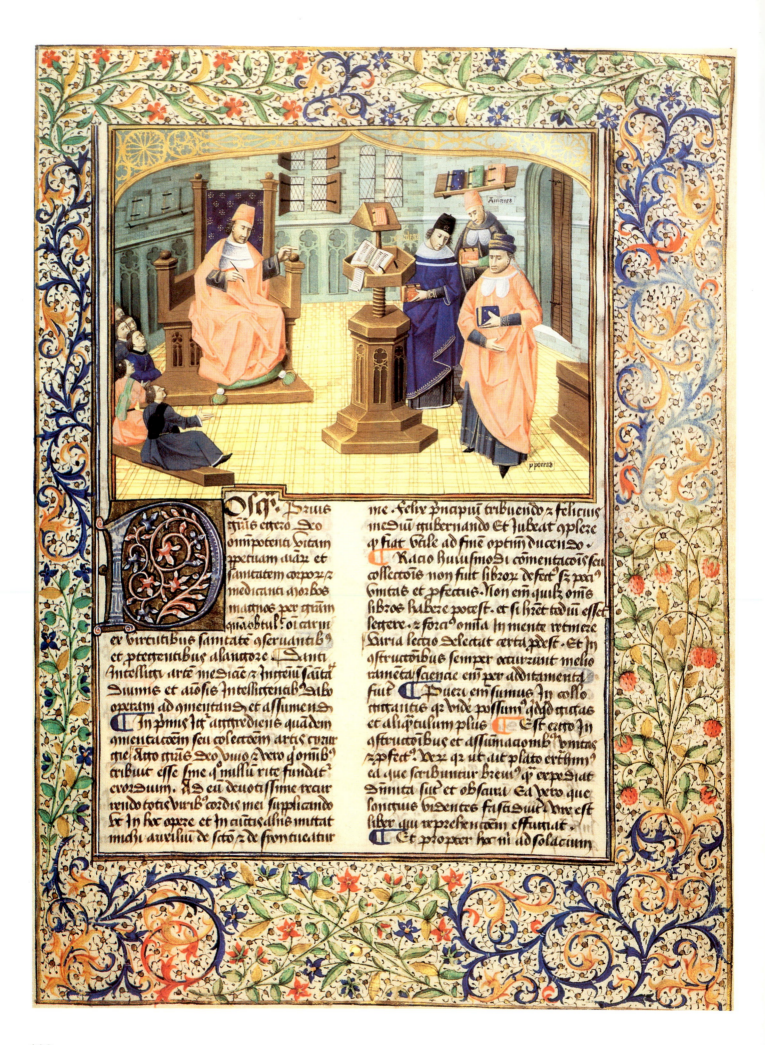

wounds, healing of harelip by freshening wound edges and then carefully suturing the defect, esophageal feeding via a silver tube, and attempts to replace prolapsed viscera by enlargement of the abdominal wound. Yperman describes both the use of ligatures to check bleeding of a wounded artery and the hemostatic value of the torsion of an artery as Lanfranc did:

> When the surgeon finds himself in the presence of a wound, from which a great deal of blood is flowing, he should examine from which part it comes. If it flows from the wound by fits and spurts, then it is evident that it comes from an artery, and in that case it is limpid and of a lighter color. If the blood flows slowly, and is of a deeper color, it comes from the common veins which nourish the body . . .
>
> Be well aware that a hemorrhage from an artery is much more dangerous than that of a vein and that such a hemorrhage is formidable if it is too large. For this reason, I would advise you immediately to stop this flow of blood if it is in your power, for it results in serious accidents and threat of death . . .
>
> Here is how one should arrest hemorrhage from veins and arteries. Those of the small veins are easily controlled by a wad of gauze applied and fixed, either dry or soaked in the blood itself, or in egg-white. Hemorrhage from a large vein is combatted in the same manner and if one does not succeed in arresting it, one may stop it in the following manner: first the finger is applied to the wad to keep it from falling and so that the blood will not flow out so easily, then water is dropped on it to cool it; the coolness counters part of the heat and thereby the blood becomes less fluid; the coolness also contracts the skin, flesh and the vessels, and so diminishes the caliber of the veins. But be careful that no water enters the veins for that will cause accidents . . .
>
> If the hemorrhage is still not arrested one should have recourse to medicaments which have hemostatic properties of various degrees . . . if you do not succeed in arresting the hemorrhage with hemostatic powders or by the means indicated earlier, it is necessary to take resort to the ligature . . . One can also resort to the following method: take a flat piece of iron with a hole in it and place it on the wound so that the hole corresponds to the injured vein; then take another piece of iron which can go through the hole, bring it to red heat and cauterize the vein through the hole . . . The arteries must be cauterized so that an eschar forms, and the cauterization should also be stronger in proportion to the size of the vein or the artery. Meanwhile care must be taken that the eschar does not fall off and that the hemorrhage does not recur. For this purpose the surest method is perhaps to seize the vein, twist it and then ligate it . . .

The most distinguished pupil of Guy de Chauliac was Peter of Argelata (?-1423), who later served as lecturer on surgery in Bologna and became the principal Italian surgeon of his time. The six books on surgery by Peter were edited by Matthaeus Moretus (circa late fifteenth century) and published in Venice (1480). Most of the contents were derived from Paul of Aegina and Guy. Peter was renowned for both his surgical operative skills and his teaching abilities. In the chapter on the treatment of the dead body he provides a graphic account of how he embalmed the corpse of Alexander V (?-1410), who was considered an anti-pope. Peter taught the "dry" treatment, or primary healing of wounds, but powdered them; he was versed in dentistry, used sutures and drainage tubes in wounds, and performed lithotomy, herniotomy, and fistula-in-ano procedures.

English surgery during the Middle Ages was not nearly as developed as in France or Italy, but certain individuals did manage to become quite prominent. Although John of Mirfield (circa second half of fourteenth century) is not recognized as a surgeon, his written comments on the relationship between medicine and surgery are enlightening. Mirfield was primarily a chaplain at St. Bartholomew's Hospital in London but also served as a physician.

In 1380 Mirfield wrote a treatise on medicine and surgery embodying much of his practical experience. This *Breviarium Bartolomei* was divided into 15 sections. The ninth section discusses wounds and bruises; the tenth is on fractures, dislocations, and sprains; and the eleventh details dislocations. Mirfield relates that a fractured rib takes 20 days for a complete union, whereas a humerus or femur takes twice as long. His chief reputation is based on the teachings and

62. *Facing page,* Guy and his predecessors. Guy is shown sitting in the lectern chair, *left.* At his feet, sitting on a bench, heads bare, are six students. On the right, wearing professorial hats and holding books in their hands, are Galen, Avicenna, and Hippocrates. Behind them other manuscripts are evident on the wall. From an illuminated manuscript of Guy's *Chirurgie,* possibly painted for le duc Charles d'Orléans, dated 1461. *(Phot. Bibliothèque Nationale, Paris, Mss, Lat 6966, f 4.)*

general observations in the *Brevarium*. These are especially relevant when his protests against the then-fashionable division of medicine and surgery are considered:

> Long ago, unless I mistake, physicians used to practice surgery, but nowadays there is a great distinction between surgery and medicine, and this, I fear, arises from pride, because physicians disdain to work with their hands, though indeed, I myself have a suspicion that it is because they do not know how to perform particular operations; and this unfortunate usage has led the public to believe that a man cannot know both subjects, but the well informed are aware that he cannot be a good physician who neglects every part of surgery, and, on the other hand, a surgeon is good for nothing who is without knowledge of medicine.

The most important medieval English surgical personality is John of Arderne (1306–1390). He was that country's first surgeon of note and, like other prominent contemporary European surgeons, probably received portions of his training in Montpellier. It is known that Arderne gained his practical surgical experience during the Hundred Years War (1339–1453), when England lost all of her possessions in France except Calais. While serving as a military surgeon in the armies of Edward III (1312–1377) and Richard II (1367–1400), Arderne was posted in Antwerp, in Algeciras, Spain, and in Aquitaine, France. He was also present at the Battle of Crecy (1346) and at the Siege of Algiers, where gunpowder was used for the first time in European military history.

In 1349 Arderne terminated his military service and established a practice at Newark in Nottinghamshire, where he remained for almost 20 years. Arderne had a particular interest in diseases of the rectum. Thus he is sometimes referred to as the father of proctology. For unknown reasons Arderne moved to London in 1370, where he lived out the remainder of his professional life.

Arderne established himself as a surgeon who took care of the upper classes, primarily nobles, knights, and clergy. In London he immediately joined the Guild of Military Surgeons. It was during the Hundred Years War that the need for military surgeons first became evident. In London the better known of these surgeons became united in a loose fellowship of 15 to 20 members. By 1369, if not earlier, they had obtained some legal recognition from the city, and the fellowship existed for another two centuries. During those 200 years temporary alliances were made with "university-trained" physicians, and struggles began with the barber-surgeons.

The earliest history of organized surgery in London and England remains conjectural. The political clout of the Guild of Military Surgeons was never substantive, and when their rules were revised in 1435, only 17 men were listed as members. With the exception of John of Arderne, none of these supposedly highly placed and learned surgeons appears to have become prominent.

Quite the opposite was seen in the development of the barber-surgeons of London. As in France, the barber-surgeons developed as a result of the clerics being forced by their superiors to abandon the practice of surgery: the barbers, who had attended to the monks in their monasteries with razors, knives, and scissors, began to perform minor surgical procedures for which the priests had been previously responsible. Over the years, these barbers were encouraged to practice surgery and perform increasing numbers of surgical operations. They soon became the "barber-surgeons," and several of them became apprentices to the English military surgeons during the Hundred Years War. Consequently, they began to learn about "major" surgery and the management of fractures and dislocations.

In thirteenth- and fourteenth-century London, guilds or companies were being established to control various types of trades. The first recorded master of the barber's guild was Richard le Barbour in 1308, although it is almost certain that the guild was in existence before that time. It rapidly became a well established and prosperous political entity within London, receiving its Royal Charter from Edward IV (1442–1483) in 1462. The barber-surgeons were allowed almost exclusive control over the practice of surgery in the city, which did nothing but harm to the smaller Guild of Military Surgeons. Although this Guild maintained some control over the practice of surgery through the mayor and aldermen, the military surgeons, too, eventually received a form of royal recognition for their services in the war in 1492 from Henry VII (1457-1509), the first Tudor king, who awarded them a badge of cognizance.

The Guild of Barber-Surgeons fought fiercely with the Guild of Military Surgeons for the total right of supervision over anyone who practiced surgery. The London city corporation sided sometimes with one group, sometimes with the other, and indecision was always present. This indecision is no more evident than in 1423, when the Guild of Military Surgeons attempted to establish an alliance with London physicians to form an Academy of Medicine. This alliance was intended to take away the licensing powers of the universities and of the Guild of Barber-Surgeons. The mayor and aldermen granted the physicians and surgeons of London the right to form a society for purposes of licensing. Whether this concept originated from a similar scheme in Paris remains un-known. Either way, two surgeons, Thomas Morstead and J. Harvey, were made masters in surgery.

As expected, the barber-surgeons became alarmed and appealed to the city corporation, attempting to show that the new academy was a denial of their privileges. The city fathers replied that they had not intended to interfere with the Guild of Barber-Surgeons and that their powers were inviolable. After these political squabbles the military surgeons stopped their overt attempts to crush their rivals, and the barber-surgeons occupied themselves with developing an educational system. The ultimate union of all surgeons in London eventually occurred much more expeditiously than in Paris, with its lengthy and conten-tious battles between the surgeons of St. Côme and the barber-surgeons.

How involved Arderne was in all the political machinations is not known. However, his surgical writings were preeminent in England for almost two cen-turies, as evidenced by the many surviving medieval manuscripts of his works. Arderne wrote many treatises, all in Latin, concerning such diverse topics as care of the eyes, venesection, sinuses, fistula-in-ano, analysis of urine, and sanitation during plagues. Not one to be ashamed of high operative fees, Arderne wrote:

> And if he see the patient pursue busily the cure, then after that the state of the patient asketh (according to the condition of the patient) ask he boldly more or less; but ever be he ware of scarce asking, for over scarce asking setteth at naught both the market and the thing. Therefore for the cure of fistula in ano, when it is curable, ask he competently, of a worthy man and a great, an hundred mark or forty pound, with robes and fees of an hundred shilling term of life by year. Of lesser men forty pound or forty mark ask he without fees; and take he naught less than an hundred shillings. For never in my life took I less than an hundred shilling for cure of that sickness.

The best-known of Arderne's manuscripts concerns anal fistula. The manu-script, originally written in 1376, described a well-authenticated surgical opera-tion for a condition that most of his predecessors and peers considered incurable. Arderne placed his patient in the lithotomy position and then threaded a ligature through the fistulous opening into the rectum, which he tied tightly to prevent hemorrhage. He then incised the outer wall of the fistula and laid open the en-tire tract. If multiple sinuses were present, Arderne painstakingly incised them. He used sponges to stop hemorrhage and avoided all corrosive or irritating dressings during the postoperative period. Arderne also recognized the role of ischiorectal abscess as the cause of anal fistula:

> . . . when there occurs an abscess in or near the anus thou shalt know it by these signs; that is by swelling, aching, burning, itching and pricking. And the patient for aching and anguish may neither sit nor lie nor sleep . . . if his low bowel be consti-pated, it should be softened so that the hardness of the stool not bring anguish in doing egestion.
> . . . an abscess breeding near the anus should not be left to burst by itself, but the surgeon should busily feel with his finger the place of the abscess, and where so is found any softness, there, the patient not knowing, carefully, be it boldly opened

with a very sharp lancette, so that the pus and the corrupt blood may go out. Or else, forsooth, the gut or bowel that is called rectum, that leads to the anus will burst within the anus . . . Which case befalling, if it only bursts within it is hard to cure, and then there will be raggedies, forsooth, if it bursts both within and without, then it can never be cured except by a surgeon fully expert in his craft. For then may it from the first day be called a fistula. Some times it befalleth some men to have only one hole appearing outward piercing through the rectum within the anus by space of one inch or two . . . And I have seen some who have seven or nine holes on one sides of the buttocks, and six or five on the other side, none of which except one pierce the rectum.

Among Arderne's many interesting clinical observations was a differential diagnosis between cancer of the rectum and simple ulceration. More important, he warned against operating for rectal cancer and discussed the great difficulty of curing it.

Arderne was scientific and methodical, yet in the manner of his time was also fond of astrology and charms. He confidently prescribed treatments based on superstition to certain of his patients. For instance, he advised epileptics to write with their own blood on a piece of parchment the names of the three Wise Men, and to soothe the Wise Men's souls by reading three Pater Nosters and three Ave Marias daily for 3 months.

Although the development of surgery remains the most interesting aspect of medieval medicine, an important adjunct was the revival of interest in human anatomy. Medieval anatomical teaching can be divided into three major periods: the Salernitans (800-1200), who confined their understanding and studies to an-

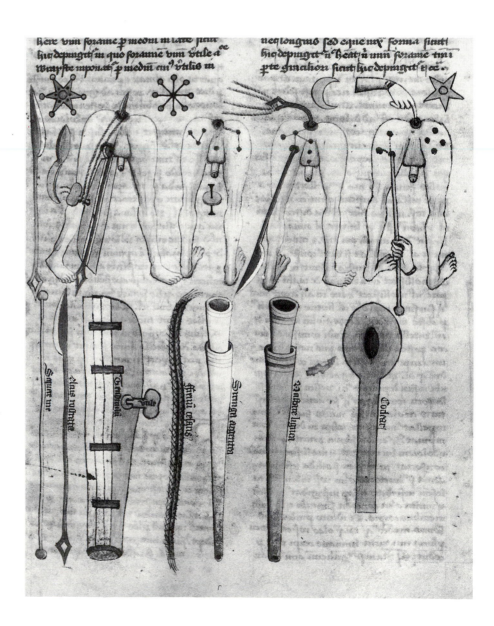

63. The first notable surgeon operating in England, John of Arderne became especially renowned for his operation for fistula-in-ano. Several illustrated medieval manuscripts of his text, which describes his operations for this and other colon-rectal complaints, have been preserved. This page from a fifteenth-century manuscript shows John's instruments and diagrams that explain how the instruments were used. *(By permission of the British Library, London, Additional MS29301, f 25.)*

112

imal dissections; the Islamic era (1300s), when anatomy lessons were obtained solely from ancient works such as Galen's; and the final period (from the fourteenth to the mid-fifteenth century), when there was a reawakening of interest in dissecting human cadavers.

The early, faltering steps toward the study of human anatomy were closely tied to the relative advancements occurring in medieval surgery. The foremost medieval dissector was Mondino de Luzzi (1275-1326), known as Mundinus. He was born in Bologna and received his university degree in medicine in 1290. He became professor of anatomy and surgery at his alma mater, although it appears that he was primarily a surgeon.

Most of the early interest in human anatomy was directed toward medicolegal purposes. Although understanding the human body was an important concept, the main social force that finally allowed dissection was the attempt to determine causes of death or to learn the nature of diseases, especially during epidemics.

64. A grisly but artistically beautiful portrayal of *The Executioner Skinning the Corrupt Judge Sisamnes* (circa 1500), painted for the courtroom of the town hall in Brügge, depicts a task undoubtedly conducted by barber-surgeons. The painting reflects a sophisticated knowledge of external human anatomy on the part of the artist, Gérard David (1450?-1523). *(Stad Brugge Stedelijke Musea.)*

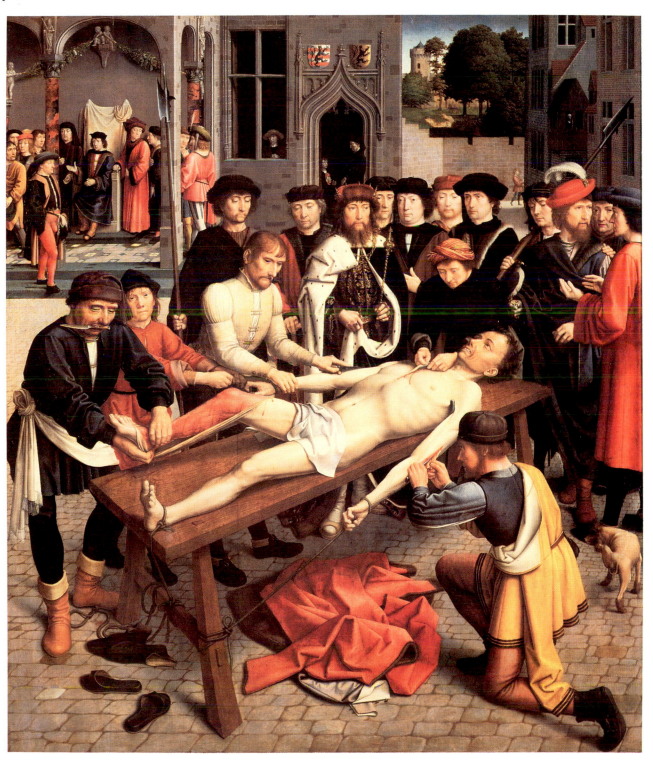

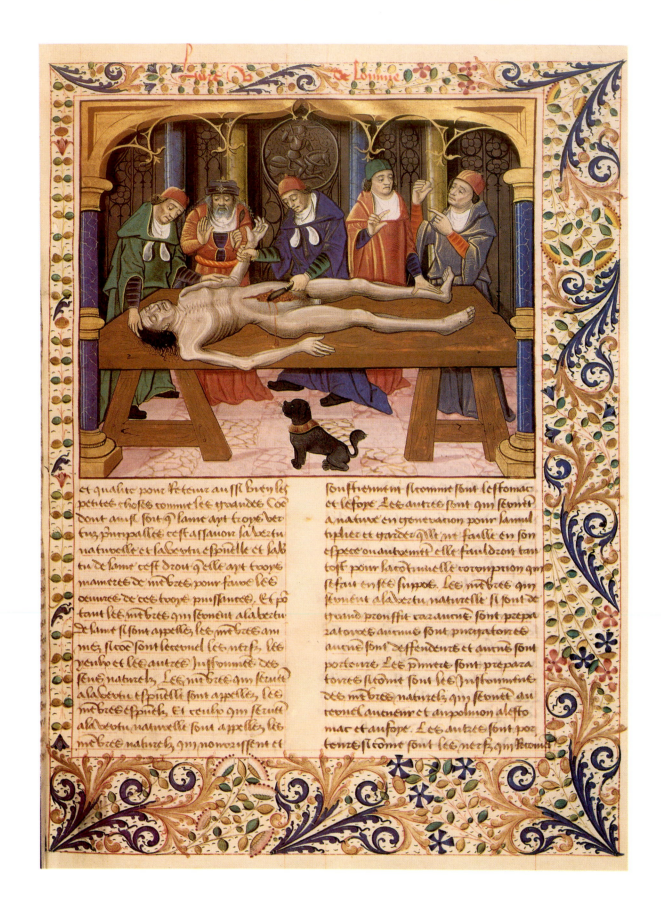

65. Anatomical dissection scene from an illuminated manuscript of the French translation of Bartholomaeus Anglicus's *De Proprietatibus Rerum.* Completed toward the end of the fifteenth century, the manuscript may have been copied from a woodcut in various previously printed editions. The well-behaved dog waits patiently for some guts to reach the floor. (*Phot. Bibliothèque Nationale, Paris, Mss, Fr 218, f 56.*)

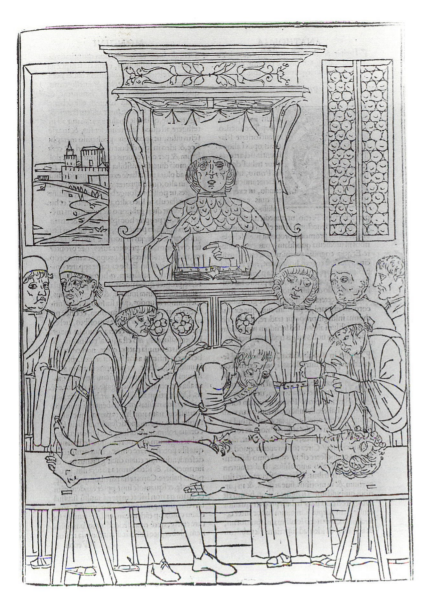

66. One of the most famous scenes of medieval medicine as it appeared in Johannes Ketham's (?-1491) *Fasciculus Medicinae* (1491). The professor lectures *ex cathedra* from the writings of Galen while a barber-surgeon demonstrates on the cadaver. The demonstration was intended to illustrate Galen's anatomical ideas, not to encourage careful observation. Not until professors began to undertake dissections personally did they begin to observe discrepancies between Galen's anatomical knowledge, based on dissections of apes, and actual human anatomy. The woodcut is by an unknown artist, perhaps from the school of Bellini. *(Jeremy Norman & Co., Inc.)*

Mundinus revolutionized the study of anatomy by personally and publicly performing human dissections. The cadavers were most often those of executed criminals. Mundinus's *Anathomia* was completed in 1316 and first printed in Padua in 1478. The work was more an instruction book in dissecting techniques than a study of gross anatomy. It served as the standard textbook of anatomy for two centuries and promulgated many of the mistakes of Galen. Included within the manual are descriptions of abdominal paracentesis, radical herniorrhaphy, and lithotomy. A detailed description is provided of the postmortem examination of two female cadavers to determine the relative size of the uterus in virgins and multiparous individuals.

After the printing press was invented, the *Anathomia* passed through 39 separate editions and translations. The work of Mundinus was continued by his pupil Niccolo Bertuccio, who was the mentor of Guy de Chauliac. By the mid-fourteenth century, the legality of public dissections was decreed at universities in Montpellier, Venice, Florence, Vienna, Bologna, Padua, Prague, Paris, and Tubingen. An anatomical theater was erected at Padua in 1445, and by the mid-fifteenth century the performance of four dissections annually was required of the Paris faculty.

The Middle Ages was a time of rediscovery in surgery. Initially restrained by general lack of surgical knowledge and skill, progress was further stifled by an outright ban on the performance of surgical operations by cleric-physicians, the only educated surgeons of the era. When both university surgeons and barber-surgeons began to perform surgery, progress resumed. This revival of surgical learning presaged the Renaissance, the Protestant Reformation, and the eventual maturation of modern surgical thought.

THE RENAISSANCE

	1450	1500	1550	1600	1650	1700

DAILY LIFE

Royal mail service in France **(1464)**
Syphilis epidemic spreads throughout Europe **(1495)**
Black-lead pencils **(1500)**
Beginnings of African slave trade **(1509)**
Coffee in Europe **(1517)**
Maritime insurance policies in Florence **(1523)**
Christmas tree at Strassburg Cathedral **(1539)**
Moscow destroyed by fire **(1547)**
Court jesters appear throughout Europe **(1549)**
Saint Andrews Golf Club, Scotland **(1552)**
Tobacco in Spain **(1555)**
Pont Neuf, oldest bridge in Paris **(1578)**
Earthquake in London **(1580)**
Life insurance policies in London **(1583)**
Forks at French court **(1589)**
Heels on shoes **(1595)**
Water closets installed in England **(1596)**

SCIENCE AND TECHNOLOGY

Christopher Columbus, Italian explorer **(1446-1506)**
Bartholomeu Dias, Portuguese explorer **(1450-1498)**
John Cabot, English explorer **(1450-1498)**
Vasco da Gama, Portuguese explorer **(1469-1524**)
Nicolaus Copernicus, Polish astronomer **(1473-1543)**
Ferdinand Magellan, Portuguese explorer **(1480-1521)**
Hernando Cortes, Spanish explorer **(1485-1547)**
Nostradamus, French astrologer **(1503-1566)**
Gerardus Mercator, Flemish geographer **(1512-1594)**
Ulissi Aldrovandi, Italian naturalist **(1522-1605)**
Walter Raleigh, English explorer, author, and courtier **(1554-1618**)
Galileo Galilei, Italian scientist **(1564-1642)**
Johannes Kepler, German astronomer **(1571-1630)**

RELIGION AND PHILOSOPHY

Desiderius Erasmus, Dutch humanist **(1466-1536)**
Niccolo Machiavelli, Italian author **(1469-1527)**
Thomas More, English humanist **(1478-1535)**
Spanish Inquisition against Jews **(1480)**
Ignatius Loyola, founder of Jesuit Order **(1491-1556)**
Francis Xavier, Spanish missionary **(1506-1552)**
First Catholic hymnal **(1537)**
Beginnings of Puritanism in England **(1560)**
Francis Bacon, English philosopher **(1561-1626)**
French Huguenots slain at Massacre of Vassy **(1562)**
John Cotton, American religious controversialist **(1584-1652)**
Thomas Hobbes, English philosopher **(1588-1679)**
René Descartes, French philosopher **(1596-1650)**

LITERATURE AND THEATER

William Tell, Swiss folk hero **(1467)**
Matteo Bandello, Italian novelist **(1485-1562)**
François Rabelais, French writer **(1494-1553)**
Everyman, English morality play **(1510)**
Miguel de Cervantes Saavedra, Spanish writer **(1547-1616)**
Edmund Spenser, English author **(1552-1599)**
William Shakespeare, English playwright **(1564-1616)**
Christopher Marlowe, English author **(1564-1593)**
John Donne, English poet **(1572-1631)**

MUSIC

Printed music **(1465)**
John Taverner, English composer **(1495-1545)**
Francesco di Bernardo Corteccia, Italian organist **(1504-1571)**
Giovanni Pierluigi da Palestrina, Italian composer **(1525-1594)**
Bartolommeo Spontone, Italian madrigal composer **(1529-1586)**
Andrea Amati, Italian violin maker **(1530-1578)**
Thomas Morley, English composer **(1557-1603)**
Claudio Monteverdi, Italian composer **(1567-1643)**
John Wilson, English singer and composer **(1595-1674)**

THE RENAISSANCE

1450	1500	1550	1600	1650	1700

VISUAL ARTS

Sandro Botticelli, Italian painter **(1444–1510)**

Hieronymus Bosch, Dutch painter **(1450–1516)**

Leonardo da Vinci, Italian artist **(1452–1519)**

Matthias Grünewald, German painter **(1465–1528)**

Hans Holbein the Elder, German painter **(1465–1524)**

Albrecht Durer, German artist **(1471–1528)**

Lucas Cranach the Elder, German painter **(1472–1553)**

Michelangelo Buonarroti, Italian sculptor **(1475–1564)**

Titian, Italian artist **(1477–1576)**

Raphael, Italian painter **(1483–1520)**

Benvenuto Cellini, Florentine sculptor **(1500–1571)**

Giorgio Vasari, Italian art historian **(1512–1571)**

Juan de Herrera, Spanish architect **(1530–1597)**

El Greco, Spanish-Greek painter **(1541–1614)**

Pieter Brueghel the Younger, Flemish painter **(1564–1638)**

Caravaggio, Italian painter **(1573–1610)**

Peter Paul Rubens, Flemish painter **(1577–1640)**

Frans Hals, Dutch painter **(1580–1666)**

Nicolas Poussin, French painter **(1593–1665)**

Giovanni Bernini, Italian sculptor **(1598–1680)**

Anthony Van Dyck, Dutch painter **(1599–1641)**

Diego Velazquez, Spanish painter **(1599–1660)**

MEDICINE AND SURGERY

Heinrich von Pfolspeundt, German **(fifteenth century)**

Niccolo Leoniceno, Italian **(1428–1524)**

Antonio Benivieni, Italian **(1443–1502)**

Hieronymus Brunschwig, German **(1450–1512)**

Thomas Linacre, English **(1460–1524)**

Giovanni de Vigo, Italian **(1460–1525)**

Jacopo Berengario da Carpi, Italian **(1470–1550)**

Symphorien Champier, French **(1472–1539)**

Hans von Gersdorff, German **(1480–1540)**

Girolamo Fracastoro, Italian **(1484–1553)**

Marianus Barolitanus, Italian **(1490–1550)**

Francisco Arceo, Spanish **(1493–1573)**

Paracelsus, Swiss **(1493–1541)**

Jean Canappe, French **(1495–1552)**

Thomas Vicary, English **(1495–1561)**

Michael Blondus, Italian **(1497–1565)**

William Bullein, English **(?–1576)**

Laurent Colot, French **(early sixteenth century)**

Caspar Stromayr, German **(sixteenth century)**

Walter Ryff, German **(mid-sixteenth century)**

Pierre Franco, French **(1500–1561)**

Dionisio Daza Chacon, Spanish **(1503–1580)**

Jean Fernel, French **(1506–1588)**

Thomas Gale, English **(1507–1587)**

Guido Guidi, Italian **(1508–1569)**

Ambroise Paré, French **(1510–1590)**

Jacques Dalechamps, French **(1513–1588)**

Giovanni Della Croce, Italian **(1514–1575)**

Andreas Vesalius, Italian **(1514–1564)**

Conrad Gesner, Swiss **(1516–1565)**

Bartholomaeus Maggius, Italian **(1516–1552)**

Felix Wurtz, German **(1518–1574)**

Bartolomeo Eustachi, Italian **(1520–1574)**

Gabriele Falloppio, Italian **(1523–1562)**

Bartolome Hidalgo De Aguero, Spanish **(1531–1597)**

Hieronymus Fabricius Aquapendente, Italian **(1533–1620)**

John Banister, English **(1533–1610)**

George Bartisch, German **(1535–1606)**

Carcano Leone, Italian **(1536–1606)**

William Clowes, English **(1540–1604)**

Gaspare Tagliacozzi, Italian **(1547–1599)**

Jacques Guillemeau, French **(1550–1613)**

Peter Lowe, Scottish **(1550–1612)**

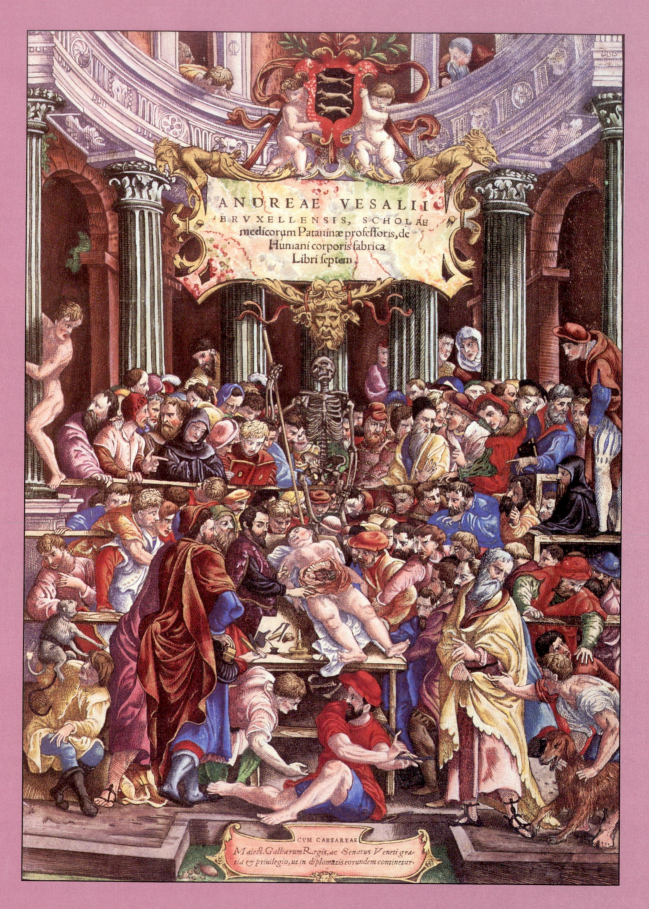

ANDREAE VESALII
BRVXELLENSIS, SCHOLAE
medicorum Patauinæ profeſſoris, de
Humani corporis fabrica
Libri ſeptem

CVM CAESAREAE
Maieſt. Galliarumq́ Regis, ac Senatus Veneti gra-
tia & priuilegio, ut in diplomatis eorundem continetur.

CHAPTER 8

THE RENAISSANCE

he European Renaissance, the great revival of learning, arts, and humanities and the growth of scientific thought that occurred from the late fourteenth to the sixteenth century, began in northern Italy, spread gradually to other countries, and marked the transition from the medieval world to modern civilization.

By the middle of the 1500s three major events had occured that predisposed European society to this rebirth of intellectualism: the invention of gunpowder, the discovery of paper and the printing press, and the voyages of discovery that revealed new worlds. These occurrences were preceded by an influx of Byzantine scholars who fled to the West after the capture of Constantinople by the Turks (1453). Most of these academicians settled in northern Italy and brought with them knowledge of the ideas of Plato and Hippocrates. These ideas in turn did much to reduce the excessive influence of the Galenists, who clung to beliefs not based on facts or scientific observation and stubbornly ignored new techniques and medications.

Gunpowder, the oldest explosive, was known to the ancient Chinese, the Arabs, and the people of India before it was introduced into Europe. In 1242 Roger Bacon (1214-1294) authored a manuscript that provided instruction on how to make it. Within a century gunpowder was being used in both cannons and blunderbusses. Such firearms made the foot soldier a more effective fighting force and equalized combatants, since a peasant could use a gun as effectively as a knight could. The knight and his armor rapidly became obsolete because the armor provided little in the way of protection from firearms. Indeed, as more deadly warfare came into existence, feudalism ceased to exist.

The discovery of paper as an inexpensive substitute for vellum or parchment contributed to the spread of Renaissance knowledge. Understandably, if a satisfactory method of manufacturing paper had not been available, it is unlikely that the invention of the printing press would have been so influential an event. It is known that the Chinese had used wood-block printing on a rudimentary form of paper as early as the eighth century. However, printing from these tediously engraved wooden blocks did not supplant the laborious method of copying manuscripts by hand because the engraving of these blocks was in itself a labor-intensive process.

There is no certainty as to the actual date of the European invention of movable type or the name of the inventor. Johannes Gutenberg (1398-1468) of Mainz is generally regarded as the strongest claimant to the honor. Gutenberg standardized the matrix size of type; his type was cast in lead from brass matrices. Gutenberg combined his movable type with two other important developments: the use of a printing press and the employment of a viscous ink that was needed to print on paper from metal surfaces.

The technique of printing had spread from Germany to Italy by the late 1460s and during the next decade appeared in every other European country.

67. *Facing page,* Vesalius personally demonstrating anatomy on the cadaver. Hand-colored woodcut frontispiece from the dedication copy of *De Humani Corporis Fabrica Libri Septem* (1543), which was presented to Vesalius's patron, Emperor Charles V. Vesalius wished to emphasize that to truly learn human anatomy, the physician must personally perform dissection. This revolutionary teaching of Vesalius was contrary to the medieval tradition, in which the physician read from Galen while his factotum did the dissecting, as exemplified in Ketham. This is the only authentically hand-colored copy of the famous woodcut. *(From the Library of Haskell F. Norman, MD.)*

68. Operations for inoperable conditions, hysterical symptoms, and nonexistent diseases have always been the province of quacks. In the sixteenth century it was widely believed that a stone in the brain caused the disturbance of reason in madmen. A quack surgeon, toward the end of his "operation," would exhibit a stone supposedly removed from the patient's skull. *Extraction of the Stone of Madness* (1557), an engraving by the Dutch painter and printmaker Pieter Brueghel the Elder (1520-1569), satirizes the surgical quackery of Brueghel's day.

Books were much cheaper than manuscripts and allowed texts to be transmitted more easily, with fewer errors. The demand for printed books was unrelenting, and because printed books were affordable, virtually every Renaissance physician and surgeon was able to purchase the medical treatises issued from these numerous presses.

With the invention of the pivot compass (circa 1400) mariners were able to steer without reference to landmarks or the stars, so great voyages of discovery and exploration were more easily undertaken. These voyages greatly increased European society's appreciation and understanding of the surrounding world.

Because of the major societal changes just described, Renaissance society began to hold a worldly rather than a religious point of view in the areas of art, literature, science, and government. A new attitude called humanism became apparent. Humans, not God, became the center of reference. There was a gradual transference of wealth and its attendant political power from the Christian church to various princes. These men took a new interest in learning and the arts, and a new age of classicism developed. The intensive study of the Greek and Roman classics was a natural consequence of this humanistic philosophy. The all-pervasive religious character of medieval education and governance had become untenable.

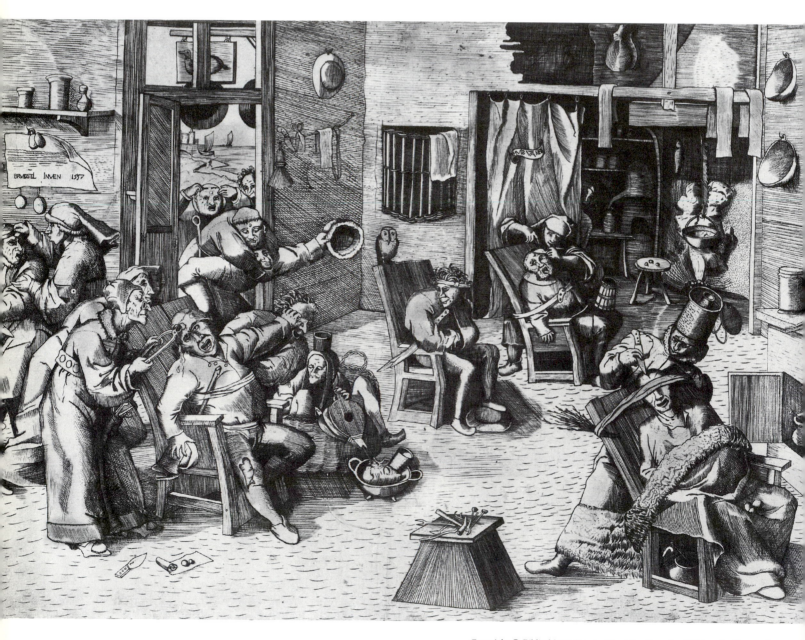

69. *The Surgeon.* Engraving (1524) by the Dutch printmaker, painter, and draftsman Lucas van Leyden (1494–1533). It has been suggested that this engraving is a subtle indictment of the barber-surgeon. He is shown wearing elegant attire, whereas his patient is portrayed as a poor country bumpkin. In the artistic language of the day the large, heavy purse below the surgeon's right arm signaled an undue preoccupation with money. *(Philadelphia Museum of Art: SmithKline Beecham Corporation Fund.)*

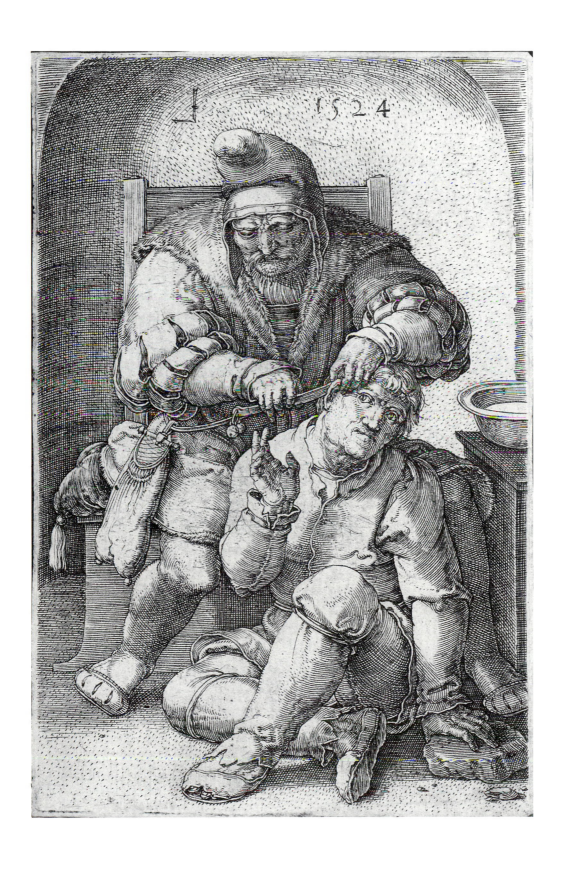

The dominant societal event of the sixteenth century in western Europe was a religious movement known as the Reformation, which resulted in the establishment of Protestantism. However, the Reformation was more than a religious struggle. It was part of the broad stream of societal change. Led by Martin Luther (1483-1546), who in 1517 nailed his *Ninety-five Theses* to the door of All Saints' Church in Wittenberg, Germany, numerous Protestant churches established themselves in England, Germany, Scandinavia, Scotland, and Switzerland. European civilization paid a great price for the Protestant victory: civil and international warfare ensued. Religious tolerance and individualism grew, but at the price of political and social disunity. The Counter-Reformation took place between 1560 and 1648. During that time the Catholic church reformed abuses within its own organization and tried to suppress Protestantism.

By the 1500s a coalescence of socioeconomic and political conditions in northern Italy, centered in towns like Bologna, Ferrara, Florence, Padua, and Pavia, brought about an inevitable burst of intellectual, educational, and creative activity. This revival of cultural learning was heightened by the appearance of many individuals with superlative credentials in the field of medicine. The medical humanists of the fifteenth and sixteenth centuries did much to further the ideals of Renaissance medicine. In conjunction with their contemporaries in astronomy, chemistry, mathematics, philosophy, physics, and zoology, as well as those in architecture, dancing, education, literature, music, painting, and sculpture, a rebirth, or renaissance, was brought to pass.

Most of the early medical humanists studied in northern Italy. Although not considered surgeons, their "opening up" of the study of medicine was to have enormous impact on the evolution of surgery. The most prominent of these early humanists was Niccolo Leoniceno (1428-1524), an amazingly erudite individual. He taught medicine at the universities of Bologna, Ferrara, and Padua.

70. This anonymous sixteenth-century engraving caricatures both barber-surgeons and their clients as monkeys. The barber-surgeons are shown performing the wide range of services the guild offered at this time: tooth pulling, haircutting, bloodletting, and wound treatment. *(Phot. Bibliothèque Nationale Paris, Ms RF 1 rés, f 66.)*

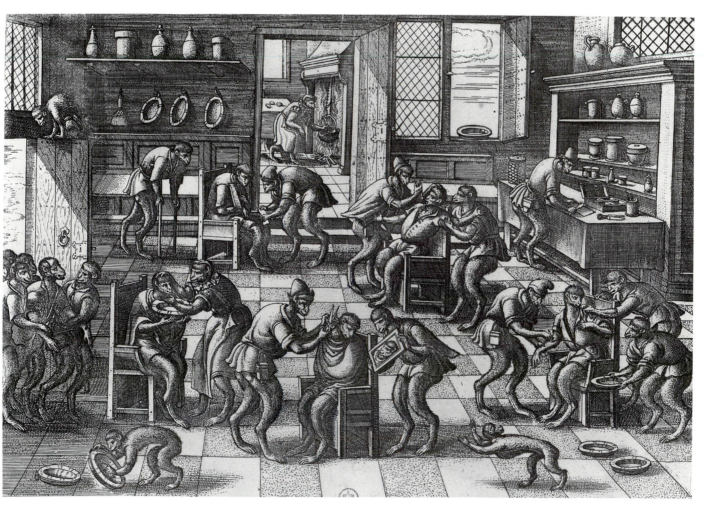

Considered one of the Renaissance's premier Latinists, Leoniceno translated the *Aphorisms* of Hippocrates and many works of Galen. Leoniceno's most important achievement concerned the correction of numerous botanical errors found in Pliny's *Natural History,* a work compiled without resort to actual examination of natural phenomena. Leoniceno refused to follow the scholastic traditions of his day and asserted that Pliny was fallible in many of his comments. This heretical viewpoint threatened many of Leoniceno's peers and led to a passionate storm of controversy. Even as his friends deserted him, Leoniceno remained adamant in his debunking of Pliny's assertions. In this regard Leoniceno set the stage for later botanist-commentators, without whom a scientifically based materia medica could never have evolved.

Thomas Linacre (1460-1524), educated in Padua and Oxford, was the personal physician to Henry VII (1457-1509) and Henry VIII (1491-1547). Linacre is best remembered for his works on grammar and his lectures on medicine at Oxford and Cambridge. Among his most influential texts were the Latin translations of Galen's treatises on hygiene, therapeutics, temperaments, natural faculties, pulse, and semeiology. These exacting translations were widely read and demonstrated to average physicians that much of their previously acquired knowledge was based on poorly translated secondhand versions of their favorite author.

Among the earliest of the French humanists was Symphorien Champier (1472-1539). Born in Lyon, he was a medical graduate of Pavia and became physician to Charles VIII (1470-1498) and Louis XII (1462-1515). Champier wrote one of the earliest and most detailed histories of medicine (1508), a widely disseminated medical dictionary, and a lengthy biography of Arnald of Villanova.

Girolamo Fracastoro (1484-1553) of Verona was physician, poet, physicist, geologist, astronomer, and pathologist. The true embodiment of the Renaissance man, he gained fame on authoring the most celebrated of medical poems, "Syphilis Sive Morbus Gallicus" (1530). In this Latin poem, which was heavily influenced by the Roman poet Ovid (43 B.C.–A.D. 17), Fracastoro provided the appellation "French disease" for syphilis. The poem recognized the venereal cause of the disease and reviewed the current knowledge of the condition and its treatment. His later treatise, *De Contagione* (1546), was a precursor of the modern theory of infection caused by invisible microorganisms.

One of the greatest medical innovators of all time, certainly among the most "bombastic," was Aureolus Theophrastus Bombastus von Hohenheim (1493-1541), generally known as Paracelsus. (It is said that Paracelsus chose his nom de plume to indicate superiority to Celsus and that the names Aureolus and Bombastus were also personal additions.) He was born at Einsiedeln near Zurich; little biographical information is available concerning his early years, and whether he truly obtained a doctor's degree in the university at Ferrara remains uncertain. However, Paracelsus did use the title of doctor as often as possible and remains one of the few physician-authors who truly advanced medicine by quarreling about its current condition.

Often portrayed as an ignorant itinerant quack, Paracelsus had an unusual knowledge of alchemy, astrology, and other occult sciences, which he had obtained from the abbots and bishops of the European countryside. He had obtained an impressive working knowledge of chemistry at the mines in western Austria and in Tyrolean laboratories. Paracelsus was an independent sort and traveled all over Europe. During his years of wanderlust, collecting information from every source, he learned a great deal about medical practice, including folk medicine. He considered himself a commoner and, like few physicians before him, became quite popular.

Paracelsus taught briefly in Freiburg and Strassburg (1525) and was shortly thereafter (1527) appointed professor of medicine and city physician in Basel. In his usual confrontational style Paracelsus began his academic career by declaring that reform was necessary relative to the works of Galen and Avicenna. Imbued with a lifelong reverence for Hippocrates, Paracelsus burned what he considered inferior works of Galen and Avicenna in a public bonfire. These actions, in addition to his lecturing in colloquial German instead of Latin, resulted in his dismissal after 18 months.

Having lost his academic post, Paracelsus resumed his itinerant life, drifting from city to city, always writing. At times he was absolutely penniless and ardent supporters were few. After practicing medicine in all the Germanic-speaking countries, he died of cancer or perhaps, according to a more glamorous myth, of a wound sustained in a tavern brawl in Salzburg. He is buried there, in the north portal of St. Sebastian's Church.

Paracelsus's teachings were a strange mixture of conceit, showmanship, senseless bombast, mysticism, astrology, and sound medical advice. He contributed to pharmacology and therapeutics, and the Paracelsian method (the use of chemical agents only in the treatment of disease) remains well known if little understood.

Paracelsus was deeply concerned about the stagnation that characterized medical thought and education. Paracelsus denounced many medical and surgical practices and subjected many ancient writers and their followers to antagonistic criticism.

The personality of Paracelsus and his contentious streak have been subjects of historical consideration from the time of his death. He was undoubtedly a vain, boastful individual. Arrogance and an intemperate demeanor did not aid his quest for legitimacy. The argumentative essence of his personality reveals, however, that he was a dedicated individual who attempted to remain true to his own principles and thought processes. Paracelsus exposed error and stirred up discussion: these are his enduring achievements. Although his individual contributions to surgery and medicine may not be of singular importance, his larger role as a reformer of medical thought remains most prominent.

The writings of Paracelsus covered all the medicine of his day. He attacked witchcraft and superstition and introduced a form of chemical therapeutics, a system based in rational chemistry with a liberal mixing of astrology and cosmology. Paracelsus discarded Galenism and the Greek humors. Physicians were taught to recognize that three basic substances, sulfur, mercury, and salt, formed the necessary ingredients of all bodies, organic and inorganic. Among other contributions to chemistry, he discovered zinc and various compounds of mercury, including calomel, and demonstrated the iron content in water. Paracelsus introduced the term *laudanum* in medicine and recognized laudanum's opioid properties.

Paracelsus bitterly deplored the separation of surgery from medicine and through his teachings attempted to bring the two disciplines together. He is known to have practiced both equally and to have signed himself "beyder Artzney Doctorn," that is, doctor in both medicines. Paracelsus probably belonged to the craft of wound surgeons and did not involve himself with operative surgery. This assumption is reasonable, since the only one of his books printed during his lifetime was a treatise on wound management, *Grosse Wundartznei* (1536).

Paracelsus's observations on wounds were remarkably incisive: deep wounds of the lungs, liver, and spleen and gunshot injuries of the head were not considered dangerous if the hemorrhage could be controlled; if control was not possible, secondary infection would prove fatal. Paracelsus described how even a small, at first insignificant injury could become serious and lead to tetanus. He strongly believed that healing was properly accomplished by nature and that interference by the surgeon could only cause serious problems. Nature healed by means of a "natural balm," according to Paracelsus, and forced suppuration was ultimately bad for the patient; all a surgeon need do was supply adequate nutrition and keep the wound clean to prevent complications. Paracelsus was blunt in stating that how to clean and detoxify wounds was not taught in the universities but could be adequately learned from nonmedical sources. The early closure of the wound was clearly indicated, although the use of sutures for this purpose was deplored.

71. *Facing page,* Aureolus Theophrastus Bombastus von Hohenheim, generally known as Paracelsus, by Quentin Metsys (1466?-1530), the Belgian painter of portraits and historical scenes. Paracelsus, most often remembered today for his contributions to iatrochemistry, now known as pharmacology, also practiced wound surgery. *(Louvre, Paris.)*

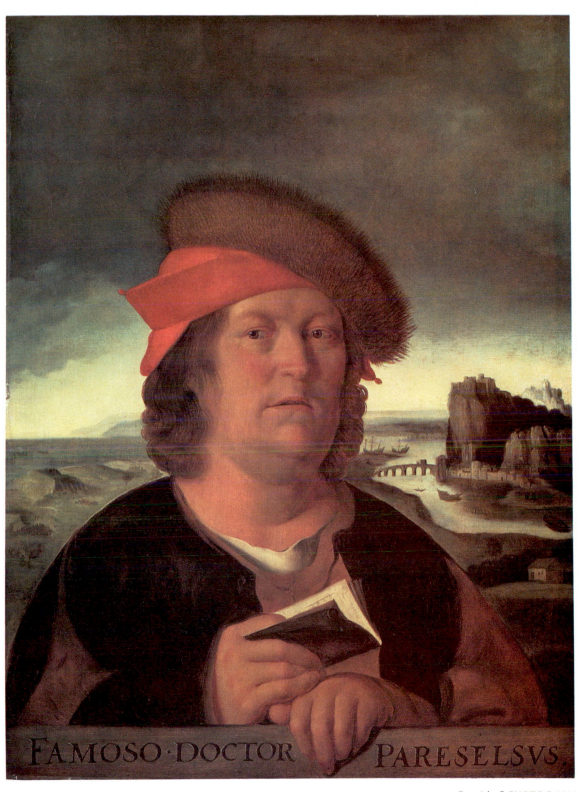

FAMOSO·DOCTOR PARESELSVS

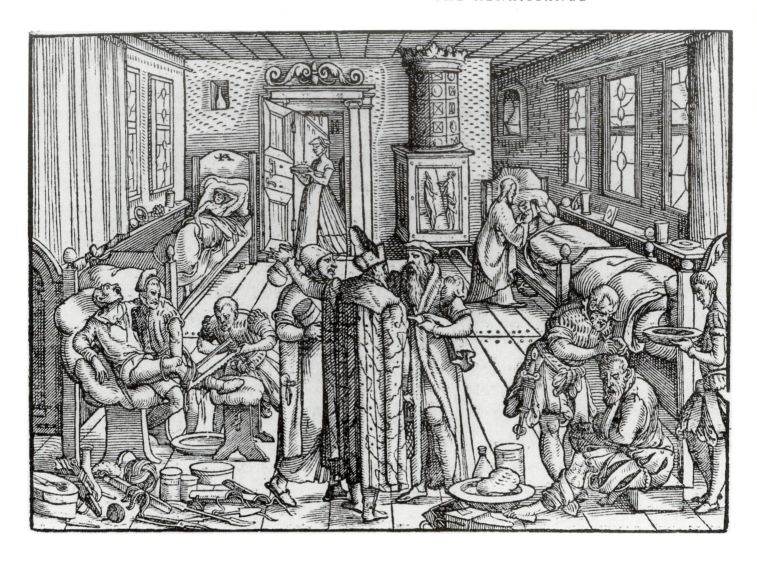

72. Woodcut showing the interior of a six-teenth-century hospital, from the title page of Paracelsus's *Opus Chirurgicum* (1565). *Foreground,* One surgeon performs an amputation, *left,* while another dresses a head wound, *right. Background,* A nurse tends to a patient, *left; right,* a patient prays to Jesus Christ. In the center foreground three physicians, one holding a urine flask, are in consultation. *(National Library of Medicine, Bethesda, Md.)*

In the *Grosse Wundartznei* Paracelsus began with a discussion of surgery be-cause he considered it the "most certain part" of medicine. He strongly rebuked those who split the two disciplines:

It is my desire to rid medicine of its most glaring errors and to teach, not according to the rules of the ancients, but on those principles which derive from the nature of things and which I have reached through my own reflections . . .

I should like to lecture to you on surgery, but first, you must understand certain things concerning medicine as a whole and the practice of surgery in particular . . . Internal medicine and surgery are based on philosophy and must not be separated except in practice; every physician must be a doctor of both medicines . . . You will not find everything written in the books of Galen and Avicenna, all of surgery has not been written, for new times bring new diseases and new books will outmode the old.

The basis of medicine is love, and not everyone can be a physician. Every surgeon should have three qualities, first as regards his own person; second, as regards the pa-tient, and, third, as regards his art. As regards his own person, the surgeon should not think he knows everything or is competent to handle all things. Not the outlay of money, nor the attendance at school, nor the reading of books will make a surgeon . . . you must learn daily from your own experience and from the experiences of others, for no matter how experienced or wise you may be, the time comes when your knowledge fails you and the patient suffers . . .

You should know the make-up of man, where the bones and other structures lie and their relation to each other . . . It is not enough that you know the externals, you must know the internals better than the externals . . .

Finally, the surgeon should know and recognize all plants and in what way they may be used, which cure, which cleanse, which act rapidly and which act slowly . . .

You should know what it is which heals a wound because without this knowledge you cannot use any medicine correctly. You should know that it is the nature of flesh, of the body, of the blood vessels, of the limbs to have within themselves an inborn balsam that heals all wounds . . . Every surgeon therefore should know that it is not he who heals the wound but the balsam in the part that heals it. If he thinks he heals it, he fools himself, and does not know his art . . . If a wound is open and unprotected, it is evident that it cannot heal. The good surgeon affords this protection by suitable dressings . . . only nature has the growing and developmental powers which make the body whole. Through food and drink this strength is preserved . . .

There are many learned men in Germany who could further medical knowledge but they are so taken up with their useless labors and with poring over old books that they cannot be made to know that the real basis of medicine is, "love thy neighbor . . ."

Medicine has become a field for the dishonest to plow, the nobleman and the merchant have much money, therefore they are cultivated. Not just the apostates, but other light-fingered folk have taken to medicine, the hangmen, poachers and others without honor . . .

Jean Fernel (1506-1588) was the leading French physician-humanist of the late Renaissance. Born in Clermont, he graduated from the University of Paris (1530). Like most of the humanists, Fernel was well trained in mathematics, philosophy, and astronomy. Much of his time was spent reluctantly serving as physician to the royal family, notably Henry II (1519-1559), his wife Catherine de Medici (1519-1589), and their sons, Francis II (1544-1560), Charles IX (1550-1574), and Henry III (1551-1589). Fernel's leading work was his *Medicina* (1554), in which he divided the study of medicine into the disciplines of physiology, pathology, and therapeutics. Many of Galen's errors in anatomy and physiology were corrected by Fernel, who also opposed intensive bloodletting.

The unfettered flowering of surgery during the Renaissance was directly related to fundamental changes in the study of human anatomy. By the end of the Middle Ages it had become apparent to physicians that further progress in the knowledge of medicine, specifically surgery, would not be attained unless scientific studies of human anatomy were made. By that time the Church's ban on human vivisection was showing some weakness. Popes Sixtus IV (1414-1484) and Clement VII (1478-1534) approved the right to study the human body. Accordingly, by the early sixteenth century there were no further major hindrances to either dissection or autopsy.

In spite of innovations in anatomy and pathology, traditional forces in surgery impeded its advance. Among these hindrances was the common custom among surgeons of keeping secret the techniques of certain operative procedures. Most commonly techniques were kept secret for surgical operations such as incision for stone in the bladder, the cure of hernia, and the treatment of cataracts. Such proprietary information was literally treated as private property, only to be handed down from father to son or sold for large sums of money to certain surgeons who swore not to reveal the details to others. It is believed that certain prominent Renaissance surgeons were obliged to pay extraordinary amounts of money to receive such privileged information.

After the work of Mundinus, a number of treatises and engraved plates containing the first crude attempts at pictorial representation of dissected parts began to appear. Not unexpectedly, these rudimentary illustrations, known as "graphic incunabula," for the most part were not based on original observation or dissection, since anatomy was still judged as a mere adjunct to surgery unworthy of consideration as a distinct discipline. Because surgery remained relatively crude and principally demanded a knowledge of the appropriate sites for bloodletting, there would have been no reason for anatomic drawings to be practical or realistic. Schematic and highly fantasized figures were adequate for the times.

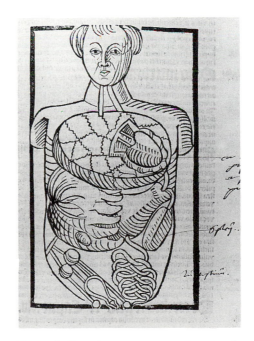

73. Early Renaissance attempts at anatomical representation were crude and highly simplified. This schematic woodcut from Magnus Hundt's (1449-1519) *Antropologium De Ho[omin]is Dignitate . . .* (1501), was the most complete published representation of the viscera up to that time. *(Jeremy Norman & Co., Inc.)*

127

74. The fetus in utero by Leonardo da Vinci, from anatomical drawings preserved at Windsor Castle in England. Although da Vinci's artistic masterpieces were anatomically advanced for his time, the anatomical drawings also reflect the limitations of his knowledge. In this case he had no knowledge of the coverings of the human fetus, and in the text on this page he also denied the presence of the fetal heartbeat. Reproduced from Leonardo da Vinci, *Quaderni D'Anatomia III* (1913). *(Jeremy Norman & Co., Inc.)*

Among the individuals who performed the most exacting human dissections were the artists of the early Renaissance. They demonstrated an increasing interest in the configuration of the body, and many studied anatomy to improve the accuracy of their drawings. In northern Italy the study of human anatomy was part of every young artist's apprenticeship. Surprisingly, these studies by artists, who were interested solely in form and function, had little noticeable effect on the progress of medical science.

The first artist known to have dissected a human body to further his artistic efforts was Donatello (1386-1486), but it was Leonardo da Vinci (1452-1519) who founded iconographic and physiologic anatomy. He admitted to performing more than 100 human dissections; among the works he left to posterity are

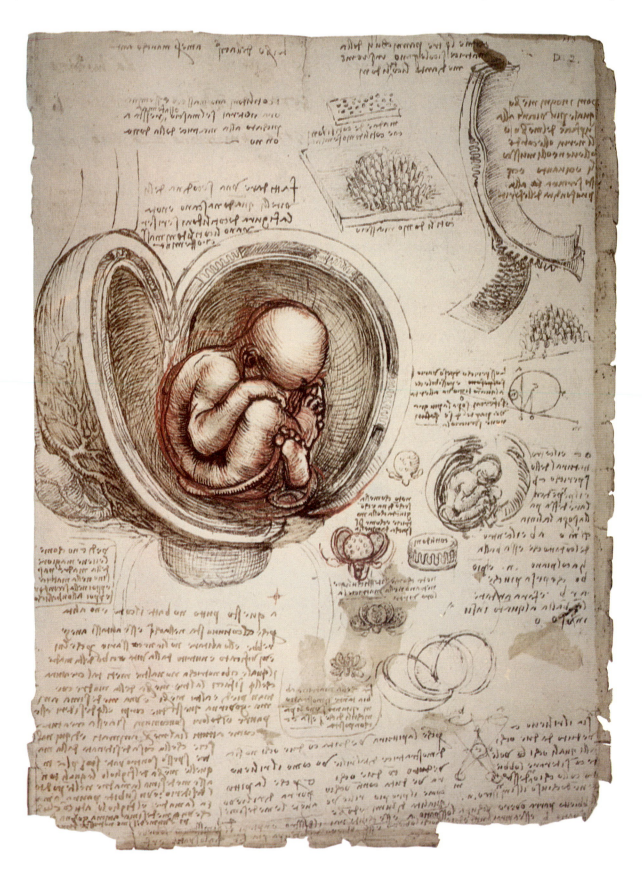

779 anatomical drawings and sketches. These illustrations, usually made beside the dissected subject, reveal an exacting acquaintance with muscular anatomy. Among the extant drawings are those representing the skeletal, pulmonary, nervous, and vascular systems, as well as detailed sketches of the cervical, thoracic, abdominal, and femoral blood vessels, deep dissections of the viscera, and cross-sections of the brain. The studies were often accompanied by annotations on physiology.

In most respects the accuracy of pictorial representation was much greater for artists than for anatomists. Da Vinci's renderings were so faithful to the dissections that anatomical nomenclature had not yet been established to guide him in naming structures. His notations of the origin and insertions of muscles, for instance, were hindered by the unavailability of proper names. Da Vinci correctly assessed the curvature of the spine, depicted the true position of the fetus in utero, and originated cross-sectional anatomy.

Among the other significant anatomical works by artists of the early Renaissance were those of Albrecht Durer (1471-1528) and Michelangelo Buonarroti (1475-1564). Durer's treatise on human proportion, *Vier Bücher Von Menschlicher Proportion* (1528), was published after his death. Written, designed, and illustrated by Durer, the work is notable for its extraordinary series of anthropometrical woodcuts. His text was the first attempt to apply anthropometry to aesthetics, and the woodcuts represent the first endeavor to employ cross-hatching to depict shades and shadows in wood engraving. Michelangelo is said to have spent more than a decade in academic pursuit of anatomical knowledge through the personal performance of dissections.

As detailed as the artists of the Renaissance were in the depiction of the human form, they were not professional anatomists. Accordingly, true scientific advances did not occur until anatomists began working with artists in collaborative publishing efforts. This transition from schematic medieval manuscript illustrations to the realistic and reproducible drawings of the Renaissance had an enormous impact on the history of surgery.

The first important modern treatise on human anatomy was authored by Gabriel Zerbi (1468-1505) of Verona, who held the chair of medicine, logic, and philosophy at the University of Padua. Zerbi's *Liber Anathomie Corporis Humani Et Singulorum Membrorum Illius* was published in Venice (1502). In this unillustrated treatise he first classified the organs into systems, described the anatomy of an infant, and detailed the gastric musculature. Alessandro Benedetti (1460-1525), Zerbi's successor at the University of Padua, founded its renowned anatomical theater (1490) and authored an *Anatomia* 7 years later. Marc Antonio Della Torre (1473-1506) taught at Padua and planned to publish a treatise on anatomy. He secured the assistance of Da Vinci to make life-sized drawings of the parts that Della Torre had tediously dissected. Although many of these illustrations were supposedly completed, Della Torre died unexpectedly, the project was never finished, and the drawings for it were presumed lost.

The first surgeon-anatomist to prepare anatomical illustrations made consistently from observations of nature was Jacopo Berengario da Carpi (1470-1550). He included Benvenuto Cellini (1500-1571) among his patients and was considered one of the most prominent physicians of his era. Berengario's eminence as an anatomist rested on early descriptions of the sphenoidal sinuses, pineal gland, auditory ossicles, and arytenoid cartilages. His numerous anatomical works (1514, 1521, and 1523) were prized for their superb illustrations. Berengario's operative skills were evident in his twice performing a rudimentary vaginal hysterectomy for prolapse of the uterus.

Although some anatomists were moving away from the teachings of Galen, others remained devoted to his ideals. Jacques Dubois (1478-1555), known as Jacob Sylvius, taught anatomy in Paris. Sylvius is best remembered for being the first to inject blood vessels with a material rendering them more visible, hence more dissectable. The Sylvian aqueduct and venous valves are mentioned in his *Isagoge* (1556). Despite his bigoted, pecuniary, and harsh personality, Sylvius attracted a large following; Andreas Vesalius was his most prominent student.

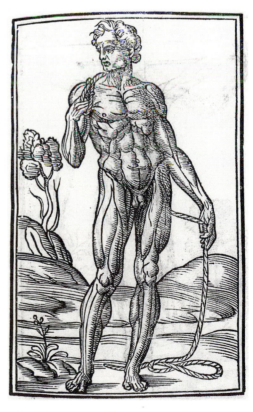

75. Berengario da Carpi was the first anatomist to publish illustrated treatises on anatomy based on his own dissections. This "muscle man" from da Carpi's *Commentaria Cu[m] Ampliissimis Additionibus Super Anatomia Mu[n]dini* (1521) is shown performing a specific action in front of a landscape background. *(Jeremy Norman & Co., Inc.)*

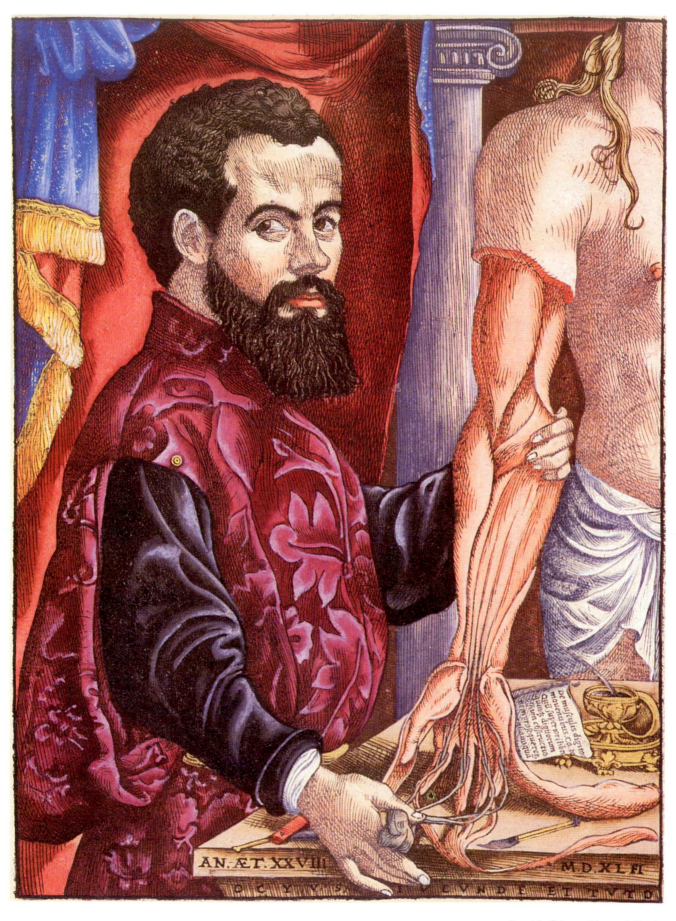

130

Few individuals have had an influence on the history of surgery as overwhelming as that of Andreas Vesalius (1514-1564). He was born in Brussels on New Year's Eve to a German family originally from Wessels on the Rhine. Four generations of his physician and apothecary forebears had extensive connections to the House of Burgundy and to the Holy Roman Emperor's court, especially that of Charles V (1500-1558).

Vesalius received his initial education in Louvain, where he underwent a thorough training in Latin, Greek, and Arabic. At 18 years of age he began the study of medicine at Montpellier and continued it in Paris. In Paris Vesalius came under the influence of Sylvius. A complex relationship evolved between them and culminated with Sylvius disparaging Vesalius and his many accomplishments.

After spending 3 years in Paris, Vesalius was directly affected by the outbreak of war between France and the Holy Roman Empire. Because he was a Roman subject, he was forced to return to Brussels. By the time he returned to Paris, Vesalius had become deeply devoted to the study of human anatomy and quite proficient in human vivisection. He eventually began to lecture in anatomy at Louvain and served as a military surgeon attached to the army of Charles V. In 1537 Vesalius accepted the Venetian senate's appointment as professor of anatomy and public prosector at the University of Padua.

Vesalius remained in Padua until 1544, when he resigned his post to become court physician to Charles V. After the emperor's abdication (1555), Vesalius continued in a similar position with Charles's successor, Philip II (1527-1598). Philip eventually moved Vesalius to Madrid, but for sundry reasons, including supposed trouble with the Inquisition, his discontent with his clinical work grew, and he planned to return to academic pursuits. In 1563 Vesalius set out on a year-long pilgrimage to Jerusalem. On his return voyage he received word of an invitation to resume his professorship at Padua, which had been vacated after the death of Gabriele Falloppio (in Latin, Fallopius) (1523-1562), but Vesalius's ship was wrecked and he landed on the tiny Peloponnesian island of Zante. There Vesalius was left to suffer a solitary death resulting from starvation and exposure.

Vesalius was a practicing surgeon and a widely recognized anatomist. In 1562 he clearly described the operation for empyema. It is related that in July 1559 he was called into consultation when Henry II of France was wounded in a jousting contest. A lance had entered the king's visor and pierced the forehead. The court physicians and surgeons extracted several large splinters of wood and dressed the wound. Couriers were sent throughout Europe to summon further experts, among them Vesalius. To determine the possible extent of the injury, experimental thrusts were made with lances into the heads of four criminals who had been decapitated. Despite all possible care, Henry II died on the eleventh day. Vesalius is said to have carried out a thorough postmortem examination, which revealed that the brain had suffered irreversible damage and that a fatal outcome had been inevitable.

The 7 years Vesalius spent in Padua left an indelible mark on the evolution of medicine and surgery. Like Mundinus, Vesalius performed dissections himself. His public lectures drew great attendance, and he was in constant demand to provide anatomical discourses and demonstrations in other Italian cities. Wide experience as the public prosector, when he taught students to dissect and inspect the parts in situ, culminated in the publication of a number of written works.

76. *Facing page,* Hand-colored version of the portrait of Vesalius in the dedication copy of his *De Humani Corporis Fabrica Libri Septem* (1543). The portrait published in the *Fabrica* is the only authentic portrait of Vesalius, and this copy is the most accurate basis for our knowledge of Vesalius's complexion and hair color. *(From the library of Haskell F. Norman, MD.)*

The first work was intended as a visual aid to supplement his lectures and included six anatomical plates *(Tabulae Anatomicae)* printed in Venice (1538). These artistic renderings portrayed the individual systems of the human body, proved immensely popular with students, and were widely plagiarized. By 1543 Vesalius had successfully attacked Galen's positions and authority, demonstrating that Galen's anatomical theories were based entirely on animal dissection.

The indefatigable efforts of Vesalius culminated in the publication of his magnificent *De Humani Corporis Fabrica* (1543) in Basel. The effect of this work was immediate and self-sustaining. At the same time, Vesalius authored an outline key to the *Fabrica,* the *Epitome,* which helped further the *Fabrica's* reputation.

77. Two views of the muscle man, from Vesalius, *De Humani Corporis Fabrica Libri Septem* (1543). Although a few of Vesalius's illustrations exist in color, these are rare. Most of Vesalius's illustrations were done in black and white. *(Jeremy Norman & Co., Inc.)*

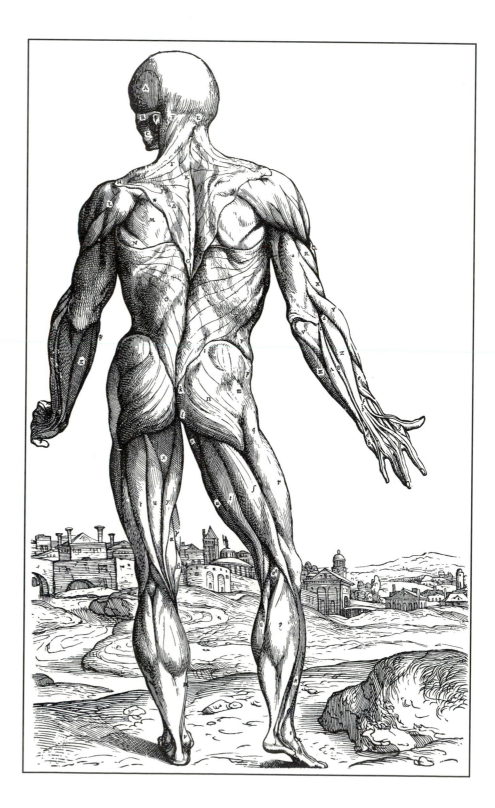

The most obvious reason for the impact of the *Fabrica* was its outstanding illustrations. For the first time woodcuts were intimately integrated with the written text. They were meant to fulfill needs that the text could only partially satisfy. Several artists, now unknown, from the school of Titian (1477-1576) in Venice produced pictures that were scientifically accurate and artistically beautiful. The many splendid woodcuts demonstrated innumerable peculiarities and minor variations in structures encountered in dissection. These illustrations, representing majestic skeletons and flayed figures set against backgrounds of landscape, were to become the standard for anatomical texts during the next two centuries.

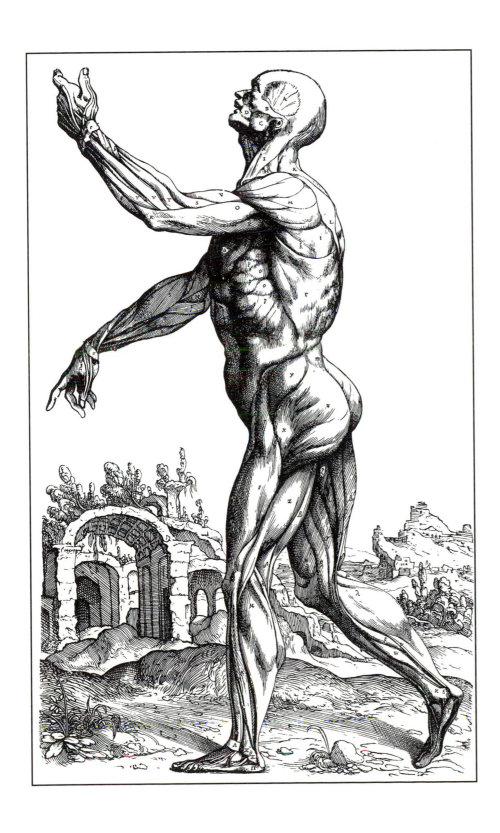

78. Woodcut frontispiece from Colombo's *De Re Anatomica Libri XV* (1559). Colombo worked with Vesalius on the *Fabrica;* the design of this woodcut, showing Colombo demonstrating at the cadaver, was clearly inspired by the frontispiece to Vesalius's work. The design of the woodcut was also believed to be influenced by Donatello's bas-relief, *The Heart Of The Miser.* *(Jeremy Norman & Co., Inc.)*

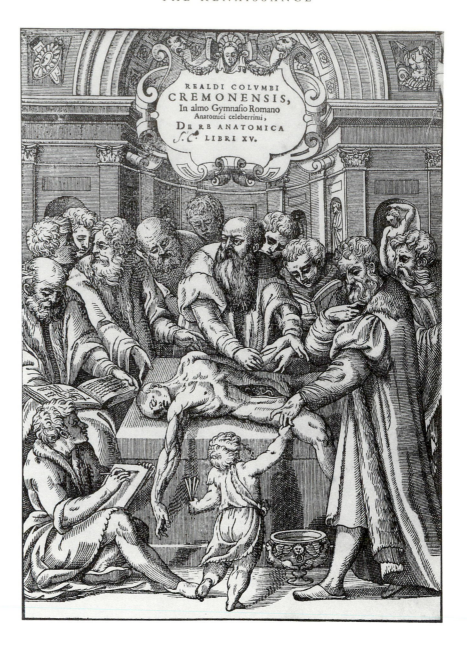

Like most other revolutionary works, the *Fabrica* attracted critics as well as sympathizers. The youthful Vesalius was subjected to unceasing vitriolic attacks for his defiance of Galenic theories. To the many criticisms Vesalius often replied with intemperate, immodest counterattacks. Not surprisingly, the deepest enmities arose between Vesalius and his unfriendly critics who supported Galenic tradition. Included in this group were Sylvius, Johann Dryander (1500-1560), Bartolommeo Eustachio (in Latin, Eustachius) (1520-1574), and Matteo Colombo (1494-1559). Disappointed, disillusioned, and embittered by these attacks, Vesalius decided to leave academic life and entered the court of Charles V. In a last fit of indignation, he burned his manuscript notes and writings and left the world of anatomy. Colombo, while continuing to make harsh attacks on the *Fabrica,* became Vesalius's immediate successor.

Colombo especially offended Vesalius because, although 20 years older than Vesalius, Colombo had served as Vesalius's assistant during the preparation of the *Fabrica.* In fact, Colombo had carried on the duties of teaching and dissection during Vesalius's absence, when Vesalius was supervising the publication of the first edition in Basel. Colombo, the most important pupil of Vesalius and his most severe critic, would himself make some important discoveries, among them the presence of pulmonary veins and the discovery that follicles of teeth could be found in a fetus, which implied that primary teeth did not form from

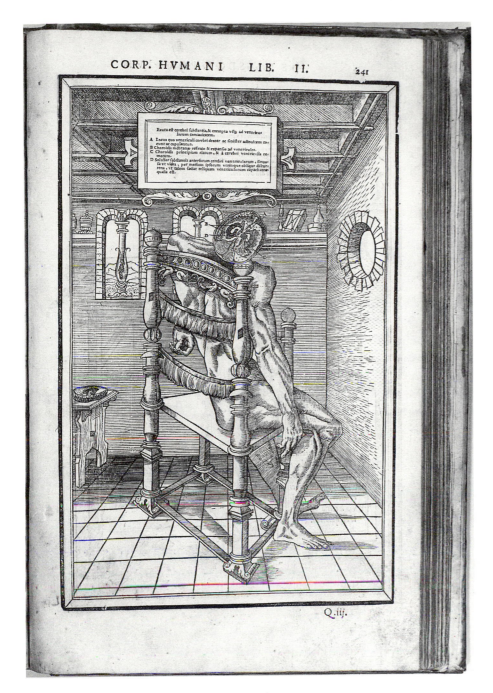

CORP. HVMANI LIB. II. 241

Q.iij.

79. Dissection of the brain. This elegant woodcut in the French Renaissance style is from Estienne, *De Dissectione Partium Corporis Humani* (1545). Estienne studied anatomy in Paris under Sylvius in 1535. One of his classmates was Andreas Vesalius. Estienne's book on human anatomy was ready for the press in 1539, but publication was delayed because of a lawsuit. Had this book been published on schedule it would have eclipsed some of the fame that followed the publication of Vesalius's *Fabrica* in 1543. *(Jeremy Norman & Co., Inc.)*

the milk the child ingested. It is suspected that Colombo plagiarized from both Vesalius and Servetus on the subject of pulmonary circulation. His book *De Re Anatomica Libri XV* (1559) was published posthumously and gave a clear description of the mode of action of the pulmonary, mitral, and aortic valves.

Although the *Fabrica* was written in Latin, its impact ultimately extended to individuals who spoke or understood only the vernacular, the everyday language of ordinary people. Galenic errors were boldly swept aside, permitting the emergence of modern medicine and surgery. Among Vesalius's greatest contribution was his research on the vascular system and the question of the circulation of blood. Although he accepted Galen's theories that the veins carry nutritive blood from the liver through the whole body, that the arteries contain blood, and that these vessels carry from the heart to tissues the blood plus the vital spirit obtained in the left ventricle of the heart, he rejected the opinion of Galen about the existence of pores in the septum of the heart:

The surface of each ventricle is extremely uneven, and beset with numerous pit-like indentations, deeply sunk in its fleshy substance. These pits, however, are not confined to the side by which the right ventricle corresponds with the left (notwithstanding it is so understood by all other anatomists), but are found over the whole ventricle surface . . .

> From these pits none which it is permitted to appreciate by the senses penetrates from the right ventricle into the left. So much are we forced to admire the diligence of the creator of all things in a healthy manner by which the blood exudes from the right ventricle into the left through passages which escape vision . . .
>
> Nor do I find even the minutest channels which would make the septum pervious, although such perforations are described by anatomical professors, who believe implicitly in the passages of blood from the right ventricle into the left. I am therefore in no little doubt as to the function of this part of the heart.

Clearly Vesalius recognized that blood must traverse from the right to the left side of the heart, but he could not explain how that occurred. In his works the pulmonary circulation is never fully described. To understand the tenor of the times and the context in which Vesalius expressed his views regarding human anatomy, one must appreciate the fate of Michael Servetus (1511-1553). Servetus, a Spanish anatomist, realized that the blood in the pulmonary circulation, after having been mixed with air in the lungs, passed into the heart. His discovery was recorded in his work the *Restitutio Christianismi* (1553). Only three known copies of this work exist: John Calvin (1509-1564) had Servetus and virtually all copies of his book burned at the stake for religious heresy.

Vesalius rendered unworkable the Galenic teachings regarding osteology and muscular anatomy. He provided a more complete account of the anatomy of the brain and was the first to describe the omentum and its connection with the stomach, spleen, and colon. Vesalius adequately described the course of the azygos and subclavian veins, as well as the mediastinum and pleura. He corrected 200 Galenic mistakes overall, including Adam's missing rib, that there is no "resurrection bone" lodged in the right great toe, and the lack of marrow in the bones of the hand.

The *Fabrica* is of interest in the history of surgery because of its many descriptions of operative cases. Vesalius advised excision of the breast for cancer and wrote about hydrocephalus and omental hernia. Vesalius's techniques for dissection are illustrated in the following excerpt from the *Fabrica,* in which examination of the recurrent nerves and the loss of voice from cutting them are described:

> And soon I begin in this way an extended dissection in the neck with a rather sharp knife which divides the skin and muscles lying under it right to the trachea, avoiding this lest the incision may deviate to the side and wound especially the principal vein. Then by grasping the windpipe with the hands, and freeing it accurately from the overlying muscles by the use of the fingers as far as the arteries lying at its side; I seek out the nerves bordering upon the sixth pair of cerebral nerves; then I note the recurrent nerves lying on the sides of the rough artery (trachea) which I sometimes intercept with ligatures, at other times I cut. And first I do the same on the other side, in order that it may be clearly seen when one nerve has been tied or cut how half the voice disappears and is totally lost when both nerves are cut. And if I loosen the ligatures the voice will return again. For this is carried out quickly and without an unusual loss of blood, and it is clearly proved how the animal struggles for deep breaths without its voice when the recurrent nerves have been divided with a sharp knife.

Vesalius's *Fabrica* stimulated wide-ranging research into human anatomy. Guilio Aranzio (1530-1589) was a prominent Renaissance anatomist who described the ductus arteriosus and the ductus venosus. In about 1541 Giambattista Canano (1515-1579) published 26 copper plates illustrating the bones and muscles of the arm and forearm. The illustrations were unsurpassed in their realism and exactitude. Canano, however, had seen unpublished woodcuts of the *Fabrica* and had been so impressed with their quality that he deliberately suppressed his own book, *Musculorum Humani Corporis Picturata Dissectio,* so few copies now exist. Charles Estienne (1504-1564), from the famous Estienne family of scholar-printers, was a pupil of Sylvius in Paris. His work, *De Dissectione Partium Corporis Humani* (1545), included illustrations of the entire external venous and nervous system.

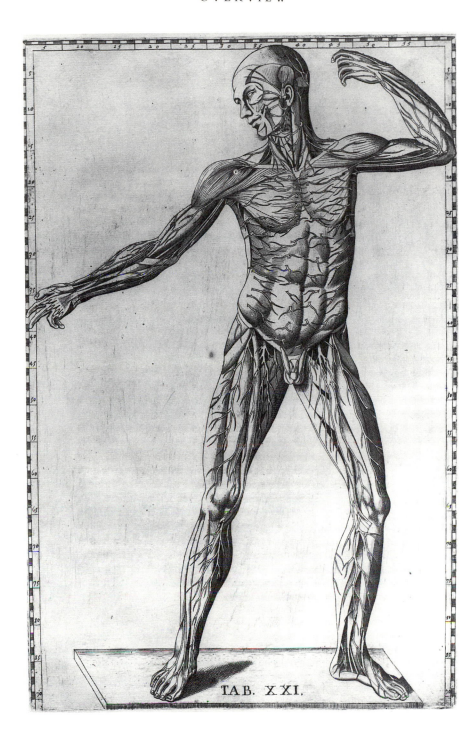

TAB. XXI.

80. Copperplate engraving from Eustachius' *Tabulae Anatomicae* (1714). The copperplates in this work were actually engraved in 1552, but for unknown reasons they remained unpublished in the Vatican Library until they were edited by Giovanni Maria Lancisi in 1714. The scales on three sides of the images provided coordinates by which any part of the body could be precisely located on the plate without recourse to identifying marks within the plate. *(Jeremy Norman & Co., Inc.)*

Two anatomists, Fallopius and Eustachius, were particularly illustrious and made striking contributions to surgical anatomy. Fallopius was Vesalius's pupil in Padua and remained loyal to him throughout his short life. He was professor of anatomy at Ferrara (1547), Pisa (1548), and Padua (1551) and was known as a careful dissector, a detailed observer, and an accurate recorder. His most renowned work is the *Observationes Anatomicae* (1561). Fallopius was the first to describe the chorda tympani and the semicircular canals. He provided a correct description of the cerebral vessels and their course, including the trigeminal, auditory, and glossopharyngeal nerves. Fallopius accurately described the circular folds of the small intestines, the sphenoid sinus, the fallopian tubes, the round ligaments, and the arteria profunda of the penis. He also clearly demonstrated how teeth formed. Fallopius enumerated all the nerves of the eye and was a versatile writer on surgical topics.

Eustachius was professor at the Collegia della Sapienza in Rome where in 1552 he completed the engravings for his *Tabulae Anatomicae*. This set of superb anatomical plates drawn by Eustachius remained forgotten and unprinted in the

Vatican Library for 162 years. In the early eighteenth century Pope Clement XI (?-1721) presented the copper plates to his personal physician, Giovanni Lancisi (1654-1720). Lancisi sought the advice of Giovanni Morgagni (1682-1771), who suggested publication, and the plates, along with notes by Lancisi, were published in 1714. Why these plates were not published in Eustachius's lifetime is unknown. Had they been printed in the mid-sixteenth century, they surely would have eclipsed some of the glory of the *Fabrica*.

Eustachius was a critic of Vesalius and of the latter's condemnation of Galen. Nonetheless, it is likely that Eustachius recognized the correctness of many of Vesalius's anatomical findings, given the many anatomical discoveries Eustachius made and presented in his *Opuscula Anatomica* (1564). His discoveries included the eustachian tube, thoracic duct, adrenal glands, and pulmonary veins and the first adequate description of the uterus. He also described the origin of the optic nerves, the cochlea, the muscles of the throat, and the abducens nerve.

Eustachius also wrote *Libellus De Dentibus* (1563), the best Renaissance treatise on the structure and function of the teeth. Eustachius, basing his work on

81. Illuminated page from the first book on pathological anatomy, Benivieni's *De Abditis Nonnullis Ac Mirandis Morborum . . .* (1507). In the early sixteenth century some printers were still influenced by the medieval manuscript tradition, which gradually diminished with the development of printing in the second half of the fifteenth century. For owners who wished to have a printed book that retained some of the elegance of illuminated manuscripts, the printer of Benivieni's book left space for hand-painted illuminated initials to be supplied at the beginning of chapters. (*Jeremy Norman & Co., Inc.*)

the dissection of fetuses and stillborn infants, was the first to study the teeth in detail. He provided an important description of the first and second dentitions, described the hard outer tissue and soft inner structure of the tooth, and attempted to explain the sensitivity of the tooth's hard structure.

In furthering the study of human anatomy, a role similar to that of the Renaissance surgeons was assumed by surgeons in the field of pathological anatomy. Without the development of both human and pathological anatomies, any evolution of the craft of surgery would have been naturally hindered. Although Morgagni is commonly held to be the direct originator of pathological anatomy, the indirect claim is more accurately awarded to Antonio Benivieni (1443-1502), a Florentine surgeon.

Benivieni was not an academician but an eminent practitioner in his native city. He was among the few medical personalities in the early Renaissance who were fresh and independent observers. Like Mondeville, Benivieni was intellectually oppressed by the authority of Greek and Arabic masters who had promulgated spurious information. His education at the universities of Pisa and Sienna was considered liberal for the times. Benivieni was a highly cultured man and maintained a wide range of friendships with many intellectuals throughout Italy. His large surgical practice provided a substantial remuneration, and after amassing a considerable fortune, Benivieni was elected to important public offices in Florence.

Throughout his surgical career Benivieni maintained voluminous, detailed patient notes. Most important, he followed up his cases with autopsies, then a rare practice. Although Benivieni considered Galen a preeminent authority, Benivieni's case reports reveal him to be a man of persistent questioning. It was Benivieni's brother Geronimo who rescued him from historical medical oblivion. Going through Benivieni's papers after his death, Geronimo came across the collection of case reports with autopsy records. Convinced of the importance of these unique observations, he turned them over to a physician friend, who prepared them for publication. In 1507 *De Abditis Nonnulus Ac Mirandis Morborum Et Sanationum Causis* first appeared in Florence. This small, 54-page volume consisted of a random series of case reports encompassing a wide variety of diseases. Of the 160 cases in the original manuscript, about 50 had been omitted. It appears that Benivieni frequently obtained permission both from the Pope and from the patients' relatives to perform postmortem examinations. The bodies were incised, not dissected, and the results are correspondingly sketchy.

Among Bienvieni's pathological reports are two instances of destructive hip-joint disease and cases of biliary calculus, mesenteric abscess, thrombosis of the mesenteric vessels, stenosis of the intestine, cancer of the pylorus, perforated large bowel, and caries of the ribs with exposure of the heart. An excerpt from the reports follows:

Case III: Stones found in the coat of the liver.

A woman of noble birth had been for long greatly tormented by pain in the region of the liver. She had consulted many physicians, but could not drive out the evil by any remedy. She therefore decided to try my help in conjunction with some others.

Thus several of us met and discussed at great length from different aspects the hidden causes of this disease. As often happens in doubtful cases, we were divided. Some thought there was an abscess on the liver, others that it was itself diseased, but I personally believed that the fault lay in the covering membrane. A few days afterward the disease took stronger hold and she departed this life, even as we had foretold by common consent from unmistakable symptoms.

I then had her dead body cut open. There were found in the lower part of the membrane round the liver, a collection of small stones varying in shape and colour. Some were round, some pointed, some square, according as position and chance had determined, and they were also marked with reddish, blue and white spots. These stones by their weight had caused the membrane to hang down in a bag a palm's length and two fingers wide. This we judged the cause of her death and decided that discussions upon what was hidden were vain and futile.

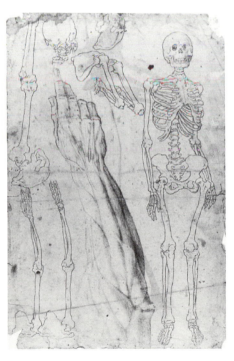

82. Original anatomical drawing by Volcher Coiter of Nuremberg (1534-1576). Coiter, who studied with Eustachius and Fallopius, made several important contributions to human anatomy and was the first to elevate comparative anatomy to the rank of an independent branch of biology. Coiter was one of the first physicians known to have drawn the illustrations for his own books. Few original anatomical drawings from the sixteenth century have survived. *(Jeremy Norman & Co., Inc.)*

It is claimed that Benivieni was the first to perform a successful lithotrity. He also recognized a case of imperforate hymen with retained menses and successfully treated the woman by incising and excising the obstructing membrane. Benivieni gained wide repute for his successful treatment of a patient with a severe inflammatory condition and attendant suppuration in the region of the submaxillary gland and the floor of the mouth. The patient was about to die of suffocation when Benivieni widely incised the inflamed area, draining the floor of the mouth, and relieved the acute submaxillary obstruction. He also reported on the plastic repair of upper-extremity burn contracture and an apparently patent omphalomesenteric duct.

During the Renaissance each country began to develop its own recognizable practice of surgery. No longer were charlatans and barber-surgeons freely roaming from one end of the continent to the other to offer their services. Each country was developing its own collection of itinerant quack surgeons, barber-surgeons, and university-educated surgeons. Thus the history of Renaissance surgery is most easily presented as the history of surgery in specific European countries.

GERMANY AND SWITZERLAND

The Reformation began in Germany in 1517. When Luther nailed his *Ninety-five Theses* to the door of a Wittenberg church, he had no intention of starting a movement that would so affect Catholicism. In 1518 Pope Leo X (?-1521) declared Luther a heretic, but Luther had many powerful protectors among the princes of Germany, who supported him to gain control of church government and church property in their lands. Three years later, the Pope excommunicated Luther. Emperor Charles V then ordered him to appear before the Imperial Diet at Worms. Once there, Luther refused to retract any of his statements. The emperor ruled against him and forbade him to preach. Luther continued to defy the Pope and the emperor and began to organize his conservative Lutheran church in 1522. Lutheranism spread rapidly through Germany and might have united the entire German-speaking world. During the bloody Peasants' War (1524-1525), however, Luther sided with the princes. Millions of disillusioned Germans then returned to the Catholic church.

In 1530 Philipp Melanchthon (1497-1560) prepared a conciliatory statement of Lutheran views called the *Augsburg Confession*. The Roman Catholics rejected it, and the Protestants banded together in the Schmalkaldic League to fight the Catholics. After several fierce battles the two sides made peace in 1555. Their treaty recognized the legality of Lutheranism in principalities of the rulers who wished it. However, no other sects were to be tolerated in the empire, an unsatisfactory arrangement that ultimately led to the Thirty Years' War, which began in 1618.

In Switzerland the 13 cantons were quite receptive to Protestantism. Ulrich Zwingli (1484-1531), a priest from Zurich, began preaching a religion of reform in 1519, and his views spread quickly throughout Switzerland and southern Germany. Differences in doctrine blocked a union between the Lutheran and Zwinglian churches.

John Calvin dominated the latter part of the Swiss Reformation. He was able to establish a powerful center for his teachings in Geneva. Calvinism spread to Germany, France, Scotland, England, and the Netherlands. Its huge success divided the Protestant world into two camps.

Both Germany and Switzerland lagged far behind in the awakening of medicine and surgery during the Middle Ages and in the great surgical renaissance which began during the fourteenth century in Italy and France. A number of reasons accounted for this backwardness, not the least of which was the sorry state of university education in central Europe. Virtually no medical progress was made in that part of Europe until the sixteenth century.

In the particular case of Germanic surgery, most individuals who practiced the art of surgery were merely simple craftsmen who, like other artisans, joined together in guilds. It was thought no more suitable for a surgeon to study books than for a carpenter or a blacksmith to do so. Since German surgeons usually had no formal education, they could neither speak nor read Latin. Their subordinate position to the physicians was long accepted, and conflict between the two groups remained minimal.

Although not as learned as their foreign colleagues, the German surgeons were well versed in the surgery of war. They were widely experienced in the growing field of military surgery, the subject of their earliest surgical works. These surgical texts were intended as practical handbooks or manuals for the use of their fellow craftsmen. They were written in the vernacular and dealt almost entirely with the treatment of wounds. Although little in them was original, for unknown reasons some of the early surgical innovations of neighboring countries first appeared in print in the German texts.

Heinrich von Pfolspeundt was a fifteenth-century Bavarian army surgeon and the earliest known German surgical writer. He composed his *Buch Der Bündth-Ertznei* in 1460. It remained in manuscript form until 1868, when it was rediscovered in Breslau, edited, and published. Pfolspeundt, a Brother of the German Order, related having participated in a number of military campaigns between his order and various Polish kings. His work reveals him to be a relatively uneducated person barely competent in his native language. However, he mentions "German and Italian Masters" from whom he had learned his skills, none of whom are historically recognizable.

83. A surgeon treating an ulcerated leg. Woodcut by Hans Weiditz, the German printmaker and book illustrator, from his famous series of illustrations for a German edition of Petrarch's *Trostspiegel In Glück Und Unglück* (Frankfurt am Main, 1584). As is typical in early illustrations of surgical procedures, the patient appears to be experiencing little discomfort. *(National Library of Medicine, Bethesda, Md.)*

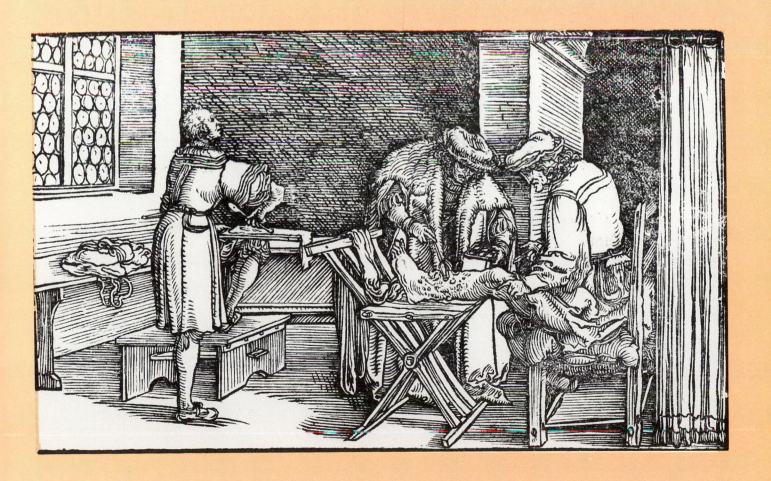

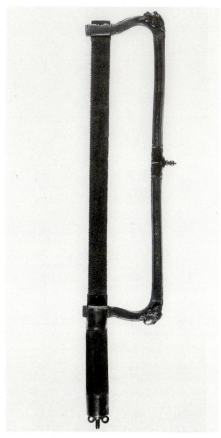

84. German amputation saw, 1571. At each end of the saw is a mask: the mask at the top reflects pain, the one at the bottom reflects calm. The inscription on the frame between the two masks may be translated, "Cruel is my form, with anxiety, distress, and great pain. When the job is done, sorrow turns to joy." *(Bayerisches Nationalmuseum, Munich, Inventory Number E772.)*

Pfolspeundt was only a wound surgeon, had no skill in major operations, and did not know how to treat fractures and dislocations. He left minor surgery to the barbers and the larger operative procedures to the cutters. His text was largely limited to discussion of the management of wounds and other injuries. Pfolspeundt's military experience provided him with a large practice in arrow wounds, and his text contains the first faint allusion to "powder-burns" suffered as a result of gunshot injuries. *Buch Der Bundth-Ertznei* is most notable for its insistence on cleanliness, including handwashing and clean bandages:

> Firstly, I advise anyone who wishes to work in this art and to heal, that he should not go to a wounded or sick person in the early morning or treat him before he has heard Mass, so far as is possible, unless there is great need, but he shall pray to the good Lord to bless the wounds, to say a Pater Noster and an Ave Maria, and confess his faith, so that strength and wisdom be given to heal the people whom he has under his hands.
>
> And he should guard himself against drunkenness when he is to treat patients, for because of it they may easily be neglected, and the doctor would be guilty of that and be punished by God. And especially, he should guard himself, if he has eaten onions or peas, or slept the previous night with an unclean woman, in the morning, against breathing into anyone's wound. Also, he should bind with clean white cloths, for if they are not clean, harm results. He should also wash his hands before he treats anyone. Also he should love healing for the sake of God, if he is able: also if the doctor knows himself to be unclean, he should not look actively into the wounds, nor should any other unclean person, else mischief and harm arises, and may even cause death of the patient. And keep people protected, or you will have to do penance before God, if you are to blame.

Regardless of his general message of cleanliness, Pfolspeundt usually poured oil of turpentine on all new wounds, looked for laudable pus, and treated wounds with healing by second intention. Most of the patients with these war injuries received strengthening drinks. The extraction of bullets by a sound was usually recommended. In addition, Pfolspeundt provided a recipe for an artificial general anesthetic consisting of opium, atropa mandragora, conium maculatum, hedera helox or arborea, lactuca, and daphne mezereum. The mixture was soaked up in sponges, which were then placed in a sealed glass bottle and dried in the sun. To produce narcosis, the medicated sponge was placed under a patient's nostrils and the patient then deeply inhaled. To awaken the patient, plugs of cotton soaked in fennel and vinegar combined with sweet-oil were put into his or her nostril.

Pfolspeundt described only a few actual operations, specifically those for harelip and rhinoplasty. The description of rhinoplasty is one of the most interesting aspects of the treatise. Pfolspeundt employed either the "Indian" method of nasal reconstruction, in which skin from the cheek or forehead was used to fashion the new nose, or a pedicled-flap technique in which skin from the arm was used. These particular methods were rarely used in central Europe during the Renaissance. According to Pfolspeundt, he learned the method from an Italian surgeon and kept it a safely guarded secret for many years.

Whether the Italian surgeon was one of the celebrated father-and-son itinerant nose restorers, the Brancas of Catania, remains uncertain. Nonetheless, the section of the *Bundth-Ertznei* on nasal reconstruction is the most detailed of the entire work and provides the only existing early Renaissance surgical text in which a satisfactory account of the Indian rhinoplastic operative method is given.

Other remarkable passages can be found in Pfolspeundt's work, for instance, instructions in a case of wounded intestine. The surgeon was told to cut through the organ at the point of injury and then introduce into the opposite ends of the divided bowel a silver tube, the margins of which had been carefully bent so as not to offer a sharpened edge. The tube could then be tied in place with a thread of green silk.

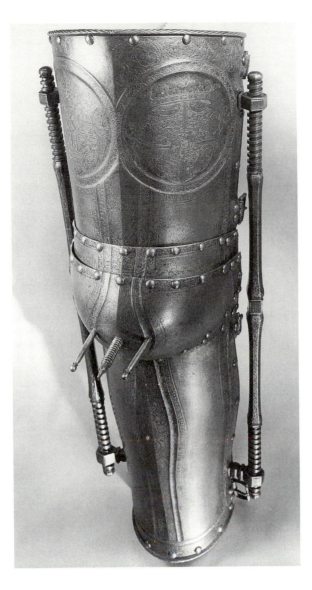

85. A sixteenth-century German orthopedic apparatus for a crooked leg, richly ornamented and probably made for a nobleman. Similar instruments are illustrated in Gersdorff, *Feldbuch Der Wundartzney* (1517). *Germanisches Nationalmuseum, Nürnberg.)*

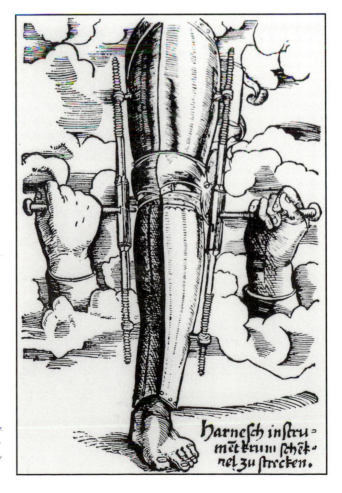

86. Woodcut from Gersdorff, *Feldbuch der Wundartzney* (1517), of an orthopedic apparatus for a crooked leg. *(Jeremy Norman & Co., Inc.)*

Within a quarter-century of Pfolspeundt lived another, more literate German surgeon, Hieronymus Brunschwig (circa 1450-1512). He was born in Strassburg and spent most of his life in the practice of wound surgery in that city. Whether he received a formal scholastic education is unknown; however, Brunschwig claims to have read or studied more than 3000 books and manuscripts during his lifetime.

In 1497 Brunschwig authored his *Dis Ist Das Buch Der Cirurgia Hantwirckung Der Wundartzny*. A remarkable publication for a number of reasons, it was the first important printed surgical treatise in German. In it Brunschwig combined a compilation of the knowledge of ancient and medieval authorities with his own extensive experience. It contained the first detailed account of gunshot wounds in medical literature and was the first extensively illustrated book on surgery. The woodcut illustrations were used not to clarify the text but to provide simple decoration. From a historical standpoint, they help portray the costumes, furnishings, and medical customs of the early German Renaissance, including a few simple operative procedures.

The *Buch Der Wundartzny* was published in numerous editions and remained popular long after the author's death. Like Pfolspeundt, Brunschwig dealt almost entirely with wound and ulcer treatment. Although he included little that was original, he did provide the first detailed discussion of the treatment of gunshot wounds. He regarded such wounds as poisoned and believed the poison could best be removed by promoting suppuration, usually via a seton made of animal hair.

The doctrine of poisoned gunshot wounds, first alluded to by Pfolspeundt and then clarified by Brunschwig, was to cause an immense amount of iatrogenic battlefield harm and handicap the work of military surgeons. As this doctrine was expanded, wounds were increasingly made to suppurate either with a hot iron cautery or with boiling oil. Consequently gangrene and pyemia were rampant during military engagements. In all fairness, Pfolspeundt and Brunschwig probably were not the first surgeons to adhere to this doctrine, although they were the first to mention it in written form.

The following important chapter headings in Brunschwig's work convey an idea of the overall character of the work:

Fatality of Wounds in Different Parts of the Body
Different Kinds of Surgical Instruments
Different Modes of Ligating Blood-Vessels
Methods of Arresting Bleeding
Treatment of Wounds Inflicted by Poisoned Arrows
Bruised or Crushed Wounds
Stab Wounds
Bites and Stings

Brunschwig quoted liberally from the writings of surgeons who preceded him and was well aware of and practiced ligation of severed vascular structures to control hemorrhage. The opening chapter contained the definition of the word *surgeon* and a description of the surgeon's duties:

It is the office of the surgeon to unite with his hand that of man's body which has been separated or which is open and make it into a whole as it had been before . . . it is necessary that the surgeon be skillful, of a moral nature, and neither too slow nor too fast in his work.

He should be faithful and careful towards the wounded and sick so that he will neither neglect nor forget anything through which the patients could suffer or be damaged . . . He himself should also not sin nor curse . . . He should not say too much except to promise health to the patients and he should talk with them pleasantly . . .

He should not quarrel or swear at the wounded or the sick and should never talk to anyone else about that which he has heard in the house of the patient. Instead he should speak to the sick and the wounded chastely and gently and always promise them recovery. But, to their good friends he should tell the truth and hide nothing . . .

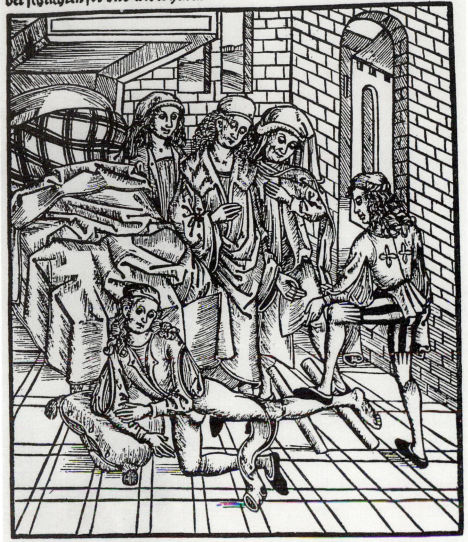

Das ander capittel des dritte dractatz wurt fagen so erm ein Bein zerbrochen ist vnd krump gehailt ist wie man das wider schlichten sol vnd wider heilen.

So einnem ein Bein zerbrochen ist vnd krump gehailt wer das einner hinckt oder vngerad das an ist vnd wil oder begert einner wider gerad zu werden alß vor so laß im machen ein wasser Bad in einner mülten do die Brotbecken teick in machen vnd Bad in dar in sey oder acht tag.

He should help the poor according to whatever they are able to pay but should ask good reward from the rich. In this manner you will achieve happiness and salvation . . . You should also wear good clothes but you should not be vain . . .

The surgeon should also know anatomy and be aware that there is a connection and a separation of the members of the body so that he knows where he should cut or cauterize . . .

You young beginning surgeons . . . When you are called to a patient if the matter appears to you too difficult or not entirely familiar do not be ashamed to send after one or two other surgeons so that they can help you and give you good advice from which you and the patient can derive great benefit . . .

I say to all surgeons if there are two or several of them that they should never quarrel before the patient for that would frighten the patient very much. Similarly, if one of the surgeons is not present one should not talk badly or derogatorily about him . . .

87. Woodcut from the earliest printed surgical book with illustrations, Brunschwig's *Dis Ist Das Buch Der Cirurgia Hantwirckung Der Wundartzney* (1497). Here the surgeon is rebreaking a limb that has healed imperfectly. *(Jeremy Norman & Co., Inc.)*

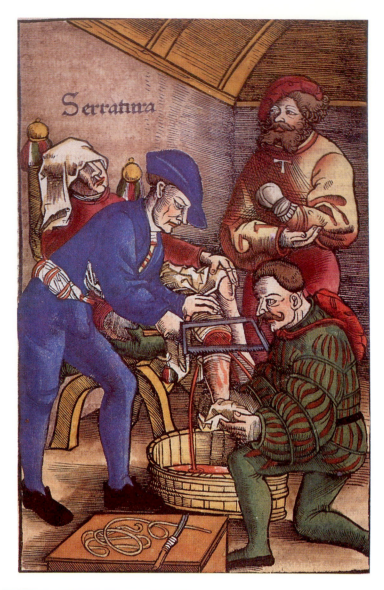

88. Amputation of a limb from Gersdorff, *Feldbuch Der Wundartzney* (1517). The surgeon cuts while his assistant holds the leg over a large bucket used for collecting blood. Behind the surgeon's assistant, *right*, an apparently happy patient wears a bladder over an amputation stump on his left forearm. The bright colors are authentic hand coloring of the period. *(Reynolds Library, University of Alabama, Birmingham.)*

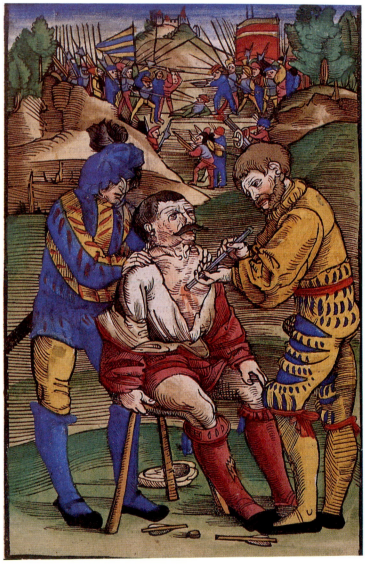

89. The military surgeon removes an arrow from a wounded soldier on the field of battle. Hand-colored woodcut from Gersdorff (1517). *(Reynolds Library, University of Alabama, Birmingham.)*

146

The last of the famous early German wound surgeons was Hans von Gersdorff (circa 1480-1540), a slightly younger contemporary of Brunschwig. Little is known of Gersdorff's early life. He gained most of his extensive experience as a military surgeon in the many futile and pointless wars of the time. Most of his career was centered in Strassburg, and he is considered an Alsatian surgeon.

In 1517 Gersdorff wrote *Feldtbuch Der Wundartzney* in vernacular German. The work is particularly valuable for its many important illustrations. These engravings offer a side glance at cultural history, especially of costumes and interiors; a battle scene depicts a cannon guarded by a trio of soldiers armed with muskets. These pictures, in particular the first rendering of an amputation in a printed surgical text, were meant to be instructive. In the engraving of the amputation the use of animal bladders is portrayed as the mode of dressing the stump.

Gersdorff is remembered for his claim to have performed more than 200 amputations for gangrene or erysipelas. After the advent of gunshot and cannon wounds, the question of how to treat such injuries became paramount to the wound surgeon. Ancient writers had advised that amputation be performed through the gangrenous portion of the limb. Later writers preferred to amputate through healthy tissue and treat the stump with boiling oil, or to use hot-iron cautery to control hemorrhage and promote suppuration. Whether Gersdorff believed such injuries to be poisoned from the outset is uncertain. There is no doubt, however, that he did employ hot oil and the cautery to cleanse out the burned powder and dead tissue. To complete the amputation Gersdorff did not suture the flaps. Instead, he brought the opposing edges together and then covered the newly formed stump with the bladder of some animal:

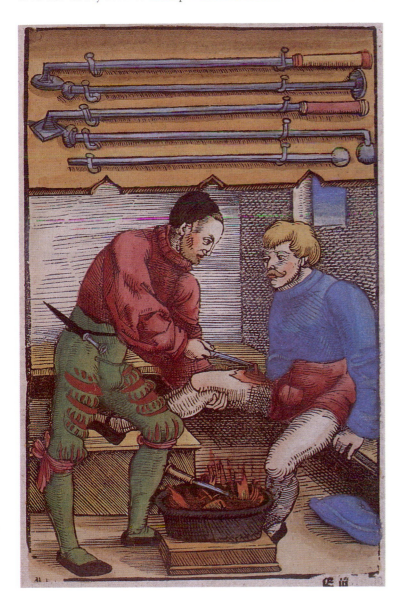

90. Treatment of a wound with cautery. Numerous cautery instruments are shown at the top of the plate. Hand-colored woodcut from Gersdorff (1517). *(Reynolds Library, University of Alabama, Birmingham.)*

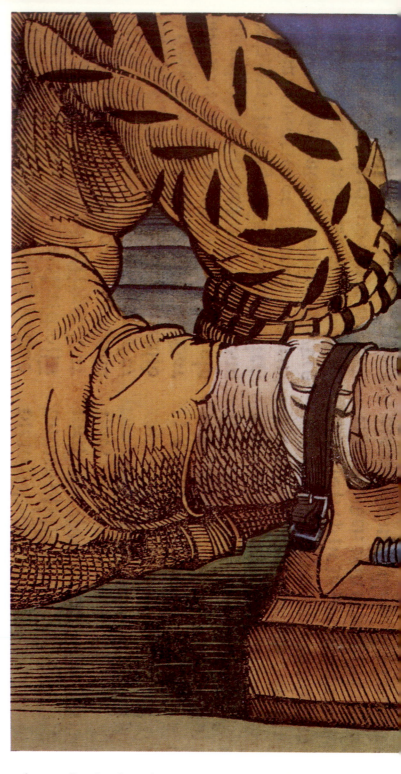

91. An orthopedic splint for a wounded leg. The artist's limited knowledge of perspective creates the impression that the patient is much larger than the artist intended. Hand-colored woodcut from Gersdorff (1517). *(Reynolds Library, University of Alabama, Birmingham.)*

If the limb must be cut off, and nothing else will help, or if it has helped but the limb cannot be preserved, you should advise the patient above all to go to confession and receive the Holy Sacrament . . .

When you are about to cut have someone draw the skin firmly back, and tightly bind the skin with a constricting band, and then tie a cord near the constricting band, leaving a space about a finger's breadth between the two, in which the incision can be made, so that the cut will be correct and even and makes a good stump. When you have made the incision, take a saw and cut the bone. Afterwards, remove the constriction, and have someone draw the skin and flesh down over the bone and pull it firmly forward. And then have a bandage ready, two finger breadths wide, which has been moistened until it is thoroughly wet, and bind it about the limb down to the incision, to keep the flesh over the wound and bind it so. And afterwards, apply the hemostyptic over it. Do not be frightened by the bleeding if it occurs, as was described before. And over the hemostyptic bind a good, thick compress.

And afterwards, take a bladder of a bull or ox or hog, which should be strong, and cut off the top widely enough so that it will go over the stump and the dressing. The bladder should be moistened, but not too soft, and draw it over and bind it firmly with a cord, then you need not worry that it will bleed.

I have never sewn a stump, but have always healed them with medicaments . . .

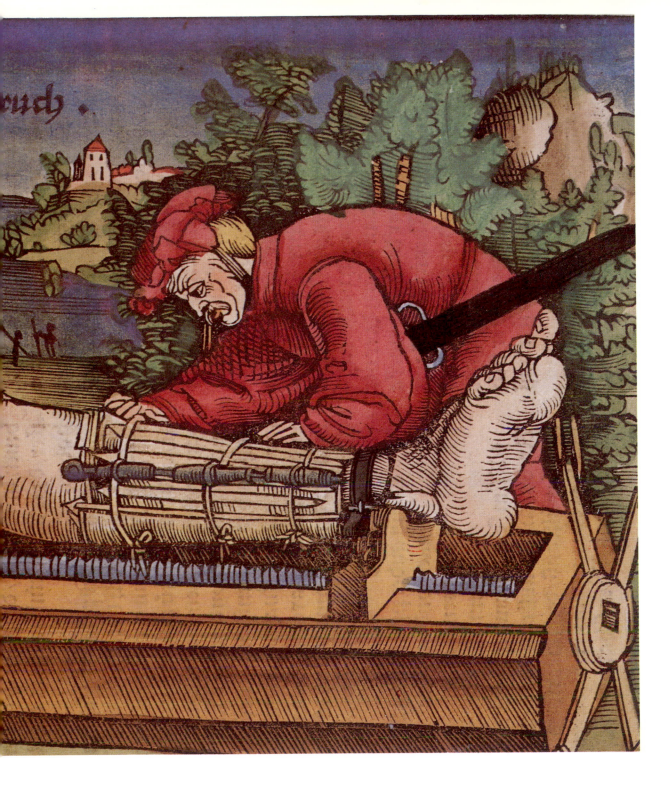

The styptic Gersdorff mentioned consisted of the following:

Take of unslaked lime two ounces, vitriol, alum, each, one ounce, of aloes to be calcined, gallnuts, colophony each a quarter of an ounce; of the residuum in the retort when you make aquafortis two and a half ounces, and the white hair of the belly of a hare or deer chopped up, and mix all together thoroughly. When you use it mix it with white of eggs . . . But if an artery rages and will not be stanched then burn it with a cautery.

Gersdorff's primary interest appears to have been surgical instrumentation. His book was full of new devices such as machines for the reduction of fractures and dislocations and for the correction of crooked limbs. His most interesting apparatus was a tripod screw-elevator for raising depressed skull fragments. Gersdorff's other innovations included giving the patient opium before an operation and awakening the patient by making him or her inhale vinegar.

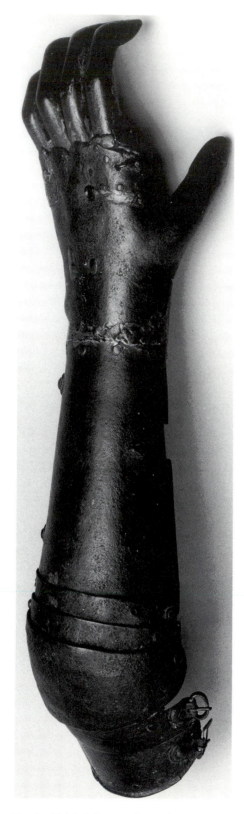

92. Artificial left arm from the sixteenth century, reputed to have belonged to a German feudal knight, Gotz von Berlichingen (1480-1562), who lost his own arm during the siege of Landshut. The artificial arm consists of an articulated wrist and elbow; the fingers are also articulated and move on a common spindle controlled by springs and ratchets, which are operated by means of a cord at the shoulder. Few other prostheses from the Renaissance period have survived. *(Reproduced by permission of the Trustees of the Science Museum, London. Inventory A121449; 26/93.)*

Walter Hermann Ryff (circa first half of the sixteenth century) deserves mention as a surgeon from Strassburg who authored a number of surgical treatises. He was of dubious moral character, having been expelled from a number of German cities. Although considered a versatile writer because he wrote treatises on surgery, hygiene, mathematics, cooking, and obstetrics, strong evidence exists that he plagiarized at least some of these works. His *Kleinere Chirurgie* (1542) and *Grosse Chirurgei, Oder Volkommene Wundartznei* (1545) are almost verbatim translations of other authors. In providing these translations, however, he compiled an interesting and varied account of Renaissance surgery. In addition, the latter work contained many detailed, highly accurate woodcut illustrations of instruments. Most of these woodcuts were printed in red and black ink.

Conrad Gesner (1516-1565) of Zurich, although not a surgeon, was considered one of the most learned medical men of the Renaissance. He studied medicine in Basel (1541) and spent much of his life as a roving practitioner in various European cities. Gesner was eventually appointed professor of natural history at Zurich (1555) and was elevated to the rank of a nobleman in 1564. Despite lifelong struggles with poverty and sickness, Gesner was inordinately industrious. He is considered one of the earliest scientific botanists and bibliographers of the Renaissance. Gesner's *Bibliotheca Universalis* (1545) was an early attempt at a systematic universal bibliography; the section on medicine, however, was never completed. His bibliographic skills are also demonstrated in *De Chirurgia Scriptores Optimi Quique Veteres Et Recentiores* (1555), a collection of surgical works from ancient writers through the writers of his own day. One of the earliest bibliographies of surgery was the list of surgeons and their works that Gesner appended to his book.

Most of the itinerant surgeons throughout Germany and Switzerland have found no place in the history of surgery because, being illiterate, they left no manuscripts or printed works. Caspar Stromayr (sixteenth century), however, was an exception. He was born in Lindau and maintained permanent residence in his native city. Stromayr's remarkable contribution to the history of surgery was his meticulously worded and beautifully written *Practica Copiosa,* which bears the date July 4, 1559. This manuscript reposed in utter solitude in the city library of Lindau until the beginning of the twentieth century. It was discovered in 1909 and eventually published in 1925. The 186 hand-colored illustrations in the manuscript are its most remarkable feature. The full-page pictures provide the most complete, detailed view of sixteenth-century surgical practice. The illustrations clarify the text and are frequently referred to in the discussion. It is possible that they were completed by Stromayr himself, but the artist remains unknown.

Stromayr was a herniotomist and cataract coucher and belonged to the group of German surgeons known as the "incisor" class. Consequently the text of the *Practica Copiosa* was devoted almost entirely to hernia repair, with a minor section on surgery of the eye. Stromayr was quite specific in differentiating between indirect and direct inguinal hernias. He emphasized the importance of removing the sac, as well as the testicle and spermatic cord, in an indirect hernia. For a direct hernia he spared the testes and recognized that the spermatic cord bore no relation to the course of the sac.

Felix Wurtz (1518-1574) was a prominent Germanic-speaking barber-surgeon. Born in Zurich, he was peripatetic in his education, receiving instruction in such diverse cities as Bamberg, Nuremberg, Padua, Pforzheim, and Rome. Having been a barber's apprentice, he must have gained extensive experience in the treatment of gunshot wounds.

Wurtz eventually returned to his native city and was enrolled in the barber's guild. Although forbidden to practice medicine, he received special dispensation, in addition to practicing his surgical skills, to prescribe various laxatives and potions. Most of his professional life was spent in Zurich; for unknown reasons he left that city in 1559 and reestablished himself in Strassburg and, later, in Basel.

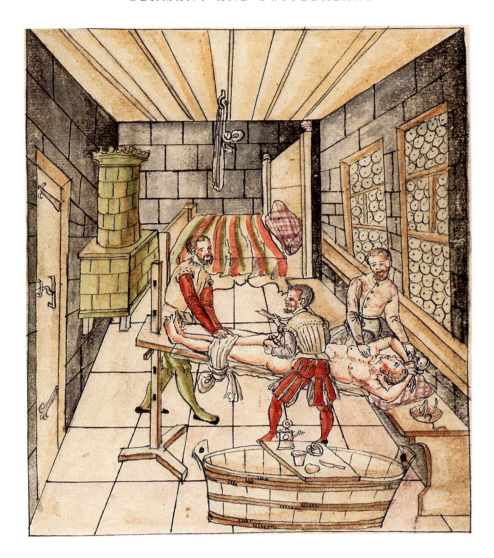

93. Original painting of the operation for hernia, by Caspar Stromayr. Reproduced from his surgical manuscript, *Practica Copiosa,* dated July 4, 1559. The bath for the patient can be seen in the foreground of the operating room. *(Ehemals Reichsstädtische Bibliothek Lindau [B].)*

Wurtz had close friendships with Paracelsus and Gesner. As a result, Wurtz closely followed the former's simple treatment of wounds and was a vigorous opponent of the common custom of placing cloth, oil, salves, or balsam on them. The following leading principles guided Wurtz in his treatment of wounds:

> Keep them as neat and clean as possible, and disturb them as little as you can; so far as may be practicable, exclude the air; favor healing under a scab; and do not give the patient a lowering diet, but feed him as you would a woman recovering from her confinement.

Wurtz's most important contribution to the craft of surgery was his *Practica Der Wundartzney* (1563). This book was written in vernacular German; many editions were published, including translations into English, French, and Dutch. Although operative surgery is not mentioned, his extensive experience in wound surgery is readily evident. Wurtz resented the criticisms directed at his clinical practices. He was adamant in promulgating the belief that current experience is of much greater value than any rule that may have been uttered by an ancient expert:

> There can be no doubt . . . that the ancients occasionally displayed great ignorance and great want of judgment, just as happens in our own time . . . How much do you suppose I care whether Galen's, or Avicenna's, or Guy de Chauliac's opinion does or does not agree with mine? Every such opinion—it should be remembered— was, at one time or another in their day, a new and therefore unproved opinion . . . In practical surgery much more importance attaches to the manner in which one carries out one's manipulations, and to the amount of experience, which one may have acquired, than to the length of time which one devotes to windy consultations.

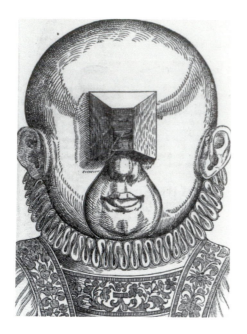

94. Mask for cross-eye. Woodcut from Bartisch, *Ophthalmolodouleia Das Ist Augendienst* (1583). In this heavily illustrated work Bartisch provided the first extensively illustrated account of any surgical specialty. *(Jeremy Norman & Co., Inc.)*

Wurtz's development of close observance of wounds and their daily changes was a most important contribution in the evolution of wound treatment. He was particularly conservative in the practice of operative surgery and emphasized this approach in his writings:

> Never, if you can help it, bereave a man of any part; for God's grace may be great upon it beyond the expectation of men.

The first great book on eye surgery, *Opthalmolodouleia Das Ist Augendienst* (1583), was written in vernacular German by George Bartisch (1535-1606). Bartisch, considered the founder of modern ophthalmology, was the first to practice the extirpation of the globe in cancer of the eye. Originally an intinerant barber-surgeon, through dint of his own personality, industry, and specialization in eye diseases and hernias, Bartisch became court oculist and surgeon in Dresden. His work is all the more striking because of the elaborate woodcuts that accompany the text, which provide a comprehensive "picture book" of Renaissance ophthalmologic surgery. Some of the woodcuts demonstrate the parts of the eye, lying successively one on top of the other, by means of superimposed flaps of the book. Among the scenes depicted are a patient, who is tied in a chair, being readied for an operation; the steps involved in cataract removal; and the perforated or stenopeic spectacles, or visors, used for strabismus.

95. Amputation scene on the title page of Walther Ryff's *Die Grosse Chirurgei* (Frankfurt, 1545). Printed in red and black, this scene appears to be a realistic depiction of the physician, the surgeon, and the surgeon's assistant. The patient, however, does not seem to feel what must have been excruciating pain. *(Jeremy Norman & Co., Inc.)*

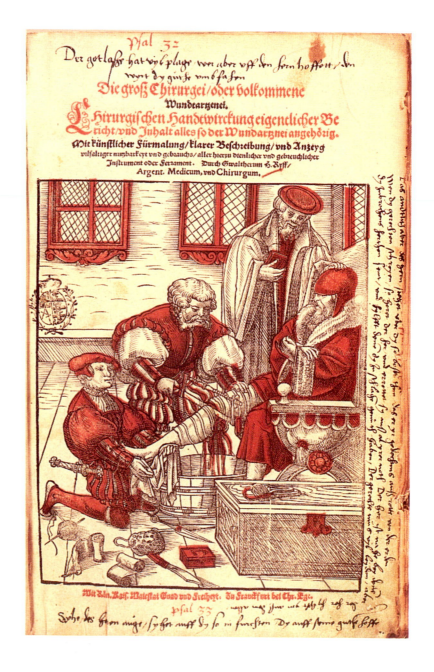

ITALY

The Renaissance in Italy was an age of repeated political invasions. In 1494 Charles VIII of France made himself Master of Naples. Although he was soon to withdraw from the area, his military action demonstrated that the separated city-states of Italy were easy to conquer. Subsequently both French and Spanish kings began to seize various pieces of Italian territory as they pleased. Over the next two centuries Italy was repeatedly invaded by monarchs and petty princes. Gradually the old families who had ruled during the zenith of the city-states died out.

In Venice, one of the era's most important trading and publishing centers, the first printed collection of the works of different writers on surgery was issued. The *Cyrurgia* (1490) contained the surgical writings of Albucasis, Avicenna, and Guy de Chauliac. A much more complete collection was the Venice folio of 1498, to which the works of Lanfranc, Roger, and Theodoric were added. The edition of 1546, considered the best, also contained the treatises of Roland and William of Saliceto.

Italian surgeons, unlike their generally illiterate Germanic-speaking counterparts, were often university educated and sometimes attained academic distinction. The vigorous rivalry between the itinerant barber-surgeons and their more sophisticated surgical peers was not readily apparent. Giovanni de Vigo (1460-1525), surgeon to Pope Julius II (1443-1513), was the first Italian Renaissance surgeon to write an account of gunshot injuries and their treatment. The son of

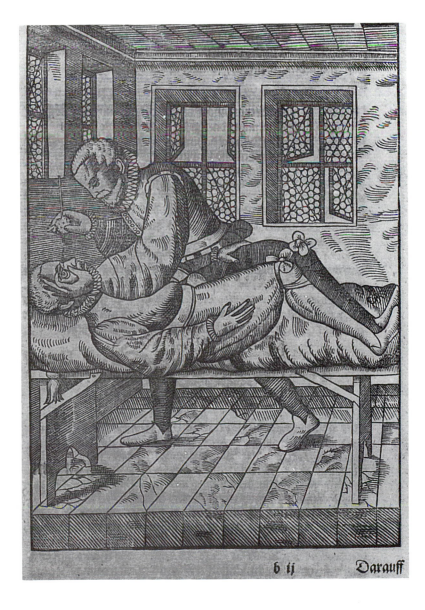

96. Couching for cataract. Woodcut from Bartisch's comprehensive account of Renaissance eye surgery, *Ophthalmolodouleia Das Ist Augendienst* (1583). *(Jeremy Norman & Co., Inc.)*

a surgeon, de Vigo became the outstanding compiler of surgical works during the early Renaissance. Consequently his masterpiece, *Practica In Arte Chirurgica Copiosa Continens Novem Libros* (1514), provides the most detailed portrait of European surgery as it existed at the end of the fifteenth century.

De Vigo's treatise, which was printed in more than 40 editions and translated into 7 different languages, was the first complete system of surgery to be found in Europe after that of Guy de Chauliac. Part of the work's great success can be attributed to its account of gunshot wounds and to the section on the "new" disease, syphilis. The treatise was best suited for a practitioner who knew little about anatomy and was not particularly interested in performing surgical procedures. De Vigo's was a surgery of ointments, salves, and plaster dressings.

De Vigo taught that gunshot wounds were poisoned burns and should therefore be treated initially with a dressing of boiling oil or an actual cautery. Much to his credit, he advocated the use of ligatures, by passing a needle beneath the vein and tightening the thread from above, for the control of hemorrhage.

Guido Guidi (1508-1569), in Latin, Vidius, followed de Vigo as the leading surgeon during the Italian Renaissance. He was born in Florence and obtained much of his professional education in his native city. Through happenstance King Francis I of France invited Guidi to improve surgery in Paris and its environs. Guidi received a great welcome from the French king, was appointed professor of surgery at the College of France, and became the king's personal physician. Guidi thus usurped the position of some of France's leading surgeons, especially Jean Tagault (?-1545), and Guidi's stay was embittered by the antagonism of the faculty of medicine at the university. In 1544 Guidi wrote *Chirurgia E Graeco In Latinum Conversa,* a translation of an illustrated Byzantine manuscript

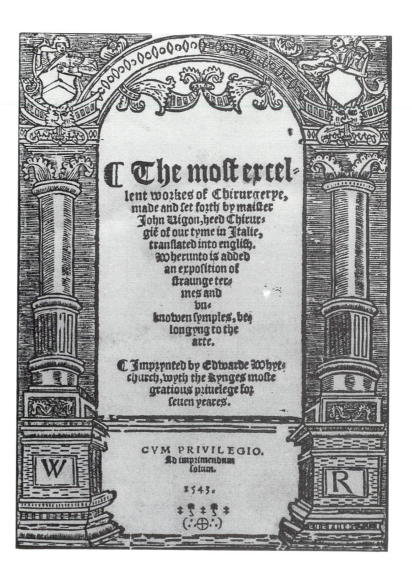

97. Woodcut title page of the first English translation of Vigo's *Practica In Arte Chirurgica* as it appeared in London in 1543. In the archaic spelling of the time, here modernized, the translation bills the author as "head surgeon of our time in Italy" and promises to add to his text "an exposition of strange terms and unknown simples (pharmaceutical remedies) belonging to the art of surgery." *(Jeremy Norman & Co., Inc.)*

154

containing surgical works of Hippocrates, Galen, and Oribasius, and added commentaries of his own. Much of the work concerned fractures and dislocations. The book's magnificent woodcut illustrations were probably redrawn by the mannerist, Primaticcio, perhaps with the participation of other Italian masters. As expected, the book was dedicated to Francis I and published with the consent of the Pope.

Guidi remained in Paris until the death of the king in 1547, when he returned to Italy as professor of philosophy and medicine at Pisa. In addition, he became a chief magistrate of that city. Guidi remained in Pisa until his death. Much of his work was published posthumously, particularly his anatomical study, *De Anatomia Corporis Humani Libri VII* (1611). Although Guidi maintains an important place in the history of surgery for his efforts in promoting surgery in France and for fostering awareness of Greek and Latin authorities, his memory is particularly preserved in the names of anatomical structures he described, such as the Vidian artery, canal, nerve, and vein.

Marianus Sanctus Barolitanus (1490-1550), known as Mariano Santo of Barletta, achieved fame as a lithotomist. He was said to have been a pupil of de Vigo and the first to have written a description of lateral lithotomy and the "apparatus magnus." The apparatus magnus was a device that allowed for the extraction of a urinary bladder calculus through an incision in the perineum after a

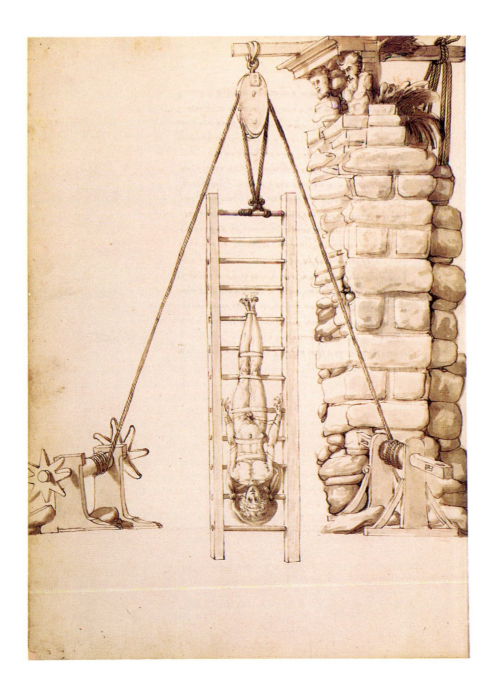

98. Reduction of a fracture or of a deviation of the vertebral column according to a method used since antiquity. For reduction of fractures Hippocrates recommended the mechanical devices used here. The patient is hung upside down to facilitate the return of the vertebrae to their normal position and is then moved up and down by the block-and-tackle system. Even in the ancient world mechanical devices were notably applied for orthopedic purposes. This manuscript drawing is part of a transcription made for Guido Guidi in Rome of a collection of surgical treatises collected from ancient and Byzantine authors by Nicétas toward the middle of the eleventh century. The painting is now attributed to Francesco Salviati. *(Phot. Bibliothèque Nationale Paris, Mss Gr 2247, f 210v.)*

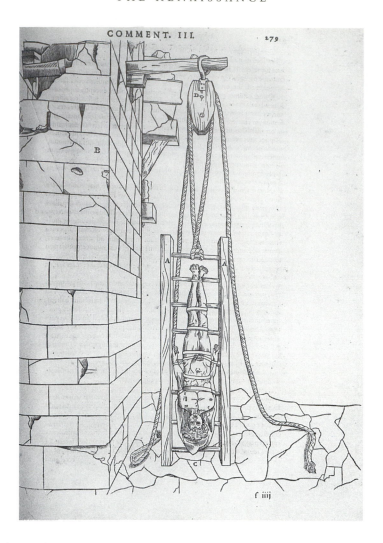

99. Around 1540 Guido Guidi made a Latin translation of an illustrated surgical manuscript. Guidi had an elegant edition of his translation published as *Chirurgia E Graeco In Latinum Conversa* in Paris in 1544. This is a page from his printed text. *(Jeremy Norman & Co., Inc.)*

grooved sound, or director, had initially been passed into the organ via the urethra. This description was given in *De Lapide Renum Liber Et De Lapide Ex Vesica Per Incisionem Extrahendo* (1535). Santo was unique in studying and writing about the operation for bladder stone and effectively legitimized that surgical procedure. As a result, he removed the operation from the hands of the wandering quacks and stonecutters who had previously monopolized its performance.

One of the most perceptive Italian surgeons of the Renaissance was Michael Angelus Blondus (Biondi) (1497-1565). In his little-known treatise *De Partibus Ictu Sectis* (1542), which was partially reprinted in Gesner's anthology, Blondus recommended the use of simple water and wetted lint in the dressing of wounds and contusions. He apparently wanted to allow nature to pursue its own course of healing and thus avoided the application of irritating drugs and other harmful substances to wounds.

Bartholomaeus Maggius (1516-1552) of Bologna wrote of gunshot wounds. He held the chair of anatomy and surgery at the medical school in his native city and later in his career accepted the position of private physician to Pope Julius III (?-1555). In the year before Maggius's death he showed experimentally that gunshot wounds were neither burned nor poisonous. In a novel series of experiments he fired balls at bags of gunpowder, which did not explode, and arrows tipped with wax or sulfur, which neither melted nor ignited. Thus Maggius disproved the traditional theory of wound combustion. These results were published posthumously by his brother in *De Vulnerum Sclopetorum Et Bombardorum Globulis Illatorum* (1552).

Giovanni Andrea Della Croce (1514-1575) propagated many concepts of de Vigo and Guidi. Della Croce was born in Venice; little information is available about his professional life. It is believed that he practiced surgery in his native city, where he was familiar with and made extensive use of the methods of Paré. Paré's methods had been brought back to Italy by Guidi and were to guide the further development of Italian surgery.

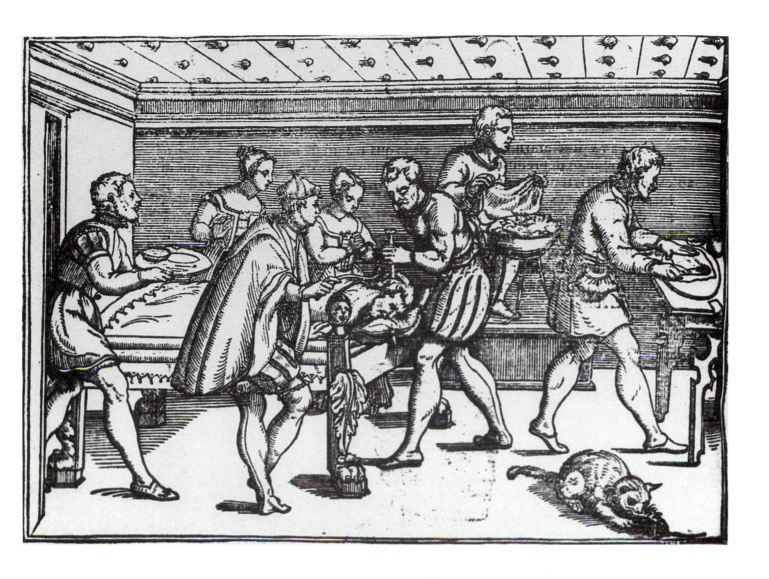

Della Croce's major written works, *Chirurgiae Libri Septem* and *Chirurgiae Universalis Opus Absolutum,* were both published in 1573. Neither work demonstrated much originality. Rather, they were compilations of previous authors arranged in historical sequence. Numerous illustrations of surgical instruments were given, and particular attention was paid to surgical techniques. Della Croce's work also contained the first illustration of a neurosurgical operation. In fashion typical of Italian surgeons of the period, Della Croce did not give Paré adequate credit for many of his concepts and techniques, partly because Italian surgeons preferred not to acknowledge the contributions of a French peer.

Carcano Leone (1536-1606) was born to wealthy parents in Milan. His medical studies were obtained in Pavia and finally in Padua, where his mentor was Fallopius. Most of Leone's professional life was spent in Milan, where he directed a medical school of his own and practiced for 28 years. Leone's reputation rests mainly on his treatise, *De Vulneribus Capitis Liber Absolutissimus Triplici Sermone Contentus,* which was published in 1583. The work concerned wounds of the head and revealed Leone's extensive knowledge of surgery and his ability to cope with such serious problems.

Gaspare Tagliacozzi (1547-1599) has been called the father of plastic surgery. He was born in Bologna into an affluent and respected family. He studied medicine in his native city, where the well-known Girolamo Cardano (1501-1576) was his mentor, and received his degree in 1570. Tagliacozzi taught surgery and anatomy at his alma mater until his death. His highly successful career included election to public office and the accumulation of a large amount of real estate and personal property.

100. This highly realistic scene of a craniotomy is the earliest depiction of a neurosurgical operation in progress. It was published in Venice in 1573 in *Chirurgiae . . . Libri Septem* by Giovanni Andrea Della Croce. The surgeon apparently had many sources of distraction in the course of the operation. *(National Library of Medicine, Bethesda, Md.)*

101. The surgeon and his book. Portrait of Gaspare Tagliacozzi, attributed to Tiburzio Passarotti. Tagliacozzi is shown with several copies of his masterpiece on plastic surgery, *De Curtorum Chirurgia Per Institionem* (1597), some with pages open to the section on rhinoplasty. The richness of Tagliacozzi's costume reflects his wealth and social status. *(Putti's Donation of the Istituto Ortopedico Rizzoli, Bologna.)*

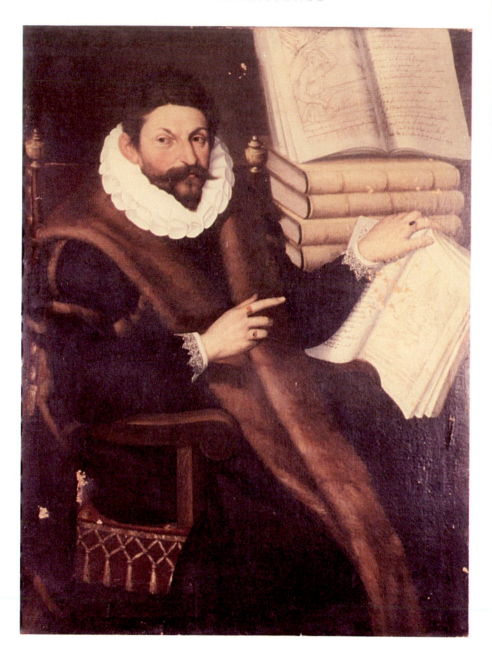

Although it would be historically incorrect to assert that Tagliacozzi actually founded the specialty of plastic surgery, he deserves credit for bringing the art of reconstructive surgery to a high level of respectability in the sixteenth century. During the late Middle Ages and throughout the Renaissance many reputable surgeons tended to shy away from performing major elective operations. For particular operations this void was filled by irregular, itinerant operators known collectively as "incisors" or "cutters." As roving mountebanks, they were able to search more widely for opportunities to operate than was the university-educated physician or surgeon. More important, they were able to escape that era's harsh penalties for surgical failure by fleeing a town before a patient died. These individuals tended to be crude, illiterate men with no code of ethics.

As in all fields of endeavor, there were exceptions to the rule: certain itinerant families developed great skill in performing individual operations and became recognized for their surgical abilities. For reconstruction of nasal and ear injuries the Brancas, father and son, of Catania, Sicily, developed an operative technique early in the fifteenth century. How these men obtained such knowledge remains historical conjecture. However, other individuals and families (such as the Bojani, Mongitore, Norcini, Pavoni, and Vivaneo families) were performing operations in the same vicinity and may have shared such information in return for learning other operative techniques.

The senior Branca took skin flaps for a new nose from the skin of the forehead. This procedure, brought to prominence by Sushruta, was known as the Indian method. Antonio, the son, refined the art by extending the procedure to the restoration of lips and ear. In so doing he apparently invented the method of obtaining skin from the arm by means of the pedicled-flap technique, which became the hallmark of Italian plastic surgery during the late Renaissance.

The need for reconstructive plastic procedures was great in sixteenth-century Italy, since facial mutilations occurred frequently as a result of traumatic injuries, dueling, and the cosmetic ravages of syphilis. As a natural consequence, pupils of the Brancas carried a knowledge of such methods to the Bojani and Vivaneo families in Calabria. It is believed that Tagliacozzi learned his operative techniques from one of these families. It has also been suggested that he was first made aware of the operation after it had been performed by Giulio Cesare Aranzio (1530-1589), professor of anatomy at Bologna.

Tagliacozzi was a careful observer and skillful in his operative techniques. In 1597 he wrote *De Curtorum Chirurgia Per Institionem*. In this volume on surgery for mutilations by means of grafting, he described in exacting detail specific operative methods, and numerous illustrations accompanied the text. The 22 full-page woodcuts depicted the individual steps of various operations through the postoperative stage, as well as Tagliacozzi's instrumentation. In most instances Tagliacozzi's treatment of nasal defects was accomplished in six sessions over 2 months. A skin pedicle from the inner upper arm was swung up and fixed to the nose. By means of an ingenious leather band the arm was tied, with the hand to the top of the head. A similar technique was developed for restoring a defective outer ear by taking the necessary skin from behind it.

As Tagliacozzi's reputation spread, his surgical clinic attracted patients and visiting surgeons from all over Europe. He was not without his critics, however, especially since the Catholic church had taken a firm stand against any improvement in human appearance, which was considered a blasphemy against God. Many of Tagliacozzi's conservative peers, including Ambroise Paré (1510-1590) and Fallopius, were relentless in their criticism of his skills and attacked his appropriation of the Branca operation.

The verbal assault on Tagliacozzi continued after his death. He was initially buried in the cloister of San Giovanni Battista in Bologna. However, his adversaries managed to convince the nuns that Tagliacozzi was in hell and would haunt the place eternally. Subsequently his body was exhumed and reburied in unholy ground beyond the walls of the city. Eventually the Tagliacotian method was lost; reconstructive surgery went into decline and was not revived until the early nineteenth century.

The last great Italian Renaissance surgeon was Hieronymus Fabricius ab Aquapendente (1533-1620). Fabricius, the most famous student of Fallopius, followed his mentor into the professorship of anatomy at Padua. Fabricius was born to a family of modest means in Aquapendente, a village near Orvieto, about midway between Rome and Siena. His academic career was marked by brilliant achievement and recognition primarily related to anatomical research.

Fabricius had so many pupils that at his own expense he built in Padua the first known permanent anatomical amphitheater. Later (1594), the Senate of Venice, which then included the city of Padua, built a larger, more elaborate structure and arranged that the name of Fabricius be affixed to its entrance. Fabricius made many anatomical and physiologic observations; the most important of these was his study of the venous valves. Although the venous valves had been described previously, Fabricius made the first complete study of their structure and function. The studies of Fabricius played an integral part in the future professional direction of his pupil, William Harvey (1578-1657), who lived in Fabricius's house while he studied medicine in Padua and was to become the dominant figure in seventeenth-century medicine and physiology.

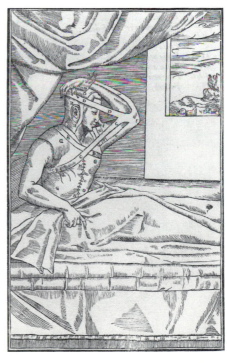

102. The so-called Italian method of rhinoplasty, reconstruction of the nose by means of a flap of skin taken from the arm, which was first described by Gaspare Tagliacozzi. The Italian method is distinct from the much older Hindu method of rhinoplasty, in which a forehead flap is pulled down. Woodcut from Tagliacozzi's *De Curtorum Chirurgia Per Institionem* (1597), which also described treatment of other mutilations by means of grafting. *(Jeremy Norman & Co., Inc.)*

159

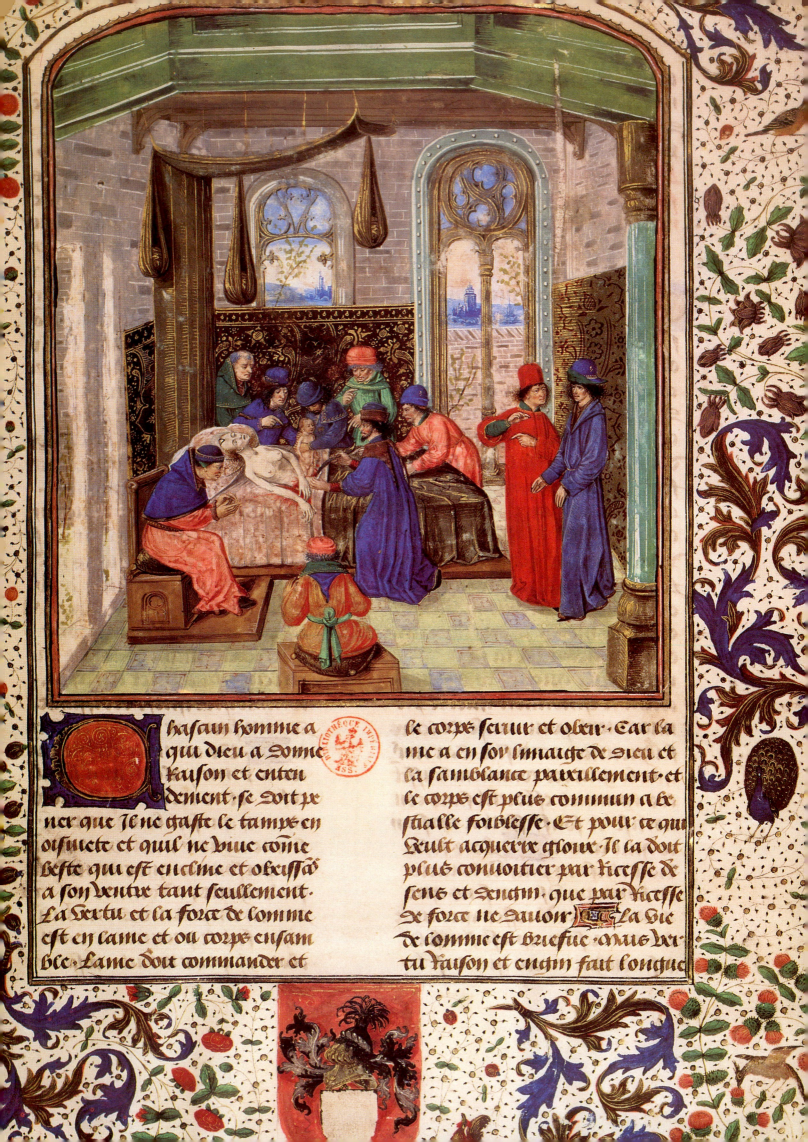

Chascun homme a
qui dieu a donne
raison et enten
dement se doit pe
ner que il ne gaste le tampz en
oisiuete et quil ne viue come
beste qui est encline et obeyssant
a son ventre tant seullement.
La vertu et la force de lomme
est en lame et ou corps ensam
ble. Lame doit commander et

le corps seruir et obeir. Car la
me a en soy ymaige de dieu et
la samblance pareillement et
le corps est plus commun a be
stialle foiblesse. Et pour ce qui
veult acquerre gloire Il la doit
plus conuoitier par richesse de
sens et scauoir que par richesse
de force ne sauoir. La vie
de lomme est briefue. mais ver
tu raison et engin fait longue

In the midst of his many endeavors Fabricius was also an influential, successful practitioner and teacher of surgery. He was reputed to be quite conservative, apparently disliking the needless use of operative therapy. Fabricius attached great importance to the teachings of Celsus and Paul of Aegina. He criticized the method of castration in hernia repair and stressed the importance of maintaining hemostasis during surgical procedures. Fabricius attempted to improve the technique of tracheotomy and referred to animal sutures in the treatment of intestinal wounds. He invented orthopedic apparatuses for the treatment of torticollis, spinal curvatures, and deformities of the feet.

Most of Fabricius's surgical thinking was recorded in his *Pentateuchos Chirurgicum* (1592), which was edited against his will by Johann Hartmann Beyer (1563–1625). The treatise contained descriptions of tumors, wounds, ulcers, fistulae, fractures, and dislocations. The work was reissued in 1617 as Fabricius's *Opera Chirurgica,* which systematically discussed all afflictions from head to foot and appropriate surgical interventions.

Cesarean section came to be recognized during the Renaissance as an important adjunct to obstetrical care and a surgical operation in its own right. Although known for at least 2000 years, cesarean section became a widely accepted procedure only because of the efforts of a Venetian monk, Scipione Mercurio (1540–1616). Much of the resistance to this surgical operation stemmed from the Church's doctrine of the preservation of life from conception.

Both Mercurio and his mentor, Giulio Cesare Aranzi (1530–1589), were interested in pelvic constriction. To study its variations, both of them dissected the dead bodies of pregnant women, and in Mercurio's work, *La Commare O Raccoglitrice* (1595), the first mention is made of pelvic contraction as an indication for cesarean section. One of the chapters provided a detailed description of the operation:

> . . . the surgeon . . . cuts along the line . . . reaching the deep fat of the abdomen by the incision, and making the incision about half a foot long, a little more or a little less . . . When the first incision is made he sees the body of the rectus muscle and he cuts it until he reaches the peritoneum; when the latter is opened one sees the uterus, which likewise must be cut, but lightly, so as not to injure the child; in cutting it one takes care to begin the incision in the upper part and make it run crosswise in order not to cut its testicles, and the epididymides, and spermatic vessels. When that has been done successfully the child is taken out at once, together with the afterbirth . . . let there be in readiness . . . the decoction of artemisia, agrimony, betony, mallow, leaves or flowers of pomegranate, and dried roses . . . sedge, and sweet-smelling bulrushes; this decoction is made in sour black wine . . . it is then strained and to the filtrate are added two pounds of . . . water . . . it is then boiled again, and in it is dipped a folded cloth . . . and when it has been so moistened the incision is fomented several times, because such a decoction has the property of stopping the flow of copious blood and strengthens the part. Then with the sponge . . . cleanse the uterus, inside and out . . . When this is done the uterus will at once return to place . . . prepare to sew up the abdomen . . . use the finger to compress the intestine . . . be careful to keep the wound covered with doubled warm cloths dipped in the decoction . . . The abdomen is sewed up with few stitches, like other sutures performed in any part of the body.

103. *Facing page,* an extraordinarily realistic painting of a cesarean section in a French illuminated manuscript from the end of the fifteenth century. While the surgeon holds his knife, one aide holds the mother's legs and the other pulls out the baby. The painting also accurately portrays a bedroom in a medieval castle. Although the operation had been performed for at least 2000 years, it was not recognized by the medical establishment until the second half of the sixteenth century. *(Phot. Bibliothèque Nationale Paris, Ms Fr cesarean section.)*

SPAIN

By the late fifteenth century most of the independent kingdoms in Spain had become united as a single, powerful country. Ferdinand V (1452-1516) and Isabella I (1451-1504), who were Roman Catholics, wanted to make Spain a wholly Catholic country, a desire that led to the beginning of the Spanish Inquisition (1480). The especially harsh regime of the Inquisition treated Jews and Islamic Moors with particular cruelty. The Spaniards persecuted the Jews and drove them out of Spain. In 1492, Spanish troops defeated the Moors at Granada, and the monarchs' wishes for a totally Catholic regime were achieved.

In 1492 Ferdinand and Isabella gave Christopher Columbus (1446-1506) the funding to make the voyage on which he discovered America. Soon afterward, Spanish explorers claimed the territories that now include Central America, South America except Brazil, Mexico, and land that was to become the states of California, New Mexico, and Texas. Spanish conquests grew especially bold during the following decades, and Spanish rule was extended to North Africa and to Naples and Parma in Italy. As a consequence of a royal marriage Spain inherited the Netherlands in 1506; Spain claimed the Philippines in 1521 and conquered Portugal in 1580.

Spain's era of glory was relatively short. The populace of the Netherlands revolted against Spanish subjugation in 1568 and declared their independence in 1581. Philip II (1527-1598) sent his armada of 130 warships to an inglorious defeat against the English (1588). By the end of the sixteenth century Spain had become little more than a second-class power.

The development of surgery in Renaissance Spain was not particularly significant, and there were few notable Spanish surgeons. Not until the sixteenth century were any signs of substantive progress evident, and most progress was made in medicine, not surgery. The first important Spanish surgeon of the sixteenth century was Francisco Arceo (Arcaeus) (1493-1573). Little information is available about his schooling and professional life. He was known to have acquired great fame for his skill in treating both surgical and internal maladies. Arceo believed in the immediate healing of a wound without suppuration, restricted the use of sutures, and is believed to have performed numerous trephinations. His most famous surgical work, *De Recta Curandorum Vulnerum Ratione,* was published posthumously in Antwerp in 1574.

Dionisio Daza Chacon (1503-?1580) was born at Valladolid, about 100 miles north of Madrid. He obtained his medical education at the universities in his native city and in Salamanca. Initially Chacon was in the private practice of medicine, but he eventually joined the army of Charles V as a military surgeon. At two seiges, at Landrecy (1543) and Saint Dizier (1544), he obtained extensive experience in the treatment of gunshot and arrow wounds. In 1545 he returned to Spain with then-Archduke Maximilian (1527-1576), cousin of Charles V, later the Holy Roman Emperor, whose personal surgeon he became. Two years later Chacon distinguished himself by rendering valuable service in his native city to victims of the plague. After he decided to remain in his hometown, he was appointed surgeon-in-chief of the hospital in Valladolid. For 6 years he served in that post, finally accepting the position of private physician to the son of Philip II. Four years later Chacon accepted the appointment as private physician to Prince Don Juan of Austria, natural brother of Philip II. Chacon accompanied the prince on various voyages and served at the battle of Lepanto (1571).

Chacon's major written work was *Practica Y Teorica De Cirugia, En Romance Y En Latin* (1600), the most exhaustive Spanish work on surgery written during the Renaissance. Chacon preferred the iron cautery, not ligatures, for his amputations. He did not consider gunshot wounds poisonous, and after 1544 he discontinued the use of boiling oil as immediate treatment.

Bartolome Hidalgo De Aguero (1531-1597) is commonly acknowledged as the father of modern Spanish surgery. He was lecturer on surgery at Seville and gained wide experience in the treatment of battlefield wounds. Like many of his

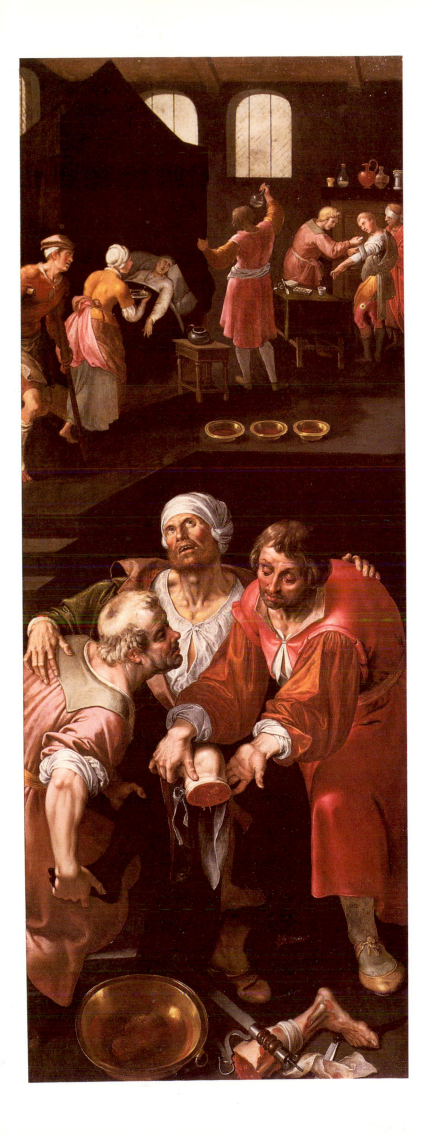

104. Sts. Cosmas and Damian are prepared to transplant the leg of an Islamic Moor onto a recent amputee. The contrast between this late sixteenth-century painting by Ambrosius Francken and an earlier version of the same legend (Plate 57) is evident. Of interest in the foreground are the amputation saw and instruments. Does the artist mean to suggest that Sts. Cosmas and Damian performed the amputation? In the background are a cripple, a patient in a sickbed, a physician examining a urine flask, and another surgeon treating a wounded man. *(Koninklijk Museum voor Schone Kunsten, Plaatsnijdersstraat 2 B-2000 Antwerpen.)*

fellow Spanish surgeons, De Aguero believed that wounds healed best by first intention. His major written work was *Tesoro De La Verdadera Cirugia, Y Via Particular Contra La Comun Opinion* (1584).

FRANCE

Before the Renaissance the French kings had gained considerable influence over the Catholic church. Consequently Francis I (1494-1547) had no interest in supporting the Reformation. Nonetheless, Protestantism did attract many followers among the lower classes. After 1540 the Protestants were severely persecuted, but the Calvinists, known as Huguenots, could not be suppressed. They gained considerable political influence, especially among the nobility and the rich merchants who joined them in protesting the persecutory rule of the crown. Ongoing conflicts between the Huguenots and Roman Catholics culminated in a series of brutal civil wars from 1562 to 1598. The most infamous attack occurred in Paris on St. Bartholomew's Day in 1572, when thousands of Huguenots were massacred.

After the coronation of Henry of Navarre as Henry IV (1553-1610), first of the Bourbon kings (1589), the internecine fighting ended. Henry, who had served as Protestant leader in the War of the Three Henrys, converted to Catholicism in 1593. Five years later, he issued the Edict of Nantes, giving the Huguenots the right to worship.

European surgery during the Renaissance owed much to France, primarily through the efforts of Pierre Franco (1500-1561) and Ambroise Paré, whose achievements were especially impressive because both men rose from poverty and neither was university educated. In the highly stratified society of the time lack of university education usually prevented individuals from obtaining important standing in medicine or surgery. Franco was trained mostly by itinerant lithotomists, cataract couchers, and herniotomists, whereas Pare emerged from the ranks of the barber-surgeons.

During the sixteenth century the barber-surgeons had clearly moved beyond the legal limitations that had earlier been placed on their clinical practice. They came to be known euphemistically as the "surgeons of the short gowns," in contradistinction to the "long-gown" or academic surgeons of the College of St. Côme. For reasons not entirely clear, the barber-surgeons' guild grew much more rapidly than the College of St. Côme. The elitist, exclusive attitude of the College restricted its membership.

During the late Middle Ages the barber-surgeons' guild, on average, had about 40 "masters," whereas an average of 10 "master" surgeons belonged to the College of St. Côme. By the late Renaissance St. Côme expanded to a membership of 30 "masters," whereas the barber-surgeons' guild grew to include almost 300 members. For the average Parisian the barber-surgeon of the "short gown" was a much more accessible, pleasant, and familiar figure than his academic "long-gown" counterpart. As a consequence, the lay public gradually elevated the barber-surgeons to the status of the "long-gown" surgeons. Eventually, although the barber-surgeons did not have equivalent social status or academic rank, the public recognized them to have superior skills.

In the sixteenth century the first teaching given in French to barber-surgeons was by Jean Canappe (1495-?1552). While serving as physician to Francis I (1494-1547), Canappe translated Guy de Chauliac's works into French (1537). Canappe's avowed purpose was to aid the barber-surgeons against the opposition of the more educated university surgeons:

> I have no thought of foisting my French translations upon those who know Greek and Latin: I interpret for others, for those who, though unacquainted with those tongues, follow the profession of surgery and who daily and unremittingly go their rounds curing maladies. Now cures are wrought by virtue to acquaintance with things, no words, things that are just as easily understood in French as in any other

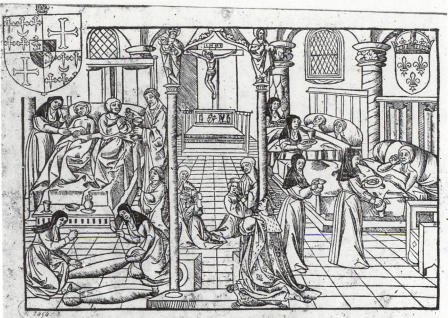

105. A ward of the Paris hospital, l'Hôtel Dieu (House of God), as it appeared on this fund-raising broadside from the early sixteenth century. Death existed closely with life in this institution run by nuns. In the foreground, *left,* two nuns in close proximity to patients in their sickbeds are shown wrapping the dead in shrouds. The text of the broadside may be roughly translated as follows:

Greetings from the Patriarch of Bourges to benefactors of the Hôtel Dieu.

Because of the poverty of the times, the nurses at the Hôtel Dieu do not have enough food to feed the patients and are asking for donations. Those people from the Hôtel Dieu who have been authorized by the church may place trunks and coffers for donations in designated churches on the designated day. Those who bring in donations will be pardoned for their sins. If those who want to bring in donations on the designated day are sick or disabled, Mass can be performed in a consecrated area of the house that is not normally used for drinking, eating, or sleeping. Anyone who interferes with this edict will be prosecuted. The designated day is from the first vespers of Easter said at noon up to and including the second vespers.

(Phot. Bibliothèque Nationale, Paris.)

language. I make bold to state that I have known many surgeons, unequipped with either Greek or Latin, but tireless in applying their minds to matters germane to their art, who were comparable, if not superior, as gauged by results, to hosts of other men, who look upon themselves as quite the thing in letters Greek and Latin. I would not have you mistake my meaning—I am not disparaging those languages nor calling them useless hindrances. I would that every student were well versed in them; it would relieve us from this labor of translation.

In attempting to elevate the status of the barber-surgeon, Canappe's efforts served as a model for the work of Paré, which would soon follow. Another French academic surgeon who authored a work expressly for the barber-surgeon was Jacques Dalechamps (1513–1588). His 933-page *Chirurgie Francoise* (1569), however, was by no means confined to the everyday practice of the French surgeons of his time. Dalechamps acknowledged Paré as the ranking surgeon in France and reproduced instruments that Paré had devised. Dalechamps's work was especially significant, since he had academic ranking, whereas Paré was a mere barber-surgeon. Dalechamps was among the first to recognize that surgical textbooks written in the vernacular were needed so that surgical training might be accessible to those who had not studied Latin as part of a university education.

The controversies in France among itinerant surgeon, barber-surgeon, and university-educated surgeon and between physician and surgeon were more intense than in any other European country. That Dalechamps could recognize Paré, a barber-surgeon, as the foremost surgeon in France, with Franco, an upstart itinerant, not far behind, was an important step in the eventual decision of the universities to make a university education available to men of the lower classes. It was obvious, at least to Dalechamps, that a positive future for French surgery depended on the outstanding barber-surgeons. The bitter rivalry between surgeon and medical practitioner was becoming so great that the profession of surgery could not afford to be divided in its own ranks by petty differences. By publicly demonstrating his recognition of these problems, Dalechamps earned his place in history as a pragmatist and realist who made a positive contribution to the advancement of French surgery.

To understand the importance of Franco, it is crucial that the role of the itinerant "cutter," or "incisor," be fully appreciated. Most medieval and Renaissance surgery concerned the dressing of wounds and the cure of ulcers. Actual operative surgery, such as herniotomy, lithotomy, nasal reconstruction, cataract couching, and anal fistulectomy, was shunned by the recognized leaders of the craft. The admittedly poor results, including frequent morbidity and mortality, could easily damage one's professional and personal reputation.

The void in surgical care was filled throughout western Europe, especially in Germany, Italy, France, and England, by groups of independent surgical entrepreneurs known as the "cutters" or "incisors." They traveled from place to place, maintaining secrecy as to their methods. Undoubtedly, many of these itinerants promised impossible cures but left behind them misery and death instead. Their fees were often ill-earned, and the itinerants frequently fled before their failures and disasters became evident.

Some of the itinerants, despite their semicriminal associations, began to attain remarkable proficiency in the performance of particular procedures. Certain families gradually gained renown throughout Europe as specialists in the surgical cure of individual diseases. Because most of these itinerant surgeons were illiterate, few of their methods were ever written down, but these crude beginnings of particular operations were eventually learned by more educated surgeons, who described them in their written works.

The Colots family, famed as lithotomists, was the earliest of the well-known itinerant surgical families. It is believed that Laurent Colot (flourished 1525) of Tresnel, France, learned the technique of lateral lithotomy from an itinerant lithotomist named Octavien Da Villa (flourished 1500). Laurent's sons, Laurent and Jean, were also practitioners of the operative procedure. A grandson, Philippe (1593-1656), continued the family tradition, as did his son Francois (1630-1706). Francois wrote an account of the method *(Traité De L'Operation De La Taille),* which was published after his death in 1727. Although the details of the Colots family's methods had been published by both Marianus Sanctus and Franco, the operation of lateral lithotomy apparently remained largely unused by other surgeons for more than two centuries as a result of the deficient education of surgeons in those times and their resistance to surgical innovation.

To the class of itinerant lithotomists belongs an unknown surgeon of the early sixteenth century from the region of Genoa. He is alluded to in written histories of that city and is said to have introduced an iron rod into the urethra and the bladder. There it struck the calculus, after which the surgeon would incise the perineum and remove the stone. Other famed lithotomists and herniotomists were the Norcinis of Italy, including Horace and Ulysses of Norsia. Eventually the Norcinis, as they were known, gained considerable experience in the diagnosis and treatment of genitourinary diseases, including urethrotomy for stricture.

The most famous of the French "incisors" was Pierre Franco (1500-1561). He was born in Provence of poor parents. Because of his background, Franco never received a formal education but was apprenticed either to an "incisor" or to a barber-surgeon. Franco was a Huguenot. To avoid the Protestant persecution he left France and accepted the office of city surgeon in the anti-Catholic city of Bern, Switzerland. He held this position and a similar one in Lausanne for 10 years.

During Franco's time in Switzerland his first major written work *(Petit Traité Contenant Une Des Parties Principalles De Chirurgie, Laquelle Les Chirurgiens Herni-éres Exercent)* was published (1556). Subsequently he returned to Orange, France, and wrote his other treatise, *Traité Des Hernies* (1561). The latter work, 544 pages in length, provided the first comprehensive survey of hernia and its operative and nonoperative therapies. Several other important surgical topics, such as genitourinary diseases, ophthalmologic difficulties, traumatic injuries, and fractures and dislocations, including amputations, were also discussed. Franco is presumed to have died shortly after his second book was published.

Franco's treatises reveal him to be a forthright, articulate, and highly religious individual. Although he rose from the ranks of the "incisors," he was adamant in his attempts to remove operative surgery (such as lithotomy and procedures for hernia and cataract) from the domain of the charlatans, itinerant quacks, and "cutters" and place it under the auspices of the regular practitioners (the surgeons of the "short" and "long" gowns). Although Franco accepted the physician's supervision of the surgeon, he was unrelenting in his attacks on those who abused the true art of surgery. He wanted to elevate operative surgery to the status of a respected part of the medical profession:

> I am sure that many will judge this work of mine as superfluous, and me overly bold . . . But I hope that if it please them to understand the reason that impelled me to do so, that they will not only find it not strange, but a work worthy of a Christian, and laudable. Not that I am unaware that the wickedness of many of our craft, accompanied by ignorance, is the reason that this part of surgery is so held in contempt: for being ignorant and knowing themselves so, they proceed nevertheless, without fear of God or man, undertaking to heal all sorts of illnesses, curable and incurable, just so that they can extort money from the poor, simple people, whom they seduce and enchant by their lies and fine words . . . who commit infinite frauds . . . after which they begin by making an incision but are unable to complete the operation . . . Which is the reason that I am constrained to recite here some of the frauds and plunderings which they commit . . .
>
> Does this not subtly despoil the poor and simple people . . . Such people no less deserve corporal punishment by the magistrate than do highwaymen. And it should be the duty of physicians and surgeons to defend their art before the courts, and not to permit further abuse of this art which is of so great importance . . . That is the reason in part, that learned physicians and surgeons call such people vagrants and abusers.

Franco was especially influential because he eagerly operated on patients with hernias and bladder stones, unlike the many well-known surgeons of France who shied away from such technical feats. Franco is believed to be the first surgeon to have described and performed an operation for strangulated hernia. He advised prompt operative intervention once it had become obvious that internally and externally administered medicines had provided little relief, whereas he believed that if the intestine had become gangrenous and the scrotum discolored, any attempt at operation was too late.

Franco usually practiced removal of the testicle as part of a herniorrhaphy. However, he was able to devise an alternative method in which the testis was spared for patients who had but one organ or who had to undergo bilateral hernia repair. His technique of closing the inguinal canal and suturing the internal ring differed only in sophistication from that of a present-day herniorrhaphy.

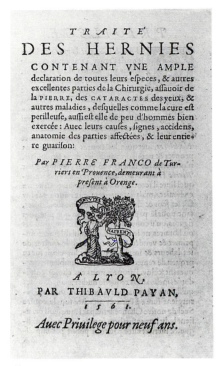

106. Pierre Franco's *Treatise on Hernias* (1561), the first comprehensive survey of the operative and nonoperative therapies for hernia. Like his contemporary, Ambroise Paré, Franco helped elevate surgery from a common trade to the beginnings of a profession. *(Jeremy Norman & Co., Inc.)*

Franco is credited with performing some of the most remarkable lithotomies of his day. He invented a forceps to aid in the crushing and removal of bladder calculus and described a number of instruments for catheterization. In 1556 he performed for the first time a suprapubic cystotomy on a 10-year-old child, a procedure that became well known as the Franconian operation for stone in the bladder:

> I will mention here an experience which I had on one occasion when I tried to remove a calculus from the bladder of a boy about ten years of age. The stone was about as large as a hen's egg and resisted all my efforts to extract it by way of the incision made in the perineum. Being in a quandary as to how I should proceed next, and the parents and friends being greatly demoralized by the suffering . . . I deliberately decided that I would make an opening above the pubic bone, and would remove the stone in this manner. Accordingly, I incised the skin above the pubes, a little to one side of the base of the penis, and carried the knife through the soft tissues down to the calculus, which I had simultaneously pushed upward by pressing the fingers of my left hand against the perineum, while at the same time my assistant made counter-pressure against the stone by firmly compressing the abdominal wall above the object. This method of extraction proved successful. In due time the wounds healed firmly and the patient was relieved of his trouble, but only after a long and most serious illness.

It appears that Franco performed the suprapubic operation only in the particular instance just described. He carefully avoided advising other surgeons to perform that operation because he was concerned about their lack of experience.

Ambroise Paré's (1510-1590) position in the history of surgery remains of supreme importance. He played the major role in reinvigorating and modernizing Renaissance surgery. Pare represents the severing of the final link between surgical thought and techniques of the ancients and the push toward the modern era. He was born in a village near Laval in northwest France, the son of a cabinetmaker. Like Franco, his formal education was meager, and he was apprenticed to various barber-surgeons. His brother Jean also became a barber-surgeon, and their sister Catherine was married to a Parisian barber-surgeon. There is historical speculation that Paré received some of his training in the shops of his brother and brother-in-law.

At 15 years of age Paré went to Paris to complete his indentured education. He attended lectures on anatomy and surgery, did a certain amount of dissecting, and served for more than 2 years as a surgeon's assistant in the leading Paris hospital, the Hôtel Dieu. From 1536 until just before his death Paré was engaged as an army surgeon, accompanying different French armies on their military expeditions or performing surgery in civilian practice in Paris.

Paré's field campaigns started in 1536, when French troops marched into the Cisalpine plain of northern Italy. After the Peace of Nice (1538) he returned to Paris, where he was married and practiced surgery. He recounted his initial experiences as an army surgeon and the inspiration for his first great contribution to clinical surgery:

> In 1536, I accompanied the large army sent to Turin by Francis the First, King of France, to retake certain castles and fortifications which were held at that time by the troops of the Emperor Charles the Fifth. My official position was that of surgeon to the foot soldiers . . . When the fighting was entirely over, we surgeons had much work to do. I had not yet had any personal experience with the treatment of gunshot wounds, but I had read in Giovanni da Vigo's work that such injuries should be considered poisoned wounds, by reason of their contact with gunpowder, and that the correct way of treating such wounds was to cauterize them with oil of sambucus that was actually boiling and to which a little theriaca had been added. At first I hesitated somewhat about carrying out this practice, but after watching the other surgeons, in order to learn exactly how they applied the boiling oil, I plucked up my courage and did exactly what they did. My supply of oil, however, soon gave out, and I then decided to use as a substitute a healing preparation composed of yolk of egg, oil of roses, and turpentine. I slept badly that night, as I greatly feared that, when I came to examine the wounded on the following morning, I should find that those whose

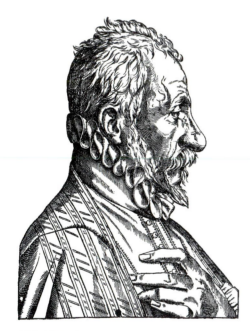

107. Woodcut portrait of Ambroise Paré, as published in the first edition of his *Oeuvres* (Paris, 1575). When his magnum opus appeared, Paré was 65 years old. For all his surgical innovations and proud achievements, Paré always attributed his success with patients to God. His motto was, "Je le pansay. Dieu le guérit," that is, "I treated him. God cured him." Although Paré knew neither Latin nor Greek, he refuted the ancients and their medical treatises. His critique of an eminent professor of the Sorbonne, Etienne Gourmelon, is brief but eminently to the point: "Surgery is to be taught by using the eyes and the hands. You, my little master, know absolutely nothing, except how to mouth your jargon from the heights of a platform." *(Jeremy Norman & Co., Inc.)*

wounds I had failed to treat with boiling oil had died from poisoning. I arose at a very early hour, and was much surprised to discover that the wounds to which I had applied the egg and turpentine mixture were doing well; they were quite free from swelling and from all evidence of inflammatory action; and the patients themselves, who showed no signs of feverishness, said that they had experienced little or no pain and had slept quite well. On the other hand the men to whose wounds I had applied the boiling oil said that they had experienced during the night, and were still suffering from, much pain at the seat of the injury; and I found that they were feverish and that their wounds were inflamed and swollen. After thinking the matter over carefully, I made up my mind that thenceforward I should abstain wholly from the painful practice of treating gunshot wounds with boiling oil.

Although other surgeons had made similar observations about the difficulties inherent in using boiling oil on fresh gunshot wounds, Paré's ability to articulate this finding in both written word and clinical practice brought him lasting fame and glory. In 1541, realizing the importance of proper credentials, he presented himself for and successfully passed a required examination to become a "master barber-surgeon" and a member of the barber-surgeons' guild.

As a result of Paré's initial battlefield experiences and the urgings of Sylvius, Paré authored a short treatise on the treatment of gunshot wounds, *La Méthode De Traicter Les Playes Faictes Par Hacquebutes Et Aultres Bastons A Feu: Et De Celles Qui Sont Faictes Par Fléches, Dardz Et Semblables* (1545). This small practical volume, written largely for Paré's fellow barber-surgeons, was the first in a lifetime of voluminous writings. Besides recounting his military tribulations, Paré described the method of tracing the course of a projectile in the body by having the patient assume the position he was in when the injury occurred.

Paré was strongly convinced of the importance of anatomy as a prerequisite to a surgeon's skills. Consequently, after his return from a second field campaign (1549), he began work on another treatise dealing with surgical anatomy. This work (*Briefve Collection De L'Administration Anatomique,* 1549) was important because it also contained sections on obstetrics in which Paré encouraged a revival of podalic version and had the courage to recommend that artificial labor be induced in cases of uterine hemorrhage.

Paré wrote an epitome of Vesalius's *Fabrica.* By making the work of Vesalius popular and accessible to surgeons, Paré had a major effect on Renaissance surgery. The influence of Vesalius is quite apparent in Paré's anatomical text, *Anatomie Universelle Du Corps Humain* (1561), especially in the illustrations.

Paré's reputation had become so great that he was begrudgingly made a member of the College of St. Côme (1554). Despite at first being refused admission because he had been a barber's apprentice and spoke not in Latin but in the vernacular, Paré gave his inaugural lecture in French and was duly mocked by the envious. His membership, championed by Dalechamps, helped bring about a later union of the barber-surgeons and the surgeons of Saint Côme.

In 1552 Paré again joined the French forces on a military expedition. Paré learned that in performing an amputation it was more efficacious to ligate individual blood vessels than to attempt to control hemorrhage by means of cauterization. In most instances, the free or cut end of a blood vessel was doubly ligated and the ligature was allowed to remain undisturbed in situ until, as the result of local suppuration, it was cast off. Paré described this work in his *Dix Livres De La Chirurgie Avec Le Magasin Des Instruments Nécessaires A Icelle* (1564).

Paré invented several new surgical instruments, including a truss for hernia, as well as artificial limbs and eyes. In addition, he bitterly condemned any surgeon, itinerant or otherwise, who castrated a patient during herniorrhaphy. Paré performed a staphyloplasty, did the first exarticulation of an elbow joint, described fracture of the neck of the femur, and suggested syphilis as a cause of aneurysm. His work in dentistry, including the reimplantation of teeth, the restoration of missing teeth, and the invention of a palatal obturator, is of major significance. Other important topics included a description of carbon monoxide poisoning and a short treatise on medical jurisprudence. Later in life, Paré wrote on nonmedical topics; a discourse on the mummy and the unicorn (1582), for instance, disposed of ancient superstitions about this therapy. His most curious work was a treatise on terrestrial and marine monsters (1573), an early contribution to teratology.

Paré's popularity was such that his position in the world of French surgery could not be ignored. In 1575 his collected works were published in vernacular French, not Latin, which raised the ire of the Faculty of Medicine of the University of Paris. The dean of the medical school attacked Paré for using French instead of Latin and invoked a seldom-used statute stating that no medical works could be published without the express approval of the faculty. Even Paré's fellow surgeons of St. Côme sought unsuccessfully to have publication banned by an act of Parliament. Paré proceeded to write a lengthy denial of the faculty's authority in his *Apologie Et Voyages* (1585), his last work, which was in many aspects an autobiography and revealed much of Paré's true nature.

108. Until Paré's death in 1590 he continued to revise his collected writings, first published in 1575. Four editions were revised by the author, and numerous reprints and translations appeared during the following century. This is the title page of the first English edition, which, as the title page advertises, was made not from a French edition but from a Latin translation. *Ambrose Parey* is the quaint, anglicized spelling of Paré's name. The figures in the operating room scene and the pharmacy shown in the upper panel are portrayed in seventeenth-century dress. At the bottom of the page Paré's instruments, as well as chemical flasks and imaginary creatures that reflect Paré's nonsurgical interests, can be seen. Like many innovators of the Renaissance, Paré combined a modern, empirical scientific spirit with true credulity. The imaginary figures in the lower right corner illustrate his treatise on teratology, in which cases actually observed are mixed with imaginary creatures reported by unreliable sources. *(Jeremy Norman & Co., Inc.)*

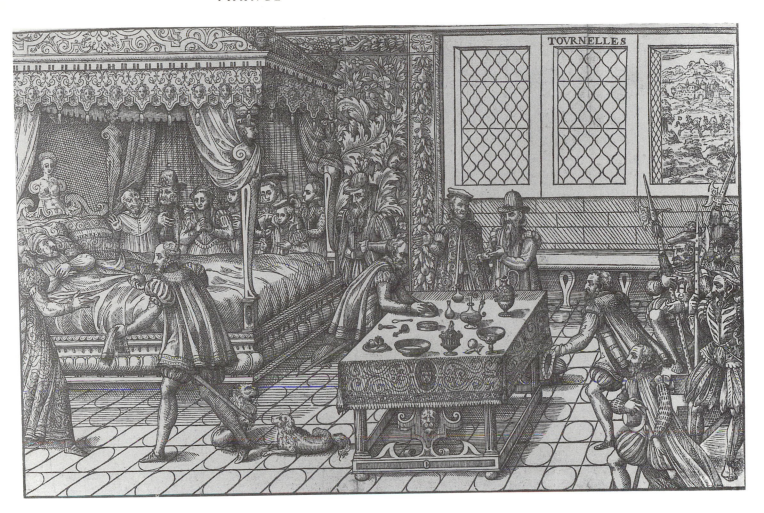

It is a tribute to Paré's remarkable career that he became chief surgeon to four successive kings of France, Henry II, Francis II, Charles IX, and Henry III, the latter giving him the additional title of Councilor to His Majesty. Viewed in the context of Paré's humble background and training as a barber-surgeon, his achievements were overwhelming. Pare demonstrated true humility in his work with his patients and in the world of healing, a humility most evident in his most remembered statement:

Je le pansay. Dieu le guérit.
I treated him. God cured him.

Pare's favorite pupil and son-in-law, Jacques Guillemeau (1550-1613), became an important French surgeon during the Renaissance. He, too, was surgeon to numerous sovereigns, including Charles IX, Henry III, and Henry IV. Guillemeau was appointed surgeon of the Hôtel Dieu and acquired fame as writer, educator, and director of the College of St. Côme. Unusually well educated for a surgeon of his time, he authored three principal works: *Traité Des Maladies De L'Oeil* (1585), the first separate book on ophthalmologic surgery published in French; *La Chirurgie Francaise* (1594), a splendidly illustrated treatise of special importance to dentistry and surgery for cleft lip; and *L'Heureux Accouchement Des Femmes* (1609).

109. Ambroise Paré with Andreas Vesalius at the deathbed of Henry II. The two men stand behind the table, Vesalius on the right. The French king suffered a lance blow above his right eye in a medieval-style tournament with the Count of Montgomery. The fatal accident occurred on June 30, 1559; despite the presence of many medical men, including Paré, the court immediately sent a messenger to Flanders for Vesalius, who was dispatched to Paris on July 2. By July 3, when Vesalius was able to examine the wounded monarch, his condition had deteriorated and Vesalius judged that he would not recover. The king died one week later. This woodcut by Jean Perrissin (circa 1570) is the only sixteenth-century image that brings together two of the greatest medical figures of the era. *(Jeremy Norman & Co., Inc.)*

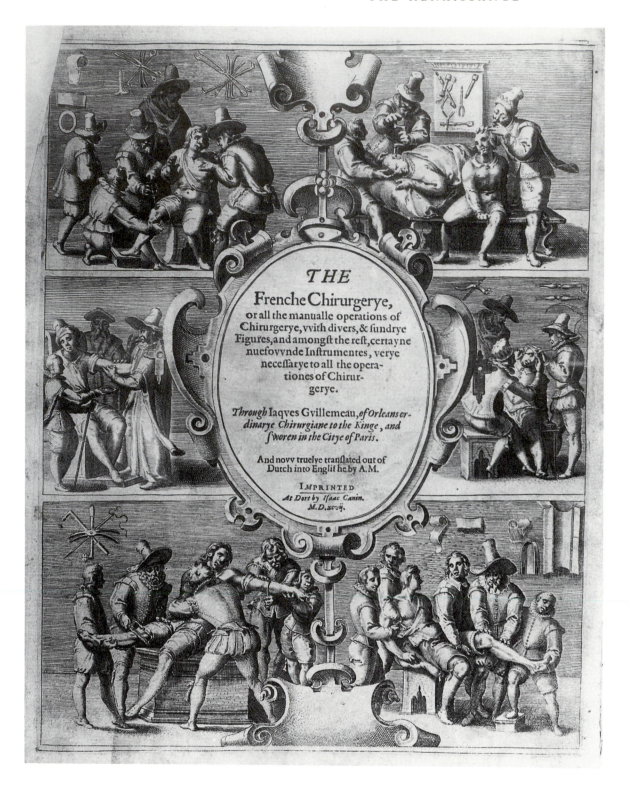

110. Paré's son-in-law, Jacques Guille-meau, learned surgery from the master and made significant contributions to surgery and dentistry himself. This is the title page of an English translation of Guillemeau's major surgical work, originally published in Paris in 1594. The translation, obviously intended for export to the English market, was published in Dordrecht, Holland, in 1597; the copperplate illustrations from the original French edition were used. The engravings on the title page are some of the best operating room scenes from sixteenth-century France. *(Jeremy Norman & Co., Inc.)*

172

ENGLAND AND SCOTLAND

In England the Reformation began with Henry VIII's quarrel with the pope over the king's right to be granted a divorce from his first wife, Catherine of Aragon (1485-1536). The pope refused such a request, and Henry broke with the Catholic church. In an exercise of defiance, parliament passed the Act of Supremacy (1534), which made the king, not the pope, head of the Roman Catholic Church in England.

Protestantism made deep inroads under Edward VI (1537-1553). Mary I (1516-1558), a zealous Roman Catholic, succeeded her half-brother Edward when he died. She and her husband, Philip II, King of Spain, tried to force Catholicism back on England. They were minimally successful, but Elizabeth I (1533-1603), Mary's half-sister, reversed Mary's policies. Elizabeth encouraged a mild form of Protestantism known as Anglicanism and broke with Spain and the pope. Her compromise solution, *Thirty-nine Articles* (1563), aimed at uniting as many English citizens as possible, but with limited effect. England would not achieve any degree of religious peace until the seventeenth century.

In Scotland, John Knox (1505-1572) led the Reformation. He persuaded the parliament to adopt a Calvinist confession in 1560. Various political considerations played a decisive role in the Protestant victory. The nobles and merchants who controlled the country wished to break off an old alliance with France in favor of England. When Mary Stuart (1542-1587), known as the Queen of Scots and a vigilant Roman Catholic, attempted to block the nobles and merchants, they drove her from the throne, eventually to be beheaded.

In Ireland the Catholic church followed all the changes that occurred in England during the reigns of Henry VIII, Edward VI, Mary I, and Elizabeth I, but

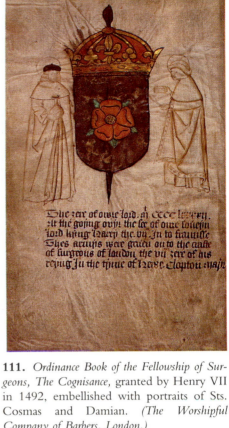

111. *Ordinance Book of the Fellowship of Surgeons, The Cognisance,* granted by Henry VII in 1492, embellished with portraits of Sts. Cosmas and Damian. *(The Worshipful Company of Barbers, London.)*

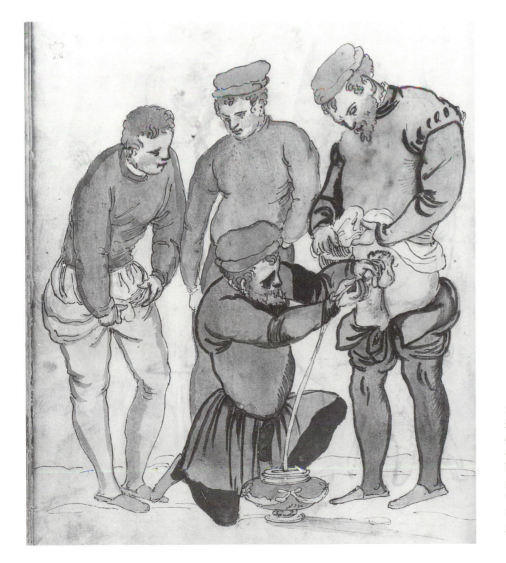

112. Sixteenth-century English manuscript illustration showing catheterization for bladder stones. Without anesthesia urethral catheterization could not have been pleasant, but as the patient on the left (holding his groin) suggests, the symptoms of the disease were probably even more painful than the relatively minor surgical procedure. *(By permission of the British Library, London, Ms 197d2, f19v.)*

173

the Irish people did not waiver in their loyalty to the pope. Protestants colonized the North, but most of Ireland remained Roman Catholic.

The growth and cultivation of surgery began in England and Scotland later than it did in the remainder of western Europe, probably because of the later appearance of medieval hospitals and universities in England and Scotland. From the time of John of Ardern to the beginning of the Tudor period (1485-1603) there were virtually no significant English surgeons, although surgical operations were being performed and surgeons had not vanished from society. The military surgeons and barber-surgeons remained active and worked amicably together, as did some university physicians and surgeons.

By the mid-sixteenth century, the number of military surgeons had remained constant, whereas the various barber-surgeons' companies grew more powerful. The London Company in 1529 published a set of rules that included an obligation to obtain a consultation in serious cases and regulations that everyone must attend the weekly lecture on surgery and that no member could take a patient who was already under the care of another.

Surgery made marked favorable progress under the Tudor autocracy. An act of Parliament in 1511, intended to control the itinerants and quacks who practiced surgery, gave the bishops the power to license practitioners and punish offenders. Thus Henry VIII provided the bishops with an independent licensing authority that extended over the dioceses of the entire country. Their authority, however, was not intended to interfere with the powers of properly authorized barber-surgeon companies or the licensing authority of the universities. By 1518 the medical licensing bodies then present in London included the universities, the bishop, the Guild of Military Surgeons, and the Guild of Barber-Surgeons.

In 1540 a momentous event in Great Britain's surgical history occurred. Under the aegis of Henry VIII Parliament passed a statute uniting the previously chartered Guild or Company of Barber-Surgeons with the small, exclusive Guild of Military Surgeons. This new Royal Commonality of Barber-Surgeons received all the previous powers granted under past British sovereigns, and more. The new charter declared that members who practiced surgery should no longer perform barber activities and that barbers should not undertake any sur-

113. *Henry VIII and the Barber-Surgeons* in 1540. Oil painting on oak by Hans Holbein the Younger, representing "the Union by Act of Parliament of the Barbers and the Surgeons to form the Company of Barber-Surgeons." The painting shows Henry VIII seated, holding in his right hand the sword of state and in his left hand a document he is handing to Thomas Vicary, his sergeant-surgeon. The Latin inscription in the painting contains a florid dedication from the barber-surgeons to the king. *(The Worshipful Company of Barbers, London.)*

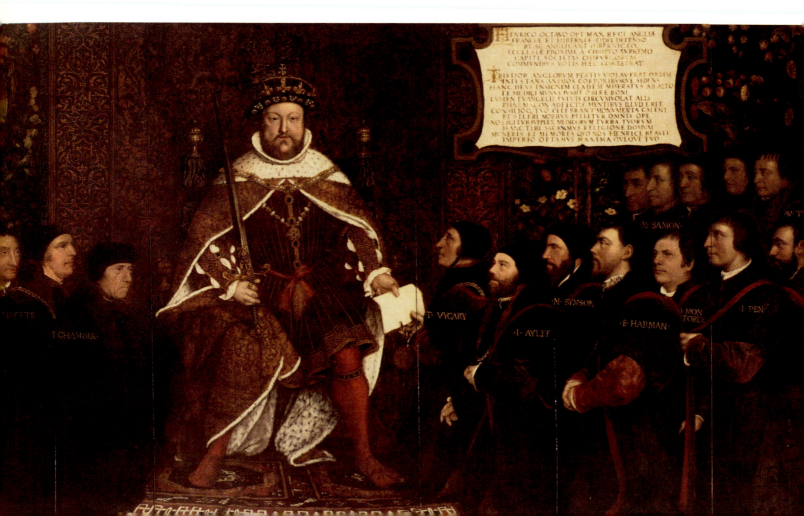

gery except dental work. The barber-surgeons of this consolidated company were permitted to place a blue- and white-striped pole in front of their offices, and the surgeons were allowed to display a gallipot and a red pole in addition.

As a result of the new royal charter a vigorous attempt was made to improve educational work. The surgical examiners instituted a series of licensing examinations, which culminated in the student receiving the Grand Diploma as a master in surgery and anatomy. Not until this diploma was granted could the student apply for the bishop's seal or license. The new company was entitled to receive the bodies of four executed criminals each year for the purpose of dissection. Thus the act of 1540 succeeded in creating for London an active educational and licensing body for the practice of surgery.

Henry VIII's personal surgeon, Thomas Vicary (1495-1561), was elected first master of the united companies. Vicary was a recognized leader in the profession, although he left behind few memorable surgical achievements or written works. He was a member of the Company of Barber-Surgeons and became a senior warden in that organization in 1528. Two years later, Vicary was made master of the company, and in 1535, chief surgeon to the king, with a grant of abbey lands. In 1548, Henry VIII transferred the management of St. Bartholomew's Hospital to the city of London and Vicary received an appointment as chief surgeon to that institution. He was entrusted with the surgical organization of the greatest hospital in Great Britain and had three surgeons working with him to effectuate his ideas.

Vicary wrote very little, but since he was the first surgeon to write in English, his works gained a wide reputation and were published in numerous editions. In 1548 he wrote an anatomical text that included chapters on surgery (*A Treasure For Englishmen, Containing The Anatomie Of Man's Body*). Vicary's greatness is found neither in his written works nor in his surgical triumphs but in his proven abilities to forward the cause of surgery through political maneuverings.

Thomas Gale (1507-1587), the most prominent British surgeon of his day, was born in London and obtained his first significant experience as a military surgeon under Henry VIII. Gale alternated his role as a military surgeon with his civilian practice for 10 years. In 1559 he was made a member of the Company of Barber-Surgeons. Gale eventually succeeded Vicary as master of the Company of Barber-Surgeons.

Gale was a prolific author who wrote in English instead of Latin. He was vigilant in his attacks on quacks and other surgical pretenders. Considered a man of high moral character, he propagated a set of ethical guidelines to aid surgeons in their practice.

The most famous of Gale's works on surgery is his four-part *Certaine Workes Of Chirurgerie* (1563). The third part of this work, "An Excellent Treatise Of Wounds Made With Gooneshot," is the most important. Gale refuted the traditional misconception that gunshot wounds were envenomed and should be treated with boiling oil:

> The usuall Gonnepowder is not venemous, nother the shotte of hoteness as is able to warme the fleshe, much lesse to make an ascar . . . Hange a bagge ful of gonnepouder on a place convenient: and then stand so far of as your peece wil shute leavell, and shute at the same, and you shall see the gonnepouder to bee no more set on fyer with the heat of the stone [used as a bullet] than if you caste a cold stone at it.

As farsighted as Gale was concerning gunshot wounds, he did not believe that traumatic injuries healed by first intention. He insisted that they be continually dressed with salves and embrocations. His treatise is replete with mentions of ointments and bizarre concoctions for such a purpose.

William Bullein (?-1576) was a close contemporary of Gale. Bullein led a tumultuous life; once he was charged with the attempted murder of a patient. Bullein was born on the island of Ely and obtained his early education at Cambridge. After traveling in Germany and Scotland, he practiced in Norwich and Durham. During the years of his practice he studied for the ministry and held a rectorate in Suffolk. He finally settled in London, where he attained considerable success and had a large practice.

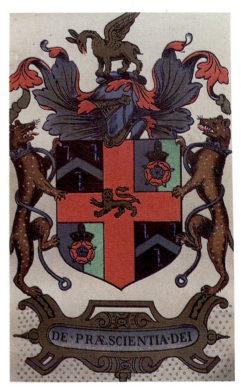

114. Frontispiece from John Flint South's (1797-1882) *Memorials of the Craft of Surgery in England (1886)* showing arms of the United Company of Barber-Surgeons, now known as the Worshipful Company of Barbers, from the grant made by Sir Gilbert Dethick in 1569 *(From the author's collection.)*

Bullein's most interesting book was *Bulleins Bulwarke Of Defence Againste All Sicknes, Sornes, And Woundes* (1579). A special part of that volume was devoted to surgery and presented a curious attempt at dialogue as the method of expression of ideas. Bullein provided a unique characterization of the requirements of a surgeon:

> He must begin first in youth with good learning and exercise in thys noble arte, he also must be clenly, nimble handed, sharpe sighted, pregnant witted, bolde spirited, clenly apparailed, pitefull harted, but not womenly affeccionated to wepe or trimble, when he seeth broken bones or bloodies woundes, neither muste he geue place to the cries of his sore paciente, for soft chyrurgians maketh fowle sores. Of the other syde, he maie not plaie the partes of a butcher to cutte, rende or teare the bodie of mannekynde. For allthough it be fraile, sore, and weake, yet it is the pleasure of God, to cal it his Temple, his instrument, and dwelyng place.

During the Elizabethan Age (1558-1603) the ablest surgeon was reputed to have been William Clowes (1540-1604). He was born at Kingsbury, in Warwickshire, and received his early medical education by apprenticeship. In 1563 Clowes accepted the position of surgeon in the English army and was immediately dispatched to Havre, France, and subsequently to Flanders. Six years later, he settled in London and became a member of the Company of Barber-Surgeons. Clowes must have gained quite a reputation because in 1575 he received an appointment to the surgical staff of St. Bartholomew's Hospital as one of its three surgeons, and six years after that appointment he was promoted to the rank of full surgeon, a position he already held at Christ's Hospital.

Clowes had considerable experience as a military surgeon. In 1585 he left his practice to serve in the army of the Earl of Leicester (1532-1588), then stationed

115. *The Surgeone's Chest,* a woodcut, with accompanying poem, from William Clowes' *A Prooved Practise For All Young Chirurgians* (1588). Similar chests containing the surgeon's instruments and medicines were taken to the battlefield. In the foreground, *right,* the surgeon, with the open chest and his instruments beside him, is treating a war wound. On the left side of the page is a battle scene. The overall composition of the woodcut is quite complex and reflects the artist's limited knowledge of perspective. *(Jeremy Norman & Co., Inc.)*

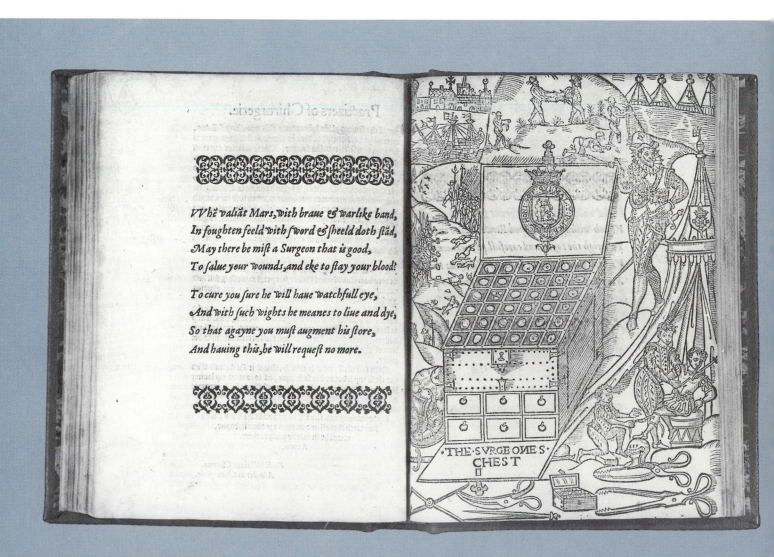

in the Netherlands. There he acquired extensive clinical experience, especially in the treatment of gunshot injuries. After returning to London in 1588, Clowes joined the English fleet that destroyed the Spanish Armada. When this task was accomplished, he returned to his practice in London and eventually became surgeon to Elizabeth I.

Of the four surgical treatises written by Clowes, the first, *A Short And Profitable Treatise Touching The Cure Of The Morbus Gallicus By Unctions* (1579), was the earliest English treatise on syphilis. In this work he demonstrated the prevalence of the disease at that time; it affected one of every 20 persons admitted to St. Bartholomew's. Clowes treated hundreds of luetic cases by using high-dosage mecurial inunctions carried to the point of salivation and facial necrosis.

The most important of Clowes's publications was *A Prooved Practise For All Young Chirurgians, Concerning Burnings With Gunpowder, And Woundes Made With Gunshot, Sword, Halbard, Pyke . . .* (1588). Clowes concentrated on wound surgery and made little mention of elective operative surgery. His treatise was full of brief case histories of patients who came under his personal care. It provided an accurate description of the various kinds of inflicted wounds and their treatment both during war and in the civilian life of Elizabethan England.

Clowes took part in the active debate about whether gunpowder and gunshot injuries were poisoned. He did not believe that such injuries were necessarily poisoned but noted that nothing ruled out poison or excrement being smeared on a bullet before it was fired. In amputations Clowes did not use the ligature but preferred astringents and caustic powders to provide hemostasis. Surprisingly, in one of the earliest forms of the flap method, he covered the stump with integument. Among the horrific injuries he reported was a case involving protrusion of the omentum and intestine through a gunshot injury of the abdomen. After making a careful examination of the eviscerated parts, Clowes decided the intestine was uninjured:

> Then with a strong double thread I did tie fast the omentum close unto the wound as possible well I might, and within a finger breadth of thereabouts I did cut off that part of the omentum that hanged out of the wound and so I cauterized it with a hot iron almost to the knot. All this being done I put again into the body that part of the omentum which I had fast tied and I left a piece of the thread hanging out of the wound, which within four or five days after nature did case forth. The thread, being fast tied, then presently I did take a needle with a double strong silk thread well waxed, wherewith I did thrust through both the abdominal wall and the peritoneum on the right side of the wound, but on the left side of the wound I did put the needle only through the wall of the abdomen. And so tied these three fast together with a very strong knot, and presently I did cut of the thread.

Clowes was a witty, interesting writer who provided unparalleled insight into the life and times of an Elizabethan surgeon. For his independent observations and open-mindedness he is best remembered.

The last of the major sixteenth-century English surgeons was John Banister (1533-1610). He was educated at Oxford and, like his close friend Clowes, accompanied English troops to Havre, France. Banister lived for a time in Nottingham but resettled in London and lectured in anatomy for the Company of Barber-Surgeons in 1581. He was one of the few individuals in London who received special dispensation from Elizabeth I to practice both medicine and surgery. Banister was strongly in favor of the reunion of surgery and medicine, and he came close to achieving that personally:

> Some of late have fondly affirmed that the chirurgeon hath not to deal in physic. Small courtesy it is to break faithful friendship, for the one cannot work without the other, nor the other practice without the aid of both.

Nonetheless, he was required to obtain a consultation with a member of the College of Physicians in dangerous cases.

Banister's written works were all published in London. Among these were *A Needefull, New, And Necessarie Treatise Of Chyrurgerie* (1575); *The Historie Of*

116. *Following pages,* John Banister lecturing on anatomy at the Barber-Surgeons Hall, London, in 1581. This remarkable painting, from the collection of the celebrated physician and connoisseur William Hunter (1718-1783), may be the only painting of an identifiable sixteenth-century English surgeon actually engaged in the business of medicine. It is a fine portrayal of how surgeons were taught anatomy at the time. The unknown artist portrayed Banister to be much larger than his students, which may have been an effort to represent Banister's higher status or may simply reflect the artist's limited skills. *(Librarian, Glasgow University Library.)*

177

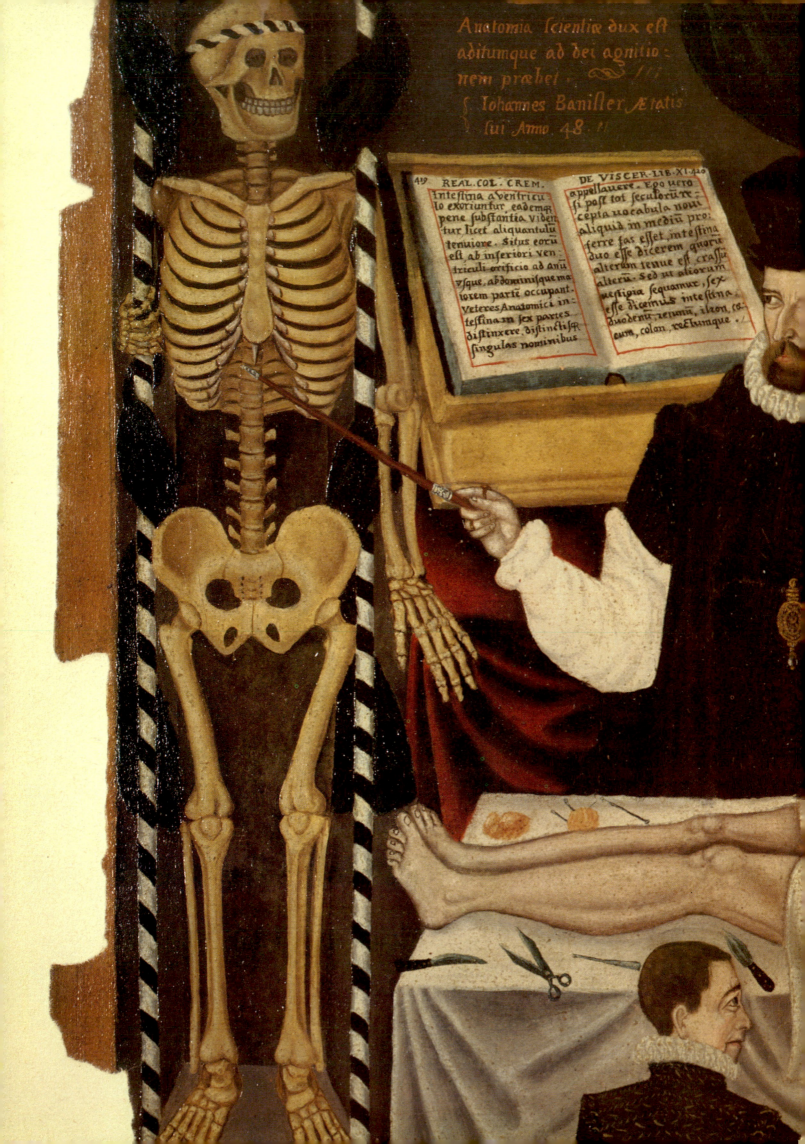

419 REAL. COL. CREM.   DE VISCER. LIB. XI. 420

Intestina à ventricu
lo exoriuntur, eademq̃
pene substantia viden
tur, licet aliquantulũ
tenuiore. Sisus eorũ
est ab inferiori ven
triculi orificio ad anũ
usque, abdominisque ma
iorem parte occupant.
Veteres Anatomici in
testina in sex partes
distinxere. Distinctisq̃
singulas nominibus

appellauere. Ego uero
si post tot seculorũ re:
cepta uocabula noui
aliquid in mediũ pro:
ferre fas esset, intestina
duo esse dicerem quorũ
alterũ tenue est, crassũ
alterũ. Sed ut aliorum
uestigia sequamur, sex
esse dicemus intestina,
duodenũ, ieiunũ, ileon, cæ
cum, colon, rectumque.

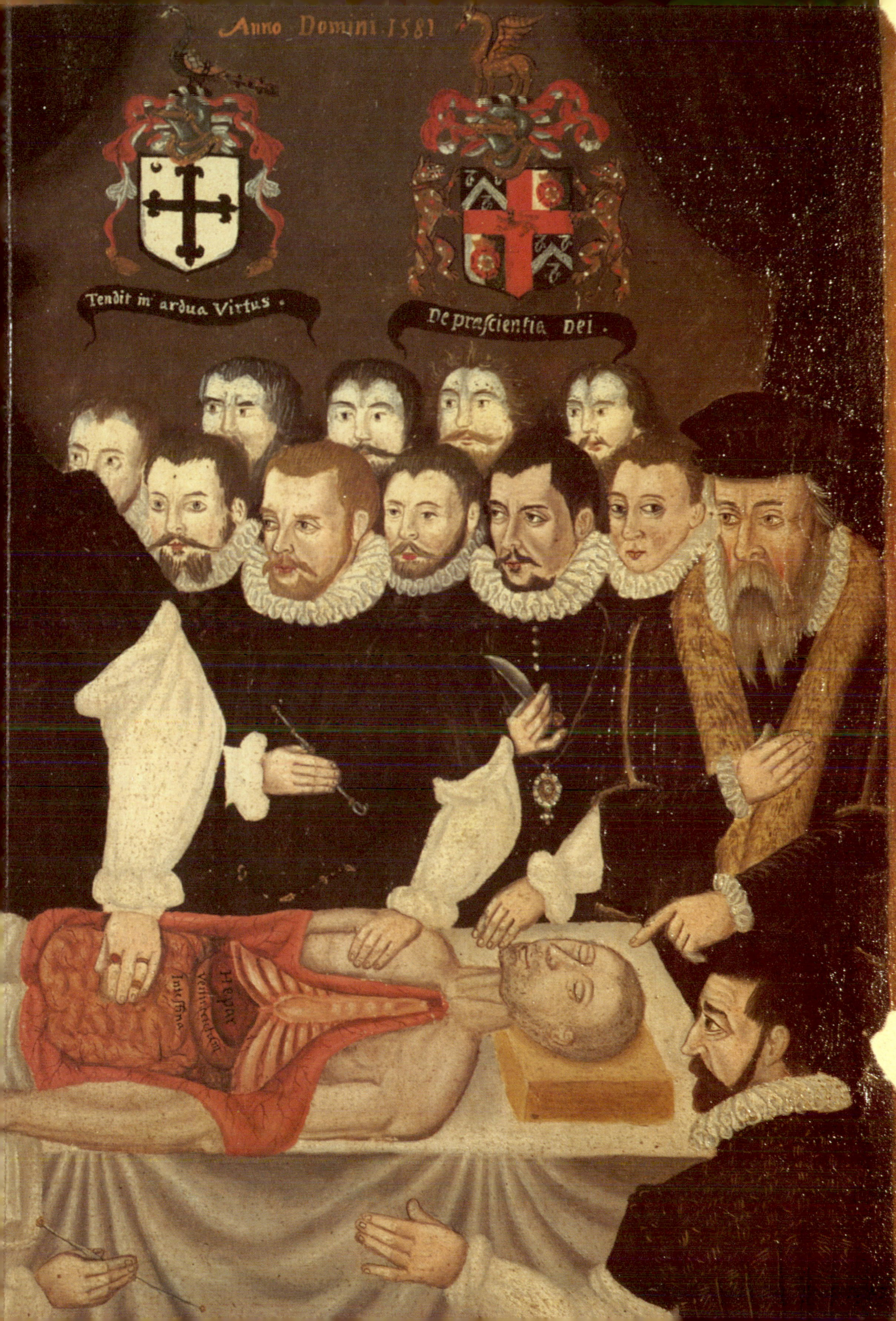

Anno Domini 1581

Tendit in ardua Virtus

De præscientia Dei

Man, Sucked From The Sappe Of The Most Approved Anathomistes (1578), a respected anatomical treatise; *A Compendious Chirurgery* (1585); and *An Antidotarie Chyrurgicall* (1589), a collection of surgical treatments.

Surgery in Scotland, as in other regions of Great Britain, was controlled by both surgeons and barbers. In 1505 James IV (1473-1513) issued a decree setting up an Incorporation of Barber-Surgeons with certain rights and privileges. The guild was to receive the body of one executed criminal each year for dissection and was also granted the monopoly of making and selling whiskey in Edinburgh. The Incorporation of Barber-Surgeons was the first legally recognized surgical entity in Scotland.

A unique relationship between physicians and surgeons developed in Glasgow. In this city alone, of all of England and Scotland, there never existed an artificial separation of medicine and surgery. In Glasgow James VI (1566-1625) granted a charter (1599) for the Faculty of Physicians and Surgeons. The creation of this new medical entity was the singular achievement of Peter Lowe (1550-1612).

Lowe was born in Errol, Scotland. He obtained his medical education in Paris and then practiced in France and Flanders. Because he had a university education, it is believed that he was a member of the Confraternity of Saint Come. Altogether, Lowe spent almost 30 years on the continent. Then, in 1596, he returned to London and, 2 years later, to Scotland. Returning to his native country with an admirable university education and a comprehensive knowledge of the surgical techniques of Franco and Pare, Lowe immediately became the most reputable surgeon in Scotland.

Having experienced in Paris the difficulties associated with the separation of physicians and surgeons, Lowe was anxious to unite all regular practitioners of medicine and surgery in his city and to control the numerous surgical quacks and charlatans. In 1598 he applied to civil and church authorities, including James VI, to establish a board that would examine the qualifications of those who wished to practice the healing arts. The following year a charter was issued to Lowe and to Robert Hamilton, a physician, to incorporate a Faculty of Physicians and Surgeons of Glasgow. This charter was the beginning of the medical school in Glasgow and gave these men and their successors the right to examine and license all practitioners of medicine and surgery in that city and the surrounding countryside. The licensed physicians and surgeons were also given the responsibility of overseeing the apothecaries and their drugs and were compelled to provide free treatment for the poor.

In addition to his political capabilities, Lowe was an author of some repute. In 1596 he provided the first English translation of the works of Hippocrates from a French version, since he was unfamiliar with Greek. Lowe's *Discourse On The Whole Art Of Chyrurgerie* (1596) was the first comprehensive and systematic work on surgery written in Great Britain. A portion of the treatise, which went through four editions, was in the form of a dialogue between Lowe and his son John regarding the surgical precepts of the Ancients. Among the important points is the first reference in English to ligation of the arteries in amputations.

Lowe is remembered for his efforts to elevate the craft of surgery from the hands of the itinerant quacks and to purge it of any unworthy individual who professed to practice it. Because of his extensive education and varied professional experiences, he was able to influence the Scottish king to effectuate needed reforms:

> I hope all honest men, especially you, who are towards his Majestie, will be earnest in purchasing of privileges and lawes, for restraining of all ignorant abusers in this Kingdome, like as is granted to men of our art, in other civill countries to the great ayd and comfort of all Kings of those parts. It pleased his sacred majestie to hear my complaint about some fourteen yeers agoe, upon certain abusers of our art, of divers sorts and ranks of people, whereof wee have good store . . . The matter being considered, and the abuse weighed by his majestie and honourable councell, thought not to be tolerated, for the which I got a priviledge under his Highnesse privie seal, to try and examine all men upon the art of chyrurgerie, to discharge, and allow in the West

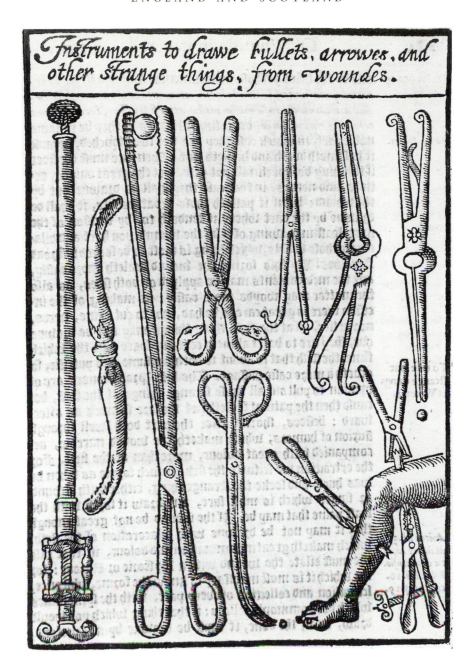

Instruments to drawe bullets, arrowes, and other strange things, from woundes.

117. "Instruments to drawe bullets, arrowes, and other strange things from woundes," from Peter Lowe's *A Discourse On The Whole Art Of Chyrurgerie* (1596). *(Jeremy Norman & Co., Inc.)*

parts of Scotland, who were worthy, or unworthy . . . such is the iniquitie of time, that abusers are commonly over-seen by such as ought to punish them: in such sort that one blinde guides another, and most commonly fall both into the ditch. In the mean time these cheaters are permitted to . . . destroy both friend and foe, ever detracting the true professors of the art. Now worshipfull brethren, in respect of those enormities with divers . . . will seek . . . to correct and punish abusers, as also to withstand the frivolous or fantasticall opinions of such as use them, and neither for request nor lucre, to admit any such ignorant abusers to professe our art.

By the end of the sixteenth century the craft of surgery in Europe had attained a tenuous but accepted and respected position within the world of medicine. Although surgeons continued to be viewed askance by their fellow physicians, the importance of a surgeon's clinical skills to an individual's health care could no longer be blithely dismissed. The importance of the surgeons' skills was especially evident in that surgeons were becoming well paid; certain individuals received enormous sums. Admittedly, large areas of medical and surgical practice remained bound up with superstition, herb therapy, and quackery. However, the true greatness of the many renowned surgeons during this era is reflected in their increasing scorn for quacks and charlatans and their application of rational empiric observations to daily practices. In essence, the humanism of the Renaissance provided surgeons with their first substantive opportunities to become respected members of the healing profession.

THE SEVENTEENTH CENTURY

| 1550 | 1600 | 1650 | 1700 | 1750 |

DAILY LIFE

Wigs become fashionable **(1600)**
Jamestown, Virginia **(1607)**
Authorized version of the *King James Bible* **(1611)**
Tobacco planted in Virginia **(1612)**
Glass industry in England **(1614)**
Black slaves arrive in Virginia **(1619)**
Patent laws established in London **(1623)**
New Amsterdam founded on Hudson River **(1626)**
Eruption of Vesuvius **(1631)**
Plague outbreak leads to passion play in Oberammergau **(1633)**
Harvard College **(1636)**
Boers settle in South Africa **(1660)**
New Jersey **(1665)**
Great Fire of London **(1666)**
Flexible fire hose **(1672)**
Dodo becomes extinct **(1680)**
First bank checks in England **(1681)**
Paper manufacturing in North America **(1698)**

> **POPULATION FIGURES (1600)**
> France 16,000,000
> Germany 14,500,000
> Poland 11,000,000
> Spanish Empire 8,000,000
> Hapsburg Empire 5,500,000
> England and Ireland 5,500,000
> Holland 3,000,000

SCIENCE AND TECHNOLOGY

Giovanni Borelli, Italian physiologist **(1608–1679)**
Blaise Pascal, French mathematician **(1623–1662)**
Robert Boyle, English physicist **(1626–1691)**
Issac Newton, English mathematician **(1642–1727)**
Jacques Bernoulli, Swiss mathematician **(1654–1705)**
Edmond Halley, English astronomer **(1656–1742)**
Daniel Fahrenheit, German physicist **(1686–1736)**

RELIGION AND PHILOSOPHY

Roger Williams, American religious controversialist **(1603–1683)**
John Locke, English philosopher **(1632–1704)**
Baruch Spinoza, Dutch philosopher **(1632–1677)**
Gottfried Leibnitz, German philosopher **(1646–1716)**
Isaac Watts, English hymn writer **(1674–1748)**
Emanuel Swedenborg, Swedish philosopher **(1688–1772)**
Voltaire, French philosopher **(1694–1778)**

LITERATURE AND THEATER

John Milton, English writer **(1608–1674)**
Samuel Butler, English satirist **(1612–1680)**
François de La Rochefoucauld, French author **(1613–1655)**
Savinien Cyrano de Bergerac, French poet **(1619–1655)**
Molière, French writer **(1622–1673)**
John Bunyan, English author **(1628–1688)**
John Locke, English philosopher **(1632–1704)**
Samuel Pepys, English diarist **(1633–1703)**
Racine, French dramatist **(1639–1699)**
Daniel Defoe, English author **(1659–1731)**
Jonathan Swift, English author **(1667–1745)**
William Congreve, English dramatist **(1670–1729)**
Joseph Addison, English poet **(1672–1719)**
Alexander Pope, English poet **(1688–1744)**

MUSIC

Antonio Stradivari, Italian violin maker **(1644–1737)**
Henry Purcell, English composer **(1659–1695)**
Giuseppe Aldrovandini, Italian composer **(1665–1707)**
Antonio Vivaldi, Italian composer **(1675–1741)**
George Telemann, German composer **(1681–1767)**
Jean Philippe Rameau, French composer **(1683–1764)**
Johann Sebastian Bach, German composer **(1685–1759)**
Domenico Scalatti, Italian composer **(1685–1757)**

THE SEVENTEENTH CENTURY

VISUAL ARTS

Rembrandt van Rijn, Dutch painter **(1606–1669)**
David Teniers the Younger, Dutch painter **(1610–1690)**
Charles Lebrun, French architect **(1619–1690)**
Guarino Guarini, Italian architect **(1624–1683)**
Jan Steen, Dutch painter **(1626–1679)**
Jan Vermeer, Dutch painter **(1632–1675)**
Christopher Wren, English architect **(1632–1723)**
Johann Fischer von Erlach, Austrian architect **(1656–1723)**
Jean Watteau, French painter **(1684–1721)**
Giovanni Tiepolo, Italian painter **(1696–1770)**
William Hogarth, English painter **(1697–1764)**

MEDICINE AND SURGERY

Nicolas Habicot, French **(1550–1624)**
Giovanni Cortesti, Italian **(1554–1636)**
John Woodall, English **(1554–1643)**
Wilhelm Fabry von Hilden, German **(1560–1634)**
Peter Uffenbach, German **(1566–1635)**
Jacques De Marque, French **(1569–1622)**
William Harvey, English **(1578–1657)**
Adrian Van Der Spiegel, Dutch **(1578–1625)**
Caesar Magati, Italian **(1579–1647)**
Marco Severino, Italian **(1580–1656)**
Gasparo Aselli, Italian **(1581–1626)**
Alexander Read, English **(1586–1641)**
Pietro De Marchetti, Italian **(1589–1673)**
Stephen Bradwell, English **(1594–1636)**
Johannes Scultetus, German **(1595–1645)**
Francis Glisson, English **(1597–1677)**
Johann Wirung, German **(1600–1643)**
Guy Patin, French **(1601–1672)**
James Cooke, English **(1614–1688)**
Thomas Wharton, English **(1614–1673)**
Paul Babette, Dutch **(? – 1675)**
Thomas Bartholin, Danish, **(1616–1680)**
Richard Wiseman, English **(1620–1676)**
Thomas Willis, English **(1621–1675)**
Jean Denis, French **(1625–1704)**
Marcello Malpighi, Italian **(1628–1694)**
Richard Lower, English **(1631–1691)**
Antony van Leeuwenhoek, Dutch **(1632–1723)**
Johann Major, German **(1634–1693)**
Robert Hooke, English **(1635–1703)**
Clapton Havers, English **(? – 1702)**
Niels Stensen, Danish **(1638–1686)**
Regner de Graaf, Dutch **(1641–1673)**
Lorenza Bellini, Italian **(1643–1704)**
Pierre Dionis, French **(1643–1718)**
John von Muralt, Swiss **(1645–1733)**
Matthaeus Purmann, German **(1649–1711)**
Charles-François Felix, French **(1650–1703)**
John Moyle, English **(?– 1713)**
Anton Nuck, Dutch **(1650–1692)**
Frere Jacques De Beaulieu, French **(1651–1719)**
Johann Brunner, Swiss **(1653–1727)**
Johann Peyer, Swiss **(1653–1712)**
Giuseppe Zambeccar, Italian **(1655–1728)**
William Cowper, English **(1666–1709)**

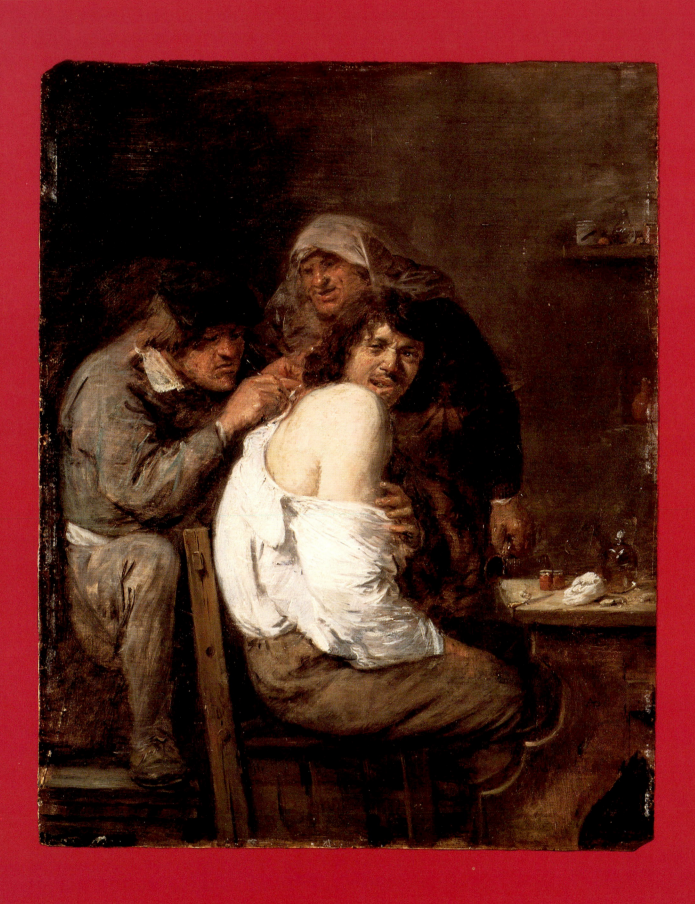

CHAPTER 9
THE SEVENTEENTH CENTURY

&

The scientific revolution of the seventeenth century represented a turning point in the history of medicine. Emphasis shifted dramatically from speculation to experimentation, and remarkable advances were made in physics and chemistry. The detailed experimental work of scientist-philosophers such as Robert Boyle (1627-1691), in his *Sceptical Chymist* (1661), and Isaac Newton (1642-1727), in *Philosophia Naturalis Principia Mathematica* (1687), provided a framework for future scientific studies.

The teaching of medicine and surgery was still heavily influenced by ancient philosophies. Initially, supporters of older influences continued to outnumber the more progressive thinkers and scientists. By the end of the century, however, the latter group was to have an overwhelming influence on the craft of surgery.

Three dominant forces from the past had to be reckoned with in the seventeenth century: Aristotelianism, Galenism, and Paracelsianism. Superstition and blind worship of ancient authors would gradually give way to observation and true scientific experimentation. An intimate relationship remained between astrology and medicine but gradually evolved into new directions of medical thought.

The great centers of medical education in seventeenth-century Europe were Leyden, Montpellier, Padua, and Paris, but the condition of medicine was vastly improved by the ambitions of royalty to establish small universities and by the formation of scientific societies. This improvement was especially evident in Germany and the Netherlands, where institutions such as Giessen (1607), Utrecht (1636), Bamberg (1648), Innsbruck (1673), and Halle (1694) were founded. Scientific societies were begun, such as the Academia Del Cimenti and the Academia De Lince in Italy. The first true botanical gardens were established at Strassburg (1620), Oxford (1621), Edinburgh (1670), Berlin (1679), and Amsterdam (1682).

Specific advances in anatomy, physiology, and medical instrumentation aided the immense flowering of medicine. The most astonishing and influential of these progressive changes was the discovery and fundamental understanding of the anatomy and physiology of the circulation of blood. The outstanding research by William Harvey of Folkestone in Kent, which concerned the continuous circulation of blood within a contained system, was the most momentous revelation in medical and surgical history since ancient classical times.

To appreciate the magnitude of Harvey's accomplishment, one must realize that the functioning of the heart and blood vessels had been a mystery since time immemorial; many physicians had investigated the problem of circulation and speculated on its solution. A complete understanding was to have an enormous impact on the craft of surgery.

Prehistoric humans must have known that blood was in motion when they cut open a live animal or saw a wounded artery or vein. Aristotle had taught

118. *Facing page, The Village Quack* (1636-1637) by the Flemish genre painter, Adraen Brouewer. The patient of this presumably uneducated barber-surgeon does not appear to be enjoying the experience, which could not have been pleasant. The old woman assistant is holding what looks like a tankard from which the patient may have attempted to obtain a fair degree of inebriation before the operation began. (Städelsches Kunstinstitut, Frankfurt am Main.)

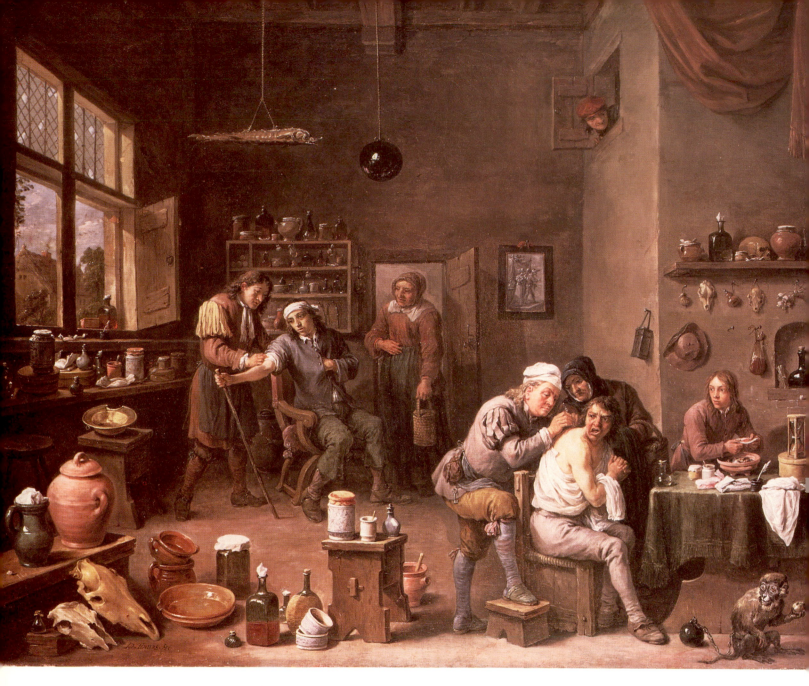

119. *The Surgeon.* Oil on canvas, by the Flemish artist David Teniers the Younger. A prolific artist best known for his genre paintings, Teniers eloquently portrayed the office of a Dutch country surgeon of the seventeenth century. In the foreground, *right,* the master surgeon is opening a boil. In the rear, *left,* a journeyman surgeon prepares a patient for bloodletting, and on the far right an apprentice holds a dressing ready for the master. Scattered all around the room are the trappings of the barber-surgeon's trade and other symbolic objects commonly understood at the time. *(The Chrysler Museum, Norfolk, Va.)*

that the heart is the center of all life. Hippocrates had believed that a "certain force" derived from inspired air entered the heart and was distributed to the remainder of the body. In observing a living heart during the second century A.D., Galen had noted that it did not contract in a simple manner. Its staggered movement suggested to Galen the forcing of blood from one side of the heart to the other through microscopic pores. Because of Galen's authority, this misconception was widely accepted for centuries.

In the sixteenth century Servetus had concluded in his *Christianismi Restitutio* (1553) that there were communications in the lungs between the pulmonary arteries and veins and had believed that there was separate transit of some but not all blood from the heart through the lungs. He is therefore credited with discovery of the pulmonary circulation. Sylvius had described the valves of the veins; further studies by Fallopius and Fabricius of Aquapendente delineated their one-way action, which proved to be an important concept that Harvey was to use to support his theory of circulation.

Vesalius had established that there were no visible communications between the right and left ventricles but did not deny the existence of "invisible" pores. Colombo, in his *De Re Anatomica Libri* (1559), had advanced a theory similar to that of Servetus regarding pulmonary circulation. Colombo had also recognized the difference in the blood's color in the right and left sides of the heart and reasoned that the blood underwent some type of change in the lungs.

Andrea Cesalpino (1524–1603), professor of medicine at Pisa, may be considered the most important of Harvey's precursors. Cesalpino actually used the term *circulation* and thought in terms of closed systemic and pulmonary circulations. In *Peripateticarum Quaestionum Libri Quinque* (1571) he proposed the existence of capillaries to connect the arterial and venous systems, which meant that there was no open effusion of blood into the tissues, as had been previously presumed. Cesalpino postulated major direct connections between larger arteries and veins and that blood originated in the heart. However, he did not visualize the venous system as an affluence returning blood to the heart. None of Cesalpino's ideas were supported by convincing experimentation or dissection, so they had no important influence upon his immediate contemporaries.

The solution of the problem of circulation was left to Harvey (1578-1657), who had a deep understanding of the entire history and literature of the subject. Harvey received his bachelor's degree from Cambridge (1597) and shortly thereafter went to study medicine in Padua, where he came under the direct influence of Fabricius of Aquapendente and his assistant, Giulio Casseri (1561-1616). Harvey must have learned from these great surgeon-anatomists the scientific methods on which he based his understanding of the circulation. Harvey brought experimental physiology to a new level of refinement that closely resembles the modern approach.

Harvey returned to England in 1602 and commenced a medical practice in London, becoming a fellow of the Royal College of Physicians 5 years later. His major affiliation was with Saint Bartholomew's Hospital, where he remained on the staff from 1609 to 1643. His reputation was quite wide, and Harvey eventually became court physician to James I (1566-1625) and, later, to Charles I

120. William Harvey demonstrating an experiment on a deer to King Charles I and the boy prince. Engraving after the painting by Robert Hannah at the Royal College of Physicians, London. *(Jeremy Norman & Co., Inc.)*

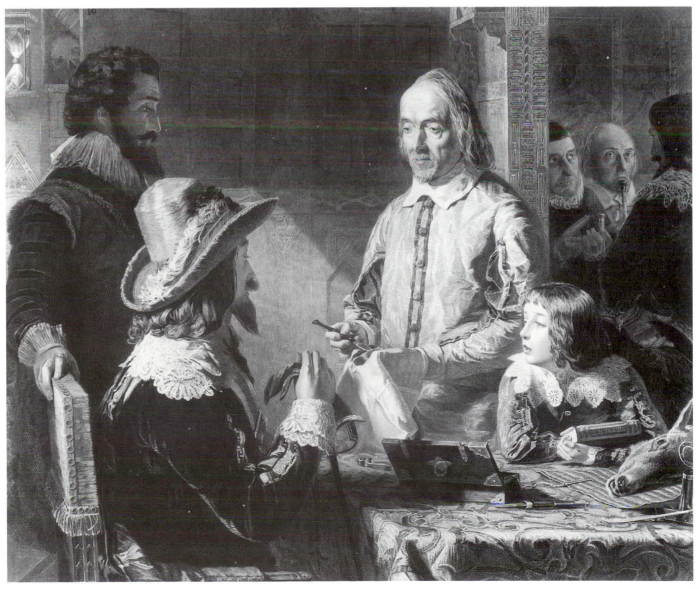

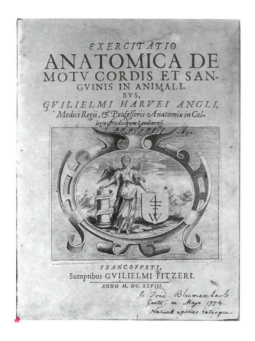

121. Title page from William Harvey's *Anatomical Experiments on the Movement of the Heart and Blood in Animals* as it was first published in Latin in Frankfurt, 1628. With this work on the circulation Harvey pioneered the modern experimental approach to physiology. This copy once belonged to the founder of anthropology, Johann Friedrich Blumenbach (1752-1840). *(Jeremy Norman & Co., Inc.)*

(1600-1649). During Harvey's years in active practice he managed to conduct a wide range of experimental research projects, including public anatomical demonstrations.

Manuscript notes of Harvey's *Lumleian Lecture* show that by 1616 he had already completed his demonstration of the circulation of the blood. After repeatedly demonstrating his experiments and delivering numerous lectures, he presented his ideas in his book, *Exercitatio Anatomica De Motu Cordis Et Sanguinis In Animalibus,* that is, *On the movement of the heart and blood in animals,* in 1628.

Exercitatio Anatomica De Motu Cordis Et Sanguinis In Animalibus has been called the most important book in the history of medicine. It is a masterpiece of sound deductive reasoning based on ingeniously simple experiments, including human vivisection, ligation, and perfusion. Harvey used inductive logic to demonstrate that the heart acts as a muscular pump in propelling the blood along the arteries and that the blood's motion is continuous and leads back to the heart via veins to form a cycle or circle:

> I began to think whether there might not be a movement, as it were, in a circle. Now this I afterward found to be true; and I finally saw that the blood, forced by the action of the left ventricle into the arteries, was distributed to the body at large, and its several parts, in the same manner as it is sent through the lungs, impelled by the right ventricle into the pulmonary artery, and that it then passed through the veins and along the vena cava, and so round to the left ventricle in the manner already indicated.

Because of Harvey's observations the study of human physiology became a dynamic science. This is most dramatically demonstrated in his use of quantitative data to prove his hypotheses. Harvey showed that the actual quantity and velocity of blood made it physically impossible for the blood to do anything other than return to the heart by the venous system. If the human heart contained 2 ounces of blood (an observation Harvey made from cadavers) and beat about 70 times per minute, then in 1 minute it pumped out 8 pounds of blood. When the number of pounds of blood pumped per minute was multiplied by the number of minutes in a day, the resulting quantity of blood pumped out of the heart in one day was enormous, far in excess of what the body could meaningfully produce from ingested food or liquids.

Harvey clearly demonstrated the functions of the valves in the veins. He did not elucidate the exact pathway by which the blood passes from artery to vein. The limitation of the lenses of that early era precluded Harvey's understanding of capillaries.

Although the work of Harvey had enormous implications for the evolution of medicine and surgery, its direct impact on the practice of seventeenth-century medicine was limited. Not unexpectedly, Harvey's book was met by the initial skepticism and outright hostility of a medical community that clung to the tenets of Galenism. Some surgeons in particular, by denying Harvey's observations and adhering instead to Galenic beliefs, attempted to remain more acceptable to the fraternity of physicians who continually denied them membership.

A great age of specialized anatomical research occurred during the seventeenth century. Individual discoveries were to have enormous impact on the conduct of surgical operations and the study of surgical pathology and physiology (see the box on p. 191). Bernardino Genga (1655-1734) wrote the first book devoted entirely to surgical anatomy, *Anatomia Chirurgica,* in 1672. Because the book contained no engravings, it played an insignificant role in the evolution of surgery.

The invention of the microscope certainly contributed to the evolution of surgery during the seventeenth century. Although a ground lens had been used as a magnifying glass during ancient times, the painstaking work of Antony van Leeuwenhoek (1632-1723) in the seventeenth century led to the production of microscopes with the power to magnify an image up to 270 times. A Delft cloth merchant, Leeuwenhoek devoted his leisure time to the study of natural history.

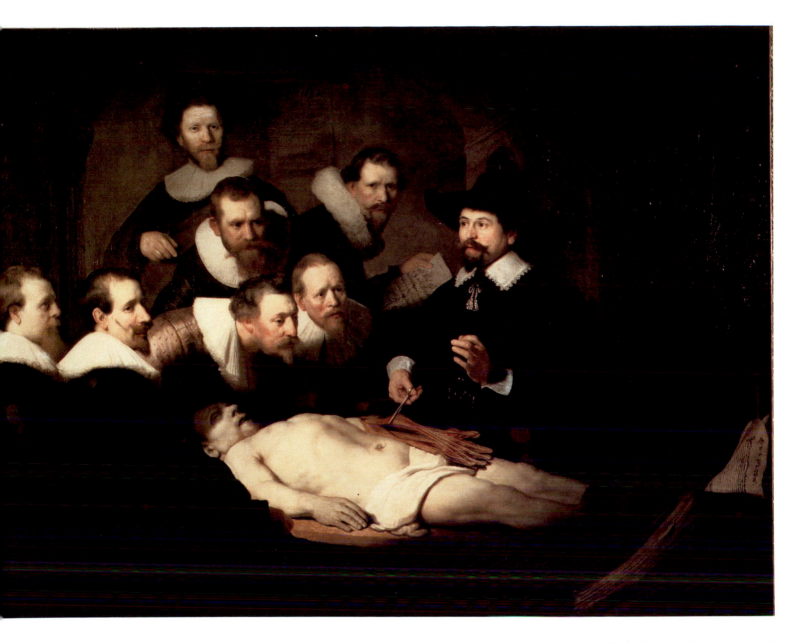

122. *The Anatomy Lesson of Dr. Nicolaas Tulp* (1593-1674), by Rembrandt van Rijn. Finished in 1632, when the artist was 26 years old, this masterpiece of medical iconography is more social commentary than medical document. Many "anatomy lessons" were painted in the seventeenth century, since dissection had been legalized. In this painting the artistic emphasis is on the portraits rather than the cadaver. The great physician and his students are all studiously posing for posterity. Ironically, Nicolaas Tulp is better remembered today for his role in this painting than for his pioneering work on beriberi or his description of the ileocecal valve ("Tulp's valve").

189

Self-taught and ignorant of Latin, he wrote more than 300 scientific papers in Dutch. Leeuwenhoek was the first to describe spermatozoa, red blood cells, the striped character of muscle, and the structure of the crystalline lens. At the time of his death he had accumulated almost 250 microscopes for which he had personally ground more than 400 lenses.

Robert Hooke (1635–1703) served at one time as a research assistant to Robert Boyle and was later employed by the newly formed Royal Society to conduct its scientific experiments. Hooke constructed one of the most famous of the early compound microscopes. His most famous work, *Micrographia* (1665), was the earliest book devoted solely to an account of microscopical observations and contained several striking illustrations. It also contained the first known reference to *cells,* a term Hooke invented.

The most outstanding of seventeenth-century microscopists was Malpighi. A professor of anatomy at Bologna, he is considered the founder of histology and biological microscopy. Although primarily remembered for his work in descriptive embryology, Malpighi's techniques for preparing tissues for examination under the microscope had enormous implications for the later development of surgical pathology.

Historical perspective permits a reflective view of the seventeenth century, with its many discoveries in anatomy, physiology, and pathology and other medical events, as a time of wonderful advancement. In truth, few of these exciting revelations were actually considered useful in daily clinical practice. Leaders in medicine placed no more than minimal emphasis on such advances as the

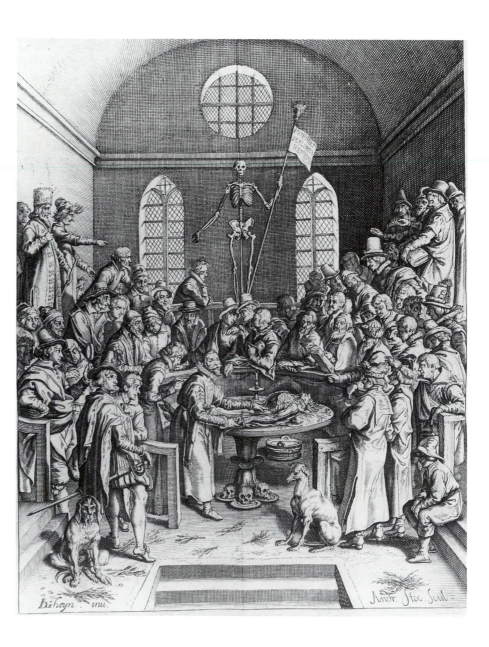

123. Anatomy as entertainment, with Pieter Paaw (1564–1617) demonstrating anatomy in his anatomical theater, the first built in the Netherlands. From Paaw's *Primitiae Anatomicae* (1615), the plate is clearly inspired by the frontispiece of Vesalius's *Fabrica* (1543), but most of the audience seems to be scarcely concentrating on the lesson. The skulls decorating the base of the dissection table are an unusual piece of appropriately macabre ornamentation. Paaw was Nicolaas Tulp's teacher. *(Jeremy Norman & Co., Inc.)*

SEVENTEENTH-CENTURY ANATOMICAL OBSERVATIONS

∞

GASPARO ASELLI (1581-1626)
Lacteal vessels (1622)

JOHANN WIRSUNG (1600-1643)
Pancreatic duct (1642)

OLOF RUDBECK (1630-1702) AND THOMAS BARTHOLIN (1616-1680)
Intestinal lymphatics and thoracic duct (1652)

FRANCIS GLISSON (1597-1677)
Capsule of the liver (1654)

THOMAS WHARTON (1614-1673)
Duct of the submaxillary salivary gland (1656)

CONRAD SCHNEIDER (1614-1680)
Pituitary membrane of the nasal chamber and sinuses (1660)

MARCELLO MALPIGHI (1628-1694)
Capillary circulation, particularly in the lungs (1661)

NIELS STENSEN (1638-1686)
Excretory ducts of the parotid gland (1662)

THOMAS WILLIS (1621-1675)
Vascular anatomy of the brain (1664)

FREDERIK RUYSCH (1638-1731)
Lymphatic valves (1665)

RICHARD LOWER (1631-1691)
Heart as a muscle (1669)

THOMAS KERCKRING (1640-1693)
Valvulae conniventes of the small intestine (1670)

REGNER DE GRAAF (1641-1673)
Ovary and follicles (1672)

JOHANN PEYER (1653-1712)
Lymphoid follicles in the small intestine (1677)

CASPAR BARTHOLIN (1655-1738)
Sublingual salivary gland and ducts (1684)

JOHANN BRUNNER (1653-1727)
Duodenal glands (1687)

ANTONJ NUCK (1650-1692)
Processus vaginalis peritonei, or Nuck's canal (1685)

CLOPTON HAVERS (?-1702)
Haversian canals (1691)

WILLIAM COWPER (1666-1709)
Female urethral glands (1699)

blood circulation hypothesis, the understanding of the physiology of respiration, and the refinement of the microscope, since none of these new developments helped the average practitioner improve a patient's state of health. Observational skills and practical experience were considered more valuable than scientific theories.

A number of new directions in medical thought became apparent during the seventeenth century as a result of tremendous advances that were made in such sciences as chemistry, astronomy, and mathematical physics. Out of these new influences grew two major modes of medical thought: iatromathematical, also known as iatrophysical, and iatrochemical.

Iatromathematical thinking essentially regarded the human body and its physiological functions as a machine that strictly obeyed the laws of mathematics and physics. Among its major adherents was the French philosopher Descartes, whose thinking about human physiology was first presented in his posthumously published book, *De Homine* (1662). He treated the human body and its pathological conditions as a material machine directed by a rational soul, which was located in the pineal body. The leaders of the iatromathematical school knew and appreciated little about the burgeoning science of chemistry. Accordingly, their efforts dwindled over the years to become nothing more than unconventional medical practices.

The iatrochemical school was a fusion of alchemy, medicine, and physiological chemistry and was practiced mainly by followers of Paracelsus, the most prominent of whom were the Belgian mystic Jean Baptiste van Helmont (1577-1644), the Leyden professor Francois de la Boe (1614-1672), and Thomas Willis in Oxford. The latter's advocacy of physiological chemistry was apparent in his qualitative examination of human urine. Willis discovered that the urine of a diabetic tasted sweet, and he was able to establish the basic principle for diagnosing diabetes mellitus and diabetes insipidus. In addition to his chemical experimentation, Willis was a superb anatomist who clarified the circulation in the brain. His *Cerebri Anatome: Cui Accessit Nervorum Descriptio Et Usus* (1664) included the most complete and accurate account of the nervous system up to that time. This important book was partly illustrated by Christopher Wren (1632-1723), who was later to become England's leading architect.

Although from the modern perspective medicine and surgery as practiced in the seventeenth century hardly appear advanced, it was a period of remarkable innovation. New therapeutic modalities were being introduced that would have enormous impact on the future development of surgical operations. The most important of these were the concept of exhaustive treatment, including bleeding and purging, and the use of intravenous injection of drugs and transfusion of blood.

Ancient authors had long imagined that the body was made up of four humors. These body fluids were believed to hold each other in balance and hence promote a healthy state; when an imbalance occurred, disease became present. Medical treatment attempted to return the humors to balance. Over the centuries emphasis was placed on all forms of draining and cleansing to ensure proper humoral balance. By the seventeenth century, this thinking was evident in the form of exhaustive treatment (i.e., bloodletting, emetics, enemas, laxatives, and sweating). Much of what is now considered therapeutic silliness was performed by barber-surgeons and their university-educated counterparts.

Bloodletting, in particular, became a source of considerable remuneration for the surgeon. Exactly when bleeding came into serious vogue remains historical conjecture. However, Tiberio Malfi's work, *Il Barbiere* (1626), the earliest book specifically devoted to barber-surgery, contained engravings detailing bloodletting, including portraits of two female barber-surgeons considered especially adept at the procedure.

124. *Facing page,* The barber-surgeon's phlebotomy, or blood-letting, stand. English, seventeenth century. The adjustable stand is carved with two bloodletting scenes. It was probably used for resting the arm during the operation. *(Reproduced by permission of the Trustees of the Science Museum, London. Inventory 602325; 28/93.)*

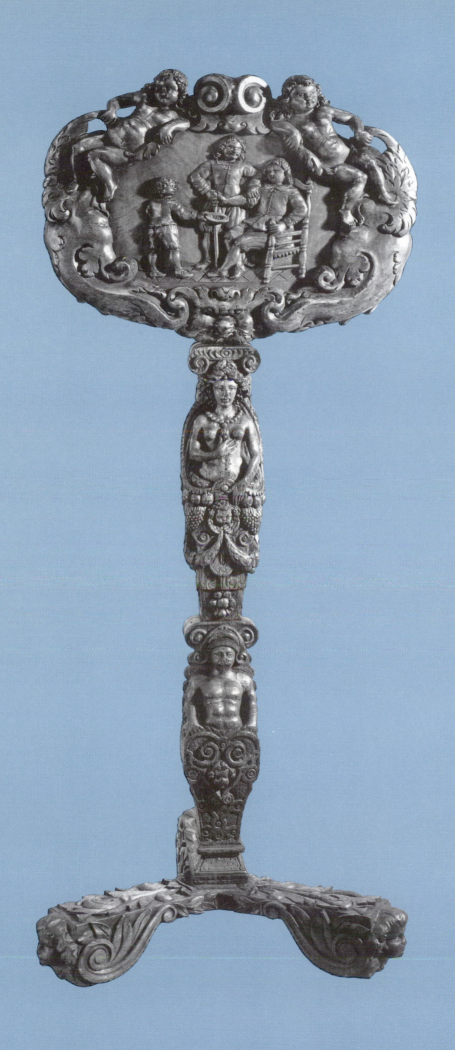

There was no easy estimation of exactly how much an individual should be bled. As a rule, the removal of approximately 500 milliliters of blood usually sufficed. However, verified accounts exist of extraordinary amounts of bleeding. A bloodletter in Yorkshire, for instance, extracted 2 liters of blood at a time if the patient was particularly corpulent. Undoubtedly, any individual would feel "different" after such therapy. The question remains, was it for better or worse?

For a surgeon, bleeding a patient had a direct salutary benefit in certain disease processes. In cases of incarcerated or strangulated hernia, bleeding was carried out until the patient became syncopal. In this way, the individual was made limp and weak, possibly to allow the surgeon a chance of reducing the herniated tissue through a narrow fascial opening.

As bloodletting became more accepted, it was used increasingly, even in healthy individuals, as a form of disease prevention. Part of the rationale for this preventive therapy is evident in the copious amounts of water and food that patients were given with it: a kind of "blood washing" was believed to occur when the amount of urination and defecation increased.

In Paris one of the major functions of surgical house officers was to bleed patients. This chore, said to consume an hour's time every afternoon, probably explains why there were more surgical interns than physician interns at the Hotel Dieu. Bleeding was also performed at the popular public baths by the bathkeeper, who often was a barber-surgeon.

Bloodletting was practiced in patients from all levels of seventeenth-century society, including the English royalty, who procured the services of a surgeon exclusively for such a purpose. Specific surgical instruments were gradually de-

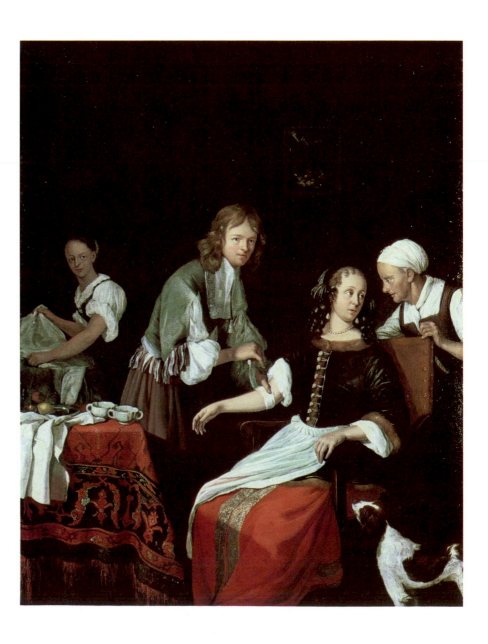

125. A surgeon bandaging a woman's arm after bloodletting. Oil painting on copper, by Jacob Toorenvliet (1635-1719). In the seventeenth century bloodletting was the most fashionable of cures. Individuals were bled for any reason and sometimes for no reason at all. Louis XIII was bled 47 times, and Louis XIV was bled 38 times. *(Wellcome Institute Library, London. Negative 16891.)*

veloped for the practice. Perhaps the most common of all such phlebotomy implements was the lancet. Lancets were usually flexible, razor-sharp, pointed blades between 5 and 7 centimeters long, in folding guards of ivory, tortoiseshell, or mother-of-pearl. These blades were used to make a small incision in a vein, from which blood was collected into "bleeding bowls." These bowls became their own art form; designs varied greatly. In general, the first "bleeding bowls" were straight sided; by the end of the seventeenth century they had become slightly convex. The usual materials for construction were silver, pewter, or ceramic. By the conclusion of the century the scarificator was being employed for bleeding purposes. The scarificator was a highly ingenious instrument consisting of a square brass, silver, or silver-plated case with slots, from which sharp, strong blades protruded and moved across, on the release of a trigger. The blades were sometimes rounded and sometimes pointed, and the depth to which they were required to incise could be regulated by a screw at the base of the instrument.

126. Barber-surgeon's sign. English, seventeenth or eighteenth century. This carved wood sign, illustrated with a bloodletting scene, was probably hung outside the office of a barber-surgeon to indicate his trade at a time when most people were illiterate. A more typical sign of the barber-surgeon was the striped pole, still sometimes found today. The pole represented the staff gripped by the patient's hand to promote bleeding, and the white and red stripes signified the tourniquet and the blood. *(Reproduced by permission of the Trustees of the Science Museum, London. Inventory A631340; MS574.)*

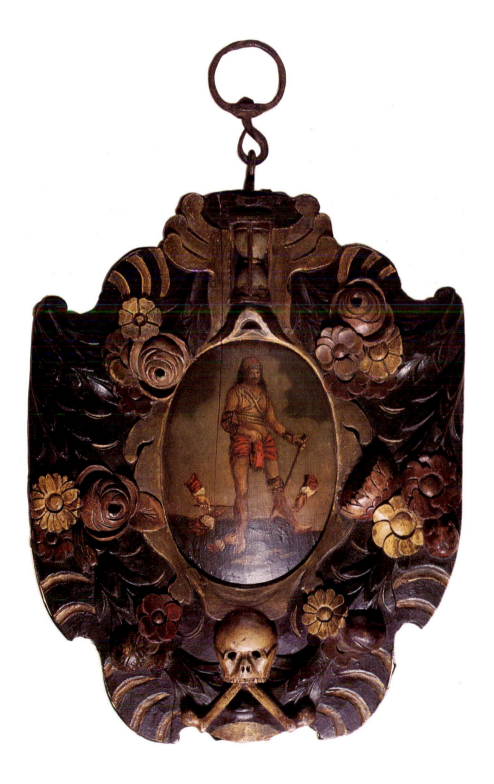

During the mid-1600s intravenous injection of drugs and transfusion of blood became medical reality. In 1656 Wren had injected wine and ale into the veins of a dog. This experiment was repeated many times; in 1665 Johann Elsholtz's (1623-1688) treatise *Clysmatica Nova* paved the way for the venous infusion of medicines.

Johann Major (1634-1693) performed the first successful intravenous injections in humans (1662). These experiments were recorded in his *Chirurgia Infusoria* (1667): the title itself suggests the surgeons' prominent role in this early research. Concurrently the earliest attempts at blood transfusion were made. When an actual blood transfusion was made from one human being to another remains uncertain. However, the vital importance of blood had been apparent since prehistoric times. The concept of using a healthy individual's blood to restore youthfulness and vitality to the aged or infirm is ancient.

One of the earliest proposals for the transfusion of blood was made by Andreas Libavius (1546-1616) in 1615. In 1628 Giovanni Colle (1558-1631) published a similar suggestion but is not known to have completed any practical experimentation. Another Italian physician, Francesco Folli of Florence, is often credited with performing the first known animal-to-animal transfusion, but he left no written record.

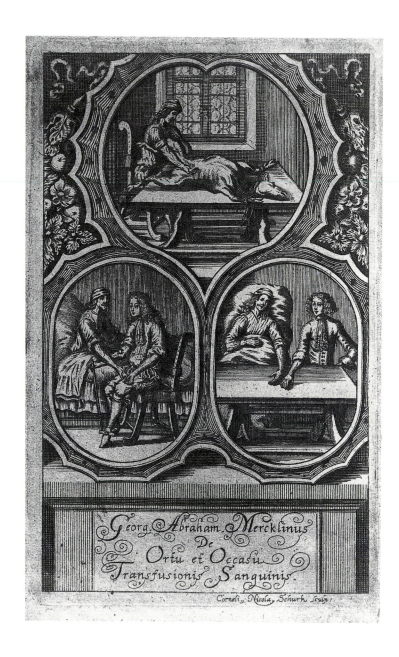

127. Blood transfusion was first practiced from animals into humans and, soon thereafter, from one human to another, without any awareness of the necessity for homogeneity of blood groups. An early portrayal of human-to-human transfusion appears in this frontispiece from Georg Abraham Mercklin's (1644-1702) *Tractatio Med. Curiosa De Ortu Et Occasu Transfusionis Sanguinis* (1679). At the top of the plate is a transfusion from an animal into a human. Both types of transfusion were considered equally effective at that time. *(Jeremy Norman & Co., Inc.)*

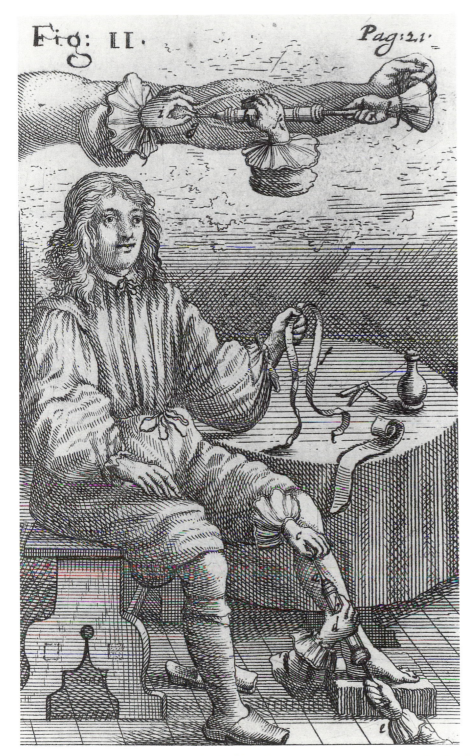

128. Much technical detail is shown in this plate from Johann Elsholtz, *Clysmatica Nova* (1665). Detail demonstrates how blood was actually transfused into an arm or a leg. *(National Library of Medicine, Bethesda, Md.)*

The first authenticated record of a blood transfusion was written by Richard Lower (1631-1691), a well-known practitioner who worked at Oxford and successfully carried out a transfusion from artery to vein in dogs in February 1665. Lower used quills for uniting the blood vessels of the two dogs, but subsequently found that the use of silver tubes connected by a piece of the cervical artery of an ox was more satisfactory.

Lower's successful transfusion of blood in dogs encouraged Jean Denis (1625-1704) of Paris to perform the first successful transfusion in a human. Before taking this bold step, Denis attempted to transfuse the blood of one kind of animal into the veins of another kind: in March 1667 the blood of a calf was transfused into the veins of a dog, without apparent ill effects. On June 15, Denis performed a transfusion in a 15-year-old boy, who had iatrogenic hypotensive shock as a result of more than 20 bleedings and various laxatives and enemas that had been administered by his physicians. Using nine ounces of lamb's blood obtained from its carotid artery, Denis performed the transfusion in the youngster, whose condition was greatly improved, with no lasting sequelae.

197

Denis's claim to priority spurred Lower to perform the first successful transfusion in a human in England. On November 23, 1667, Lower and Edmund King (1629–1707) successfully transfused the blood of a sheep into a Bachelor of Divinity student at Cambridge. A few days later the renowned Samuel Pepys (1633–1703) met the subject of this experiment at a dinner party. Pepys recorded in his famous diary an account of the meeting:

> I was pleased to see the person who had his blood taken out. He speaks well, and did this day give the Royal Society a relation thereof in Latin, saying that he finds himself much better since, and as a new man, but he is cracked a little in his head, though he speaks very reasonably and very well. He had but 20s. for his suffering it, and is to have the same again tried upon him: the first sound man that ever had it tried upon him in England, and but one that we hear of in France, which was a porter hired by the virtuosoes.

Records of the Royal Society show that the divinity student did, indeed, undergo a second transfusion on December 14, which apparently went well, without any serious side effects. Lower continued his experimentation with blood and in 1669 injected dark venous blood into the lungs of an animal. He correctly concluded that its consequent bright red color was due to the blood absorbing some of the air passing through the lungs. Lower described this final project in his monograph *Tractatus De Corde Item De Motu & Colore Sanguinis Et Chyli In Eum Transitu* (1669). Because the patients who had received the first

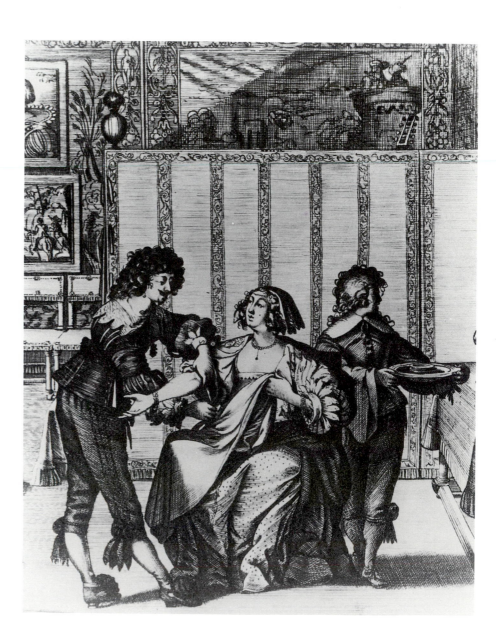

129. *The Bloodletting,* by Abraham Bosse (1602–1676). Bosse has included much valuable detail concerning both the furnishing and decor of the room and the costumes of this elegant, fashionable barber-surgeon, his assistant, and the wealthy patient. *(National Library of Medicine, Bethesda, Md.)*

transfusions did not receive too much blood, they did not die. Although other physicians did perform a few further animal experiments, little more was heard of blood transfusion in England for more than a century.

After the triumphs of Denis, blood transfusion rapidly came into vogue in Paris, but setbacks were not long in coming. A Swedish baron had become ill during a visit to Paris in the summer of 1667. As a last resort, Denis gave this young man a large transfusion of calf's blood on July 24, but the transfusion failed and the baron died the following day. In 1668 one of Denis's patients died after the third of a series of transfusions. The distraught and infuriated widow instituted legal proceedings against Denis in a case that aroused great emotion. A verdict was rendered against Denis, and it was directed that neither he nor any physician could perform a transfusion without the express permission of the Faculty of Medicine of Paris. Since this conservative Faculty had always been opposed to the whole idea of transfusion of blood, no permissions could ever be obtained. In 1670 the practice of transfusion was forbidden by law in France.

The cultural and social aspects of seventeenth-century medicine and surgery suggest it to have been a time of individual scientific endeavor rather than of concerted advancement of science. Each country took a different approach to its professional communities, especially in the sponsorship of scientific societies. The French government, through the Academie Royale Des Sciences, which was founded by Louis XIV, was a staunch supporter of its leading scientists and physicians. Conversely, in England the Royal Society was organized as a private group without true government backing.

Most surgeons were not well compensated, although certain prominent individuals were well off. The medieval custom of paying a lifetime annuity for a successful operation remained somewhat in vogue. According to records of a Frankfurt tariff of 1668, a German barber-surgeon received 10½ marks for setting a fractured arm, 31 marks for repairing a dislocation of the elbow or knee joint, or, if the result was poor, half as much. Operative results often regulated fees; a surgeon charged 31 marks for amputating an arm, 51 marks for a lithotomy, or half that amount if the patient died. At least, the overt problem of being put to death for a mortality no longer existed for surgeons in the seventeenth century.

As in every previous century of human existence, the major medical problems, other than those resulting from wars, were not of a surgical nature. Epidemic disease continued to extract a huge price: bubonic plague remained a serious problem and in London (1665) killed almost 70,000 persons; similar numbers of persons died in other large cities such as Milan (1630), Vienna (1679), and Prague (1681). No country in Europe escaped this scourge of the seventeenth century. To compound the problem, substantive public health reforms and attempts at improving sanitary conditions were few.

The first well-known written ridicules of the healing arts were published during the seventeenth century. Jean Poquelin (1622-1673), better known as Moliere, was unrelenting in his sarcasm toward the weaknesses and foolish actions of the physicians and surgeons of France. He had little use for the medical profession, against whom he carried a lasting grudge. Although physicians bore the major brunt of his pen, surgeons and their pedantic teachings were also made to look foolish. Moliere's farces such as *L'Amour Médecin* and *Le Malade Imaginaire* remain popular to this day.

Surgery in the seventeenth century did not keep pace with the progress in anatomy and physiology. In comparison to the extensive development of the medical literature, the literature of surgery seems quite meager. Surgeons had not yet achieved the social and academic status of physicians, and bitter antagonisms were still apparent in particular countries.

GERMANY AND SWITZERLAND

The overriding societal event in seventeenth-century Germany was the Thirty Years' War (1618-1648). The last of the great religious wars of Europe, the Thirty Years' War began as a civil war between the Protestants and Roman Catholics in the German states. Germany became the battlefield where Catholic Austria, often allied with Spain, fought the Protestant Danes, Swedes, and Dutch (1625-1635). Catholic France entered the war to fight against Catholic Austria, putting the interests of the kingdom of France above those of the Church (1635-1648).

The war, a sad chapter in European history, ended with the signing of the Peace of Westphalia in 1648. The treaty stripped most of the power from the Holy Roman Emperor and permitted France to acquire Alsace and Lorraine;

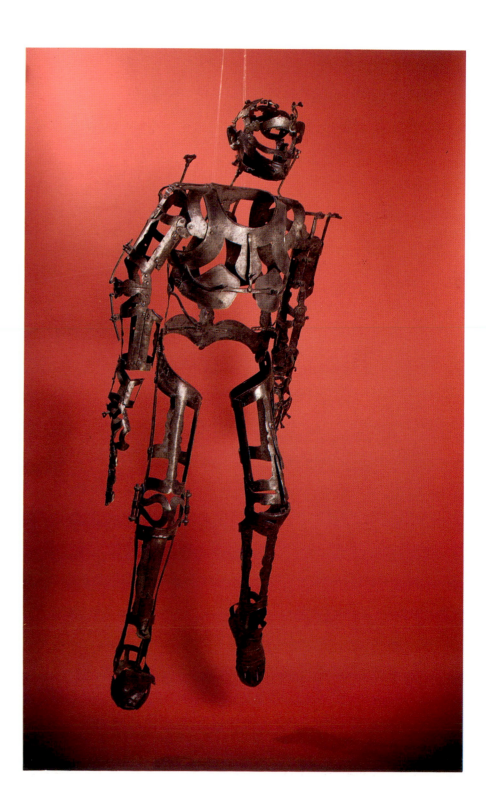

130. Suit of orthopedic armor, seventeenth-century Germany. *Left,* Frontal and, *right,* rear views. The armor is shown suspended. It is fully articulated and measures approximately 5 feet from head to toe. Each arm and leg demonstrates a different type of metal splint available at the time. Although the purpose of these steel splints was medical, they were undoubtedly fabricated by a company whose usual work was to produce armor for military purposes. Few other examples of this sort of instructional device have survived. *(Jeremy Norman & Co., Inc.)*

Sweden gained control of the mouths of the Elbe, Oder, and Weser rivers. In addition, Calvinism was granted equal status with Catholicism and Lutheranism.

As a result of the war Germany was left in a pitiable condition. It is estimated that almost half of the populace had been killed or wounded. Ruin was everywhere: whole cities, villages, and farms had disappeared.

For unknown reasons the surgeons of Germany did not gain or appear to use as much knowledge from their experience during the Thirty Years' War as did those in France. The barber-surgeons in Germany continued to reign supreme; their various guilds contained men of ability and independent thought.

The most prominent seventeenth-century German surgeon was Wilhelm Fabry von Hilden (Fabricius Hildanus) (1560-1634). He was born in Hilden, not far from Dusseldorf, the son of a relatively well-to-do court clerk. A series of personal misfortunes confronted von Hilden as an adolescent. His father died in 1570, his stepfather just 3 years later. Shortly thereafter, von Hilden was

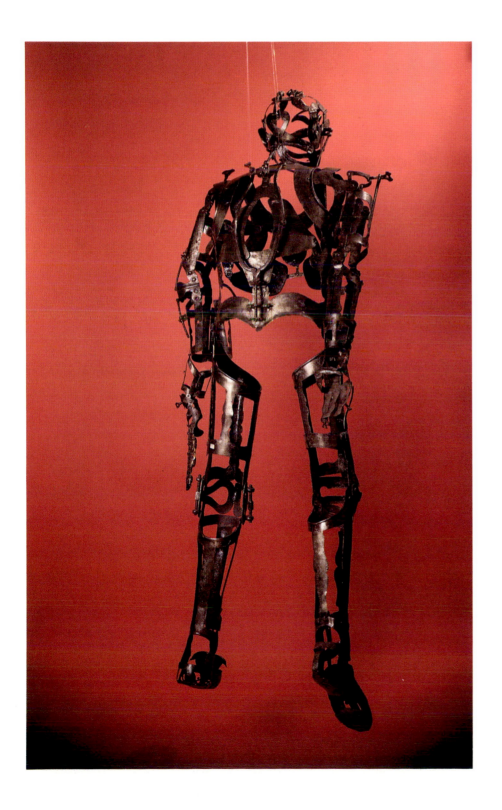

131. Orthopedic armor from the *Opera Chirurgica* of Girolamo Fabrici (1533-1619), as published in Leiden, 1723. This engraving was first published in the early seventeenth century and could have been the model for the armor illustrated in the preceding plate, which bears a striking resemblance to it. *(Jeremy Norman & Co., Inc.)*

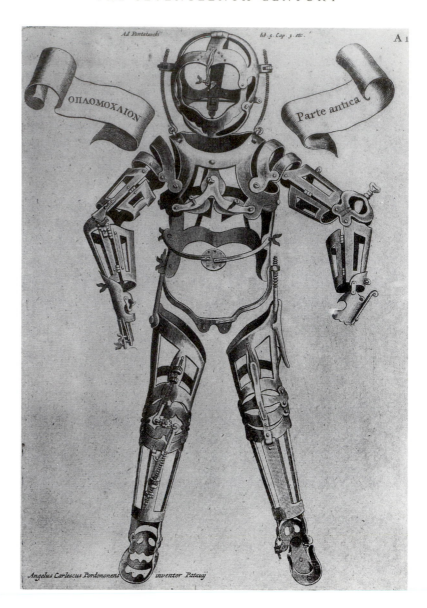

struck by the bubonic plague, which left him bedridden for months. Having little in the way of financial means, he was forced to forego the formal study of medicine and become an apprentice in the "lesser" craft of surgery.

For more than a decade von Hilden was initiated into the art of surgery by a thorough apprenticeship under a succession of skilled and experienced wound surgeons and barber-surgeons. From 1576 to 1580 he commenced his training under the wound surgeon Dumgens in Neuss. Next, he entered the service of Cosmas Slotanus, a pupil of Vesalius and the first barber-surgeon of the Duke of Cleves. In 1585 von Hilden spent time with the German barber-surgeon Bartisch at Metz. Shortly thereafter, he traveled to Geneva and began to work with Jean Griffon, a distinguished wound surgeon. After a few years, von Hilden returned to his native city and to Cologne (1591-1596), where he established a clinical practice. Although not considered a true itinerant surgeon, von Hilden was peripatetic in his career and eventually settled for varying periods of time in Bern, Geneva, and Lausanne.

In Cologne von Hilden wrote the first of his many important works. The *De Gangraena Et Sphacelo* (1593) was the earliest surgical treatise in which a surgeon recommended amputation above the gangrenous or injured part. Von Hilden stated that in gangrene of the foot the site of amputation should be four to five fingers' breadth below the knee, whereas, if the gangrene extends above the knee, the incision must be as close to the gangrene as possible, yet always made in healthy tissue. To control hemorrhage during an amputation, von Hilden devised a kind of tourniquet by means of a ligature tightened by a stick of wood. He also advised that arteries be individually ligated.

Von Hilden is remembered for his method of amputating with a red-hot knife. He considered this method to have three advantages: it is less painful; because the muscles are more completely retracted, the bone could be divided higher up; and the loss of blood is decreased when either a separate cautery or a ligature is used. His traditional bent is also evident in his advocacy of a "weapon salve" to aid healing, an atrocious mixture of mummy powder, earthworms, iron oxide, pig brain, and moss from the skull of a man who had been hanged under the sign of Venus. Oddly, this concoction was not directly applied to the wound but to the weapon that caused it.

Despite von Hilden's lack of a university education, he was well versed in the classics; all his writings were in Latin, with subsequent translations into German. The most admirable characteristics of his professional life were his careful observation of his patients and his detailed recordings of his comments. From this wealth of clinical material von Hilden began to publish several monographs in 1606; these were followed by collections of case reports in series of 100 each. All these works were eventually collected in a massive six-volume set, *Observationum Et Curationum Chirurgicarum Centuriae* (1606-1641), von Hilden's most important work and for many decades the best collection of case records available. Among his most original ideas was the use of a magnet to extract an iron splinter from the eye, an idea first suggested to him by his wife.

In 1607 von Hilden authored the first book *(De Combustionibus)* devoted entirely to burns. In his essay he described three degrees of burns and also discussed the proper treatment of gunshot wounds. In so doing, much discussion was brought forth regarding the heating of the bullet by its passage out of the gun and through the air. In addition, he discussed the possibility of poisoning of the wound as a direct result of the gunpowder itself.

Among the important recommendations of von Hilden was the first suggestion in Germany for a field chest of drugs for army use, in *Neu Feldt Arztny Buch Von Kranckheiten Und Schäden* (1615). Von Hilden's advice was taken after his death, when the government began to supply such chests as standard military equipment.

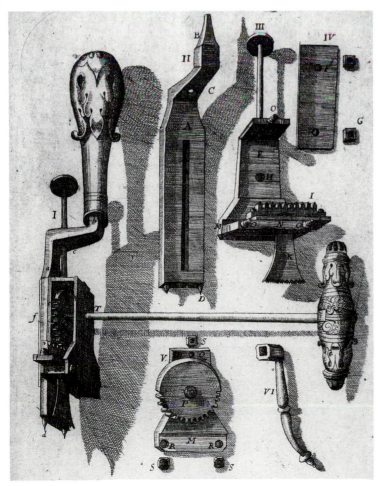

132. Instruments for drilling through bone. Plate 5 in the first edition of Scultetus, *Armamentarium Chirurgicum* (Ulm, 1653). Scultetus's illustrated handbook of surgical instruments and operations was not published until after his death. Nevertheless, it became the best-selling illustrated surgical manual of the seventeenth century. Although the first edition was published in folio format (14 by 9 inches), all the formats of later editions and translations were smaller, perhaps because surgeons found a lighter manual easier to carry. Of the 43 plates in this book, the first 20 represent detailed illustrations of the instruments Scultetus used, together with explanatory text describing the operations for which each was used. The elaborate ornamentation shown on the instruments illustrated by Scultetus seems to have been expected by purchasers of fine-quality goods in that Baroque age, and ornamental variations appear on some surviving instruments from the period. Purchasers of the book could take it to an instrument maker in their city and order instruments to be made: at that time most surgical instruments were made to order. Until the nineteenth century few instrument makers maintained inventories of surgical instruments for sale. *(Jeremy Norman & Co., Inc.)*

Von Hilden, also a well-known lithotomist, wrote *Lithotomia Vesicae* in 1628. In it he detailed his many operations for stone in the male bladder, for which he normally used a lateral perineal incision. He was accustomed to remove the stones in women via the vagina or the urethra.

Von Hilden displayed genius in the invention of instruments and technical aids and became one of the seventeenth century's most eloquent supporters of the empirical craft of surgery. His reputation endured long after his death.

Peter Uffenbach (1566-1635) compiled a surgical anthology of sixteenth-century writers, *Thesaurus Chirurgiae,* in 1610. Although little is known about Uffenbach, his work provides one of the best summaries of the surgical knowledge at the time.

The most important surgical work from the Thirty Years' War was Raymund Minderer's (1570-1621) *Medicina Militaris, Seu Libellus Castrensis* (1620), in which the author furnishes a detailed account of seventeenth-century military surgery in Germany.

An important early seventeenth-century German surgeon was Johannes Scultetus (1595-1645). He was born in Ulm but obtained his medical education in Padua, where he received his medical degree in 1621. Scultetus served in the military during the Thirty Years' War but in 1625 returned to his native city in the capacity of city physician.

Like increasing numbers of seventeenth-century surgeons, Scultetus was quite liberal in his indications for surgical intervention, as is evident in his famous *Armamentarium Chirurgicum* (1653), which became the most popular surgical text of the seventeenth century. Although published posthumously by his nephew, the work was published in numerous editions and translations in practically every European country. The work, literally a "picture book" of seventeenth-century surgery, displayed all the ingenious, complex devices that Scultetus created. Scultetus is best remembered eponymically for describing a position for herniotomy and castration in which the patient is on an inclined plane with the head lower than the legs; and for inventing a bandage with several overlapping tails, which is usually applied on the thorax or abdomen.

Matthaeus Purmann (1649-1711) was born in the northern part of Germany at Luben in Silesia. He was not university educated; instead he received his surgical training from a wound surgeon in Gross-Glogau. From 1675 to 1679 Purmann served as a military surgeon in the army of Frederick William (1620-1688), the elector of Brandenburg (Prussia). Purmann's military experience was extensive and included treating men who had been seriously injured by a new device, the glass grenade.

After the Peace of Saint Germain, Purmann settled in Halberstadt as city wound surgeon. He developed a thriving practice involving not only surgical problems, but also the difficulties of treating victims of the plague. In 1690 Purmann resettled in Breslau, where he served as chief surgeon.

Like von Hilden, Purmann wrote his many works in Latin with subsequent translations into German. His most important treatise is *Der Rechte Und Warhafftige Feldscher (The Proper Army Surgeon)* (1690). Purmann's rational approach to many aspects of military surgery is belied by his strong advocacy of "weapon salve" and the "sympathetic powder," a magic powder that was sprinkled on the already-used wound dressings before they were replaced on the wound. The additive action of the sun was believed to release a kind of healing power. Purmann provided exacting instructions regarding the use of a weapon salve:

> Take the weapon or instrument wherewith the patient was wounded, while it is bloody, or instead of it a stick put into the wound that it may be bloody. Anoint it with the unguent about a hand's breadth, and wrap it up in a clean linen rag or paper, your hands being very clean and then lay the weapon or stick in a place neither too hot nor cold; two or three days after anoint it again, and so for four or five times till the wound is well. The patient in the mean time must keep the wound clean, and cover it with a fine linen rag, without applying any medicine to it.

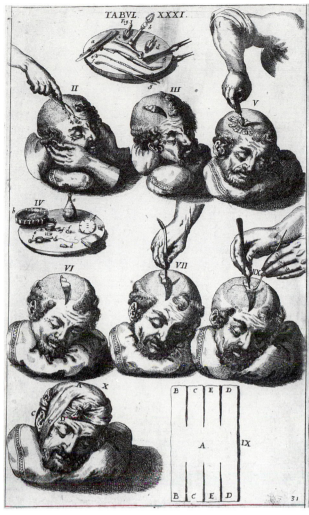

133. Plate 31 in Scultetus's *Armamentarium Chirurgicum* (1653) illustrates the immensely practical value of his manual and may explain why it was such a tremendous international surgical best-seller. Within the illustration itself all the instruments necessary to perform the craniotomy are shown. The plate shows the stages of the operation and the postoperative bandage. Brief explanatory text is keyed to guide letters in the plate. *(Jeremy Norman & Co., Inc.)*

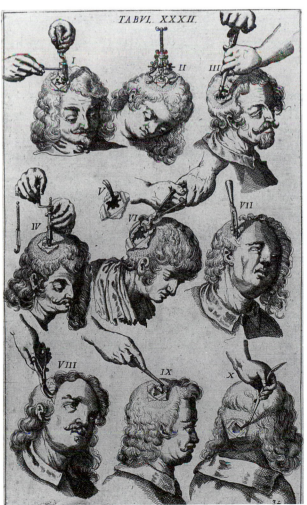

134. Plate 32 in Scultetus's *Armamentarium Chirurgicum* (1653) shows how some drilling instruments were to be used in craniotomies. As is usual in the illustrations from early surgical manuals, the patients, experiencing the full impact of the operations before the existence of anesthesia, do not seem to be suffering much. *(Jeremy Norman & Co., Inc.)*

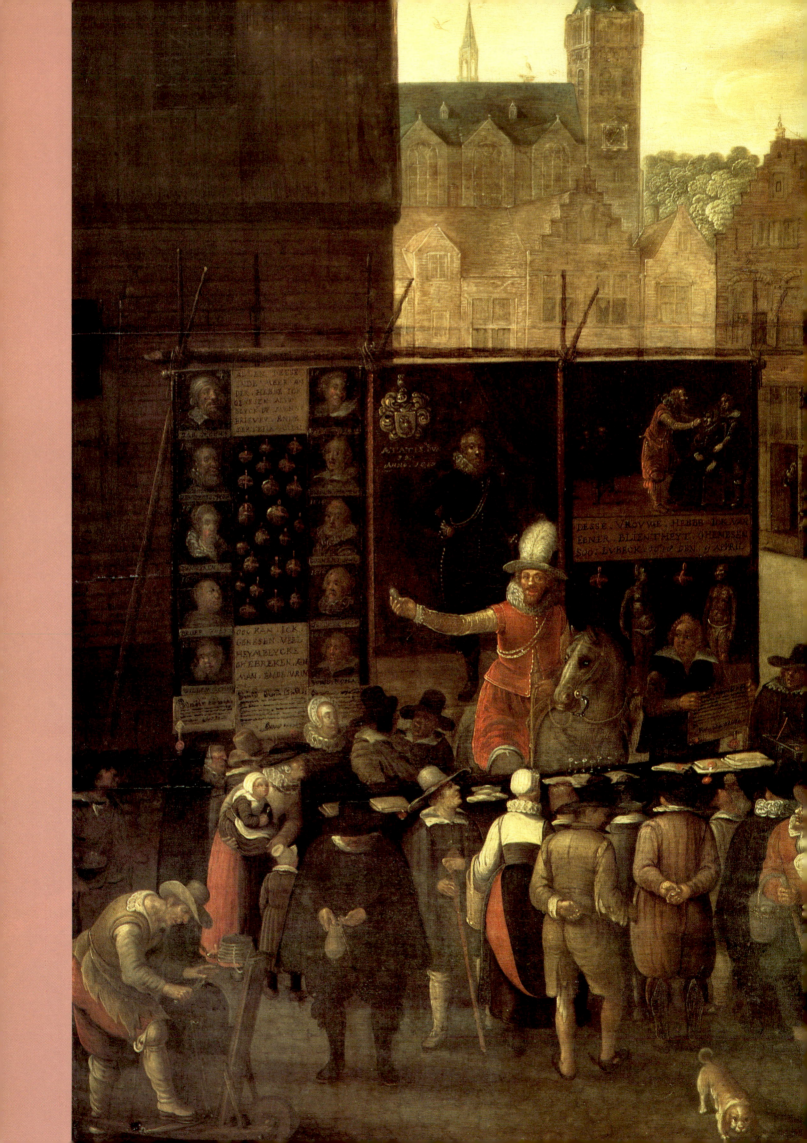

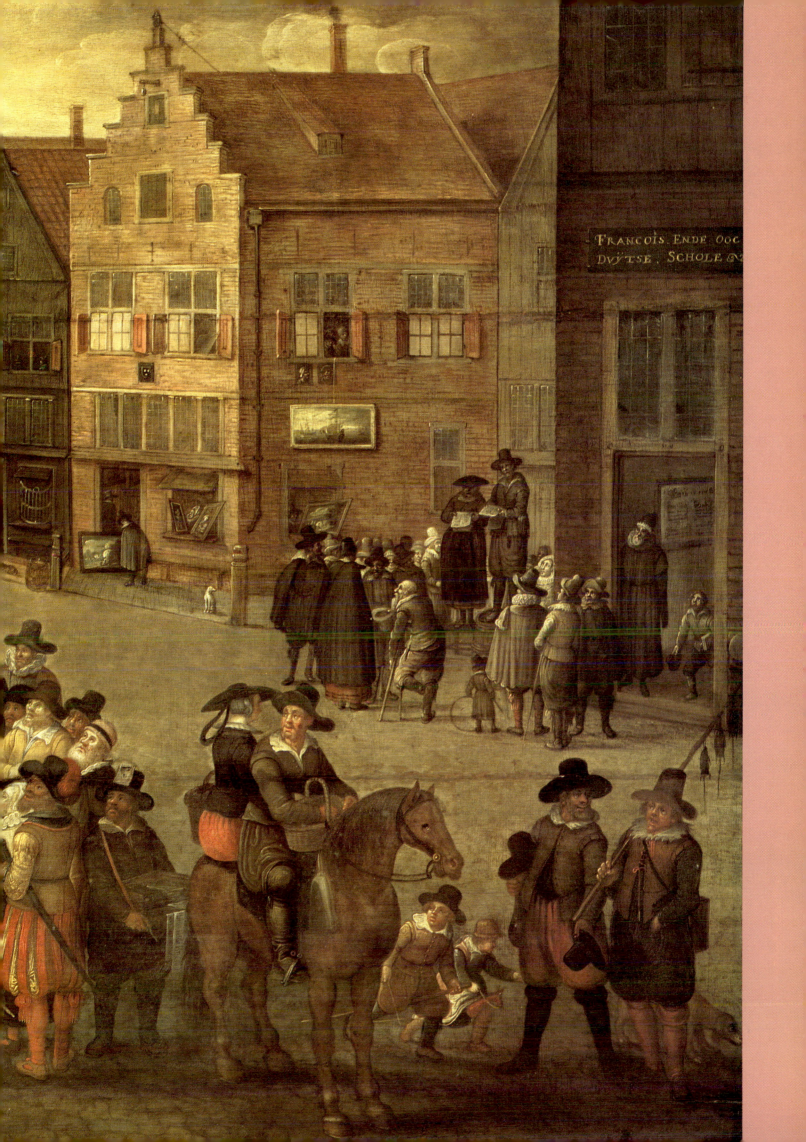

135. *Preceding pages,* an itinerant surgeon appears on horseback before a billboard advertising his skills in performing operations for lithotomy, hernia, and cataract. During the sixteenth and seventeenth centuries many surgeons may have obtained their patients by this kind of "medicine show." Portion of an anonymous painting from the northern Netherlands, first half of the seventeenth century. *(Rijksmuseum-Stichting, Amsterdam.)*

Among Purmann's important writings are *Chirurgischer Lorbeerkranz* (1685), *Funfzig Sonder-Und Wunderbare Schusswundkuren* (1693), *Chirurgia Curiosa* (1694), and what some regard as his magnum opus, *Grosse Wundartzney: Chirurgia Magna* (1692-1705). In all these works he continually stressed the importance of understanding anatomy for the proper practice of surgery.

Purmann appears to have performed all the important operations known or proposed during his time. In 1668 he performed the first recorded blood transfusion in Germany.

John von Muralt (1645-1733), a Zurich anatomist-surgeon, deserves mention. He studied at several of the major universities in Europe and in 1671 returned to his native city. Establishing a thriving practice, von Muralt soon anounced public lessons in anatomy, with demonstrations on the bodies of criminals and of persons dying from "remarkable diseases" in the hospitals. In 1677 von Muralt authored his *Vade Mecum Anatomicum,* which included a number of chapters on surgical techniques. Among the more elaborate techniques was a method of amputation in which skin flaps were used.

ENGLAND, SCOTLAND, AND IRELAND

The seventeenth century was a time of great political instability in England. What began with the glorious reign of Elizabeth I soon became unsettled after her death in 1603. James VI of Scotland was the immediate heir and became James I of England, the first of the Stuarts. England and Scotland were joined in a personal union under one king but were ruled as separate kingdoms. James I was not a popular ruler and assassination attempts, including one led by the infamous Guy Fawkes (1570-1606), were made on his life.

Under James's son Charles I (1600-1649), the struggle between the king and Parliament became quite bitter. Charles ruled as an absolute monarch and did not call any parliamentiary sessions from 1629 to 1640. Civil war broke out in 1642; men who supported the king were called Royalists or Cavaliers. Parliament's greatest support came from the Puritans, who attempted to force their strict beliefs on the populace. Oliver Cromwell (1599-1658), one of the Parliament supporters, led the Puritan army to a series of smashing victories. Charles fled to Scotland but was soon turned over to the Puritans and beheaded.

England became a commonwealth, or a republic, ruled by a committee of Parliament. Cromwell ended that form of government in 1653, and the country became known as a protectorate, with Cromwell the Lord Protector. Actually Cromwell was a dictator who ruled until his death. Cromwell's son Richard (1626-1712) was subsequently chosen Lord Protector but had difficulties handling the affairs of state. George Monk (1608-1670), a general, helped Charles II (1630-1685) restore the Stuarts as rulers of England.

Under Charles II the country turned against the Puritans and their strict beliefs. Many Puritans fled the country to settle in America. After the death of Charles II, his brother James II (1633-1701) came into power. James II wished to restore Roman Catholicism and absolute rule to the king. He was eventually forced to abdicate (1688), at which time Parliament invited his daughter Mary II (1662-1694) and her husband, William III (1650-1702), ruler of the Netherlands, to become king and queen. Parliament simultaneously passed an act requiring the king and queen of England to be members of the Church of England. William and Mary assumed the throne, and Parliament passed the Bill of Rights (1689), which ensured basic civil rights for the people.

As England became increasingly isolated politically from the rest of western Europe and, consequently, the western European universities, English surgeons had to rely on the teaching organized by various barber-surgeon companies and English universities. The activity of barber-surgeon companies was reaching its zenith. In Bristol, London, Newcastle, Norwich, York, Edinburgh, Glasgow, and Dublin students not only were apprenticed but also went through a regular course of anatomy that included dissections, surgical lectures, and examinations.

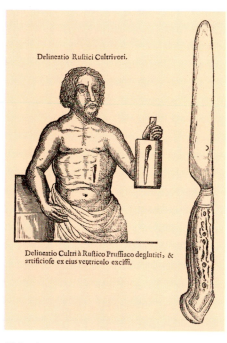

Delineatio Rustici Cultrivori.

Delineatio Cultri à Rustico Pruffiaco deglutiti, & artificiofe ex eius veutriculo exciffi.

136. An unusual case in the history of seventeenth-century surgery. This woodcut shows a Prussian who somehow swallowed an entire knife in 1640 and lived to tell the tale because his surgeon, Daniel Beckher (1594-1655) of Koenigsburg, was able to locate the knife in the patient's stomach by means of a magnet and to remove it, leaving a large scar. The operation was so sensational that the patient and his knife were painted, and the King of Prussia retained the blade as a souvenir. From Beckher, *Cultrivori Prussiaci Curatio Singularis* (1640). *(Jeremy Norman & Co., Inc.)*

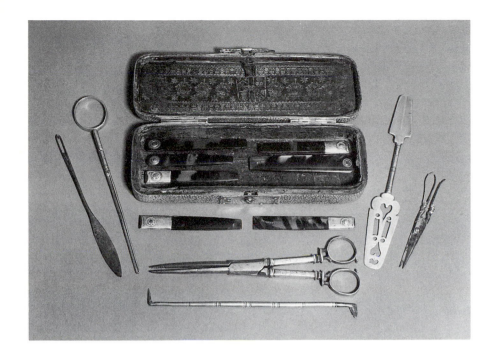

137. English surgical instrument case, late seventeenth century. The case, made of silver-mounted shagreen (fish skin), bears the arms of a Barber-Surgeons' Company. It contains scissors, a tongue depressor, forceps, probes, and lancets. The double-edged blades of the lancets are placed between tortoise shell covers united with inverted screws. The lancets were used to open veins during bloodletting. The various sizes and shapes of lancets were used on veins of different sizes and locations. *(Reproduced by permission of the Trustees of the Science Museum, London. Inventory A608302; 913/82.)*

The London barber-surgeons' company, to further enhance their political clout, obtained a second Act of Parliament in 1604 and received a new charter in 1629, which mandated that no one could practice surgery in London and Westminister until he had passed an examination by four examiners in the presence of two or more master barber-surgeons. Furthermore, no ship was permitted to leave the Port of London until its naval surgeon and the surgeon's chest and instruments had been examined by two officials of the company. In an apparent attempt to appease the universities, apprentice surgeons could not commence training until they could readily understand Latin.

In 1695 an unusual quarrel arose in London that illustrated the increasing activity of the surgeons who were not members of the Company, but instead were attached to hospitals and their medical schools. The London barber-surgeon's company complained that surgeons at St. Thomas' Hospital pretended to qualify surgeons in 6 to 12 months. The surgeons at St. Thomas replied that they took no apprentice for less than 7 years but they did allow other men's apprentices, who had served as country surgeons, to dress wounds for them. To satisfy the concerns of the London barber-surgeon company, however, the surgeons of St. Thomas agreed to insist on certification of their apprentices' previous work; the hospital surgeons also accepted the proviso that such persons should not practice in London except when admitted to the company. Thus for a time the London barber-surgeon's company maintained its authority over one of the hospital schools that would soon grow to major importance.

By the middle of the seventeenth century it was becoming evident that an English surgeon, if sufficiently educated and devoted to his craft, could reach a position of equality with the best physicians in the community. In many respects this changing attitude was brought about by the increasing numbers of well-known English surgeons and their erudite writings.

John Woodall (1556-1643) can be considered the link between sixteenth- and seventeenth-century English surgery. Little is known of his early life or his medical education and training. Woodall did serve with the troops of Elizabeth I in France in the aid of the French king, Henry IV. Later Woodall traveled through Germany, France, and Holland and also served as surgeon to a colony of English merchants near Posen, Poland. In 1604 Woodall was sent to Russia under the auspices of James I to interview Boris Godunow (1551-1605), Czar of Russia, regarding a possible commercial agreement to provide England with additional trade routes.

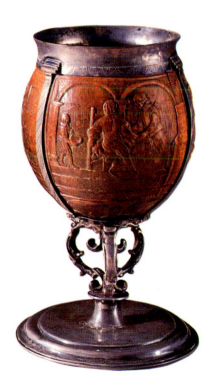

138. Coconut cup mounted in silver, made at York, England, by M. Gill, late seventeenth century. The coconut palm was new to Europe in the seventeenth century. The scenes carved in the coconut depict shaving and bloodletting, the skills of the barber-surgeon. *(Reproduced by permission of the Trustees of the Science Museum, London. Inventory A641076; MS573.)*

After returning to England, Woodall was appointed the first surgeon-general of the newly reorganized East India Company (1612), which provided him with the power to appoint all surgeons and mates to the company's ships. The East India Company opened the vast realm of India to British trade and was important in making India part of the British Empire. Its charter, provided by Elizabeth I, provided it with sole trade rights to all of the Indian and Pacific Oceans. Shortly thereafter, Woodall joined the London barber-surgeons' company and was honored with an appointment as surgeon to St. Bartholomew's Hospital. Woodall remained on staff for more than 20 years. In 1633 he was elected Master of the Barber-Surgeons and became one of the company's best-known examiners.

Woodall wrote a number of important treatises. *The Surgeons Mate* (1617) was one of the earliest books on naval medicine. The East India Company considered the work so important that it compelled each ship's surgeon to own a copy. In it were descriptions of a surgeon's chest, uses of instruments, and other sound advice for a ship's surgeon. Woodall was an early advocate of the use of limes and lemons as a preventive measure against the development of scurvy:

> I find we have many good things that heal the scurvy well on land, but the sea chirurgeon shall do little good at sea with them, neither will they indure. The use of the juices of lemmons is a precious medicine and well tried, being sound and good, let it have the chief place, for it will deserve it . . . it is to be taken each morning, two or three spoonfuls . . .

Woodall was a conservative surgeon in performing amputations, although he demonstrated that such an operation could be completed through the ankle joint. Nonetheless, his surgical experience was said to include hundreds of amputations. When an amputation was performed for gangrene, he suggested the incision be made through dead rather than living tissue. Woodall never used a cautery during an amputation but did refer to the use of ligatures in his text.

Among the more highly educated of seventeenth-century English surgeons was Alexander Read (1586-1641). He was born at Aberdeen, studied at Oxford, and received some of his surgical training in France. Like Banister, Read was one of the few who vigorously advocated the union of medicine and surgery. An individual of his word, Read was both a fellow of the Royal College of Physicians and lecturer at the Company of Barber-Surgeons. In the tradition of Vicary and Clowes, Read gave lectures at the barber-surgeons' guild house every Tuesday. Portions of talks given from 1632 to 1634 were published as *The Chirurgicall Lectures of Tumors and Ulcers* (1635). Three years later, *A Treatise of the First Part of Chirurgerie,* which contained portions of his lectures on wound care, was issued.

Read defined a wound as a "solution of continuity" caused by an external instrument. Healing was believed to be produced by agglutination in the case of those healed by first intention, in which no ointments or salves were placed. To accomplish healing, the wound edges were brought together gradually so that the deep and superficial portions fit snugly together. The reapproximation was accomplished by bandaging or dry stitching (strips of cloth or plaster were glued to the flesh and their free edges drawn together by threads), or by stitching with needles.

In 1638 Read wrote the *Manuall of the Anatomy or Dissection of the Body of Man.* He was quite interested in surgical anatomy; his experimentation with animals included the removal of a dog's spleen. Read recognized the following methods of maintaining hemostasis: (1) application of pledgets of lint moistened with white of egg or vinegar and water; (2) individual ligation of an artery or vein (although Read disapproved of ligatures in amputations); (3) transverse section of a bleeding vessel, which was lifted up by a hook and twisted; (4) cauterization or escharotics; (5) application of wound-healing medicines such as aloes; (6) opening a vein on the opposite side of the body while bandages are applied to the extremities; and (7) application of cold to the entire body or administration of a large dose of opium.

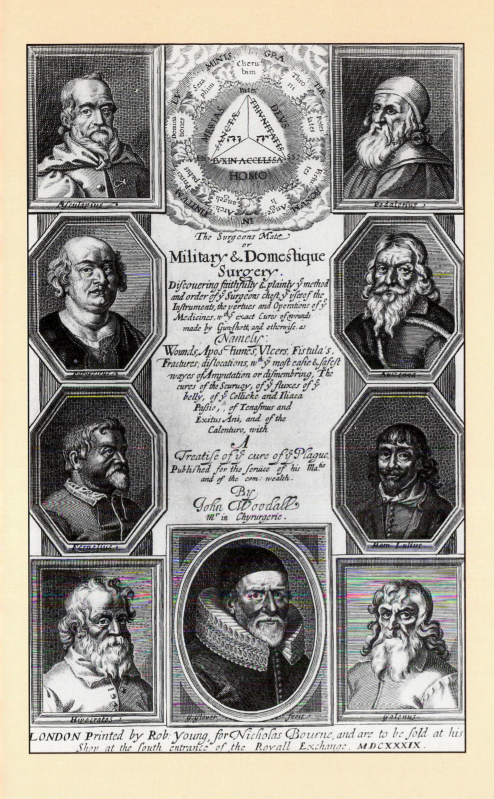

139. Engraved title page by G. Glover of the second edition of the first textbook for naval surgeons, John Woodall's *The Surgeon's Mate* (London, 1639). Surgeon-general of the East India Company, Woodall had a captive audience for his treatise; it was made required reading for all surgeons in the company. The textbook also found a much wider market because it contained innovative work on the treatment of such conditions as scurvy, gangrenous limbs, and gunshot wounds. The title page contains fanciful portraits of great physicians of the past such as Aesculapius, Hippocrates, and Galen. Beneath the emblem of the Holy Trinity and Woodall's name is, presumably, an authentic portrait of Woodall himself. *(Jeremy Norman & Co., Inc.)*

In 1633 Stephen Bradwell (1594-1636) wrote *Helps for Suddain Accidents Endangering Life,* the earliest known book on first aid from a surgeon's standpoint. Although little biographical information is available on Bradwell, he is not known to have distinguished himself as a clinical surgeon. His two other treatises were about the plague and dealt more with internal medicine than with surgical techniques.

James Cooke (1614-1688) lived in Warwick, where he was known as a general practitioner. In 1648 he wrote *Mellificium Chirurgiae,* which became a favorite textbook for surgeons, midwives, and naval surgeons. It was extremely practical, including such items as the contents of a surgeon's chest and overall medical and surgical therapeutics. Although the writing style was dull, the book was printed in numerous editions.

The most imaginative and best-known of English seventeenth-century surgeons is Richard Wiseman (1620-1676). He was devoted to the political cause of the Royalists and remained a staunch monarchist throughout his life. Some historical discrepancies exist concerning events in his early life; there is evidence that he was of illegitimate birth. Wiseman received his initial surgical training as an apprentice to a barber-surgeon around 1637. This particular mentor must have been a naval surgeon because Wiseman, while completing his services, entered the Dutch navy as a sea surgeon. At that time the Netherlands was in the process of fighting for its freedom from Spain. More than 80 years of struggle eventually ended in a Dutch victory in 1648.

Medical and public health conditions aboard a fighting ship left much to be desired. Undoubtedly, Wiseman gained much experience in handling the wounded. His naval service continued until just after the outbreak of England's civil war, when he returned to his homeland and joined the Royalist forces under Charles I. Initially Wiseman was a staff surgeon under the command of the Prince of Wales, son of Charles I, later to become Charles II. The military campaign was one of successive defeats and withdrawals. Wiseman always remained loyal to the prince and was eventually appointed his personal surgeon and, in reality, confidant.

In 1649 Charles I was beheaded, and the prince, now King Charles II, fled to Scotland with Wiseman in attendance. In 1651 the Scots declared Charles II their king, but Cromwell defeated his army and Charles II fled to France. During this campaign Wiseman was captured by Parliament's army during the battle at Worcester and placed under arrest. He did not regain his freedom until 1652, when he settled in London. Almost immediately, Wiseman joined the company of barber-surgeons, which gave him the right to practice. On suspicion of disloyalty he was rearrested and incarcerated in the Tower of London.

The length of Wiseman's imprisonment and reasons for his release are unknown. However, the political climate in London must have been less than inviting. Wiseman left England and took service in the Spanish navy for 3 years.

The English populace grew dissatisfied with the protectorate, and Charles II was invited to return and was crowned king in 1660. Shortly after the restoration, Wiseman was appointed by Charles II to be surgeon-in-ordinary to the royal household. In 1664 Wiseman became a member of the barber-surgeon's court of assistants and, a year later, master. Wiseman was eventually promoted to be sergeant-surgeon to the king and awarded a pension of 150 pounds a year, to commence in March 1671.

Wiseman played a pivotal role in the struggle of English surgeons for equality with physicians. His surgical writings reflected these beliefs and constituted a record of wide clinical experience, both at sea and on land. In 1672 he wrote *Treatise Of Wounds.* Four years later, the treatise was enlarged and printed in an expanded folio volume as *Severall Chirurgicall Treatises* (1676). There are eight of these treatises, each comprising a separate chapter on tumors, ulcers, diseases of the anus, the king's evil, wounds, gunshot wounds, fractures and luxations, and

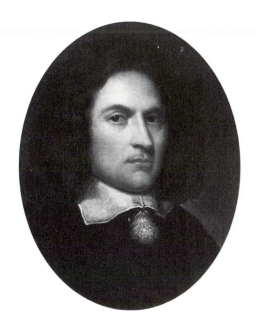

140. Painting of Richard Wiseman, derived from the miniature portrait by Samuel Cooper and owned by His Grace the Duke of Rutland. *(Reproduced by kind permission of the President and Council of the Royal College of Surgeons of England.)*

lues venerea. The work covered more than 600 surgical cases and is considered the first "modern" English text on surgery, even though it did not contain a single illustration or diagram. It was well written, logically arranged, and comprehensive. Wiseman, skillful surgical technician, was at his best in describing injuries and their treatment. He emphasized that the decision to amputate should be made promptly because during battle the patient was less sensitive to the pain of the operation. Wiseman amputated from above the diseased part and widely employed primary amputation in the treatment of gunshot wounds of the joints. On the other hand, he strove to preserve limbs, if any reasonable hope of salvage existed:

> In the heat of fight, whether it be at sea or land, the chirurgeon ought to consider, at the first dressing, what possibility there is of preserving the wounded member; and accordingly, if there be no hope of saving it, to make his amputation at that instant, while the patient is free of fever.

Wiseman provided the first description of tuberculosis of the joints. He is known to have investigated scrofula, or swollen glands of the neck, usually caused by tuberculosis. The treatment of scrofula, also termed "the king's evil," provides insight into the seventeenth-century belief in supernatural healing. As pragmatic as Wiseman was regarding virtually all aspects of seventeenth-century clinical surgery, he accepted the traditional belief that the king's touch could cure scrofula:

> But when upon trial the chirurgeon shall find the contumaciousness of the disease, which frequently deluded his best care and industry, he will find reason of acknowledging the good of God; who hath dealt so bountifully with this nation in giving the kings of it, at least from Edward the Confessor downwards (if not for a longer time), an extraordinary power in the miraculous cure thereof . . . I myself have been a frequent eye-witness of many hundreds of cures performed by his majesty's touch alone, without any assistance of chirurgery; and those, many of them, such as had tired out the endeavors of able chirurgeons before they came thither.

The lure of the sea was becoming a boon for surgeons in seventeenth-century England. As the country's political strength and corresponding naval needs increased, so did the necessity for sea surgeons. In 1686 John Moyle (?-1713) authored a little-known but quite practical work, *An Abstract of Sea Chirurgery*. Although scant information is available on Moyle, he describes himself on the title page as "sometime a sea chirurgeon in his majesties service."

A fascination with the sea is evident in Moyle's three-part work. The *Abstract* discussed the fitting out of the sea chest and the choice of proper medicines and bandages according to the type and length of voyage and the ship's destination; gave instructions on how a surgeon should act during battle and at other times; and listed miscellaneous directives regarding "the physical office imposed on him."

Moyle taught nothing of civilian surgery. He assumed that the reader was already a competent practitioner on land. The stark details of operating in the low-ceilinged, cramped spaces below deck in dim light supplied by candles are dramatically described. The actual surgical techniques described by Moyle are quite crude. Ligature is not mentioned; cautery and pressure tamponade are used in its place. Moyle's practical abstract, in contrast to a work like Wiseman's, is invaluable for demonstrating how the average surgeon of the seventeenth century performed surgery.

James Yonge (1646-1721) was born in Plymouth and apprenticed to a naval surgeon. He was present at the bombardment of Algiers by the English navy (1662) and subsequently made several voyages to Newfoundland and the western coast of Africa. In 1670 he settled in his home city and was appointed surgeon to the Naval Hospital at a salary of 5 shillings a day. Four years later, Yonge was appointed deputy surgeon-general of the English navy.

In his surgical treatise, *Currus Triumphalis, E Terebintho* (1679), Yonge provided the first account of a flap operation for amputation, as opposed to the old circular method:

> The ligatures and gripe being made after the common manner you are with your catlin, or some long incision-knife, to raise a flap of the membranous flesh covering the muscles of the calf, beginning below the place where you intend to make excision and raising it thitherward of length enought to cover the stump. Having so done turn it back under the hand of him that gripes; and, as soon as you have severed the member, bring this flap of cutaneous flesh over the stump and fasten it to the edges thereof by four or five strong stitches and, having so done, clap a dossil of lint into the inferior part, that one passage may be open for any blood or matter than may lodge between.

Yonge also provided one of the earliest printed descriptions of a tourniquet:

> . . . Very useful in amputations, especially above the knee; that is to say a wadd of hard linnen cloth, or the like, inside the thigh a little below the inguen, then passing a towel round the member; knit the ends of it together, and with a battoon, a bedstaff, or the like, twist it, till it compress the wadd or boulster so very strait in the crural vessels that their bleeding when divided by the excision, shall be scarce large enough to let him see where to apply his restrictives.

ITALY

Few seventeenth-century Italian surgeons were commensurate in rank with those of the previous four centuries. There was little political activity in Italy to suggest any formal organization of surgeons. Although barber-surgeons and itinerant surgeons were present, their activities did not appear to rival those of their counterparts in other European countries.

Giovanni Cortesi (1554-1636) was one of the earliest students of Tagliacozzi. Cortesi succeeded his mentor as professor of surgery at Bologna. Cortesi's best-known work, *Tractatus De Vulneribus Capitis* (1632), discussed wounds of the head. Little in his book is unique, however, and its influence on the evolution of Italian surgery was minimal.

The most notable Italian surgeon of the seventeenth century was Caesar Magati (1579-1647). He was born at Scandiano in the Duchy of Reggio and received his degree of Doctor of Medicine from the University of Bologna (1597). Magati then departed for Rome to devote himself to the study of anatomy and surgery. After returning to his native region, he commenced practice and developed an excellent reputation. In 1612 Magati was offered the professorship of surgery at the University of Ferrara. He held this position for a number of years, but poor health caused him to resign his post. For unknown reasons Magati decided to become a Capuchin monk, although he continued with a modicum of surgical work. In 1647, his illness, as well as suffering caused by bladder calculi, which had became acute, forced him to visit Bologna in the hope of obtaining relief via a surgical operation. The operation proved unsuccessful, and Magati died shortly thereafter.

Magati had an enormous impact on Italian surgery in a number of discrete ways. His only book, *De Rara Medicatione Vulneram, Seu de Vulneribus Raro Tractandis, Libro Duo* (1616), was quite well received. He urged the simple, expectant treatment of wounds by bandages moistened in plain water, without ointments. The process of cicatrization, he insisted, is not effected by the efforts of the surgeon but is fundamentally the work of nature. Therefore, he argued, bandages should not be renewed too often. He vehemently protested against the practice of introducing wicks and pledgets of lint into wounds. Magati also affirmed that gunshot wounds were not poisoned. The impact of his doctrines lasted well into the next century.

Marco Severino (1580-1656) was a famous anatomist and surgeon who taught at the University of Naples. Severino is alleged to have saved the lives of

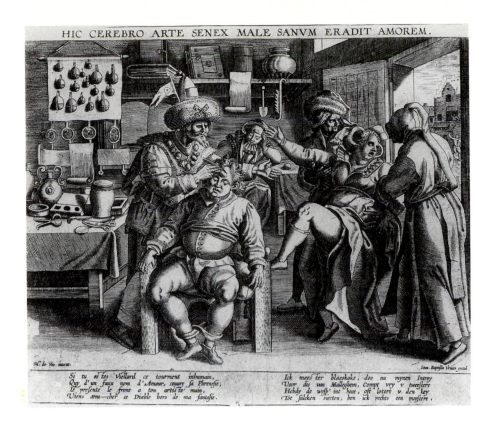

141. Removing the "stone of madness." Seventeenth-century engraving by Jean-Baptiste Vrints, after Maerten de Vos. The headline above the print may be translated, "With this brain surgery an old man mistakenly eradicates a healthy passion." While the patient's wife is clearly protesting, the quack surgeon, wearing a curious hat and a necklace of stones apparently removed from previous patients, operates on the old fool. Hanging on the wall, *left corner,* may be additional "stones of madness" that the quack has collected. The caption below the print may be translated, "To an old man love is an inhuman torment, concealing madness. Here is my forehead. Come, with your skilled hand remove this demon from my mind." *(Wellcome Institute Library, London.)*

numerous patients during a severe epidemic of diphtheria (1610) by performing tracheotomies for obstructed airways. To accomplish the operations he constructed a tubelike instrument and a trocar to keep the incised opening free for passage of air. Severino was the author of a surgical treatise, *De Recondita Abscessum Natura Libri* (1632), the first textbook of surgical pathology and the first treatise to include illustrations of pathological lesions with the text. In it he described abscesses, buboes, granulomas, neoplasms, and other disease processes.

Pietro De Marchetti (1589-1673) wrote the best-known surgical text of the seventeenth century in Italy. His *Observationum Medico-Chirurgicarum Rariorum Sylloge* (1664) contained many valuable clinical observations and strange case histories. Marchetti was succeeded as professor of surgery at Padua by his son Domenico, who is said to have successfully performed a nephrotomy for renal calculi in 1633.

During the seventeenth century it was considered dangerous to suture divided tendons, as the elder Marchetti observed:

Nerves and tendons must never be sutured, for this practice is often followed by fatal tetanus. The ingenious surgeon should rather remedy deformities by appropriate splints, as I did in the case of a distinguished Marshal of France, of the family of Montmorency. He received a sword cut on the right wrist, dividing the extensor tendons of the thumb. When the wound healed the thumb was drawn across the palm of the hand, so that he could not hold sword, dagger or lance, and was entirely incapacitated for the profession of arms, apart from which he declared life was not worth living. So he consulted me about amputating his hand, to which I could in no wise consent, but devised an iron case to hold the thumb out, fixed by two cords to bracelets round the wrist, and so he was able to hold and use all kinds of weapons.

Giuseppe Zambeccari (1655-1728) was born near Florence, studied at Pisa, and was especially influenced by Lorenzo Bellini (1643-1704), his professor of anatomy. In 1704 Zambeccari succeeded his mentor as professor of anatomy and held the position until his death. Zambeccari was one of the first surgeons to perform extensive animal experimentation to further the craft of surgery. In 1680 in a small booklet he described his numerous experimental operations on the cecum, eye, gall bladder, kidney, liver, mesenteric veins, omentum, pancreas, and spleen. By means of his experiments on dogs Zambeccari was able to demonstrate that the spleen is not essential to life and that after splenectomy the animal does not undergo a change in personality. By experimentally removing a kidney, Zambeccari strongly influenced the evolution of renal surgery.

NETHERLANDS

By the middle of the seventeenth century the Netherlands had become one of the recognized centers of surgical and anatomical teaching. Both Leyden and Amsterdam were beginning to attract students from all over Europe. The most illustrious of the teachers was Paul Barbette (?-1675), son of a Strassburg surgeon, who studied in Montpellier and Paris but finally settled in Amsterdam. Barbette was the first to suggest laparotomy for intestinal obstruction. After performing splenectomy on dogs, he recommended its performance in humans. He is also said to be among the earliest to have described femoral hernia. Barbette's *Chirurgia* (1658) went through 10 editions; his *Opera Omnia Medica Et Chirurgica* (1672) was printed 22 times.

Adrian Van Der Spiegel (1578-1625), known as Spigelius, was born in Brussels and studied at Padua. There he remained, lecturing and writing on anatomy, until he succeeded Guilio Casseri (1561-1616) in the chair of anatomy. Spigelius is especially noted for his trephinations of the skull. He is eponymically linked with an abdominal hernia through the semilunar line and with the caudate lobe of the liver. Among his most important works are *De Semitertiana Libri Quatuor* (1624), in which is found the first extensive account of malaria, and a posthumously published edition of his collected writings, *Opera Quae Extant Omnia* (1645).

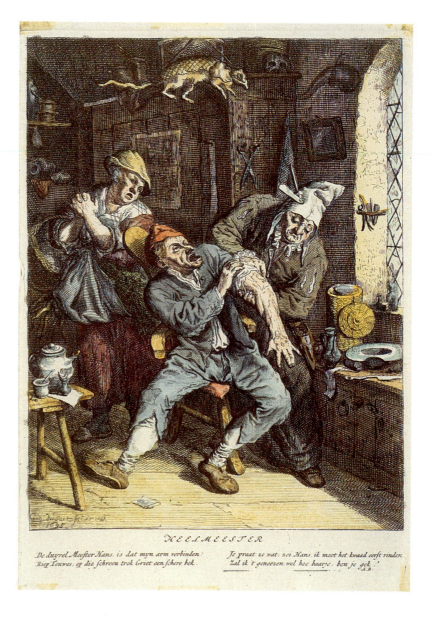

142. *The Village Surgeon* (1695), an etching by Cornelis Dusart (1660-1704). Unusual in its realistic depiction of the patient's discomfort, the print shows the surgeon, undignified in demeanor, with a lancet tucked into his cap and a probe in his hand, performing a minor operation on his patient's arm. Among the depicted artifacts of the barber-surgeon's trade are an instrument case strapped to the surgeon's belt and various medical and dental instruments on racks on the wall. On the window ledge is a barber's bleeding bowl; its semicircular notch allowed it to be brought close to the neck for shaving or close to a limb for bleeding. The operation is taking place near the window, the only good source of light in the room. *(Boston Medical Library.)*

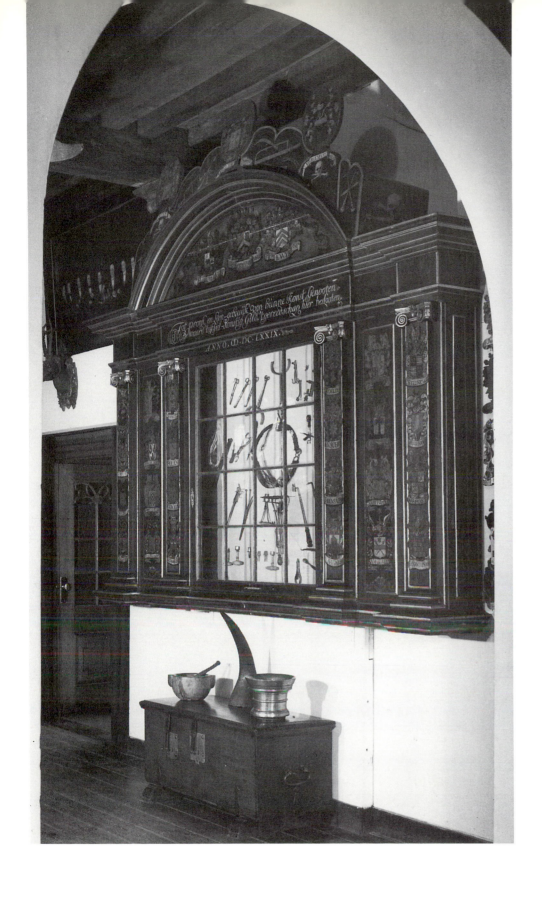

143. The original instrument cabinet of the Surgeons' Guild of Leiden, Netherlands, 1679. It contains a complete set of seventeenth-century surgical instruments willed to the guild in 1687 by one of its members. Because surgical instruments were particularly expensive at the time, it is possible that the Surgeons' Guild allowed its members to borrow the valuable instruments for operations. *(Municipal Museum "De Lakenhal," Leiden, The Netherlands.)*

217

FRANCE

The uncontrolled power of the French kings and their court and ministers grew steadily during the seventeenth century. France became an internationally strong nation, largely through the efforts of able ministers. Among the most prominent was Duc de Sully (1560-1641), who served Henry IV (1553-1610). Louis XIII (1601-1643) succeeded Henry IV but was only 9 years of age, so his authority was turned over to Cardinal Armand Richelieu (1585-1642). Richelieu accomplished more than any other individual to strengthen and solidify the French monarchy. Louis XIV (1638-1715), the "Sun King," succeeded his father and had a reign that lasted more than 70 years. However, his many military misadventures impoverished the French state, causing Jean Colbert (1619-1683), Louis XIV's controller of finances, to implement a strict internal economic program previously proposed by de Sully.

The official status of the barber-surgeon's guild in Paris greatly improved during the first portion of the seventeenth century. In 1603 the government of that city authorized the title of the guild to be "barber-surgeons" rather than simply "barbers." Concurrently, master barber-surgeons were given the legal right to treat all kinds of wounds. Three decades later, Louis XIII reaffirmed the enabling statutes of his "dear community of master barber-surgeons" and recognized the community as "the principal source of the knowledge and practice of this art in all our kingdom." Higher aspirations had earlier prompted the guild to attempt to change the name to "surgeon-barbers." This effort, in addition to one in 1643 to curtail subordination to the medical faculty, ended in failure.

Surprisingly, some master barber-surgeons left the guild to join the ranks of the Confraternity of St. Côme. Among these were the distinguished Nicolas Habicot (1550-1624), author of a text on anatomy (1610), and Jacques De Marque (1569-1622), who wrote *Traicté Des Bandages De La Chirurgie* (1618). However, most barber-surgeons did not wish to give up their barber's work in exchange for admission to the more elite organization.

In 1613, revolutionary-minded members of both the College of St. Côme and the barber-surgeons' guild attempted to unite the two companies, and the royal government gave its approval to this venture. However, a majority of the academic surgeons of St. Côme disavowed the union, thereby ending the agreement. More than 40 years later, the same plan for unification was proposed and met a far warmer reception from the academic surgeons, including the provost of St. Côme. On October 1, 1655, the surgeons of both the "long gown" and "short gown" put aside their centuries-old rivalry and signed a contract of union.

In joining forces with the barber-surgeons, the academic surgeons had an obvious economic incentive. As the membership of the prosperous guild of barber-surgeons increased, the guild threatened the viability of the much smaller company of academic surgeons. The inescapable fact was that it was difficult to make a living by practicing only "surgery." Without the mix of "barber's work," such as bloodletting and wound care, the economic stability of a practicing surgeon was seriously threatened. On a more practical level, barber-surgeons commanded much higher fees than did their academic counterparts. The affiliation of the barber-surgeons' guild with the Parish Church of St. Sepulchre was fortuitous, since that church was patronized by more and richer merchant guilds, which allowed for greater prosperity in patient referrals, than was the Church of St. Côme, with which the academic surgeons were affiliated.

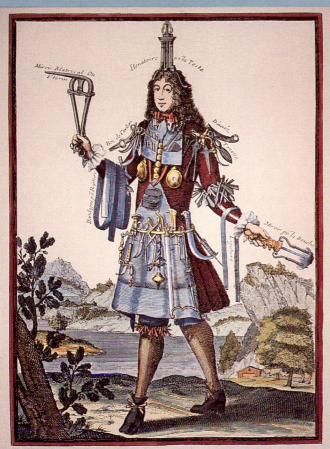

Habit de Chirurgien

144. *The Surgeon (left)* and *The Physician (below)*, as caricatured in the late seventeenth-century French series of prints of trades by Larmessin. This series was widely popular during the eighteenth century. In these typical characterizations the surgeon is shown as the technician of the scalpel, whereas the physician is depicted as the scholar of medical thought. *(Jeremy Norman & Co., Inc.)*

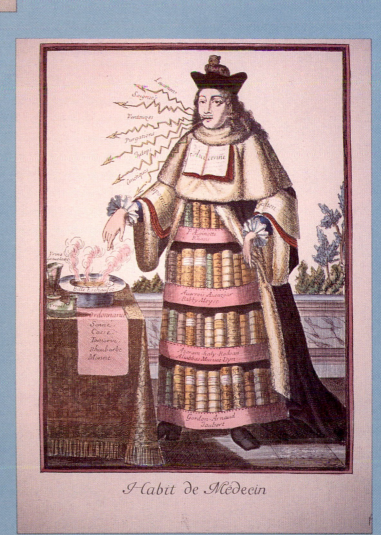

Habit de Médecin

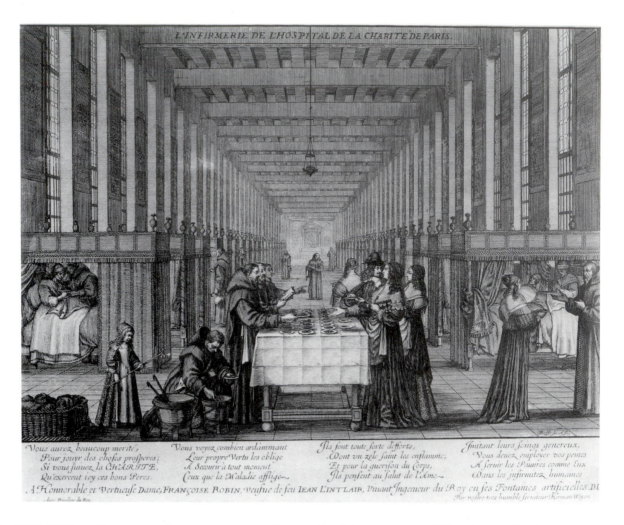

L'INFIRMERIE DE L'HOSPITAL DE LA CHARITE DE PARIS.

Vous aurez beaucoup merité,
Pour jouyr des choses prosperes;
Si vous suiuez la CHARITE,
Qu'exercent icy ces bons Peres.

Vous voyez combien ardamment
Leur propre Vertu les oblige
A Secourir à tout moment
Ceux que la Maladie afflige

Ils font toute sorte d'efforts,
Dont vn zele saint les enflamme;
Et pour la guerison du Corps,
Ils pensent au salut de l'Ame

Imitant leurs soings genereux,
Vous deuez employer vos peines
A seruir les Paures comme Eux
Dans les infirmitez humaines

A Honnorable et Vertueuse Dame, FRANÇOISE ROBIN, Veufue de feu IEAN L'INTLAIR, Viuant Ingenieur du Roy en ses Fontaines artificielles. DI...

145. Anne of Austria (1601-1666) visiting the great hospital ward of La Charité in Paris. Engraving after a gouache in the Musée Carnavelet, Paris, circa 1635 by Abraham Bosse. The ward was divided into private rooms by the drawing of curtains around each bed. This innovation put an end to the medical promiscuity typical among patients during the Middle Ages. *(Philadelphia Museum of Art, SmithKline Beecham Fund Corporation.)*

In many respects the small, elitist company of Parisian academic surgeons constituted an anomaly in the seventeenth century. There were no equivalents of the College of St. Côme in other French cities, where barber-surgeon guilds were the only formal surgical organizations. Furthermore, there were no companies of "pure" surgeons to be found in any other European country. In London the small company of surgeons had merged with the affluent barber-surgeons a full century before. In other countries, especially Germany, surgery was virtually controlled by barber-surgeons and itinerants or empirics. It was only in the major Italian university center that surgeons received medical degrees and assumed respected faculty positions. Nonetheless, even in Italy the barber-surgeon remained predominant.

The surgeons of St. Côme accomplished no great things for surgery; in fact, they contributed little of theoretical or practical value during their 350 years of existence. The major failure of these academic surgeons was their unwillingness to commit their work and knowledge to writing. Their intention was to keep surgical techniques from falling into the hands of the barber-surgeons, but the result was severe limitation of the influence of the surgeons of St. Côme on the future evolution of French surgery.

During the second half of the seventeenth century a strengthening of the united surgical guild was evident. There was a marked increase in its prestige in the eyes of the public, as well as a definite movement to separate the practice of surgeons from that of barbers. At the same time, the Faculty of Medicine was concerned about their potential loss of control over the united surgical community. Their indignant feelings are summed up in a revealing letter written by Guy Patin (1601-1672), the curmudgeonly dean of the Paris medical faculty:

> We are now at odds with our barber-surgeons who wish to unite with the surgeons of St. Cosmas, our ancient enemies. Those of St. Cosmas are miserable rascals, nearly all tooth-pullers and very ignorant who have attached the barber-surgeons to their string, by making them share their halls and their pretended privleges . . . They talk

of giving degrees of bachelors of licentiates and other such ceremonies and vanities, altogether indecent for such booted lackeys. The cause will be plead in one month and I believe that all the audacious designs of this temerarious riffraff will be bridled and regulated . . .

Are these surgeons of St. Cosmas not amazing? They had permission from the king about three hundred years ago by which they were given leave to assemble together. They claim from the word "license" that they were allowed to make licentiates in surgery, which however they have never undertaken to do heretofore . . . And they would produce for us doctors ignorant of Latin who would not know even how to read or write. We do not attempt to obstruct their being surgeons of St. Cosmas or that others unite with them. But we would only have a company of barber-surgeons, as we have had until now, which would be dependent on our Faculty, and would take every year an oath of fidelity in our schools before our Dean . . . and pay us every year a certain sum for the rights which we have in their functions. But we oppose robes, bonnets, licenses, nor any similar abuses . . . They are already sufficiently vainglorious and stupid without furnishing themselves with any such paraphernalia.

Thus the medical faculty brought and won its case before the Parisian government, which ruled that the new group of surgeons was subordinate to the physicians, as the barber-surgeons' guild had been. In a final sign of subordination, all indications of the academic status of the surgeons of the long gown were deemed no longer applicable to the new group. In the 1670s further legislation ordered the united surgical community to provide financial and honorary signs of deference to the Faculty of Medicine.

As surgery evolved in Paris, it became evident that attempts to make surgeons beholden to physicians could not be easily implemented because there were simply not enough medical doctors to supervise the surgeons. How could medical doctors possibly be physically present whenever a surgeon needed to make a clinical decision or perform an operation? On a practical level the physicians had no knowledge of surgical procedures and could not possibly guide the surgeon during a case.

By the end of the century the growing prestige of the Paris surgeons was evident. A new surgical amphitheater had been constructed in the city (1694) to offer public anatomy and operative courses to large audiences. This building offered visible evidence of the growing affluence and prestige of the united surgical guilds. More important, several prominent surgeons, including Pierre Dionis (1643-1718) and Charles-François Felix (1650-1703), were regarded with much favor by Parisian society.

Despite the growing prestige of Parisian surgeons, few of them actually performed major operations. In the 1690s, of the approximately 400 to 500 master surgeons, perhaps 5% practiced the bold, often new procedures such as lithotomy. Most surgeons earned a livelihood by completing minor surgery, which included treating abscesses; applying external medications to various skin ailments, bruises, and cuts; reducing incarcerated hernias; removing foreign objects; setting fractures; and treating skin tumors, venereal diseases, and ulcers. Realistically, this kind of work was not sufficient to provide a livelihood for the entire surgical community. By the end of the century certain surgeons had a growing disdain for what they regarded as socially demeaning work, so surgeons in Paris increasingly began to turn to the practice of internal medicine.

Because surgeons outnumbered physicians, it was not difficult for surgeons to usurp the physicians' practice of internal medicine. Equally important, surgeons were more accessible economically and socially to persons of modest means. Most surgeons tended to be comparable in social status to the artisans, the middle and lower classes, and the small-scale merchants, who made up a much greater portion of the populace than the wealthy patients of the Paris physicians.

By the final years of the seventeenth century it was evident that Paris barbers and surgeons were going their separate ways. The departure of the barbers reflected tangible alterations in the nature of surgery, which would become more evident in the next century.

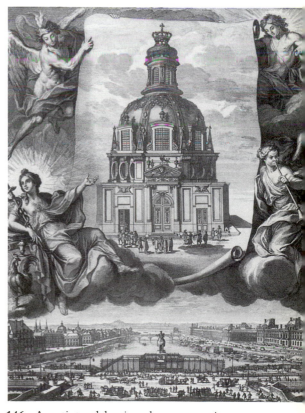

146. Aquatint celebrating the construction of a new amphitheater in 1694 by the Royal Company of Master Surgeons of Paris. The amphitheater greatly advanced the teaching of surgery. Surgery is allegorized by the figure on the lower left. (*National Library of Medicine, Bethesda, Md.*)

Because French surgery was in confusion, little surgical progress was achieved until the end of the seventeenth century. Consequently, many seventeenth-century French surgical treatises have been forgotten. The known important works of the century are listed in the box below. Charles Le Clerc's *La Chirurgie Complete* (1695) was a quiz-compend that passed through 18 editions. Among other things, it mentioned the use of vitriol buttons for achieving hemostasis and a method of 24-hour-long manual compression as treatment for aneurysms used at the Hôtel Dieu.

The influence of Dionis in reestablishing the prominence of French surgery cannot be underestimated. In 1673 Louis XIV ordained that anatomical demonstrations and certain operations be publicly held in the Jardins du Roy free of charge so that students of surgery might benefit. The chosen director of this program was Pierre Dionis (1643-1718), who in an introduction to one of his later textbooks wrote:

> The king, better inform'd than any in his Dominions, of whatever can contribute to the good of his subjects, by a particular declaration, which he caused to be verified and registred in his presence in March, 1673, ordered, that the demonstrations of anatomy and chirurgical operations shou'd be annually held in his Royal Garden gratis, and with the doors open, in order to furnish young students in chirurgery with the means of perfecting themselves in their art, which his majesty has always looked on as one of the most necessary in a state.

The king's declaration proved to be of utmost importance to surgery, for it marked the beginning of true surgical teaching in France and the starting point of the great French school of surgeons that would lead world surgery for more than a century. The political "power play" of the medical faculty—to unite the barber-surgeons and academic surgeons and thus humiliate the academics—was finally answered by royal decree, which increased opportunity for future instruction in surgery. The public demonstrations, as well as those presented by master

---

SEVENTEENTH-CENTURY FRENCH SURGICAL TREATISES

∾

JEAN GIRAULT
Chirurgie Francoise (1610)

GUILLAUME LOYSEAU
Observations Medicinales Et Chirurgicales (1617)

JOSEPH COVILLARD (?-1660)
Le Chirurgien Opérateur (1633)

RENÉ MOREAU (1587-1656)
Epistola De Laryngotomia (1646)

LEONARD TASSIN (?-1687)
La Chirurgie Militaire (1673)

NICOLAS DE BLEGNY (1652-1722)
L'Art De Guerir Les Hernies (1676)

SCRIPION ABEILLE (?-1697)
Le Parfait Chirurgien D'Armée (1695)

M. DE LA VAUGUION
Traité Complet Des Opérations De Chirurgie (1695)

CHARLES LE CLERC (1644-1700)
La Chirurgie Completè (1695)

surgeons other than Dionis, such as Georges Mareschal (1658-1736), surgeon of the Charité hospital and personal surgeon to Louis XIV; and Jean Mery (1645-1722), chief surgeon of the Hôtel Dieu, came to fascinate Parisian society.

Dionis strongly advocated that the most important subject for a surgeon to learn was human anatomy. Accordingly, the first important text Dionis wrote was *L'Anatomie De L'Homme* (1691), which immediately became one of the most popular medical texts and was translated into numerous languages, including Chinese. The courses in anatomy and surgery that Dionis taught became so popular that the original royal decree had to be amended:

> For the space of eight years I have performed those in the Royal Garden, to which the concourse of students was so great, that the largest hall destin'd for them would not hold one half of the auditors; which obliged us to prepare seal'd tickets which we distributed to chirurgeons apprentices, that they alone might enter, and to avoid confusion by the exclusion of those who were plac'd to serve their time in barber shops, and of those whose bare curiousity drew then thither.

It is clear in Dionis's statement that the exclusion of "barbers" from the ranks of Parisian surgeons had begun. In essence, the barbers were excluded by the only criterion possible, that of educational fitness.

The most important work of Dionis is *Cours D'Operations De Chirurgie,* first published in 1707. The book provided an outstanding description of surgical conditions as they existed in Paris in the late seventeenth century. Dionis indulged in descriptions of surgical history, providing excellent discussions of itinerant surgery for hernia and bladder calculi. Although Dionis described major operations in a systematic manner, he also inveighed against surgical quacks and charlatans.

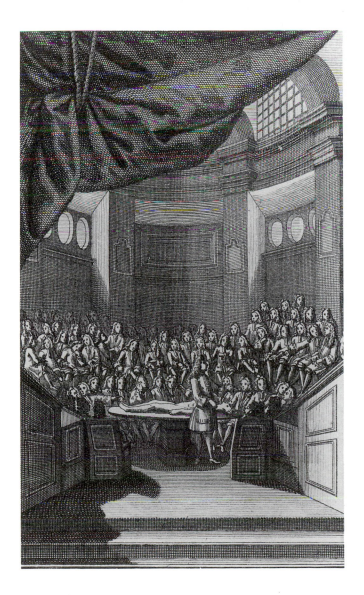

147. View of the interior of the Parisian surgical amphitheater, as published in Pierre Dionis's *Cours D'Operations De Chirurgie* (1707). Dionis was among the most influential early teachers of surgery in the new facility. *(National Library of Medicine, Bethesda, Md.)*

223

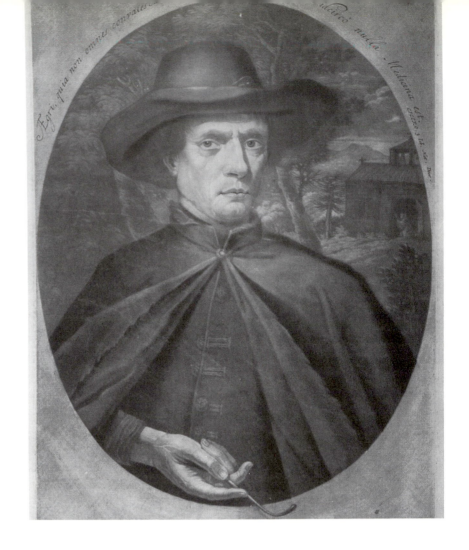

148. Frère Jacques De Beaulieu, the wandering lithotomist who distributed his operative fees to the poor. Aquatint by Pieter Schenk after Pool, published in Leiden circa 1750. *(Jeremy Norman & Co., Inc.)*

One of the most colorful stories Dionis told concerned the wandering lithotomist Frère Jacques De Beaulieu (1651-1719), who began as a bungling experimenter and eventually was recognized as a master of the operation. De Beaulieu was a French Franciscan monk who learned the art of operating for bladder calculi from an itinerant Italian surgeon. De Beaulieu traveled about the French countryside offering to treat gratuitously all persons affected with calculi. Unlike most itinerant surgeons, who zealously guarded their secret surgical methods, De Beaulieu made it a rule to operate in the presence of one or more physicians or surgeons and was always willing to provide instruction to those who wished to learn his method. Although De Beaulieu never asked for remuneration, he was always pleased to receive a written testimonial of what he had done for a given individual. Of the monies he received from the wealthy, De Beaulieu retained only that required for his most basic support and for the purchase of instruments. The remainder he distributed to the poor.

In 1697 De Beaulieu visited Paris and sought permission to demonstrate his lateral method of cutting for bladder calculi at the Hotel Dieu and Charite hospitals. He supposed that in view of his established reputation the request would prove acceptable to the surgeons of the city, but the chief surgeons of those institutions protested heatedly. The hospital administrators, however, granted De Beaulieu's request, and during the spring of 1698 he performed there almost 60 lithotomies.

De Beaulieu had mixed results in his lateral operation; nonetheless, the public treated him with due consideration. Eventually the jealous Paris surgeons, led by Mery, succeeded in discrediting De Beaulieu. Clearly the Parisian surgeons had ulterior motives in forcing De Beaulieu to leave the city. However, they used clear-cut scientific criteria, including anatomy, clinical statistics, postmortem examinations, and technical considerations, to accomplish their objective. Thus they were able to emphasize the difference between a surgeon who was well versed in anatomy, as Dionis advocated, and a mere half-educated itinerant. De Beaulieu, who was the most compassionate of individuals, was forced to resume his wanderings through Europe and eventually died unknown and impoverished. The very profession he had wished to improve had no use for the well-intentioned outsider.

Charles-François Felix (1650–1703), a prominent French surgeon of the seventeenth century, served as the king's "Premier Surgeon," a role that would figure prominently in the declining power of barber-surgeons. For centuries the king had employed his own personal, or premier, surgeon. Although the individual in that position was in royal employment and could be considered the most prominent surgeon in France, he usually held no special jurisdiction over the College of St. Côme or the various barber-surgeon guilds in the kingdom. Rather, it was the king's "Premier Barber" who served as chief of all communities of barber-surgeons.

After the 1655 ruling that united the two surgical organizations, leadership of the new entity passed into the hands of the premier barber. The royal government later came to consider it inappropriate that a barber be the chief of the only Parisian surgical guild. Consequently, in August 1668 the king's council ordered the premier barber to sell his dominion over the art of barber-surgery to the premier surgeon, Felix. During the ensuing decade a series of royal edicts and decrees reinforced and occasionally extended the premier surgeon's authority over barber-surgeons.

By 1686 Louis XIV had suffered from a painful anal fistula for many years. Various physicians had tried to cure him by using numerous medicines and laxatives, but to no avail. It became obvious to all involved that a surgical operation would be necessary. Charles-François Felix, a court surgeon and son of the previous premier surgeon, was chosen to perform the surgery. He had never operated for fistula previously, so he practiced on patients in the city's charity hospitals. A silver bistoury, a narrow-bladed knife used for making incisions, was constructed for the momentous occasion. At 7 o'clock on a November morning Felix proceeded to cut twice with the bistoury and eight times with scissors. The king was said to have behaved with great courage throughout the ordeal and continually encouraged Felix in his nerve-racking task. In testimony to the king's resolve, that very evening he insisted on holding a council and the next morning received ambassadors. Because Felix did not want the wounds to heal too quickly, he operated three times again in December. In January the king promenaded in the Orangerie at Versailles to demonstrate his complete recovery and to show his thanks for the public's well-wishes.

The fistula operation performed on Louis XIV dramatically illustrated the curative powers of surgery. The procedure forever became one of the competent surgeon's technical skills. Felix himself was inundated by requests from courtiers and sycophants who, knowing they had no pathological condition, nonetheless entreated him to perform the same operation on them. Felix received a magnificent reward from the king that included 300,000 livres, a country estate, and noble rank.

The surgical community shared in Felix's success, as evidenced by its growing acceptance in French society. Felix eventually was named premier surgeon, and his role in redefining French surgery became dominant. In 1699, for example, despite the opposition of a majority of barber-surgeons, he imposed new statutes on the Paris guild. Felix was in an ideal position to secure royal legislation and then to oversee its implementation. The revenues accruing to his office were immense, including dues from all the communities of barber-surgeons in France. Felix was virtually king of French surgery.

During the last decades of the seventeenth century Felix helped lay the groundwork for a unified French surgical profession. He ensured that power became more centralized in his office, where he was surrounded by an elite group of Paris surgeons he himself chose, supposedly on the basis of merit. The ascendancy of the premier surgeon enabled French surgery to become the domain of an elite meritocracy, which would prove more efficacious than a national surgeons' guild for teaching and research. French surgery was thus prepared for its zenith during the next century.

THE EIGHTEENTH CENTURY

	1650	1700	1750	1800	1850	1900

DAILY LIFE

Yale University **(1701)**

First evening paper in London **(1706)**

Princeton University **(1746)**

Mutineers of H.M.S. Bounty land on Pitcairn Island **(1789)**

Union College (Schenectady, New York), first nondenominational college in the United States **(1795)**

Metric system adopted **(1795)**

Rosetta stone **(1799)**

> ### POPULATION FIGURES (1700)
> France 19,000,000
> England and Scotland 7,500,000
> Hapsburg Empire 7,500,000
> Spain 6,000,000

SCIENCE AND TECHNOLOGY

Anders Celsius, Swiss astronomer **(1701-1744)**

Benjamin Franklin, American inventor **(1706-1790)**

Henry Cavendish, English chemist **(1731-1810)**

Joseph Priestley, English chemist **(1733-1804)**

Charles Coulomb, French physicist **(1736-1806)**

Luigi Galvani, Italian physiologist **(1737-1798)**

Joseph Guillotin, French inventor **(1738-1814)**

Antoine Lavoisier, Franch chemist **(1743-1794)**

Alessandro Volta, Italian physicist **(1745-1827)**

John Dalton, English chemist **(1766-1844)**

Andre Ampère, French physicist **(1775-1836)**

Humphrey Davy, English chemist **(1778-1829)**

Jons Berzelius, Swedish chemist **(1779-1848)**

Michael Faraday, English chemist **(1791-1867)**

RELIGION AND PHILOSOPHY

John Wesley, English theologian **(1703-1791)**

David Hume, Scottish philosopher **(1711-1776)**

Jean Rousseau, French philosopher **(1712-1778)**

Immanuel Kant, German philosopher **(1724-1804)**

Noah Webster, American lexicographer **(1758-1843)**

Arthur Schopenhauer, German philosopher **(1788-1860)**

LITERATURE AND THEATER

Samuel Johnson, English author **(1709-1784)**

Thomas Paine, American author **(1737-1809)**

Marquis de Sade, French novelist **(1740-1814)**

Johann von Goethe, German writer **(1749-1832)**

William Blake, English poet **(1757-1827)**

Robert Burns, Scottish poet **(1759-1796)**

William Wordsworth, English poet **(1770-1850)**

Jane Austen, English novelist **(1774-1817)**

Washington Irving, American author **(1783-1859)**

Jacob Grimm, German folklorist **(1785-1863)**

George Byron, English poet **(1788-1824)**

Percy Shelley, English poet **(1792-1822)**

John Keats, English poet **(1795-1821)**

MUSIC

Joseph Haydn, Austrian composer **(1732-1809)**

Wolfgang Mozart, Austrian composer **(1756-1791)**

Ludwig von Beethoven, German composer **(1770-1827)**

Gioacchino Rossini, Italian composer **(1792-1868)**

Franz Schubert, Austrian composer **(1797-1828)**

VISUAL ARTS

Francois Boucher, French painter **(1703-1770)**

Thomas Chippendale, English cabinetmaker **(1719-1779)**

Joshua Reynolds, English painter **(1723-1792)**

Josiah Wedgwood, English pottery manufacturer **(1730-1795)**

Francisco de Goya, Spanish painter **(1746-1828)**

John Turner, English painter **(1775-1851)**

Jean Ingres, French painter **(1780-1867)**

Ferdinand Delacroix, French painter **(1799-1863)**

MEDICINE AND SURGERY

Herman Boerhaave, Dutch **(1668-1738)**

Johann Rau, Dutch **(1668-1719)**

Jacobus Winslow, Danish **(1669-1760)**

John Munro, Scottish **(1670-1738)**

Jean-Louis Petit, French **(1674-1750)**

James Douglas, Scottish **(1675-1742)**

John Douglas, Scottish **(?-1743)**

Martin Naboth, German **(1675-1721)**

Dominique Anel, French **(1678-1725)**

François La Peyronie, French **(1678-1747)**

Zabdiel Boylston, United States **(1679-1766)**

THE EIGHTEENTH CENTURY

1650	1700	1750	1800	1850	1900

MEDICINE AND SURGERY

Claudius Amyand, English **(1680–1740)**
Giovanni Santorini, Italian **(1681–1737)**
Giovanni Morgagni, Italian **(1682–1771)**
Lorenz Heister, German **(1683–1758)**
Abraham Vater, German **(1684–1751)**
Henri Le Dran, French **(1685–1773)**
Abraham Titsingh, Dutch **(1685–1776)**
Simon Krueger, Danish **(1687–1760)**
Claude-Nicolas Le Cat, French **(1700–1768)**
Samuel Sharp, English **(1700–1780)**
Gerard van Swieten, German **(1700–1772)**
Edward Nourse, English **(1701–1761)**
Jean Baseilhac, French **(1703–1781)**
John Ranby, English **(1703–1773)**
Chevalier Taylor, English **(1703–1772)**
Linnaeus, Swedish **(1707–1778)**
John Pringle, English **(1707–1782)**
Albrecht von Haller, Swiss **(1708–1777)**
William Heberden, English **(1710–1801)**
Hughes Ravaton, French **(mid–eighteenth century)**
William Bromfield, English **(1712–1792)**
William Shippen, United States **(1712–1801)**
Percival Pott, English **(1714–1788)**
John Bard, United States **(1716–1799)**
Joseph Warner, English **(1717–1801)**
Olof Acrel, Swedish **(1717–1806)**
William Hunter, Scottish **(1718–1783)**
Pierre Brasdor, French **(1721–1797)**
Pieter Camper, Dutch **(1722–1789)**
Antoine Louis, French **(1723–1792)**
Johann Meckel, German **(1724–1774)**
Ferdinand Leber, German **(1727–1808)**
Giovanni Brambilla, Italian **(1728–1800)**
John Hunter, Scottish **(1728–1793)**
Samuel Croker-King, Irish **(1728–1817)**
Sylvester O'Halloran, Irish **(1728–1807)**
Charles White, English **(1728–1813)**
John Jones, United States **(1729–1791)**
Raphael Sabatier, French **(1732–1811)**
Alexander Monro (*secundus*), Scottish **(1733–1817)**
Caspar Wolff, German **(1733–1794)**
Don Antonio Gimbernat, Spanish **(1734–1816)**
John Morgan, United States **(1735–1789)**
William Hey, English **(1736–1819)**
Carl Siebold, German **(1736–1807)**
William Hewson, English **(1739–1774)**
Henry Callisen, Danish **(1740–1824)**
Jean Sigault, French **(1740–?)**
Nicolas Saucerotte, French **(1741–1812)**
William Withering, English **(1741–1799)**
August Richter, German **(1742–1812)**
William Blizard, English **(1743–1835)**
François Chopart, French **(1743–1795)**
Pierre-Joseph Desault, French **(1744–1795)**
Henry Park, English **(1744–1831)**
Benjamin Rush, United States **(1745–1813)**
François Chaussier, French **(1746–1828)**
Benjamin Bell, Scottish **(1749–1806)**
Edward Jenner, English **(1749–1823)**
Henry Cline, English **(1750–1827)**
Guillaume Pellier De Quengsy, French **(1751–1835)**
William Dease, Irish **(1752–1798)**
John Warren, United States **(1753–1815)**
Thomas Kast, United States **(1755–1820)**
Everard Home, English **(1756–1832)**
Matthew Baillie, English **(1760–1823)**
John Bell, Scottish **(1763–1820)**
John Abernethy, English **(1764–1831)**
Xavier Bichat, French **(1771–1802)**

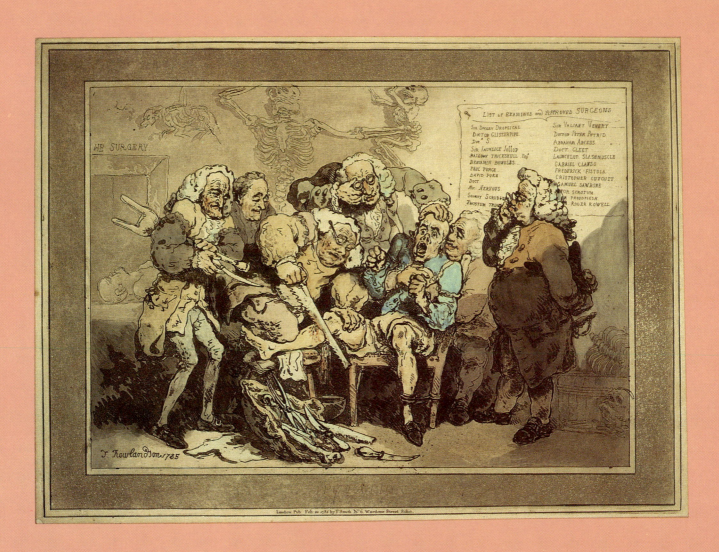

THE SURGERY.

LIST of EXAMINED and APPROVED SURGEONS

J. Rowlandson 1785

CHAPTER 10

THE EIGHTEENTH CENTURY

During the eighteenth century, struggles for a balance of power swept over all of Europe. The most important conflicts, known as the wars of succession, were disputes concerning inheritance of or succession to particular thrones. The social impact of these wars, which often altered the direction of governments, was staggering, and the development of surgery was affected in the countries involved.

The four consequential succession wars were those of Spain (1701-1713), Poland (1733-1735), Austria (1740-1748), and Bavaria (1778-1779). In addition, the Seven Years' War (1756-1763) involved nearly every nation in Europe and extended to America. While Prussia and Austria fought for control of Germany, Prussia's ally, England, and Austria's ally, France, battled for control of the seas and of the territories in North America. When the Seven Years' War finally ended, Prussia had become the leader of the German-speaking states and England had driven the French out of North America (in the French and Indian War).

Internal changes in each European country reflected much socioeconomic and political dissent. Medical theories and systematization dominated eighteenth-century thought. A tendency toward formalism transformed the various theories, however idealistic, into rational but excessively rigid methodologies. The eighteenth century is also known as the Age of Enlightenment, a European philosophical movement characterized by rationalism, an impetus toward learning, and a spirit of skepticism and empiricism in social and political thought.

The lessons of the seventeenth century had led humanity away from blind faith in authority to a new belief in human progress. Eighteenth-century physicians, like their seventeenth-century counterparts, were seldom able to keep abreast of the dazzling scientific advances, especially in fields outside of medicine, and in medicine few of the startling experimental discoveries in physics and chemistry were put into practical use for the treatment of patients.

Eighteenth-century medicine reflected an age of classification, categorization, grouping, and arrangements. The greatest of the classifiers was the Swedish physician and naturalist, Carl von Linné (Linnaeus) (1707-1778), who invented the system of binomial nomenclature and attempted to furnish each living thing with a generic or family name (genus) and a specific or given name (species). It was Linnaeus in his *Systema Naturae* (1735) who termed the human being *Homo sapien*.

Despite Linnaeus's invaluable contributions to natural history, his voluminous medical classifications, in a practical sense, proved worthless. They did little to advance the cause of medicine and provided no pragmatic benefit to patients. Much more applicable work was performed by the greatest medical systematist after Galen, Albrecht von Haller (1708-1777). Born into an aristocratic Bern family, he was considered a child prodigy. Haller began his study of medicine under Hermann Boerhaave (1668-1738) in Leyden. Haller received his medical

149. *Facing page, The Amputation,* 1785. Hand-colored etching, aquatint, and stipple engraving by Thomas Rowlandson. Rowlandson's lack of respect for and dislike of the medical profession frequently found expression in his caricatures. A group of elderly, unhealthy surgeons are in the act of amputating the perfectly healthy leg of a young, terrified patient who is strapped to his chair. One of the surgeons holds a wooden leg, which will soon be needed. The operation is taking place in a dissecting room littered with skeletons. A "List of Examined and Approved Surgeons" on the wall includes such names as Christopher Catgutt and Peter Putrid. *(Boston Medical Library.)*

150. Portrait of Albrecht von Haller (1757), engraved by P.F. Tardieu after the painting by E.J. Handmann. *(Jeremy Norman & Co., Inc.)*

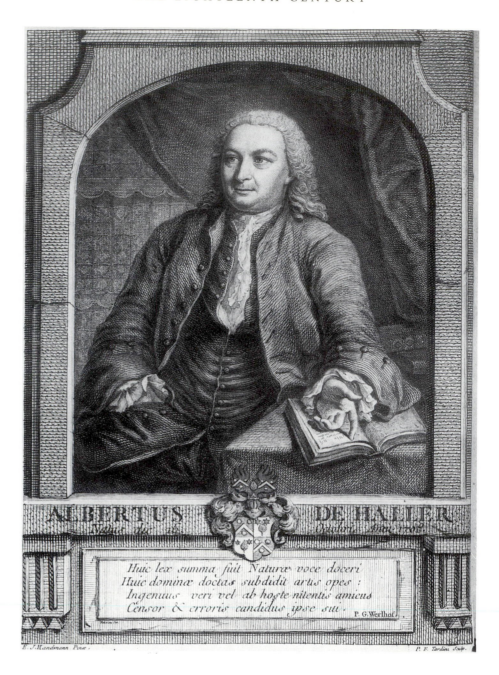

degree in 1727; for his thesis he disproved the contention of Georg Coschwitz (1679-1729), eminent surgeon and anatomist, that there was a secondary salivary duct. Haller accomplished this by dissecting the structure in question and proving it to be a blood vessel. To broaden his educational horizons, Haller traveled to London and Paris. Shortly thereafter he returned to Switzerland and enrolled in Johann Bernoulli's (1667-1748) course in mathematics in Basel.

Haller had clearly received a well-rounded education. In 1731 he began to practice medicine in his native city. Two years later he wrote his first of several momentous anatomical studies. His work raised jealousy in his colleagues, who prevented him from obtaining the position of director of the Bern city hospital. Eager to gain some type of affiliation with a university, Haller applied for the professorship of history at the University of Bern. Once again he was refused, this time on the basis that the chair in history should not be occupied by a physician.

George II (1683-1760) of England had established a new university at Göttingen in the early 1730s. Haller was offered and accepted the chair in anatomy and surgery at the university, where he taught from 1736 to 1753. He gained a tremendous reputation, especially for his teaching skills and physiological experimentation. He taught all branches of medicine, grew one of Europe's outstanding botanical gardens, and published a multitude of works.

Haller became homesick and in 1753 was elected as a public health official in Bern. He resettled there and for the next 23 years had a period of intense literary activity.

Haller compiled his two-volume *Bibliotheca Chirurgica* (1774) during the final years of his life. The first serious attempt at a comprehensive, critical bibliography of all prior surgical texts, monographs, and treatises, the *Bibliotheca Chirurgica* ensured Haller's place in surgical history. Haller also prepared separate bibliographies of botany (1771), anatomy (1774), and medicine (1776). In each of these massive compilations the contents were arranged chronologically, from the days of medieval manuscripts to Haller's own time. Authors were given numbered sections, and their names were followed by brief descriptions of their educations and professional backgrounds; each author's writings were then listed, with the titles, places, dates, of publication, and sizes of the books accurately transcribed. The index to the two volumes, reflecting the magnitude of the bibliography, occupied nearly 50 pages and cited 5000 authors. Haller personally commented on 95% of the important surgical works.

Although Haller is acknowledged as one of the greatest surgical bibliographers, it is alleged that he never performed a surgical operation on a living person: his surgical teachings were purely theoretical. Nevertheless, Haller's many bibliographical observations helped place the literature of surgery on a firm foundation, and his *Bibliotheca Chirurgica* is considered one of the most important written works in the history of surgery.

The leading physician of the early eighteenth century was Haller's mentor, Boerhaave. Through his presence the university at Leyden became one of the premier medical centers in Europe. Boerhaave was an outstanding clinical teacher, and his bedside instruction method was unique on the continent until 1745.

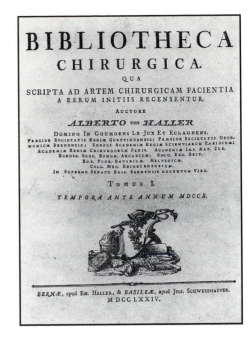

151. Haller's *Bibliotheca Chirurgica* was the first attempt at a comprehensive, critical bibliography of surgical literature. *(From the author's collection.)*

EIGHTEENTH-CENTURY DISCOVERIES IN PHYSIOLOGY

∾

STEPHEN HALES (1677-1761)
Measurement of blood pressure (1733)

JOHN WALSH (1725-1795)
Observations on the electric property of the torpedo fish (1773)

CHARLES BLAGDEN (1748-1820)
Demonstration of the importance of perspiration in the maintenance of constant body temperature (1775)

EDWARD STEVEN (1755-1834)
Isolation of human gastric juice (1777)

ANTOINE LAVOISIER (1743-1794) and PIERRE LAPLACE (1749-1827)
Invention of an ice calorimeter (1780)

LUIGI GALVANI (1737-1798)
Theory of animal electricity, or galvanism (1791)

ARMAND SÉQUIN (1768-1835) and ANTOINE LAVOISIER (1743-1794)
Ability to measure human metabolism (1789)

WILLIAM CRUIKSHANK (1745-1800)
Demonstration that carbon dioxide is given off by the skin (1795)

Hermann Boerhaave (1668-1738) was educated not only in medicine but also in the arts, including music and literature, and he taught chemistry, physics, and botany. Boerhaave was one of the earliest to propose that a medical student follow up a patient's fatal illness with a postmortem examination. Boerhaave's work was complemented by that of Bernard Albinus (1697-1770), one of the most renowned anatomist-illustrators of his day and director of instruction in dissection at Leyden. Albinus had studied with Bidloo and Boerhaave and held the chairs of anatomy and surgery (1718) and medicine (1745) at Leyden.

The writings of Boerhaave were enormously influential, especially *Aphorismi De Cognoscendis Et Curandis Morbis* (1709), *Methodus Discendi Medicinam* (1726), *Elementa Chemiae* (1732), and *Opera Omnia Medica* (1742). Through the efforts of Boerhaave and other prominent eighteenth-century medical practitioners, the internal medicine practice of that century appeared to be superior to its surgery, primarily because the efforts at categorization made by the systematists resulted in the publication of specialized medical texts, the introduction of many new

EIGHTEENTH-CENTURY DISCOVERIES IN CLINICAL MEDICINE

WILLIAM COWPER (1666-1709)
Aortic insufficiency (1706)

FRIEDRICH HOFFMANN (1660-1742)
Chlorosis (1730) and rubella (1740)

JOHN FREKE (1688-1756)
Myositis ossificans progressica (1740)

THOMAS CADWALADER (1708-1779)
Lead colic and lead palsy (1745)

JAMES LIND (1716-1794)
Scurvy (1753)

NICHOLAS ANDRY (1658-1742)
Infraorbital neuralgia (1756)

LEOPOLD AUENBRUGGER (1722-1809)
Percussion of the chest as a diagnostic measure (1761)

ROBERT HAMILTON (1721-1793)
Linking of orchitis with parotitis or mumps (1761)

JOHN HILL (1714-1775)
Association between tobacco and cancer (1761)

GIOVANNI MORGAGNI (1682-1771)
Mitral stenosis and heart block (1761)

FRANK NICHOLL (1699-1778)
Aortic aneurysm dissection (1762)

FRANCIS HOME (1719-1813)
Diphtheria (1765)

WILLIAM HEBERDEN (1710-1801)
Varicella and variola differentiation (1767)
and angina pectoris (1772)

FRANCESCO FRAPOLLI (?-1773) and FRANCOIS THIERRY (1719-?)
Pellagra (1771)

WILLIAM HEWSON (1739-1774)
Blood clotting and lymphocyte (1771)

MATTHEW DOBSON (1731-1784)
Sugar diabetes (1776)

JOHN FOTHERGILL (1712-1780)
Facial neuralgia (1776) and migraine (1777)

JOHN LETTSOM (1744-1815)
Alcoholism (1779)

WILLIAM WITHERING (1741-1799)
Digitalis (1785)

JOHANN FRANK (1745-1821)
Diabetes insipidus (1794)

MATHEW CAREY (1760-1839)
Yellow fever (1793)

MATTHEW BAILLIE (1760-1823)
Pulmonary tuberculosis (1793) and chronic obstructive pulmonary emphysema (1797)

EDWARD JENNER (1749-1823)
Smallpox inoculation (1798)

drugs, and the accurate description of previously unappreciated pathological entities. Outstanding eighteenth-century discoveries in physiology and clinical medicine are listed in the boxes on pp. 231 and 232.

As important as clinical medical observations were for the eighteenth-century surgeon, anatomical teachings continued to be invaluable. The general anatomical treatises and atlases (see the box on p. 234) were mostly topographic and iconographic. Important individual anatomical observations were also made (see the box on p. 236).

Despite the progress made in the art and technique of surgery during the eighteenth century, only by the end of the century did surgeons as a group begin to rise above their traditional social status as technicians or craftsmen to receive acceptance as professionals on a par with physicians. The acceptance of surgery as a scientific profession equal to medicine occurred at various times in different countries, and it is difficult to pinpoint when surgery ceased being regarded as merely a technical mode of treatment and assumed its place as a branch of scientific medicine firmly grounded in principles of physiology and pathology. The greatest surgeons of the past, like Galen and Vesalius, had advanced both sciences, surgery and medicine. Their enormous fame and prestigious social positions derived more from their achievements in medicine than from those in surgery. Paré was the great exception, a barber-surgeon who rose from obscurity to appointment as surgeon to the king. Paré's achievements as surgeon and writer brought him recognition equal to that of any physician. By the second half of the eighteenth century other surgeons would claim equal rec-

152. An operation scene in a hospital. Pencil drawing and gray wash over chalk, by William Hogarth. An apparently unfinished study by the great English satirist. While a scullery maid holds a candle, a surgeon performs an operation on the bedridden patient's leg. The surgeon's assistant, *left*, holds the instrument box while a physician studies the patient's urine in a urine flask held up to the light. *(The Pierpont Morgan Library, New York, III, 35.)*

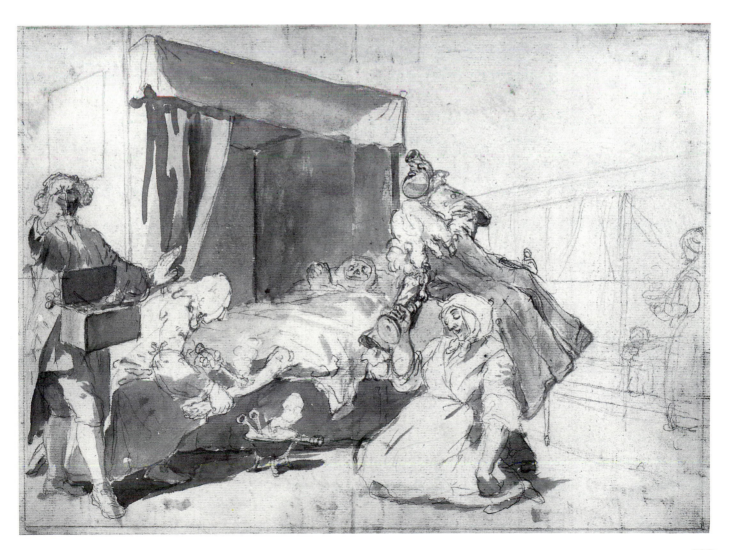

EIGHTEENTH-CENTURY ANATOMICAL TREATISES AND ATLASES

General Treatises and Atlases

FREDERIK RUYSCH (1638-1731)
Thesaurus Anatomicus (1701-1716)

GIOVANNI SANTORINI (1681-1737)
Observationes Anatomicae (1724)

ABRAHAM CHOVET (1704-1799)
A Syllabus or Index, of All the Parts That Enter the Composition of the Human Body (1732)

JACOBUS WINSLOW (1669-1760)
Exposition Anatomique De La Structure Du Corps Humain (1732)

JOSEPH LIETAUD (1703-1780)
Essais Anatomiques (1742)

SAMUEL SOEMMERRING (1755-1830)
Vom Baue Des Menschlichen Körpers (1791-1796)

Specialty Atlases

ANTONIO VALSALVA (1666-1723)
Ear: *De Aure Humana Tractatus* (1704)

WILLIAM CHESELDEN (1688-1752)
Bones: *Osteographia* (1733)

GEORGE EISENMANN (1693-1768)
Uterus: *Tabulae Anatomicae Quatuor Uteri Duplicis* (1752)

BERNARD ALBINUS (1697-1770)
Bones and muscles: *Tabulae Sceleti Et Musculorum Corporis Humani* (1747)

JOHANN ZINN (1727-1759)
Eye: *De Ligamentis Ciliaribus* (1753); *Descriptio Anatomica Oculi Humani* (1755)

ANTONIO SCARPA (1747-1832)
Ear: *De Structura Fenestrae Rotundae Auris Et De Tympano Secundario Anatomicae Observations* (1772); *Anatomicae Disquisitiones De Auditu Et Olfactu* (1789); *Den Penitiori Ossium Structura Commentarius* (1799)

EDUARD SANDIFORT (1742-1814)
Duodenum: *Tabulae Intestini Duodeni* (1780)

PAOLO MASCAGNI (1752-1815)
Lymphatics: *Vasorum Lymphaticorum Corporis Humani Historia Et Ichnographia* (1787)

SAMUEL SOEMMERRING (1755-1830)
Cranial nerves: *De Basi Encephali Et Originibus Nervorum Cranio Egredientium* (1778)

ognition. One surgeon who undoubtedly received full scientific and social acceptance for his enormous accomplishments in surgery, comparative anatomy, and other fields was John Hunter (1728-1793), and there were many others. By the end of the eighteenth century, surgeons as a group had transformed themselves from technical craftsmen to professionals grounded in science like their physician counterparts. No longer were they just barber-surgeons on a par with roving charlatans and quacks. Surgeons had become scientific as well as technical innovators.

The close relationship that had been established between surgeons and anatomical research continued during most of the eighteenth century. Thus many of the period's outstanding anatomical and surgical discoveries were made by so-called surgeon-anatomists. Among the most important of these were William Cheselden (1688-1752); the Monros: father Alexander (primus) (1697-1767), son Alexander (secundus) (1733-1817), and grandson Alexander (tertius) (1773-1859); Percival Pott (1714-1788); William Hunter (1718-1783) and his brother John (1728-1793); the Meckels: father Johann (1724-1774), son Philipp (1756-1803), and two grandsons, Johann (1781-1833) and his younger brother August (1790-1829); Pierre-Joseph Desault (1744-1795); and Antonio Scarpa (1747-1832). Through their combined efforts the role of surgery in the rise of modern medical thought would be ensured.

In many respects the study of general anatomy was considered less interesting than the new fields of pathological anatomy, comparative anatomy, and embryology. Giovanni Morgagni (1682-1771) literally founded pathological anatomy with his monumental two-volume *De Sedibus, Et Causis Morborum Per Anatomen Indagatis Libri Quinque* (1761). For more than 50 years (1715-1771) he held the chair of anatomy at Padua and helped move pathology from a purely descriptive study to one based in scientific theory.

Morgagni was born in Forli and studied medicine in Bologna, where he came under the tutelage of Valsalva and in 1701 received the degree of Doctor of Medicine. Almost from the outset of his medical studies Morgagni's chief interest was in the study of the human body. As time passed, he became increasingly interested in the changes that take place in organs and tissues as the result of injuries and diseases. He scrupulously maintained case histories and autopsy findings. Morgagni was in the habit of constantly writing down, in the most painstaking detail, as many departures from the normal appearance as he could recognize.

In contrast to the poorly organized but first systematized pathological anatomical work (1679) of Theophile Bonet (1620-1689), Morgagni's effort was both methodical and accurate. His book consisted of a series of 70 letters in which approximately 700 cases are reported and clinical symptoms are correlated with postmortem findings. Morgagni made pathology a genuine branch of modern medicine by clearly defining such entities as hepatic cirrhosis, renal tuberculosis, heart block, syphilitic lesions of the brain, and pneumonic solidification of the lung. He resolved many misunderstandings. For example, he demonstrated that a brain abscess was a cause, not an effect, of suppuration in the ear. Morgagni showed that paralysis in half of the body was the result of an injury in the opposite brain hemisphere. Although he never practiced surgery, Morgagni improved surgery by investigating the results of ligating various blood vessels. He also described several malignant tumors and provided instructions for operating on them.

Among the prominent eighteenth-century pathologists was Matthew Baillie (1760-1823). Like Morgagni, he was not a surgeon but enjoyed a lengthy association, through his research, with several renowned English surgeons including his uncles, the Hunters. Baillie was physician to George III (1738-1820) and one of the leading practitioners in London. His *Morbid Anatomy* (1793), which was accompanied by an atlas that contained a series of engravings (1799-1803), was the first systematic, illustrated textbook of pathology to treat the subject as an

EIGHTEENTH-CENTURY ANATOMICAL OBSERVATIONS

WILLIAM COWPER (1666-1709)
Bulbourethral glands (1700)

MARTIN NABOTH (1675-1721)
Cysts and glands of the uterine cervix (1707)

ADAM THEBESIUS (1686-1732)
Coronary valves (1708)

ALEXIS LITTRE (1658-1726)
Male urethral glands (1719)

ABRAHAM VATER (1684-1751)
Ampulla of the bile duct (1720)

FRANCOIS DU PETIT (1664-1741)
Vasomotor nerves (1727)

JAMES DOUGLAS (1675-1742)
Peritoneum (1730)

FRANCOIS POUPART (1661-1709)
Inguinal ligament (1730)

JACOBUS WINSLOW (1669-1760)
Foramen between the greater and
lesser sacs of the peritoneum (1732)

ANTONIO VALSALVA (1666-1723)
Aortic sinus (1740)

HARTWIG TAUBE (1706-?)
Carotid body (1743)

JOHANN LIEBERKÜHN (1711-1756)
Intestinal crypts (1745)

JOHANN MECKEL (1724-1774)
Sphenopalatine ganglion (1748)

JEAN DESCEMET (1732-1810)
Posterior elastic layer of the cornea (1758)

DOMENICO COTUGNO (1736-1822)
Cerebrospinal fluid and pathways (1764)

FELICE FONTANA (1730-1805)
Venous sinus of the sclera (1765)

JEAN PETIT (1674-1750)
Lumbar triangle (1774)

HEINRICH WRISBERG (1739-1808)
Intermediate nerve (1777)

ALEXANDER MONRO (SECUNDUS) (1733-1817)
Communication of the lateral ventricles of the brain
and the third ventricle (1783)

PIETER CAMPER (1722-1789)
Superficial fascial layer of the abdomen (1784)

ANTONIO GIMBERNAT (1734-1816)
Ligament in the crural arch (1793)

ANTONIO SCARPA (1747-1832)
Nerves of the heart (1794)

independent science. Illustrated with magnificent copper plate engravings after drawings by William Clift (1775-1849), the textbook displayed the morbid appearance of each organ in succession.

The beginnings of modern embryology and comparative anatomy received considerable impetus from the research of Caspar Wolff (1733-1794). He worked in Berlin and is best remembered for his description of the embryological mesonephros. Wolff observed in great detail the early processes of embryonic differentiation and declared invalid the concept of "preformation." His firm stand against the accepted theory that the embryo was preformed and encased in the ovary was upheld by his staunch promulgation of the doctrine of epigenesis. According to the hypothesis of epigenesis, the embryo developed from a single form as a result of division, and organs were subsequently formed from blastodermic layers.

Because surgery did not evolve separately from medicine, it is necessary to have an understanding of the social, economic, and intellectual climate in which eighteenth-century medicine was practiced to fully appreciate the surgical tenor of the times. The full impact of the cardinal features of eighteenth-century clinical medicine—the introduction of routine postmortem examinations, new methods of testing that yielded more precise diagnoses, and the use of preventive inoculation—would not be apparent until the following century.

During the eighteenth century several attempts were made to employ new instruments of precision in the diagnosis of disease. Before watches had hands to record the seconds, John Floyer (1649-1734) invented his pulse-watch, which divided the minute, and wrote the two-volume *The Physician's Pulse-Watch* (1707-1710). Floyer's invention was an attempt to obtain the pulse rate by timing its beats with a watch that ran for exactly 1 minute. Floyer's work, however, received little respect; the revival of the old Galenic tradition of specific pulses (i.e., that each individual disease had a particular pulse rate) entirely masked his intention.

In 1740 George Martine (1702-1741) introduced the concept of clinical thermometry in his *Essays Medical and Philosophical*. James Currie (1756-1805) applied Martine's ideas in clinical practice and made original observations on the use of cold-water packs in the treatment of fever *(Medical Reports, 1797)*, but his ideas, like Floyer's, were soon neglected.

The social status of the eighteenth-century physician was, for the most part, excellent. In some countries physicians carried swords; in others the people commonly showed their respect by lifting their hats to physicians. In England the well-known, fashionable physician wore a powdered wig, a coat of red satin or brocade, short breeches, stockings and buckled shoes, and a three-cornered hat and often carried a goldheaded cane. Surgeons usually did not receive the same respect as physicians. Nonetheless, many well-known surgeons were resplendent in their finery.

As the profession of medicine became more organized, scientific and medical societies flourished. Among the most important for the surgeon were the Paris Academie de Chirurgie (1731) and the Royal College of Surgeons of London (1800). The great modern medical libraries had their beginnings early in the eighteenth century, including the Biblioteca Lancisiana at Rome (1711) and the library of the Faculty of Medicine at Paris (1733). Physicians, too, particularly Richard Mead (1673-1754), Hans Sloane (1660-1753), and William Hunter (1718-1783), were engaged in book collecting and acquired massive private libraries. Medical periodicals were being published with greater frequency.

Medical education, especially anatomical instruction, was being well taught in numerous European cities. Chairs of anatomy had been established in Great Britain at Edinburgh (1705), Cambridge (1707), Glasgow (1718), Oxford (1762), and Dublin (1785). The hospital medical school had its beginnings in such institutions as Guy's Hospital (1723), the Edinburgh Hospital (1736), the

153. Surgical instrument set in decorated leather case, eighteenth century. The set of steel instruments with ebony handles includes an amputation knife, a saw, and a selection of trephination instruments. *(Reproduced by permission of the Trustees of the Science Museum, London. A600887; 27/93.)*

Meath Hospital (Dublin, 1756), London Hospital Medical School (1785), and St. Bartholomew's (1790). Apart from hospital medical schools, many new hospitals were established in most principal British cities or provinces, and such famous institutions as the Charite in Berlin (1710) and the Allgemeines Krankenhaus in Vienna (1784) were also founded.

Eighteenth-century surgery was not without its critics: Thomas Rowlandson (1757–1820) accomplished with water colors and aquatint engravings what Molière had accomplished with the pen. Among Rowlandson's many caricatures were those of surgical operations, dissections, and the surgeon's daily existence. His titles, such as "The Persevering Surgeon," were especially biting.

The first tentative reforms toward public health, surgical cleanliness, hospital salubrity, and surgical statistics were being considered. George Baker (1722–

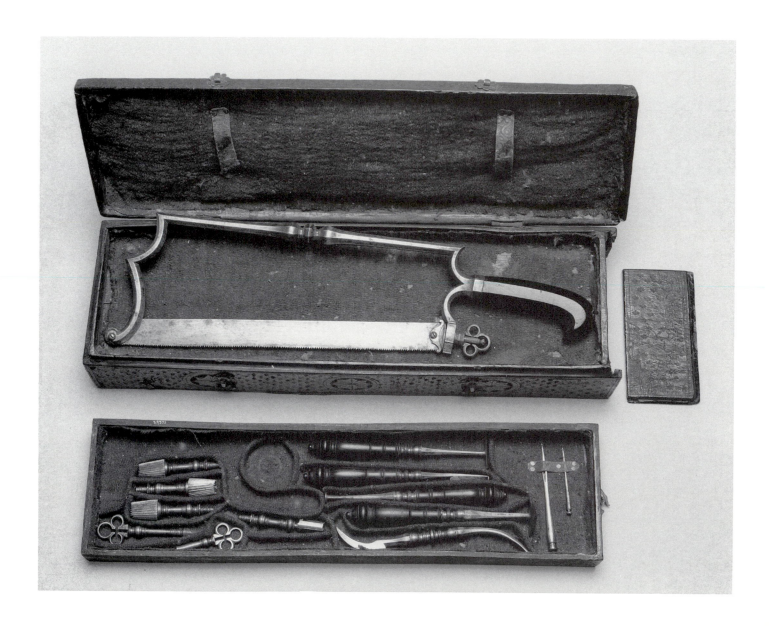

1809) demonstrated the association of large pieces of lead used in vats and cider presses with colic and other health-related problems. John Pringle (1707-1782), one of England's leading surgeons, proposed the first modern principles of military sanitation, especially in the ventilation of hospital wards. Both Pringle and Stephen Hales (1677-1761) were instrumental in securing better ventilation for those confined in ships, jails, barracks, and mines. The efforts of reformer John Howard (1726-1790) were paramount in changing the medical management of prisons, hospitals, and charity hospitals, especially in the eradication of vermin vectors and the attendant typhus fever. Johann Frank's (1745-1821) nine-volume *System Einer Vollstandigen Medicinischen Polizey* (1779-1827) was the first systematic treatise on public hygiene.

The impact of surgery was evident in the field of military medicine. Much of the history of surgery had been made in military ventures, and in the eighteenth century the administration of military medicine became a function of government. Army hospitals were placed under military regulation by the French in 1718 and by the English in 1762. Schools of military medicine were founded, including the prestigious Prussian Pèpiniére (1785) and the Austrian Josephina (1785). At the battle of Fontenoy (1745) a sophisticated treatment system was used to care for the wounded: they first received treatment on the front line from regimental surgeons; then the wounded were transferred to ambulance stations, where major operations such as amputations were performed. After surgery the wounded were transported to general hospitals in nearby cities. By 1750 the English army was using "flying," "fixed," and "convalescent" hospitals.

At the end of the 1700s the necessary role of surgery within the context of medicine had become clearer. No less of a respected authority than Boerhaave stated:

> Whoever therefore has so thoroughly understood the diseases already described, and laid before his eyes, as to be well acquainted with their several causes, nature, effects, and method of cure; and has applied all these particulars to the internal and unseen parts of the body; and compared them with the actions of the sound parts, and afterwards with the several appearances of internal diseases, will find that what is internal corresponds exactly with what is external; that external diseases, which fall under the surgeon's care, ought first to be treated of; and that otherwise nothing regular or just could be performed or advanced in the practice of physick.

Boerhaave's proclamation demonstrates the increasing interdependence of internal medicine and surgery, which had been cultivated in the common ground of eighteenth-century pathological anatomy and experimental physiology. At long last, physicians and surgeons had knowledge in areas that were essential to both disciplines. For thousands of years surgeons had attempted to rely on an objective anatomical diagnosis. With the advent of pathology, physicians were able to regard disease from a perspective that had long been prevalent among surgeons. However, because surgery, to make its most impressive gains, still awaited the advent of anesthesia and antisepsis, eighteenth-century internal medicine appeared to yield more dramatic results, for example, in diagnosis and treatment.

FRANCE

Louis XV (1710-1774), the great-grandson of Louis XIV, became his successor in 1715. The reign of Louis XV lasted for almost 60 years, and the French populace came to hate the king for his laziness and prodigal ways. Surprisingly the nation revolted not against Louis XV but against his well-intentioned but ineffectual grandson, Louis XVI (1754-1793). His reign was marked by the French Revolution, which lasted from 1789 to 1799.

The revolution began when Louis XVI called a meeting of the rarely used National Assembly to direct them to provide money for his bankrupt government, and it ended when Napoleon Bonaparte (1769-1821) became first consul of France. During the intervening 10 years thousands of nobles and aristocrats, including Louis XVI and his queen, Marie Antoinette (1755-1793), were guillotined. Many revolutionary leaders, including Georges Danton (1759-1794) and Maximilien Robespierre (1758-1794), achieved brief notoriety and then were condemned to die by guillotine. When the revolution had ended, power had passed from an absolute monarchy to a great and growing middle class.

After the execution of Louis XVI on January 21, 1793, the throne passed in name only to his son Louis XVII (1785-1795). However, the young dauphin was taken from his mother in that year and placed in prison. He was never to see his mother, Marie Antoinette, again: she was beheaded on October 16. The young king died 2 years later, on June 8, as a result of abuse and the sheer neglect by his guards. Although the Bourbon kings would be restored to their throne after the defeat of Napoleon, feudal government had been abolished. The revolution did not make France a democracy, but it did manage to create a limited monarchy.

Eighteenth-century European surgery achieved great prominence in France. At the beginning of the century new patterns of surgical education and training were apparent. Two kinds of apprenticeships were available. The first was a formal arrangement for a period of 2 consecutive years, in which the apprentice's family and the master surgeon agreed to a legal contract, or brevet. The young man would provide certain services and obedience to his mentor; the surgeon agreed to provide education and training, as well as food, shelter, and other basic needs. The family paid the master surgeon a fee according to his reputation and paid the city's surgical guild a fixed amount. For families unable to afford a brevet apprenticeship, another type of apprenticeship, known as *garçons chirurgiens* or *serviteurs chirurgiens,* existed. The garçon's relationship to the surgeon was more like that of a domestic servant to a master. The teenager served for at least 6 years in return for room, board, and the opportunity to learn the surgeon's craft without paying a fee. This type of apprentice was in a much more menial position than was the brevet apprentice and had less freedom to attend hospitals and public lectures. More important, a master surgeon could have only one apprentice at a time but was not restricted as to the number of garcons.

Regardless of educational tract, neither the brevet apprentice nor the garcon was likely to learn how to perform major operations from the average Parisian master surgeon. In many instances military service provided greater experience in operative techniques. Accordingly, the Paris surgical community's statutes of 1699 recognized the importance of such service by awarding the equivalent of 1 year of apprenticeship to young surgeons who served during an army campaign.

Several renowned Parisian surgeons offered practical training beyond minor surgical operations. These surgeons received fee-paying students, or pensionnaires, in addition to the one apprentice permitted them. The pensionnaire differed from the apprentice in that he did not enter into a binding agreement with the master surgeon, nor did he hope to fulfill an entrance requirement of one of the guilds. He was simply allowed to accompany the distinguished master surgeon in his daily routines. The pensionnaires tended to be wealthy students from outside Paris and from foreign countries. Most were already graduates of medical school and came to Paris to strengthen their surgical training.

Once an apprentice or a garcon had completed his service, he began the final stage of surgical training, the journeyman or compagnon stage, which usually lasted for 7 years. During that time the journeyman received a small stipend. Most compagnons hoped to become eligible for the mastership and were not allowed to practice surgery on their own. Those who chose not to move to the provinces, where a surgical mastership could be acquired with much greater ease, usually left their masters after a few years and commenced independent practices illegally in Paris. None of these individuals could realistically hope to become a Paris master surgeon unless he were a son or a son-in-law of such a master or had political connections in the royal court or a hospital. It is estimated that there were 2000 such illegal practices in Paris in 1731.

The best of the young surgeons sought to serve under surgeons who worked in hospitals. In this way they were able to accompany the surgeons on hospital rounds and receive special access to hospital functions, including surgical operations. Some of the most prestigious hospitals, such as the Hôtel Dieu, had informal, loosely organized training programs.

By the first decades of the eighteenth century, many French surgeons, especially in Paris, had begun to realize the value of a liberal education in addition to training in their craft. Thus young eighteenth-century surgeons, unlike their predecessors, were beginning to receive a university education as a preliminary step toward formal surgical training. In this educational environment, job opportunities were enhanced and the professional milieu emerged in which numerous French surgical triumphs would occur.

154. *A Barber-Surgeon (left)* and *The Barber's Wife (right)*. Two engravings by Martin Engelbrecht from a series on trades and professions. The barber-surgeon is portrayed with a trephine appropriately on his head, a barber's bowl around his neck, and a pan in his hand. His elegant costume is bedecked with other tools of the barber and the surgeon. *(Bibliothèque des Arts Décoratifs, The Louvre, Paris.)*

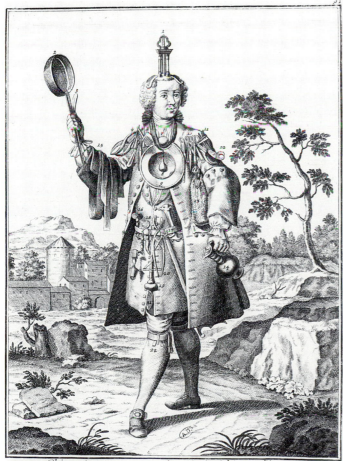

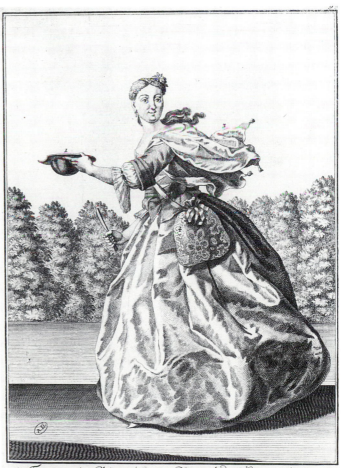

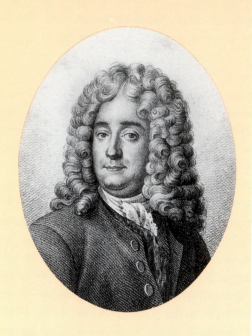

155. Georges Mareschal, First Surgeon to Louis XIV and Louis XV. Engraving by Ambroise Tardieu after a painting at l'Ecole de Médecine de Paris. *(Historical Collections, College of Physicians of Philadelphia.)*

The actual transformation of French surgeons from practitioners of guild mentality to well-educated professionals can be traced to 1715. In that year the 55-year reign of Louis XIV came to an end when he died of gangrene in his lower extremity. The premier surgeon Georges Mareschal (1658-1736), successor to Felix, cared for the king during his final illness. A significant turning point in the relationship between surgeons and physicians occurred because Mareschal was highly regarded and because his treatment of the king was deemed more appropriate than that of the premier physician Gui-Crescent Fagon (1638-1718). Before 1715 the premier surgeon had always been deferential toward the premier physician. After the king's premier physician, Fagon, was forced to leave his post, the physicians never again dominated their surgical counterparts.

Mareschal began a public campaign after 1715 to improve the status of the Paris surgical community. Arguments occurred with increasing frequency between the Royal Company of Master Surgeons and the medical faculty. In 1719 two of the administrators of the surgical community publicly insulted representatives of the medical faculty when the latter attempted to preside over the reception of new candidates for surgical mastership.

Mareschal was the son of an Irish soldier of fortune who had been forced to leave Great Britain and take refuge in France. He died in poverty, leaving Mareschal a penniless 13-year-old orphan. He was soon apprenticed to a provincial surgeon, and after his training he settled in Paris. Despite his lack of funds and political connections, Mareschal managed to become a master surgeon, surgeon-in-chief at the Charité hospital during the 1690s, and premier surgeon from 1703 until his death.

For French surgery 1715 was an auspicious year not only because of Mareschal's triumph, but also because it was the year that François La Peyronie (1678-1747) decided to permanently settle in Paris. La Peyronie was born at Montpellier, the son of a well-to-do master barber-surgeon. Unlike many of his peers, he was the recipient of an extensive liberal arts education at a Jesuit college. La Peyronie embarked on a surgical career that included wide practical experience gained in several provincial hospitals. During the late 1690s he spent time as Mareschal's pensionnaire at the Charité and attended private courses in mathematics and natural history.

La Peyronie returned to Montpellier, where he began to lecture on surgery and anatomy and was named a surgeon to that city's Hôtel Dieu. He was professionally successful in treating several prominent members of the nobility and the clergy. In 1704 La Peyronie became surgeon-major of the army that Claude Villars (1653-1734), a French general and, later, marshal of France, was assembling in the Cevennes region of the country.

In 1714 La Peyronie was asked to return to Paris to treat a nobleman. The lifesaving therapy La Peyronie administered and his politically powerful relationship with Philippe, Duke of Orléans (1674-1723), led La Peyronie to a number of prestigious surgical posts. Philippe was quite important, since he acted as regent of France until Louis XV came of age. Thus La Peyronie enjoyed a close relationship with the young king from 1719 until 1747.

Under the regent's patronage La Peyronie became a demonstrator at the Jardin du Roi and chief surgeon at the Charité hospital. In 1719 he was nominated as successor-designate to the premier surgeon, his mentor, Mareschal. La Peyronie actually assumed most of the 61-year-old Mareschal's surgical practice and served with Mareschal as premier surgeon until the latter's death.

La Peyronie's incisive thinking ultimately freed French surgery from the grasp of the domineering physicians. Because both Mareschal and La Peyronie were much stronger politically in their relationship with Louis XV than was the new premier physician, Francois Chicoyneau (1672-1752), they were able to secure rulings from the king that were favorable to the surgical profession and enhanced their own power. Clearly, Mareschal needed the stimulus of the younger La Peyronie to provide the momentum for prosurgical legislation and to direct the surgical community's growing rebellion against the medical faculty.

La Peyronie did not write any major surgical treatises but is eponymically remembered for his description of fibrous cavernitis of the penis. He was a man of immense intellectual and scientific accomplishment who also had a great desire to uplift the position of French surgeons. La Peyronie recruited promising young provincial surgeons to come to Paris and supported them with his own funds. Two of his most prominent protégés, François Quesnay (1694-1774) and Antoine Louis (1723-1792), wrote some of the most devastating polemics against the Paris medical faculty and were at the forefront of the articulation of goals by their surgical peers.

In an especially humiliating affront to the physicians of Paris, La Peyronie willed his entire estate, worth more than 1.5 million francs, to the surgical communities of Paris and Montpellier. These funds would prove instrumental in making Paris the surgical mecca of Europe in the mid-eighteenth century.

With the complete trust of the regent and young Louis XV, Mareschal and La Peyronie accomplished final liberation of surgery from the domination of the medical faculty. In September 1724 both men petitioned the king to endow five public lectureships in surgery and anatomy at the amphitheater of St. Côme. Thus the royal government, not the surgeons of St. Côme, officially supported and financed surgical instruction. The premier surgeons were appointed administrators of the courses and were allowed to name the five instructors. Mareschal and La Peyronie decided to make the positions lengthy tenured posts rather than lectureships that rotated among the masters of St. Côme. In 1725 the five "royal demonstrators" were named: Jean-Louis Petit (1674-1750) taught surgical principles; Antoine Andouille taught osteology and bone diseases; César Verdier (1685-1759) was the anatomist; Sauveur-François Morand (1697-1773) lectured on surgical diseases and operations; and Jean Malaval discussed surgical therapy. Public affirmation of the surgeons' competence as teachers, which became evident in the escalating popularity of the courses, refuted any pretensions on the part of the medical faculty that physicians alone had the competence to teach.

Highly displeased with the king's ruling, the medical faculty went into revolt. Despite the king's order expressly forbidding any public demonstration against the surgeons, the physicians marched on St. Côme. In the midst of a driving sleet, wearing their full academic regalia, they threatened to break down the doors of the amphitheater. The assembled crowd suddenly turned on the supercilious physicians and forced them away without regard for their red velvet robes and furs.

Two important events firmly placed the surgeons on an equal social and scientific level with their physician peers. First, in 1731 Mareschal and La Peyronie petitioned the king to establish a society that would meet once a week to hear and discuss presentations of papers on surgical topics. This society became known as the Royal Academy of Surgery and consisted of the 70 leading master surgeons in Paris. Its initial president was Mareschal, who was succeeded by La Peyronie and, later, Germain-Pichaut De La Martinière (1696-1783). The Academy attempted to advance surgical knowledge by gathering, reviewing, editing, and publishing clinical observations submitted by surgeons from all countries.

The Academy was clearly elitist by organization, and several hundred Paris master surgeons had no voting privileges, nor did they contribute to the weekly meetings. Thus the Academy was able to strengthen its position within Paris and erode the political base of the guild organization of surgeons.

The most important function of the Academy was its yearly publication of *Memoires* from 1743 until 1774. These lengthy review articles were highly praised and valued for their wealth of practical information. Indeed, after the initial volume's publication in March and at La Peyronie's instigation, a royal declaration was set forth on April 23, requiring future candidates for the Paris surgical mastership to take a master of arts degree from a French university. The preamble to the declaration stated that the public courses and the publication of the *Memoires* demonstrated that master surgeons had made a convincing case that young surgeons, to profit fully from lessons at the Academy, ought to have knowledge of Latin and an understanding of philosophy.

A second major step in the evolutionary process of eighteenth century French surgery concerned the second provision of the Royal Declaration of 1743, which declared that henceforth Paris master surgeons were forbidden to work as barbers. Conversely, barber's work would be considered an inferior profession and would belong solely to the barber-wigmakers. Therefore, when the last few Paris barber-surgeons retired from practice, such an occupation would become extinct.

From 1743 until 1750 the medical faculty and the members of the Academy of Surgery participated in a series of legal battles and diatribes. In some instances the disagreements were quite petty; at another level serious educational, social, and economic issues were being debated. The surgeons, among themselves, were asking important questions about the actual educational requirements of future surgeons. Most important, the French public finally viewed surgeons as being on the same societal level as the physicians, and their debates as equally important.

A halt was put to the constant internecine squabbling between physicians and surgeons when the king's council put forth decrees in April 1749 and July 1750. These rulings declared that any signs of subordination by the surgeons to the medical faculty were to be abolished or rendered meaningless. Higher educational standards for Paris surgeons would be enforced, including the obtaining of master of arts degrees. Nongraduate or "unlettered" surgeons, although not prohibited from practicing, would be relegated to a secondary status in the surgical community. Only the most experienced house officers from the major Parisian hospitals and surgeons of the king's household would be promised full privileges as master surgeons without regard to university education. Finally, the surgical community of Paris was recognized as a college separate but equal in academic rank to the medical faculty of the university. These higher standards were the probable cause of a decline in the membership of the Parisian surgical company from a maximum of 280 masters in 1755 to only 192 master surgeons in 1789.

The transformation of French surgery from a craft guild to a liberal profession was complete in 1750. In the second half of the eighteenth century Paris would showcase the talents of its surgeons, and that city became the mecca for surgeons from throughout the civilized world who sought further education and training.

As the practice of surgery flourished, a number of innovations were begun within the structure of surgical education. The Paris College of Surgery commenced a dissection school with practical instruction in anatomy and surgical operations, and a clinical research and teaching hospital was constructed. The sophistication of surgical education in Paris was soon known throughout France. In most other provinces royal surgical schools were opened, bringing an eventual end to the medieval concept of apprenticeship.

As both public and royal support for the surgeons grew, support for the physicians declined, especially during the 1760s and 1770s, when La Martinière obtained legislation for the acquisition of property and the construction of new facilities for the College. As the king's premier surgeon, he exerted enormous political pressure on various governmental officials, and more than 600,000 francs were furnished for the buildings. On December 14, 1774, the cornerstone of a complex of buildings devoted exclusively to the surgical community was laid by Louis XVI. Spacious and sumptuous, these structures dwarfed those of the medical faculty, which were dilapidated and soon to be demolished. The most spectacular section was the nucleus of a splendid surgical library unmatched in Europe, with a collection of 800 books from the days of the Confraternity of St. Côme plus 132 volumes donated in the bequest of La Peyronie.

Four major hospitals in Paris played crucial roles in the evolution of surgery in the 1700s: the Hôtel Dieu, the Charité, the Hôpital General, and the Invalides. The Hôtel Dieu was the oldest of Parisian hospitals, dating back to at least the thirteenth century. It received indigent male and female patients of all ages; normally between 2000 and 3000 patients at a time received treatment,

156. *Facing page,* Louis XVI placing the foundation stone of the Ecoles de Chirurgie at Paris in 1774. Drawing by G. de St.-Aubin in the Musée Carnavalet, Paris. *(Cliché photothèque des Musées de la Ville de Paris.)*

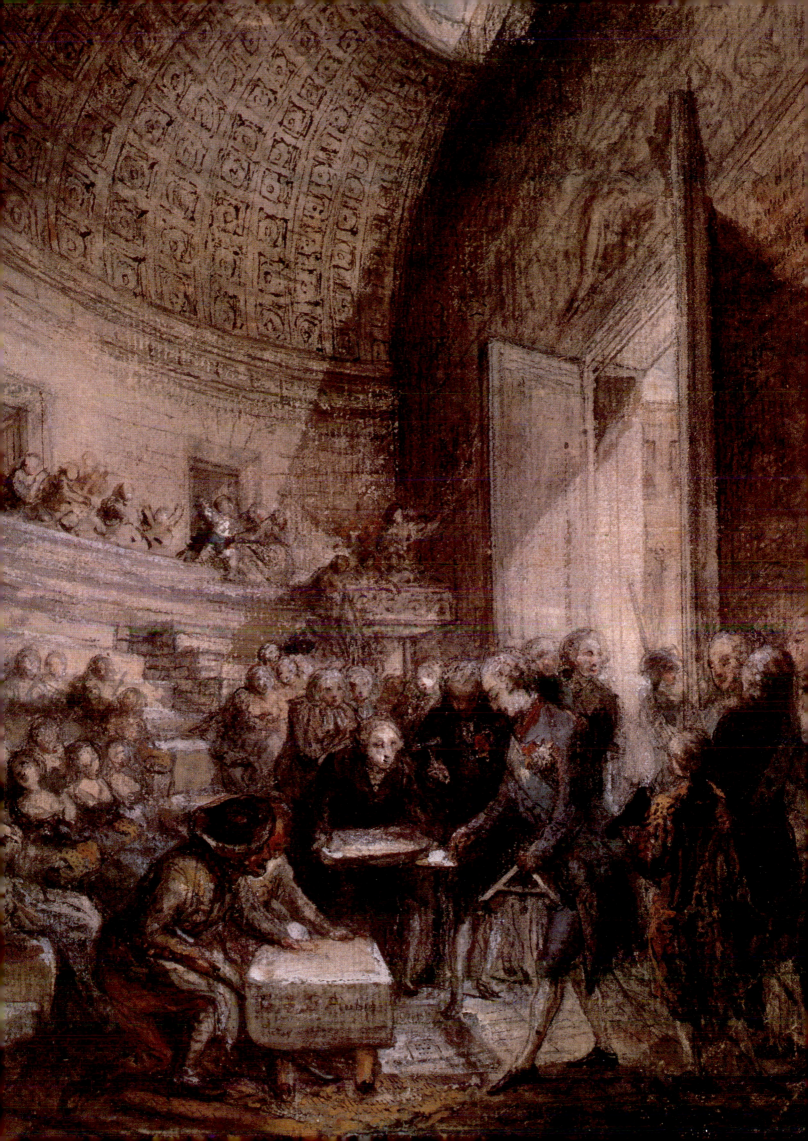

although the number of beds never exceeded 1200. The euphemistically termed "large beds," slightly over 4 feet in width, were intended for four patients simultaneously.

The Charité hospital was founded in 1602 and contained almost 200 beds, each for an individual patient. The physically immense Hôpital General was established by the king in 1656 for the avowed purpose of clearing Paris of beggars and other indigents. Its 10,000 patients lived in wretched conditions. The Invalides was a 500-bed military hospital founded in 1674. Patients with a wide range of medical and surgical conditions were admitted, and the minister of war had direct control of admissions and daily administration.

The Paris College of Surgery gave its official approval to a formalized type of hospital surgical training in new statutes in 1768. These statutes declared 2 years of work in a major hospital to be equivalent, in terms of qualifying for a surgical mastership, to 3 years of services in private practice. The medical faculty were not as enamored with hospital service as the surgeons were, so the number of surgical house officers was 10 times that of medical trainees. Thus working in Parisian hospitals became an attractive means of obtaining previously unavailable practical experience for surgeons from throughout Europe and America.

In the expansive academic atmosphere created by political successes the practice of surgery and the personal well-being of surgeons flourished. Many notable surgeons participated in the advancement of knowledge and technique, and their cumulative observations and numerous literary contributions culminated in an impressive surgical hierarchy.

157. The Hôtel des Invalides, founded by Louis XIV as a hospital for his soldiers and today the resting place of Napoleon. The design of the hospital and its adjoints was begun by Libéral Bruant and continued, along with the magnificent church visible in back, by his pupil Jules Harddouin Mansart, the favorite architect of Louis XIV. The Mansart dynasty of architects was prominent in the seventeenth and eighteenth centuries, and Jules was responsible for many French architectural achievements, including parts of Versailles, the Place Vendôme, and the dome of Les Invalides. The design Les Invalides influenced the conception of other buildings in Europe, such as the Royal Naval Hospital at Greenwich, England, designed by Sir Christopher Wren. *(National Library of Medicine, Bethesda, Md.)*

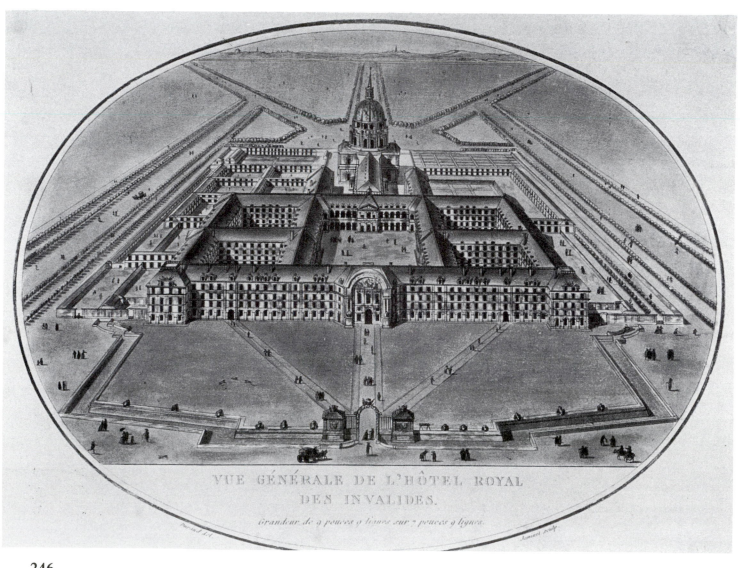

VUE GÉNÉRALE DE L'HÔTEL ROYAL
DES INVALIDES.

Grandeur de 9 pouces 9 lignes sur 7 pouces 9 lignes.

The leading French scientific surgeon of the first half of the eighteenth century was Jean-Louis Petit (1674-1750). He was born in Paris and by his sixteenth birthday was a well-respected dissector. His precocious understanding of anatomy was aided by the guidance of Alexis Littre (1658-1726), a renowned anatomist and surgeon who lived in the Petit home. Littre described the male urethral glands, was the first to suggest inguinal colostomy in intestinal obstruction, and is eponymically linked with both parietal and diverticular hernias.

In 1692 Petit joined the surgical staff of the army. He was present at the siege of Namur and served through all the succeeding campaigns until 1697, when he was placed in charge of the military hospital at Tournay. After leaving the army, Petit resumed the regular study of medicine, obtaining his master of surgery (Ch. M.) degree in March 1700.

Petit's reputation as a bold, skillful surgeon attracted large number of students to his home, where he organized a private school. Many of his pupils became the leading physicians and surgeons of Europe. Petit was one of the founding members of the Academy of Surgery and later served as its director. He became internationally famous: he was invited to Poland and Spain to treat nobility and royalty.

Petit was the originator of many important surgical methods. He invented the screw tourniquet, performed the first successful operation on the mastoid cells for mastoiditis (1736), and greatly improved the technique of circular amputation by incising the skin and muscles at different levels instead of using the "guillotine" approach. His most important written works include *L'Art De Guerir Les Maladies Des Os* (1705) and the posthumously published three-volume *Traité Des Maladies Chirurgicales Et Des Operations* (1774-1783). Petit provided the first accurate account of osteomalacia, clearly understood the differences between the compression and concussion of the brain, and conducted original investigations into the formation of thrombi in wounded arteries, specifically in relation to hemostasis and amputations.

The most renowned of Petit's pupils and the closest to Petit in age was Dominique Anel (1678-1725). He was born in Toulouse, studied at Montpellier and Paris, and served with the French army in Alsace. Anel's professional life included postgraduate studies in Vienna, teaching positions in Rouen and Genoa, and eventual practice in Paris. Among his surgical triumphs was the ligation of a traumatic brachial artery aneurysm, and he devised a new operation for lachrymal duct fistula, in which a fine-pointed syringe was used. Anel was the first to catheterize a lachrymal duct (1713), and his reputation as an ophthalmologist was unsurpassed.

When Petit assumed the directorship of the Academy of Surgery (1731), Sauveur-François Morand (1697-1773) was named its first secretary. Although he was not well educated, Morand was an ingenious surgeon. His most remarkable accomplishments include one of the earliest recorded successful operations for temporosphenoidal abscess (1752) and the first description of cleidocranial dysostosis (1760).

Morand was succeeded as secretary by Antoine Louis (1723-1792), who became permanent secretary. His organizational abilities contributed greatly to the success of the Royal Academy of Surgery and its marked influence on the progress of French surgery. As a young surgeon, he had already challenged the supremacy of physicians and had became a leading advocate for Paris surgeons. In 1749 Louis completed his service at the Salpêtriére, a division of the Hôpital General, and was legally entitled to automatic reception into the College of Surgery. He instead asked to become the first surgical candidate to sustain a public examination and to present in Latin his thesis on whether the transmission of malaria was hereditary. This symbolic act was a moment of triumph for surgeons because it demonstrated that surgeons were as liberally educated, especially in Latin, as their physician peers. In 1757 Louis was appointed surgeon to the Charité. Although he authored many works, including numerous surgical treatises, he is best remembered as a learned historian, an editor, and a critic. Louis was also a pioneer of French medical jurisprudence: he presented a classic discussion of the differential signs of murder and suicide in cases of hanging.

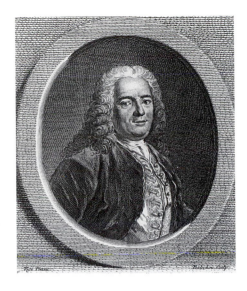

158. Jean Louis Petit in 1742. (*Historical Collections, College of Physicians of Philadelphia.*)

159. Advertising card of Jacques Songy, coustelier at Paris, 1732. This elegant flyer for the surgical-instrument maker shows about 20 different instruments made by Songy for surgeons and barbers, along with his trademark, a stag. In the upper left corner a winged putto brandishes a scalpel. (Jeremy Norman & Co., Inc.)

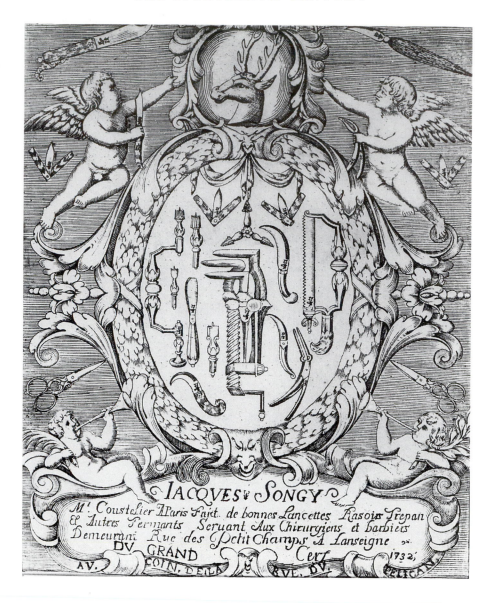

Nicolas Andry (1658-1742) was born in Lyon and was originally a clergyman. His place in the evolution of French surgery is curious, since he was not a surgeon. Instead, Andry was dean of the medical faculty, author of the first textbook on medical parasitology (1700), and an unfriendly personality who constantly battled with surgeons. His only contribution to surgery was the two-volume *L'Orthopédie Ou L'Art Prévenir Et De Corriger Dans Les Enfants, Les Difformités Dur Corps* (1741), the first book on *orthopedics*, a term that Andry himself introduced. Andry advised attention to proper posture in the prevention and correction of spinal curvature. Andry's was also the first work on diseases of children to mention chlorosis.

Henri Le Dran (1685-1773) was among the most distinguished early members of the Academy. He was the son of a surgeon and received his education in Paris. In 1724 Le Dran was appointed one of the four surgeons to the Charité, and he eventually became its chief of surgery. He established a school of anatomy there, and from his studies came a prominent text on the operation of lithotomy (1730). Four years later, Le Dran was appointed chief surgeon to the French army and his observations were described in *Traité Ou Reflexions Tirées De La Pratique Sur Les Playes D'Armies A Feu* (1737). In 1742 Le Dran authored a treatise on operative surgery. His most important contribution to surgery is found in a paper on cancer, in which for the first time the humoral theory of oncogenesis is discarded and the lymph theory is proposed. Le Dran was a celebrated teacher and had many pupils from Germany; the most prominent of these was Haller.

Claude-Nicolas Le Cat (1700-1768) was a surgeon from Rouen who became surgeon-in-chief of the Hôtel Dieu in that city. He initially wanted an ecclesiastical career but, following the urging of his father, himself a prominent surgeon, decided to study surgery. In 1724 Le Cat went to Paris and became politically affiliated with the archbishop of Rouen as his personal physician and surgeon. When the post of surgeon to the Hôtel Dieu of Rouen was vacated (1731), Le Cat "won" the post. He was especially skilled in writing lengthy essays, for which he received a number of honors from the Academy of Surgery. Although Le Cat was a prolific writer, only his works on lithotomy (1752) had more than a minimal influence.

Among the accounts of lithotomy that Le Cat described were the methods of Jean Baseilhac (1703-1781), also known as Frère Jean de St. Côme. He was born at Poyestruc, in the region of Hautes-Pyrenees. Both his father and grandfather were masters in surgery, and he received his early surgical training from his grandfather and an uncle. In 1724 Baseilhac settled in Paris, where he became a surgeon's pensionnaire. Two years later he became one of the regular house officers at the Hôtel Dieu in Paris. Having completed his term of service, Baseilhac was appointed personal physician to the bishop of Bayeux in Normandy. The clergyman died in 1728 but in his will left Baseilhac enough money to pursue a regular course of instruction at the school of St. Côme and to procure the usual complement of surgical instruments.

160. Hernia trusses, from an unpublished eighteenth-century English translation of the *Treatise on Bandages* by the French surgeon Henri-Fançois-Michel Disdier (1708-1781). *(Boston Medical Library.)*

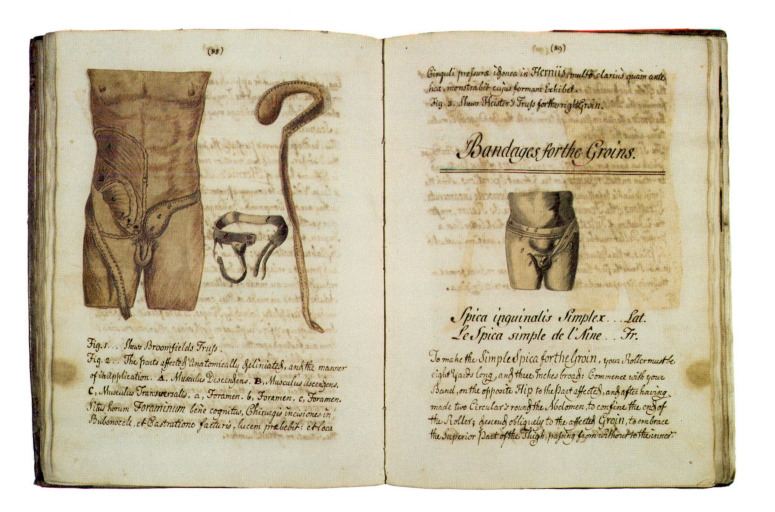

In 1740 Baseilhac decided, for unknown reasons, to become a member of the Feuillants branch of the Franciscan monks. Although the clergy were not permitted to practice surgery, an exception was made in his case and he was granted the special privilege of practicing surgery among the indigent. Circumstances allowed Baseilhac to stop performing general surgical operations and to specialize instead in lithotomy. He was of the opinion that the method of De Beaulieu was preferable to the more complicated procedure of the academic surgeons. Subsequently Baseilhac devised a concealed lithotome that he claimed would lessen the danger of making a perineal incision in the improper place or of too great a length.

In 1753 Baseilhac established near the St. Honoré gateway in Paris a special hospital for lithotomy patients. The poor classes were not expected to pay any fee, and money was often given to these individuals when they were discharged. Records from that institution show that Baseilhac and his nephew Pascal Baseilhac performed more than 1000 lithotomies before Jean Baseilhac's death.

Pierre Brasdor (1721-1797) was professor of anatomy and operative therapy at the College of Surgeons and a major contributor to the *Memoires* of the Academy. He is eponymically linked with a treatment of aneurysm by ligation of the artery immediately distal to the lesion. Brasdor never actually performed the technique but is given credit for providing the initial hypothesis. Most of his innovative operative techniques concerned surgery on bones and amputations.

Hugues Ravaton was a respected military surgeon who authored one of the eighteenth century's best treatises on gunshot injuries. His *Chirurgie D'Armée* was issued in 1767, and the four-volume *Pratique Moderne De La Chirurgie* in 1776. He also was among the first to perform amputation by means of the double-flap method.

Raphael Sabatier (1732-1811) was born in Paris, the son of Pierre Sabatier, one of the earliest members of the Academy. Raphael Sabatier was a pupil of Petit and at 24 years of age was appointed professor of anatomy at the Academy. In 1773 Sabatier was made a member of the Parisian Academy of Sciences. Most of his operative innovations were in ophthalmology, although he did recommend the resection of the head of the brachial os. In his later years Sabatier was named one of Napoleon's personal surgeons. His numerous literary contributions included the three-volume *Traité D'Anatomie* (1764) and the mammoth *De La Medécine Operatoire* (1796).

Jean Sigault (1740-?) studied surgery in Paris and received his mastership in 1770 despite his presentation before the Academy (1768) of a treatise that proposed substituting the section of the symphysis of the pubis for cesarean section. The master surgeons promptly rejected his proposal, with little discussion. In 1777 Sigault created a sensation when he performed a successful symphysiotomy to deliver the infant of a woman in labor whose pelvic deformities prevented vaginal delivery. The Paris Faculty of Medicine took special pride in this surgical achievement because of Sigault's prior rejection by the Academy, because he had quietly joined their institution, and because the innovation appeared to be a triumph for the faculty in a field traditionally dominated by surgeons. During the ensuing controversy the College of Surgery discredited the operation for a second time. However, the Sigault affair demonstrated the medical faculty's willingness to encourage surgery within its own ranks.

François Chopart (1743-1795) was born in Paris, where he received all of his surgical training, including service as an intern at Hôtel Dieu. In 1768 he received a prize from the Academy for his treatise *Memoire Sur Les Lésions De La Tête, Par Contrecoup*. Two years later Chopart was awarded his master of surgery degree, which was soon followed by an appointment as professor of practical surgery. In 1782 he was chosen to succeed Toussaint Bordenave (1728-1782) as professor of physiology. Chopart, with Pierre Desault (1744-1795), wrote the two-volume *Traité Des Maladies Chirurgicales Et Des Operations Qui Leur Conviennent* (1795). Chopart is remembered for his description of a disarticulation at the midtarsal joint, leaving only the astragalus and calcaneum, with the soft parts of the sole of the foot to cover the stump.

In addition to the construction of a new complex of buildings devoted exclusively for the surgical community of Paris, the hospice of the College of Surgery was also established in 1774. In many respects, the hospice further accentuated the elitism of certain Paris master surgeons, who now had their own private hospital in which clinical research, education, and major operative surgery could be carried out. The general problems of medical educational reform, including the lack of organized clinical instruction, could now be left to others.

The French Revolution played such a tremendous part in reshaping the lives of French citizens that, not unexpectedly, surgeons and surgical thinking were also profoundly affected by the upheaval. The necessity for change in the French health care system was increasingly apparent during the final years of the old regime. Before the revolution, reformers had begun to castigate the costs and corruption of medical and surgical practices.

From 1789 to 1793 politics was thought to hold the key to health. Accordingly, physicians and scientists flocked to the side of the revolutionaries, believing that the funds for the new science of health would come from Church properties confiscated in late 1789. The concept of professional unification as a way to create this new health care delivery system became a subject of lively debate. A Committee of Health was established within the revolutionary movement, and the question put: "Will all the parts of the healing art be practiced by the same individual or by several?" In October 1790 a majority of the committee members voted that physicians and surgeons should be given the same education and undergo the same examinations. There was an inevitability in this change, since social distinctions such as the traditional superiority of physicians over surgeons ran counter to any revolutionary notion of equality and fair play.

Neither the old guard of Paris surgeons nor the medical faculty had much chance to prevent unification. Public instruction at the Paris College of Surgery persisted through 1794, but the College became a shell of its former self. The surgical institutions of the old regime in Paris were so closely linked to the discredited monarchy that there was no possibility of their remaining in an unaltered state. Universities and their medical schools were shut down in 1791, not because issues had been resolved but because paranoia caused the radicals to fear that counterrevolutionary plots might be conceived in the halls of academic freedom.

In 1792 the revolutionary assembly formally dissolved all religious corporations and secular congregations of men or women. Furthermore, the assembly annulled the charters of all guilds, corporations, and scientific societies. On August 18, 1792, a law passed by the legislative assembly abolished simultaneously the Faculty of Medicine and the College and the Academy of Surgery. The effect of the law would prove to be catastrophic both for society and for the armies of the revolution.

The foreign wars that engulfed revolutionary France for the remainder of the eighteenth century and beyond posed devastating problems for the understaffed and poorly supplied medical corps. The number of military deaths resulting from epidemics increased, and the decaying medical situation was further complicated by shortages of bandages, medicines, and beds and by growing graft among suppliers.

Where the French once had an impressive military medical complex, charlatans again interfered, and the death rate among wounded soldiers reached staggering proportions. Military surgeons were in short supply, and inexperienced physicians were pressed into service without adequate clinical knowledge. Their training was pathetic, and they created havoc on the battlefield.

Occasional instances of surgical successes included Pierre Percy's (1754-1825) use of "flying hospitals." As chief surgeon of the revolutionary armies, he organized groups of three mounted surgeons, a crew of litter bearers, and specially designed ambulances to remove the injured from the battlefield. Each "flying hospital" carried its instruments and a supply of bandages, lint, brandy, vinegar, bread, wine, salt, and bouillon.

Until 1795 surgeons who volunteered for military service had been given much latitude in their daily activities and had ranked as upper-echelon officers. In that year they were completely subordinated to the military command and their pay and prestige were reduced. Bakers, butchers, and other service personnel were considered equally valuable.

Because of the continuing shortage of properly trained physicians and surgeons, particularly in the French army, Antoine Fourcroy (1755-1809), a chemist, and François Chaussier (1746-1828), a Dijon surgeon and anatomist, were asked by the National Convention to prepare a plan to ensure the maintenance of an adequate army health service. Accordingly, their plan, which was enacted into law in December 1794, called for the creation of what were essentially military medical schools in Paris, Montpellier, and Strassburg. From each French district a youth not yet conscripted was selected by the government to be trained at its expense at one of the schools. The institutions emphasized military surgery; little attention was given to theories of medicine or nontraumatic surgery. After a 3-year course of education and training the young graduate was immediately posted to a regiment in the field.

With the abolition of degrees in medicine and surgery (1790-1791) and the dissolution of all academies (1793), the creation of the Ecole De Santé (School of Health) in 1794 marked the total unification of medicine and surgery in France. Educational requirements for the practice of either medicine or surgery were to be identical, and only one degree, that of Medicinae Doctor, would be awarded. By the same ruling the new Paris School of Health inherited the alma mater of the former faculty and the medical College and Academy of Surgery. The new school in Paris opened its doors on January 20, 1795, and the destinies of the disciples of St. Côme and the medical faculty of Paris became inextricably intertwined.

Pierre-Joseph Desault (1744-1795), a surgeon-anatomist, provided most of the dynamism of late eighteenth-century French surgery. He was born in the small village of Magny-Vernois in the Haute-Saône, the youngest of seven siblings. His parents were peasants with little family income. Most of his early education was received in a school run by Jesuits in the nearby village of Lure. Desault received his early surgical education from one of that village's barbersurgeons. He then served 3 years at the Belfort military hospital, where he had the opportunity to perform numerous anatomical dissections and gained practical experience with patients.

Desault's name appears among those of students registered for public courses at the College of Surgery in Paris in the mid-1760s. Concurrently he began to give private lessons in anatomy and operative surgery, a common practice among young surgeons. Desault's overwhelming success, however, was unexpected. Despite his poor teaching presence, the clarity of his ideas and the precision of his knowledge brought large crowds of students and the concomitant jealousy of several Parisian master surgeons. Prior regulations that medical teaching could be given only at the Faculty of Medicine or the College of Surgery were invoked, and Desault was ordered to desist. However, these restrictions were circumvented when La Martinière and Louis supported Desault, even to the point of themselves attending some of his sessions.

By 1776 Desault had achieved marked success, and La Martiniere selected him to be the first candidate to present a thesis in the newly constructed buildings of the College of Surgery. Even before this official recognition as a master surgeon, Desault had been appointed professor at the Ecole Pratique. This post in turn led to a consultantship at the hospice of the College of Surgery, where Desault also served briefly as chief surgeon.

Desault initiated profound changes in the teaching of surgical anatomy. Anatomy was to be learned in the dissection amphitheater, according to Desault, and should not be limited to knowledge of the body's structure, which he considered useless unless it was connected with knowledge of bodily functions. Desault clearly recognized alterations that are produced in part by disease or by accidental injuries and also the influence exerted by these lesions on neighboring

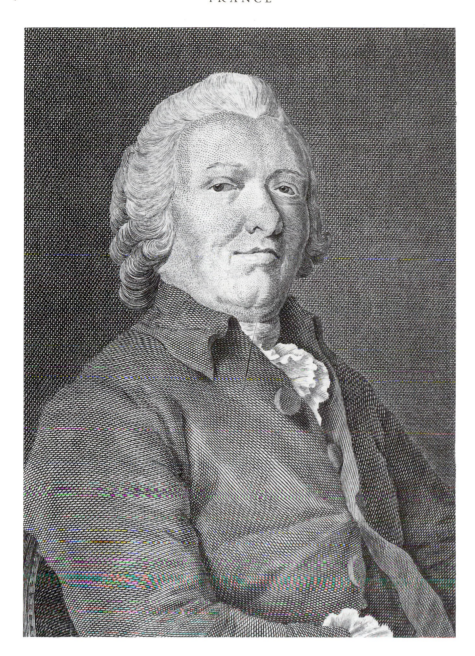

161. Engraving of Pierre-Joseph Desault (1791) by L.J. Cathelin after a drawing by Charles Nicholas Cochin. *(Historical Collections, College of Physicians of Philadelphia.)*

tissues or organs. Most of his major contributions to surgery stemmed from his anatomical studies. These contributions included the technique of ligating blood vessels, especially the femoral artery, for the treatment of popliteal aneurysm and the placement of a bandage for fracture of the clavicle, in which the elbow is bound to the side, a pad having been previously placed in the axilla.

Although the recognition of Desault as an outstanding surgeon came later than his reputation as an anatomist, within a few years he had advanced from novice to one of the foremost clinical surgeons in France. In 1782 he was appointed chief surgeon to the Charité, and 6 years later he attained the equivalent position at the Hôtel Dieu.

Before Desault, clinical instruction at the Hôtel Dieu had been informal at best. The chief surgeon's role had been quite limited, and the burden of learning rested on each student's individual initiative. Foremost among the educational difficulties for surgeons was the absence of a separate operating room. In a short time Desault managed to found the first true surgical clinic in Paris and was presenting surgical lessons in a new hospital surgical amphitheater.

Desault's greatest impact on the evolution of surgical education and training resulted from his introduction of the clinical surgical lesson. His classes were extremely popular, drawing students from all of Europe and America. These physicians and surgeons, including Jean Corvisart (1755-1821), Dominique-Jean Larrey (1766-1842), Marc-Antoine Petit (1766-1811), and Xavier Bichat (1771-1802), would promulgate Desault's teaching methods during their careers.

Events in the revolution overtook Desault at the pinnacle of his success. Denounced by one of his many personal rivals, he was arrested in May 1793 and incarcerated in the Luxemburg quarter of Paris. Trumped-up charges were brought against him, including his supposed refusal to treat political patients wounded in a shooting during the preceding August. A popular outcry against his detention compelled his release after only 4 days, but the incident plagued him for the remainder of his life.

With the closing of all institutions of higher education Desault, who remained fearful of future arrests, was psychologically prevented from completing any further meaningful work in surgery. In December 1794 he received the important professorial chair of clinical surgery in the new Ecole De Santé. However, he remained unhappy with the changes that had occurred, especially with the combined teaching of surgery and medicine in the same institution.

During 1794 the young Louis XVII was languishing in prison. Desault was called to treat him and lavished the 9-year-old dauphin with all his attention. In so doing, Desault himself became violently ill with sepsis of unknown origin and died on June 1, 1795. Whether Desault might have been the victim of some type of palace intrigue that culminated in his own murder is a fascinating conjecture. Bichat, one of Desault's students, performed an autopsy to disprove rumors that Desault's death was caused by poisoning; no poison was found.

Despite his outstanding reputation, Desault provided little in the way of a written legacy. A surgical text that he coauthored with Chopart gave Desault little pleasure because he played a minor role in its preparation. Desault started the first surgical periodical, the *Journal De Chirurgie* (1791-1794), which presented his views in articles written by his most distinguished pupils. His most famous work was the three-volume *Oeuvres Chirurgicales* (1798-1803), which appeared after his death under the editorship of Bichat.

Of all the students of Desault, the most distinguished was Xavier Bichat (1771-1802). Although the training of Bichat was exclusively that of a surgeon, his scientific interests embraced all of medicine, especially descriptive anatomy, histology, and tissue pathology. He was born in Thoirette in the Jura, the son of a provincial surgeon. His initial surgical apprenticeship was taken in his native region. He then worked in Lyon for more than a year (1791-1792) with Marc-Antoine Petit and Louis-Vincent Cartier (1768-1839), both students of Desault. The outbreak of the 1793 war between France and most of its surrounding neighbors, collectively known as the First Coalition, interrupted Bichat's education. He served in the French army, holding positions at several military hospitals, where he received much practical training.

Bichat journeyed to Paris in 1794, where he joined the crowd of students who were regularly following the practical instructions given by Desault. The latter, aided by recommendations from Petit and Cartier, was quick to perceive the young surgeon's potential. Desault was so measurably impressed by Bichat that he invited Bichat to live with him and take charge of his private surgical practice. Furthermore, Bichat acted as his corresponding secretary, answering for him all the requests for advice that came to him from every district of France. Bichat also assisted Desault at all his operations in private practice.

During the last year of Desault's life Bichat was also entrusted with the editorship of the *Journal De Chirurgie,* which had begun to languish because Desault lacked the time and desire to carry out the duty. Bichat, at 23 years of age, authored all three final volumes of the journal.

After Desault's death Bichat's interests gradually shifted from surgery to internal medicine. Although he gave up the practice of surgery, he remained convinced that the discipline illuminated general medical principles:

> . . . devoted for some time to the study of medicine, then to hospital practice, I can no longer concern myself with surgery except insofar as it is an essential basis for all medical knowledge, an important means of analogy in a multitude of difficult cases, and a guide without which the physicians would often proceed haphazardly.

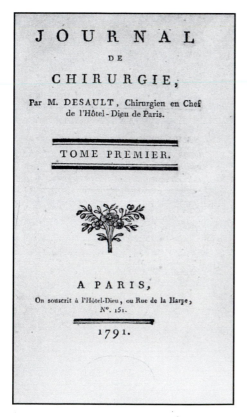

162. Title page of the first volume of the world's first journal devoted specifically to surgery, a periodical whose publication ended after only four volumes because of the death of Desault, its editor, in 1795. *(Jeremy Norman & Co., Inc.)*

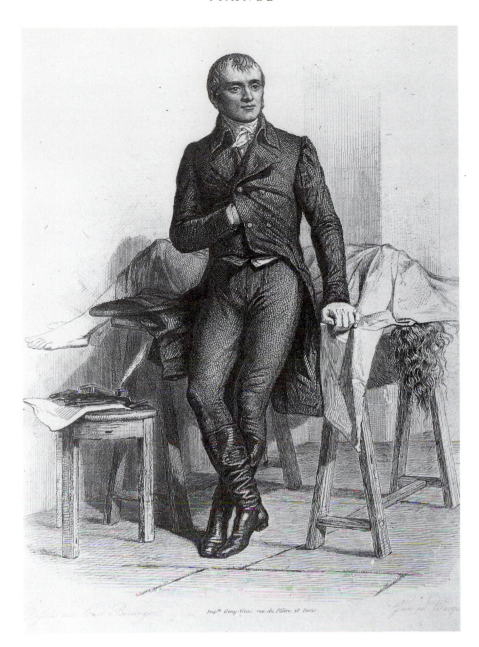

163. Xavier Bichat at the dissection table. Following the fashion of the time, Bichat has affected the mannerisms of Napoleon in his hairstyle and in the placement of his right hand inside his coat. *(Historical Collections, College of Physicians of Philadelphia.)*

Bichat's *Recherches Physiologiques Sur La Vie Et La Mort* (1800), *Traité Des Membranes* (1800), four-volume *Anatomie Generale* (1802), and five-volume *Traité D'Anatomie Descriptive* (1801-1803) opened up entirely new fields for anatomists, physiologists, and pathologists. He emphasized tissues as the units of which organs were composed, introduced the terms *animal* and *vegetative system* to descriptive anatomy, and is eponymically linked with many anatomical and descriptive terms. At the age of 31 years Bichat died of either typhoid fever or tubercular meningitis.

In eighteenth-century France admirable advances were made in several surgical specialties. The Faculty of Medicine had been interested in pursuing research regarding head injuries. A group of "physiological" or "neurological" surgeons brought the techniques in cerebral and spinal surgery to the forefront. François du Petit (1664-1771) authored two short reports in 1718 and 1719 that demonstrated the effects of cervical sympathectomy on the eye, and showed that contralateral paralysis is complete only when the corpus striatum on either side is injured. Anne Charles De Lorry (1726-1783) performed a series of suboccipital and spinal punctures in dogs and cats and concluded that the medulla was an area central to vital bodily functions. Nicolas Saucerotte (1741-1812) was a skilled lithotomist and military surgeon who noted that cerebral wounds are most dangerous at the base of the brain and least so in the frontal area. He also provided the first known clinical description of acromegaly.

Surgery of the eye was widely practiced in France by Antoine Jan-Maître (1650-1730), Michel Brisseau (1676-1743), Dominique Anel (1678-1725), Pierre Demours (1702-1795), and Jean Descemet (1732-1810). Jacques Daviel (1696-1762) originated the modern method of treating cataract by extraction of the lens during the 1740s and 1750s in Paris. Valentin Hauy (1745-1832) founded the first school for the blind, and to him belongs the honor of being the first to emboss paper as a means of reading for the blind. In 1789 Guillaume Pellier De Quengsy (1751-1835) authored the two-volume *Precis Ou Cours D'Operations Sur La Chirurgie Des Yeux,* the first separate book on ophthalmic surgery.

164. The modern method of treating cataract by extraction of the lens, as first described by its inventor, Jacques Daviel. By the time Daviel published this paper in the second volume of the *Mémoires De l'Académie Royale De Chirurgie* (1753), he had already tested his method on 206 patients and had success in 182. *(Jeremy Norman & Co., Inc.)*

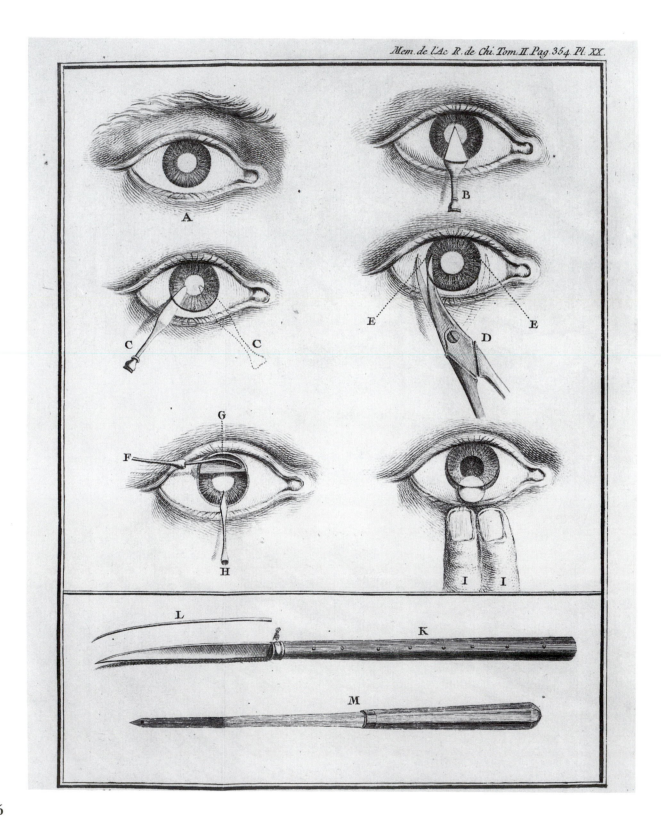

GREAT BRITAIN AND IRELAND

After the death of William III in 1702 there were no immediate heirs to the English throne. William's wife, Mary II, had died almost a full decade before him; her sister Anne (1665-1714) assumed the royal crown. The reign of Queen Anne is called the Augustan Age because its cultural leaders—in particular, the writers Jonathan Swift (1667-1745), Joseph Addison (1672-1719), and Alexander Pope (1688-1744)—sought to reproduce in England the political stability and classical art of Rome under Emperor Augustus. During most of Anne's rule (1702-1714) true political power was wielded by John Churchill (1650-1722), the Duke of Marlborough, who had defeated the French at Blenheim in 1704.

During Anne's reign the 1707 Act of Union joined Scotland to England and Wales and named the new kingdom Great Britain. Commercial prosperity was great, and Parliament became the unquestioned, supreme power in the country. In 1713 the Peace of Utrecht ended the War of the Spanish Succession, giving Gibraltar to Great Britain.

Although Anne had 14 children, none survived her, and she was succeeded by her second cousin, George I (1660-1727), her closest Protestant relative. A German prince of the House of Hanover, George I could not speak English, although he was the great-grandson of England's King James I. George I took almost no part in government affairs, leaving most decisions in the hands of the Whig party. Robert Walpole (1676-1745) led the Whigs in Parliament and is considered the first prime minister of Great Britain.

George I's son George II (1683-1760) became king in 1727. Like his father, George II spoke little English and had only a passing interest in national affairs. Yet, during his reign Great Britain became one of the world's great colonial powers. In 1757 Robert Clive (1725-1774) defeated the Bengals at Plassey, and the empire of British India was established. Two years later, James Wolfe (1727-1759) defeated the French under Louis Montcalm (1712-1759) at the Battle of Quebec.

William Pitt the Elder (1708-1778), through his position as paymaster-general of the armed forces, was largely responsible for Great Britain's success in building colonies. In 1760 George III (1738-1820) succeeded his father as ruler. He took a far greater part in governing Great Britain than did the previous members of the House of Hanover. Pitt was appointed prime minister in 1766, but his inability to manage the affairs of state led to his resignation in October 1768.

George III tried to destroy the power of the Whig aristocrats by choosing Frederick North (1732-1792) as his prime minister. George III was quite nationalistic, and North and his Tory party, along with the king, decided that the American colonies should help redress the huge debt caused by the Seven Years' War. The British government was prepared to collect the new taxes by force. The American colonies rallied to the cry that "taxation without representation" was unjust. War broke out, and France sided with the colonists. The Whigs, led by William Pitt the Younger (1759-1806), opposed the conflict. The fighting ended when Charles Cornwallis (1738-1805) surrendered the British forces at Yorktown in 1781. North resigned shortly thereafter, and Pitt was appointed prime minister in December 1783.

The Industrial Revolution greatly changed the lives of the British in the mid-1700s. After such inventions as the spinning jenny (1767) and the steam engine (1769), Great Britain became the world's first important industrial nation. Coal mines were expanded to provide fuel for factories, and great industrial cities such as Birmingham and Manchester grew rapidly.

The English had governed Ireland since the thirteenth century, and the English monarch held the title "King of Ireland." However, the Irish populace never really accepted English rule. In the late 1700s British leaders decided to make Ireland part of a United Kingdom. The Irish Parliament was naturally unenthusiastic about this decision, and a rebellion led by Theobald Tone called for complete Irish independence from British rule and equal rights for persons of all religions. After months of bloodshed the British defeated the rebellious Irish populace. As a result of Tone's rebellion the British government passed an Act of Union (1800), which dissolved the Irish Parliament and united Ireland and Great Britain.

The socioeconomic conditions in eighteenth-century Great Britain were wretched. The population of London at midcentury was 750,000, or 10% of the total population of England, Wales, and Scotland. Filth abounded; sanitation was practically nonexistent, although a public health network was in its infancy. Travel was difficult: a coach ride from London to Edinburgh took from 1½ to 3 weeks, depending on weather conditions. Overcrowding, prostitution, unruly mobs, and all types of petty and major crimes were common in London. The dangers of the plague still existed, and 5-year infant mortality was as high as 50%. Much of the infant mortality was attributed to malnutrition.

Although scientific advances were being made in medicine and surgery, both the education and licensing of physicians were becoming unregulated. Before the century ended, no qualifications would be necessary for the practice of surgery in Great Britain. For various social and economic reasons, British society and government opted for unlicensed practice instead of an improved and regulated form of medical organization. The development of medical schools and hospitals, which increased dramatically during the century, proved to be the sole factor in fostering quality medical education.

The abdication of governmental control over medical practice and the absence of any public guarantee of an individual's professional credentials inevitably led to an increase in surgical charlatans and quacks. In the seventeenth century local authorities had made attempts to control their activities, but eighteenth-century Great Britain proved to be a fertile environment for charlatans.

The long list of surgical quacks was led by Chevalier Taylor (1703-1772), a supposed eye surgeon. His mother was an apothecary in Norwich. Taylor had actually worked for a time with Cheselden at St. Thomas's Hospital and had invented a cataract needle and other ophthalmological instruments. In 1727 he authored a 74-page monograph, *An Account of the Mechanism of the Eye,* which was dedicated to Cheselden. Taylor was said to be a clever buffoon who had given up all pretense to a respectable practice. Usually clothed in black and wearing a long, flowing white wig, Taylor was quite articulate and had a modicum of surgical skill. He lectured throughout the country, expressing himself in sentences with inverted syntax and a Latin gibberish. Taylor called his self-made language "true Ciceronian," but he was poorly understood. His autobiography, published in two volumes (1761), remains one of the curiosities of eighteenth-century surgical history.

Among the other ophthalmological impostors were William Read (?-1715), who authored *A Treatise of the Eyes* (1706), and Thomas Woolhouse (1650-1734), who wrote a 350-page work, *Dissertationes Ophthalmicae De Cataracta Et Glaucomate* (1719). Mrs. Mapp, an acclaimed and quite affluent bonesetter, and Joanna Stevens, who trumpeted a recipe to cure bladder calculi, were famous female impostors. The latter was so successful that in 1739 Parliament actually attempted to buy her formula for the then-astronomical sum of 5000 pounds. The recipe was eventually obtained by Parliament and was found to contain a mixture of eggshells, garden snails, soap, seeds, hips, and haws. In each one of Stevens's "certified" cured cases, the calculi were later found in the patient's bladder during postmortem examination.

The first great social achievement in eighteenth-century British medicine was the revival of hospitals. English hospitals had been secularized at the time of the Reformation and had gradually lost their identity and general purpose. Only St. Bartholomew's and St. Thomas's survived in London as general hospitals, each with approximately 300 beds. New infirmaries founded in the eighteenth century were modeled along the lines of the two existing institutions. Most were initially small and were supported by public subscriptions. Once their usefulness

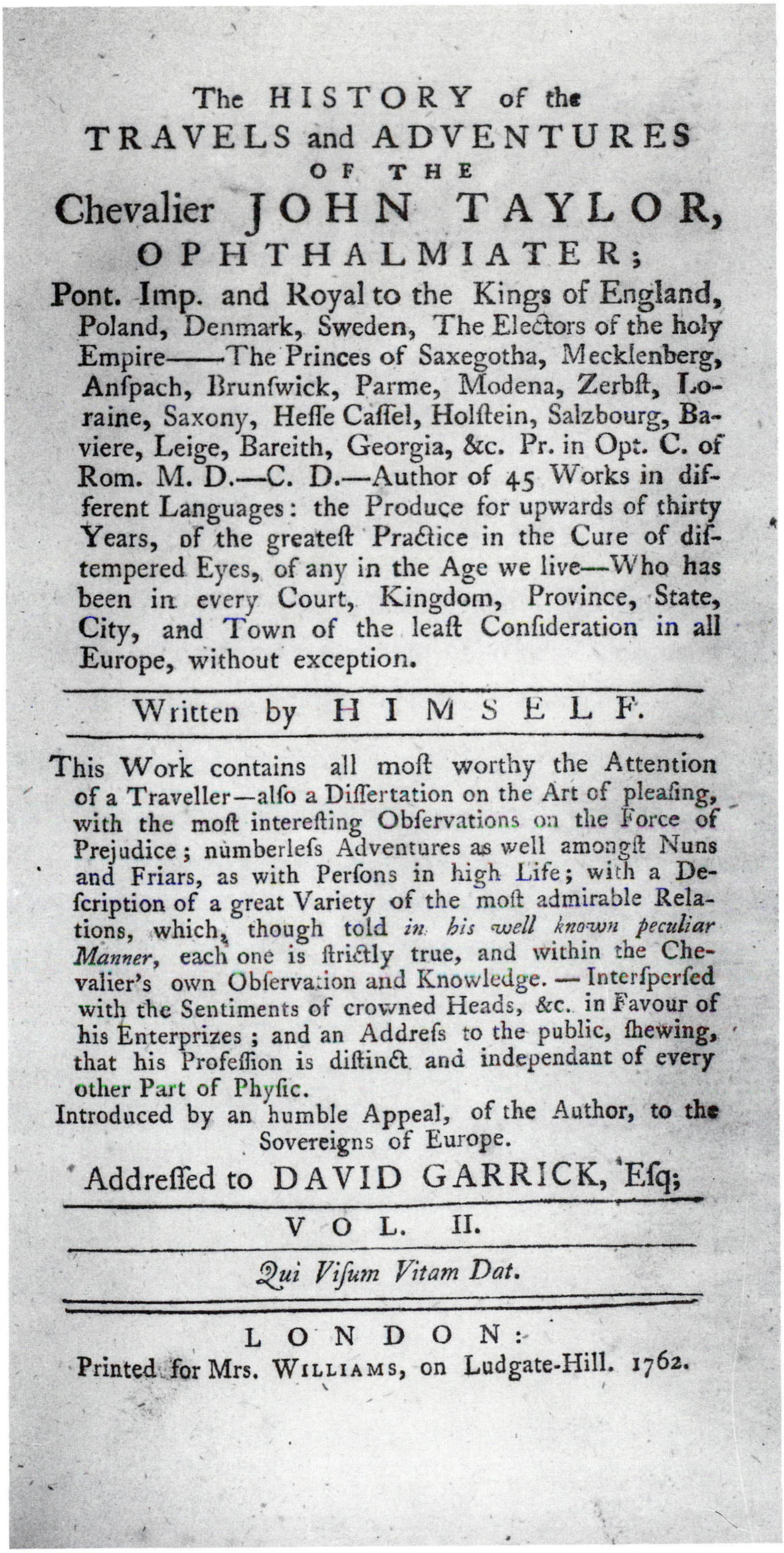

The HISTORY of the
TRAVELS and ADVENTURES
OF THE
Chevalier JOHN TAYLOR,
OPHTHALMIATER;

Pont. Imp. and Royal to the Kings of England,
Poland, Denmark, Sweden, The Electors of the holy
Empire——The Princes of Saxegotha, Mecklenberg,
Anspach, Brunswick, Parme, Modena, Zerbst, Lo-
raine, Saxony, Hesse Cassel, Holstein, Salzbourg, Ba-
viere, Leige, Bareith, Georgia, &c. Pr. in Opt. C. of
Rom. M. D.—C. D.—Author of 45 Works in dif-
ferent Languages: the Produce for upwards of thirty
Years, of the greatest Practice in the Cure of dis-
tempered Eyes, of any in the Age we live—Who has
been in every Court, Kingdom, Province, State,
City, and Town of the least Consideration in all
Europe, without exception.

Written by HIMSELF.

This Work contains all most worthy the Attention
of a Traveller—also a Dissertation on the Art of pleasing,
with the most interesting Observations on the Force of
Prejudice; numberless Adventures as well amongst Nuns
and Friars, as with Persons in high Life; with a Description of a great Variety of the most admirable Relations, which, though told *in his well known peculiar
Manner*, each one is strictly true, and within the Chevalier's own Observation and Knowledge. — Interspersed
with the Sentiments of crowned Heads, &c. in Favour of
his Enterprizes; and an Address to the public, shewing,
that his Profession is distinct and independant of every
other Part of Physic.
Introduced by an humble Appeal, of the Author, to the
Sovereigns of Europe.

Addressed to DAVID GARRICK, Esq;

V O L. II.

Qui Visum Vitam Dat.

L O N D O N:
Printed for Mrs. WILLIAMS, on Ludgate-Hill. 1762.

165. The ophthalmological quack Chevalier Taylor had considerable scientific
knowledge of ophthalmology but, like most
ambitious quacks, was driven by greed and
ambition to treat cases that were incurable
during his time. Taylor's numerous publications were unabashed self-advertisement.
The verbose title page of his autobiography
includes, as one might expect, many exag-
gerations. Taylor traveled throughout Europe with great fanfare in a brightly painted
carriage decorated with paintings of the eye,
usually leaving a town before the disastrous
results of some of his operations were discovered. *(Jeremy Norman & Co., Inc.)*

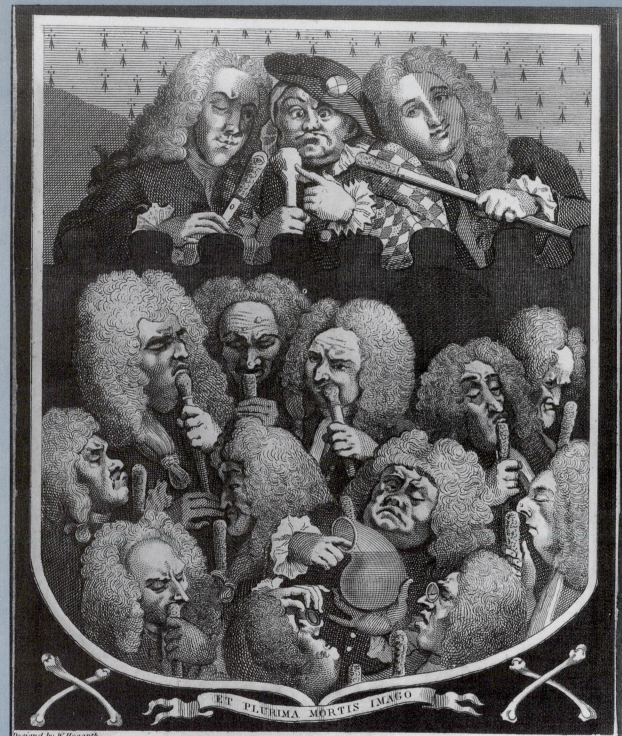

ET PLURIMA MORTIS IMAGO

Design'd by W. Hogarth.

The Company of Undertakers

Beareth Sable, an Urinal proper, between 12 Quack-Heads of the Second and 12 Cane Heads Or. Consultant. *On a · Chief · Nebulæ, Ermine, One compleat Doctor issuant, checkie sustaining in his Right Hand a Baton of the Second. On his Dexter and Sinister sides two Demi-Doctors, issuant of the Second, and two Cane Heads issuant of the third; The first having One Eye couchant towards the Dexter side of the Escocheen the second Faced per pale proper & Gules, Guardent. With this Motto.* Et Plurima Mortis Imago.

A Chief betokeneth a Senatour or Honourable Personage, borrowed from the Greeks, and is a Word signifying a Head; and as the Head is the Chief Part in a Man, so the ... in the Escocheon should be a Reward of such only whose High Merits have procured them Chief Place, Esteem, or Love amongst Men ... Italian ... the bearing of Heads in Armes (saith Upton) doth import some Excellence.

London Publish...

was appreciated, however, the hospital movement grew markedly and these undersized houses were replaced by large, magnificently equipped buildings. Nonetheless, overcrowding and lack of effective sanitation resulted in dreadful septic complications of operative wounds.

As more hospitals and operating amphitheaters were constructed, British surgery entered a new era. Prior training of surgeons had occurred primarily on the battlefield, but a succession of men were now being trained in civil practice and in the new hospitals. Among the new London hospitals were the Westminster Infirmary (1719), Guy's Hospital (1721), Saint George's Hospital (1733), London Hospital (1740), and Middlesex Hospital (1745). In Dublin there was the Jervis Street Hospital (1728), and in Scotland, the Edinburgh Royal Infirmary (1729) and the Aberdeen Hospital (1739).

Eventually medical schools were affiliated with the new hospitals, and they evolved in tandem. Still, until 1734 no British physician was permitted to lecture on anatomy in a hospital dissecting room, and another 30 years passed before a series of systematic lectures on surgery was delivered in a hospital.

In Great Britain the barber-surgeon companies were in full power at the beginning of the century. In many instances the surgeons in the various companies were increasingly involved in the financial management, which caused discontentment among the nonsurgical members. As long as the legal monopoly of barber-surgical practice continued, however, both parties were forced to resolve their petty differences in amicable ways.

166. *Facing page, The Company of Undertakers,* an engraving by William Hogarth. This print was originally intended to have been called *Quacks in Consultation.* It offers a coat of arms for physicians above a Latin motto that may be translated, "Everywhere the image of death." The elaborate caption is couched in heraldic terms. The upper division of the shield depicts three famous English quacks of the period. On the left is the notorious quack oculist, Chevalier John Taylor, his cane decorated with an eye. In the center is the famous bonesetter, Mrs. Sarah Mapp, her cane decorated with a bone. On the right is Dr. Joshua Ward ("Spot Ward," for a port wine birthmark on his face). Ward was known for his famous pill, a preparation of antimony and arsenic, which produced a violent diaphoretic reaction in the patient and led in about equal measure to miraculous cures or death. *(Jeremy Norman & Co., Inc.)*

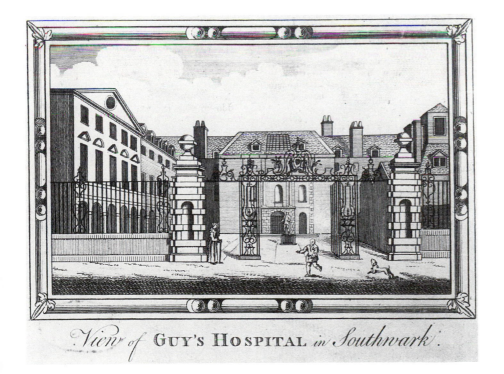

View of GUY'S HOSPITAL in Southwark.

167. Eighteenth-century view of Guy's Hospital, founded opposite St. Thomas's Hospital in 1724 by Thomas Guy, a bookseller of humble origins who made a vast fortune in publishing and other investments. A bachelor of almost comic frugality in his personal expenditures, Guy was a model of generosity to others and a noted philanthropist. His will, which provided for many beneficiaries, was notable enough to be published three times in 1725. Guy's Hospital, which received the bulk of his estate, was intended to house 400 sick people who were thought incurable or curable only by extensive treatment. Guy also specified that the hospital could accept up to 20 lunatics. *(National Library of Medicine, Bethesda, Md.)*

168. *The Reward of Cruelty,* engraved after a drawing by William Hogarth, 1751. This engraving, the last in Hogarth's series, *The Four Stages of Cruelty,* alludes to the English law, which as a deterrent to crime, offered the freshly executed bodies of criminals to the Barber-Surgeons' Company for dissection. These dissections were advertised to the public and frequently became grisly spectacles. Here we see the criminal fresh from the scaffold, the noose still around his neck. The gleeful surgeons are clearly relishing their gruesome task, bones are boiling in the caldron, and a dog is about to eat the criminal's heart.

The scene of this print is believed to be a composite based on the Cutlerian Theater of the Royal College of Physicians in Warwick Lane and the old Barber-Surgeons' Hall. Because the surgeons had separated from the barbers in 1745, the surgeons were no longer allowed to use the dissecting theater of the Barber-Surgeons' Company; their new theater, close to Newgate Prison and convenient for receiving criminals, was not opened until August 1751. *(Jeremy Norman & Co., Inc.)*

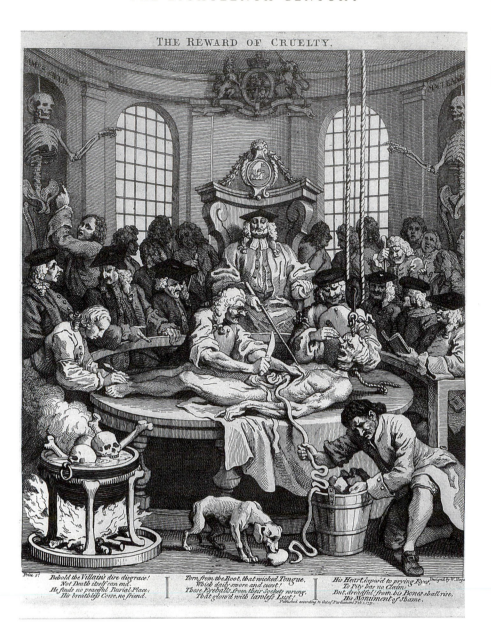

THE REWARD OF CRUELTY.

The London Company of Barber-Surgeons had controlled surgery in the metropolis for almost two centuries, but changes were taking place within its ranks that would have enormous historical repercussions. Although at the beginning of the century the barbers outnumbered the surgeons by 20 to 1, the greater part of the company's income was coming from the surgeons. As the number of hospitals increased, so did the number and, correspondingly, the importance of surgeons. The two sections of the company had obviously diverged in status and interests, and their separation was inevitable.

In other British cities similar difficulties were encountered. In Glasgow the barbers had no power to promulgate regulations, so they resisted paying fees to the company. In 1701 they appealed to the city council through the union of guilds to be separated from the surgeons. The council found in their favor, and after much infighting the surgeons renounced any claims to the day-to-day aspects of the barbers' practices. Separation was achieved in 1719. In Bristol violent disputes took place between the two sections of the barber-surgeon company. In 1742, without the authority of any legislation, the Bristol surgeons simply left the company.

At the beginning of the eighteenth century, very little competent surgical instruction was available in England or Scotland; the best of what little there was existed in London. The London Company of Barber-Surgeons acted as the bellwether for most of the country, and its dissolution had enormous impact on the future of British surgery and on the craft of surgery in England and Scotland. The final divorce between the London barbers and surgeons was orchestrated primarily by two men, William Cheselden and John Ranby (1703-1773).

Cheselden (1688-1752) was the leading British surgeon during the first half of the eighteenth century, and his work ushered that country's surgical education and training into a new era. He was born at Somerby, near Burrow-on-the-Hill, Leicestershire, where he received his early education. Cheselden soon migrated to London, where he came under the influence of James Ferne, a surgeon on the staff of St. Thomas's Hospital. Cheselden became a bound apprentice for 7 years (1703 to 1710). During these years he also studied anatomy with Cowper, who had begun the country's first private lectures on the subject. In December 1710 Cheselden was admitted to the London Company of Barber-Surgeons, and in January 1711 he received full certification to practice as a surgeon. He was elected a fellow of the Royal Society of London in the following year.

In London the surgical educational system was gradually improving, and the demand for better anatomical teaching had been answered through a system of private schools. Since hospital appointments were difficult to obtain and practices slow to develop, Cheselden began giving private courses in anatomy in 1711. In that year he authored in Latin a 31-page syllabus to serve as a guide for his lectures. Two years later Cheselden wrote his first major text, *The Anatomy of the Human Body,* which was to be published in 13 editions and become the standard medical student's textbook of anatomy for almost a century. He illustrated the book with some of his own drawings and included surgical references to enhance its practicality.

The success of Cheselden's anatomical lectures brought him into direct conflict with the Company. Apparently, after anatomical demonstrations had been given at the barber-surgeon's hall, Cheselden occasionally would take an undissected part home to use in his own private lectures. When the Company heard of this, they summoned him to a special meeting in March 1714. He was accused of teaching anatomy in his home at times that conflicted with public dissection at the Company hall. Because Cheselden was a superior teacher, his lessons drew students away from the barber-surgeons. He was warned not to teach at home again, and he promised not to commit the offense in the future. This event, which occurred relatively early in his career, demonstrated the political strength of the barber-surgeons; it is likely that Cheselden's displeasure with this show of pique later strengthened his resolve to separate surgeons from barbers.

Cheselden's greatest literary work remains in anatomy, although he was known primarily as a surgeon. In 1733 his *Osteographia, or the Anatomy of the Bones* was published. Considered one of the most outstanding productions of eighteenth-century anatomists, the work contained full, accurate descriptions of all the human bones. The accuracy of the plates resulted from the innovative use of the camera obscura by Cheselden and his assistant, Gerard Van Der Gucht (1696-1776), and from the former's personal intervention in the drawing and engraving process. The work was an absolutely luxurious production in its day. It was issued only for subscribers in 300 copies for the British market and 100 for the remainder of Europe.

Most of the anatomical research that was incorporated into the *Osteographia* was accomplished after Cheselden's appointment to the surgical staff of St. Thomas's Hospital (1719). Although he was turned down for this position many times, his eventual nomination allowed him to demonstrate his many technical abilities. Foremost among these was his interest in lithotomy, for which he received teaching appointments as "first lithotomist" at Westminster Hospital, St. George's Hospital, and St. Thomas's. Cheselden's fame as a lithotomist increased, especially after the publication of *A Treatise on the High Operation for the Stone* (1723).

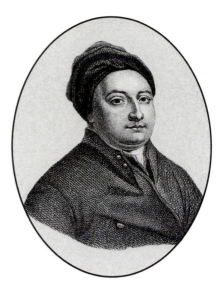

169. Portrait of William Cheselden wearing his turban, engraved by Ambroise Tardieu after the painting by Jonathan Richardson. Formal eighteenth-century paintings typically show figures wearing powdered wigs. This portrait of Cheselden without a wig is unusual; however, Cheselden may have preferred the turban to a wig. Routine wearing of wigs required keeping the hair quite short, and in the cold climate of England it was for both practical and aesthetic considerations that turbans were worn when the wig was off. *(Historical Collections, College of Physicians of Philadelphia.)*

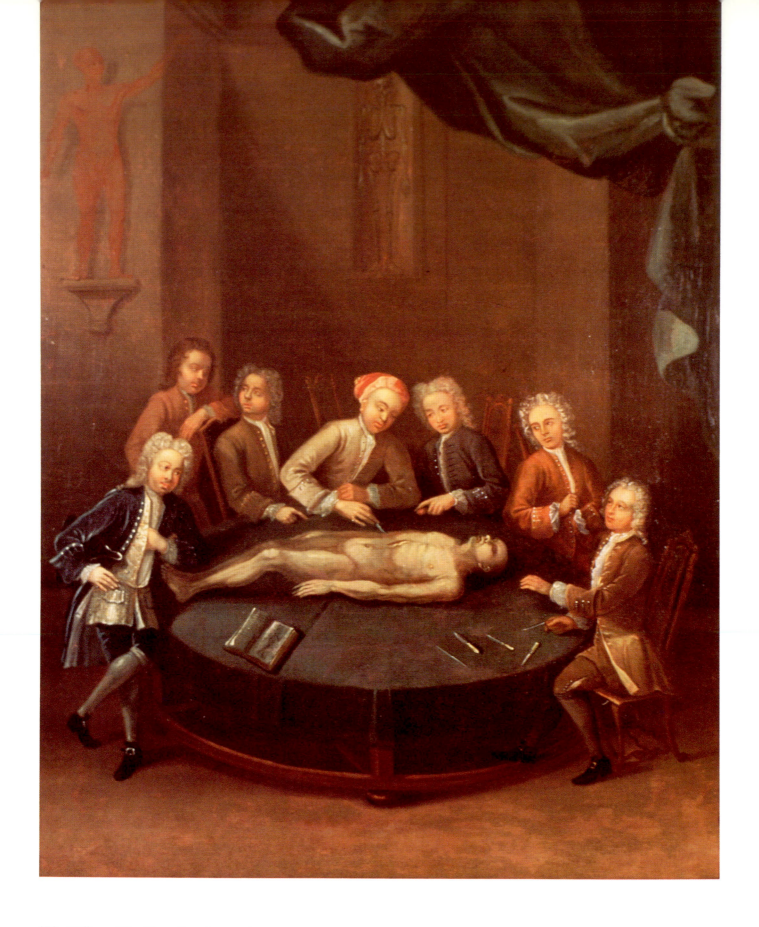

170. William Cheselden dissecting at the Barber–Surgeons' Hall, circa 1730. An anonymous oil painting by an artist of limited skill. Cheselden is wearing his turban; the rest of the surgeons are wearing wigs. *(The Trustee of the Wellcome Trust, London.)*

At the beginning of the eighteenth century in London, lithotomy, an operation that had long been used, incorporated a midline perineal incision. This method was fraught with frequent, serious complications and an unacceptably high death rate. John Douglas (?-1743), lithotomist at Westminster Hospital and a brother of James Douglas, the renowned anatomist, had revived the suprapubic or "high" operation in his *Lithotomia Douglassiana* (1720). Cheselden was impressed with Douglas's success and soon had a larger series than that of Douglas, with a lower mortality. Cheselden acknowledged his indebtedness to Douglas, but Douglas accused Cheselden of plagiarizing his work and became Cheselden's lifelong enemy. Douglas's intense hatred was only exacerbated when the overseers of Westminster Hospital chose Cheselden over Douglas to be "first lithotomist." Douglas, in a display of "literary violence," authored his *Animadversions on a Late Pompous Book, Intituled, Osteographia* (1735).

Cheselden has always been regarded as the eighteenth century's cleverest and most expeditious stonecutter because of his championing of the lateral incision. The operation of lithotomy was a difficult one, and patients with bladder calculi submitted to it only when the discomfort became unbearable. Until Cheselden's time the operation was usually performed by means of a large incision in the midline of the groin, dilation of the bladder neck, and forcible extraction of the stone with forceps. This surgical operation often took as long as an hour and, in the absence of anesthesia, must have been a painful ordeal for both patient and surgeon.

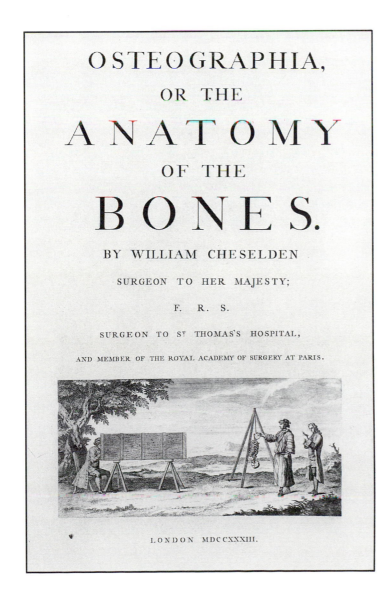

171. Title page of Cheselden's *Osteographia,* showing Cheselden drawing bones through the camera obscura. He was the first to use this instrument to gain precision in his anatomical illustrations. This work is among the most beautiful atlases of bone anatomy ever published. *(Jeremy Norman & Co., Inc.)*

172. Whimsically portrayed skeleton of an ape, perhaps an orangutan, from Cheselden's *Osteographia*. Engraved, probably from Cheselden's own drawing, by Jan van der Gucht. Cheselden's book emphasized human osteology but included some beautiful comparative osteological studies. *(Jeremy Norman & Co., Inc.)*

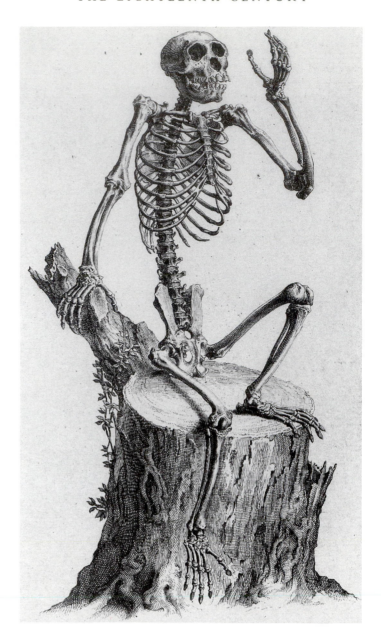

The hazards of both the "high," or suprapubic, and the midline perineal approaches to lithotomy caused Cheselden to abandon these methods by the mid-1720s. Having heard of the lateral perineal incision developed by the French itinerant lithotomist Frère Jacques De Beaulieu, Cheselden chose to adopt this method and to improve upon it. Within 3 years he could report brilliant results with less than 10% mortality. His success relied heavily on cadaver dissection, which helped him understand the anatomy, and on maintaining hemostasis during postoperative care.

Cheselden became an internationally acclaimed surgeon; important individuals traveled long distances to be placed under his care. Cheselden's operative dexterity in using the lateral incision was astounding: the average procedure lasted no longer than a minute or two. He was made a member of the French Academy of Sciences and the first foreign member of the Paris Royal Academy of Surgery. Cheselden's methods remained the standard by which any lithotomy was measured for more than 150 years. Cheselden provided a modest account of his struggles with lithotomy:

What success I have had in my private practice, I have kept no account of, because I had no intention to publish it, that not being sufficiently witnessed. Publickly in St. Thomas's Hospital I have cut two hundred and thirteen; of the first fifty only three died; of the second fifty, three; of the third fifty, eight; and of the last sixty-three, six. Several of these patients had the small pox during their cure, some of which died, but I think not more in proportion than what usually die of the distemper; these are not reckon'd among those who died of the operation. The reason why so few died in the two first fifties was, at that time few very bad cases offered; in the third, the operation being in high request, even the most aged and most miserable cases expected to be sav'd by it; besides, at that time, I made the operation lower in hopes in improving it, but found I was mistaken . . . One . . . bled to death by an artery into the bladder, it being very hot weather at that time. But this accident taught me afterwards, whenever a vessel bled that I could not find, to dilate the wound with a knife, till I could see it. Now if Jacques or others, who of late have been said to have performed this operation, whether by design or chance, did not take care to secure the blood-vessels, which as yet has not been supposed, whatever their dexterity in operating might be, their success at least can be not secret, for many of their children and most of their men patients must have bled to death. If I have any reputation in this way, I have earn'd it dearly, for no one ever endured more anxiety and sickness before an operation, yet from the time I began to operate, all uneasiness ceased; and if I have had better success than some others, I do not impute it to more knowledge, but to the happiness of a mind that was never ruffled or disconcerted, and a hand that never trembled during any operation.

Among Cheselden's many clinical interests was ophthalmology. In his first anatomical text he provided detailed descriptions of the structure of the lens and described several of his initial ophthalmological operative experiences. He is credited with being the first to have made an artificial pupil where inflammation had destroyed the natural pupil. This iridotomy was among the most important contributions to ophthalmology during the eighteenth century.

As Cheselden's reputation grew, his friendships with great men of literature also flourished. Among the most prominent was Pope, who was a patient in Cheselden's house and memorialized the surgeon in this poem:

Late as it is, I put myself to school,
And feel some comfort not to be a fool,
Weak though I am of limb and short of sight,
Far from a lynx and not a giant quite;
I'll do what Mead and Cheselden advise,
To help these limbs and to preserve these eyes.
Not to go back is somewhat to advance,
And men must walk at least before they dance.

While still in the prime of his life, Cheselden decided in 1737 to retire from the staff of the three hospitals in which he had been so active. He obtained a sinecure at the Chelsea Hospital, which was primarily a home for elderly persons. He lived and worked there in semiretirement from 1737 until his death. During those years Cheselden's involvement in the formation of a new surgical society was most important to him.

In 1738 Cheselden became a member of the court of assistants of the Company of Barber-Surgeons and almost immediately was nominated as one of the 10 examiners. Six years later he became junior warden of the company. During his tenure in office, on December 20, 1744, the surgeons announced without any prior warning that they wished to permanently separate from the barbers. As expected, the barbers requested that the status quo be maintained. Parliament appointed a committee to consider the matter. Cheselden's actions were clearly behind much of the controversy, since the chairman of Parliament's committee was none other than his son-in-law, Charles Cotes, who was also a prominent physician, and Cheselden donated 550 pounds toward payment of the expenses incurred by the proceedings. The committee upheld the petition of the surgeons, and a bill was brought into Parliament that would make the surgeons of London and the barbers of London two separate corporations. Parliament passed the bill, to which the royal signature was affixed on May 2, 1745. Thus was born an independent Company or Corporation of Surgeons.

The formal separation was greatly aided by John Ranby, who served as sergeant surgeon to George II. As a close friend of the sovereign, Ranby undoubtedly performed persuasive lobbying. Ranby had been sworn a foreign brother of

Benjamin Germain,

Surgeons Instrument - Maker,

AT THE

Saw and Crown, without *Bishopsgate,*

L O N D O N ;

(*Late Apprentice to Mr.* Wigglesworth,
in the Minories)

MAKES and Sells all Sorts of Surgeons
Inftruments; alfo Razors, Sciffars, Lancets,
Pen-Knives, Fleams and Horfe-Sciffars, Table-
Knives and Forks, Gardeners and Cooks Knives,
of all Sorts; and Mounts the beft Blades, in Silver
or Agate Hafts, &c. Likewife Shagreen and
Fifh-Skin Cafes, good Hones, and all Manner of
Cutlery Ware.

N. B. Lancets and Razors, &c. carefully Ground
and Set.

173. Advertising card of Benjamin Germain, Surgeons' Instrument Maker, London, circa 1750. Germain featured his surgical instruments in this flyer. He also offered just about any other object of cutlery that could be purchased at the time. *(Boston Medical Library.)*

the Company of Barber-Surgeons in 1722 and, in holding the office of sergeant surgeon, had joined a lengthy list of reputable physicians, including Vicary, Clowes, and Wiseman. Although not a prolific writer, Ranby did author the 44-page *Method of Treating Gunshot Wounds* (1744). In gratitude for his assistance the new Company of Surgeons named Ranby its first master.

In 1745, surgical techniques in Great Britain were not markedly different from those in the rest of Europe. Although surgical education and training were more organized in France, the major operations performed on both sides of the English Channel were quite similar. Few surgeons confined their practice solely to surgery. To do so in the days before antisepsis was understood and before effective anesthetics were available would have meant financial ruin, since so few "minor" or "major" surgical operations were actually carried out.

Although the Company had a wonderful chance to advance the cause of British surgery, advances were minimal. The act of Parliament in 1745 entitled those who had satisfied the Court of Examiners to practice without hindrance anywhere in Great Britain, and apprenticeship was no longer specifically required. Many foreign nationals who were practicing surgery in London were admitted to the new Company without inquiry regarding their training. In 1749, surgeons retiring from the armed forces were granted freedom to enter civilian practice, specifically exempting them from any evidence of true apprenticeship or training. Thus it became impossible to ensure that a young surgeon would acquire surgical training in a systematized fashion based on some type of apprenticeship.

The Company dragged on in an uninspired existence for 45 years. Early difficulties led to financial and administrative irregularities that were not readily overcome. Surgeons were excellent technicians but were unprofessional in their business dealings. Company master John Gunning, in a speech to the Court of Assistants in 1790, criticized every aspect of the Company's daily management. About their actual building he uttered his most famous words:

> You have in it a theater for your lectures, a room for a library, a committee room for your Court, a large room for reception of your community, together with the necessary accommodation for your clerk. But how great soever your intentions were I am sorry to observe they have been but ill executed. Your theater is without lectures, your library without books is converted into an office for your clerk, and your committee room is become his eating parlour; and is not always used even in your own common business, and when it is thus made use of it is seldom in a fit or proper state . . . If, gentlemen, you make no better use of the Hall than what you have already done, you had better sell it and apply the money for the good of the Company in some other way.

Even the hoped-for teaching of anatomy on a limited basis failed to flourish in the new Company. Some of the most renowned surgeon-anatomists of that era lived in London, namely Percivall Pott (1714-1788), William Hunter, and John Hunter, and the excellence of their private anatomy lessons drew students away from the Company's courses.

The control of the Company had gradually passed into the hands of the 10 members of the Court of Assistants, who were also examiners. In most instances these examiners were appointed for life and were the only regular attendants at meetings. The Court of Assistants had passed a self-serving regulation that an examiner had to be called in for mandatory consultation by a private surgeon when a patient was dying or an amputation was planned. In this way a financially lucrative reward was ensured for virtually every examiner.

During its first 50 years of existence the Company of Surgeons was nothing more than a bloated, inefficient examining body. Members took the imponderable position that if a "satisfactory" final examination was carried out, teaching must have occurred at some level. Thus young apprentices were forced to obtain private teaching from members of the Company without any form of organizational support from the Company.

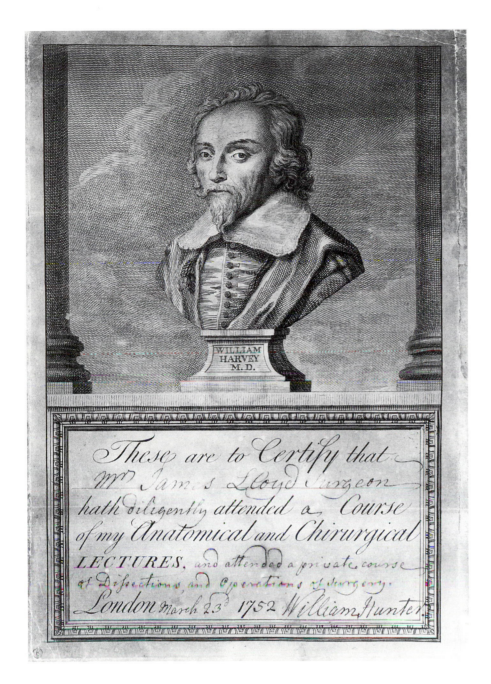

174. Certificate filled out and signed by William Hunter at his Great Windmill Street School that "Mr. James Lloyd, surgeon," had "dilgently attended a Course of my Anatomical and Chirurgical Lectures, and attended a private course of Dissections, and Operations of Surgery, March 23, 1752." Lloyd (1728-1800) was a prominent member of the medical community in Boston, Massachusetts. Like many American physicians and surgeons of the eighteenth century, he received his training abroad. *(Boston Medical Library.)*

Clearly, the individualistic attitude of most Company surgeons resulted in petty quarrels, tardy publications, and a general lack of cohesiveness and created an untenable educational environment. Nonetheless, the art of surgery, existing outside the Company, continued to be consolidated and advanced by means of careful clinical observations and superb teachers in private settings.

Because the Company of Surgeons failed to adequately organize surgical education, effective licensing was nonexistent. Two types of programs assumed much of the responsibility for education. First were the private schools of anatomical and surgical instruction. The most prominent of these was the Windmill Street School under the auspices of the Hunters, Baillie, and Cruikshank. In the absence of any great public medical institution, these schools provided excellent instruction but were decidedly transient and had no licensing powers.

The many new hospitals and the schools of medicine and surgery that were evolving with them represented the second type of educational institution for surgeons. The surgeons attached to these hospitals had the opportunity to take their apprentices with them while performing surgical operations. In this way the initial efforts to provide systematic teaching, including bedside instruction,

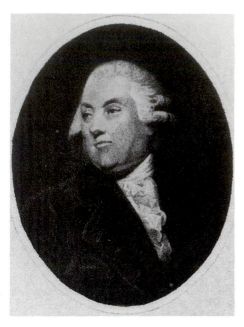

175. Percivall Pott. *(Jeremy Norman & Co., Inc.)*

were made. Schools naturally evolved from such individual entrepreneurship, and the emerging surgical educational system was of enormous benefit to the student. The apprentice's physical presence in a hospital also helped increase the overall efficiency of the institution's patient care.

St. Bartholomew's Hospital allowed anatomical lectures under the direction of Edward Nourse (1701-1761) in 1734. Percivall Pott began his series of discourses on surgery there in 1765. Two decades later John Abernethy (1764-1831) taught not only surgery and anatomy but also physiology. At St. Thomas's Hospital Cheselden began his lecture series on anatomy in 1720. However, the governors of that hospital had previously taken the matter of teaching under their own purview when they passed a regulation forbidding pupils or surgeons to dissect without permission of the institution's treasurer (1703). A formalized anatomical school was functioning at St. Thomas's by 1780. At the London Hospital the entry of the first "house" pupil occurred in 1742; William Blizard (1743-1835) formalized its medical school in 1785, patterning it after the medical faculty in Edinburgh. The medical school at Guy's Hospital opened in 1769, when a resolution passed by the governors called on all surgeons of the institution to give occasional lectures to the students.

Although there were many teachers of surgery in eighteenth-century London, the two most outstanding individuals were Percivall Pott (1714-1788) and John Hunter (1728-1793). Pott was born on Threadneedle Street in that city. When Pott was a young boy, his father passed away and the family was left with little financial means. A distant relative assumed the fiscal responsibility of providing for Pott's education, and the adolescent was apprenticed to Nourse in 1729 for the sum of 200 pounds. In addition to a private surgical practice, Nourse organized anatomy lectures in his home on Aldersgate Street. Pott served during his 7-year apprenticeship as Nourse's primary assistant in preparing cadavers for public demonstrations of dissection.

At the age of 22 years, after having successfully passed the examination for a Grand Diploma, Pott was admitted to the Company of Barber-Surgeons. He continued to assist his mentor both at surgical operations and with his private lectures. In addition, Pott opened his own office for the practice of surgery in London when he rented a house on Fenchurch Street, where he lived with his mother and half-sister. Three years later, in 1739, he changed his address to Bow Lane.

Like many of his contemporaries, Pott's initial efforts to receive a hospital appointment met with failure. However, he was nominated assistant surgeon at St. Bartholomew's in 1745, and full surgeon 4 years later. He remained in that position for the next 38 years. At his retirement Pott said that he had served the institution "as a boy and a man" for half a century.

In the winter of 1756 Pott was riding his horse to the hospital when he was thrown off and suffered a supposed compound fracture of the lower part of the fibula and tibia. Realizing the gravity of the injury, Pott refused to let himself be moved until a proper mode of transportation had been secured. He lay on the cold pavement while waiting for the arrival of two "chair men" and their poles. Pott purchased a door, to which the poles were nailed. He reclined on the improvised stretcher and was carried to his home. A multitude of his fellow surgeons were called, all of whom recommended immediate amputation, which was then the accepted treatment for such an injury. Pott agreed, but just as the instruments were being prepared, Nourse arrived and decided to attempt to save the leg by reduction. In time the injury healed properly, and Pott retained his leg without any evidence of disability. The story may be apocryphal, but a lengthy recuperation may have stimulated Pott's interest in medical writing because from that year on, he produced a steady flow of surgical texts that brought him international recognition.

In *A Treatise on Ruptures* (1756) Pott refuted many of the old theories concerning the causes of hernias and methods of treatment. He was the first to describe "congenital hernia" and became embroiled in a bitter academic feud with the Hunters, who demanded priority for tracing the anatomy of congenital rup-

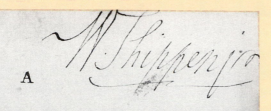

A
TREATISE
ON
RUPTURES.

BY

PERCIVALL POTT,

SURGEON to St. Bartholomew's-Hospital.

Chirurgia non quidem medicamenta atque victus ratio-
nem omittit, sed manu tamen plurimum præstat;
estque ejus effectus inter omnes medicinæ partes evi-
dentissimus.   A. CORN. CELSUS

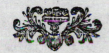

LONDON:
Printed for C. HITCH and L. HAWES, at the
Red-Lion, Pater-noster-Row. M.DCC.LVI.

176. The title page of Pott's *Treatise on
Ruptures* (1756) includes a Latin quotation
from Celsus that distinguishes surgery as
"working with the hands" from medicine as
"prescribing medicines and regimens." The
placement of this Latin quotation on Pott's
title page indicates that by the eighteenth
century many surgeons could read Latin. In
previous centuries knowledge of medical
Latin was generally limited to physicians.
This particular copy was owned by the illustrious American surgeon, William Shippen.
(Jeremy Norman & Co., Inc.)

tures. Pott denounced the so-called radical cure of hernia, although he was known to have performed numerous "conservative" operations for strangulation.

In 1760 Pott authored his *Observations on the Nature and Consequences of Wounds and Contusions of the Head, Fractures of the Skull, Concussions of the Brain*. This treatise showcased Pott's extensive knowledge of surgical literature, which allowed him to systematize the treatment of head injuries. He described the signs by which extradural hematoma can be differentiated from extradural abscess. One characteristic of the latter is the puffy tumor, a circumscribed swelling of the scalp indicating either an underlying osteitis of the skull or an extradural abscess. Pott explained, among other clinical points, the lucid interval that precedes the coma of extradural hemorrhage. In his *Practical Remarks on the Hydrocele or Watry Rupture* (1762) he provided a classic description of hydrocele.

Pott's methods for treating fractures and dislocations became standard after the publication of *Some Few General Remarks on Fractures and Dislocations* (1765). In that work he stressed the necessity for the immediate setting of a displaced fracture and the need for relaxation of the muscles so that the reduction could be successfully performed. Splints, when used, should immobilize the joints above and below the fracture site and be well padded. From personal experience Pott realized the gravity of the decision to amputate in cases of compound fractures and weighed the chances of saving a limb against the attendant hazard of death from infection. It is in his work on fractures and dislocations that the classic description of a Pott's fracture is found:

> When the fibula breaks within two or three inches of its lower extremity, the inferior fractured end falls inwards towards the tibia, that extremity of the bone which forms the outer ankle is turned somewhat outward and upward, and the tibia having lost its proper support is forced off from the astragalus inwards, by which means the weak bursal or common ligament of the joint is violently stretched if not torn, and the strong ones which fasten the tibia to the astragalus and os calcis are always lacerated, thus producing a perfect fracture and a partial dislocation to which is sometimes added a wound in the integuments . . . All the tendons which pass behind or under, or are attached to the extremities of the tibia and fibula or os calcis, have their natural direction so altered that they all contribute to the distortion of the foot and that by turning it outward and upward.
>
> It is extremely troublesome to put to rights, still more so to keep it in order, and unless managed with address and skill is very frequently productive of lameness and deformity ever after . . . But if the position of the limb be changed, if by laying it on its outside with the knee moderately bent, the muscles forming the calf of the leg and those which pass behind the fibula and under the os calcis are all put in a state of relaxation and non-resistance, all this difficulty and trouble do in general vanish immediately, the foot may easily be placed right, the joint reduced, and by maintaining the same disposition of the limb everything will in general succeed very happily.

Chirurgical Observations Relative to the Cataract, the Polypus of the Nose, and the Cancer of the Scrotum (1775) included the first description of an occupational cancer. By detailing cancer of the scrotum in chimney sweeps, Pott was the first to trace the origin of a type of cancer to a specific external agent, in this case the carcinogenic agents in the chimney soot. In this 1775 monograph Pott also described senile gangrene, or insufficient blood supply to the legs.

The best known of Pott's works are his two volumes on spinal diseases: *Remarks on That Kind of Palsy of the Lower Limbs, Which Is Frequently Found To Accompany a Curvature of the Spine* (1779) and *Farther Remarks on the Useless State of the Lower Limbs in Consequence of a Curvature of the Spine* (1782). His name is eponymically linked with tuberculous caries of the spine, which were described from a clinical standpoint in the first text. Pott depicted the condition of the collapsed vertebrae and spinal curvature but failed to appreciate the relationship between the ensuing paralysis and the deformity. Pott believed he had found a cure for this usually hopeless condition by creating superficial abscesses in the back. Of course, Pott did not understand the pathological and bacteriological features of tuberculosis. Among Pott's other monographs are those on lachrymal fistula (1758) and fistula-in-ano (1765).

Pott always remained quite active in the organizational affairs of the Company of Surgeons. In 1753 he was elected one of the first masters of anatomy; 3 years later he was appointed to the Court of Assistants; and eventually he was named to the Court of Examiners. In 1765 he succeeded Robert Young as governor of the Company.

John Hunter (1728-1793) is considered one of the most influential surgeons of all time. He extended the horizons of surgery, medicine, and science. Because of Hunter surgery came to be regarded as a branch of scientific medicine firmly backed by physiology and pathology. Hunter was born on a small farm in Scotland, not far from Glasgow. The youngest of 10 children, he was considered a poor student who was never interested in the educational process. He dropped out of school at 13 years of age, and the likelihood of future success was slim.

In 1748 he wrote to his older brother William to ask whether he might come to join William in London. William was quite the opposite of his youngest brother: he was studious and reserved and had already established his reputation as an obstetrician and anatomist. William agreed to his brother's request, and the younger Hunter was given the task of preparing anatomical dissections.

John Hunter demonstrated an amazing aptitude for the anatomical sciences. Within a year he was able to instruct some of his brother's students in the rudiments of anatomy. At the same time, John began to attend with great interest some of his brother's lectures on surgery. In the summer, when no teaching was done, he worked with Cheselden at Chelsea Hospital. In 1751 he enrolled as an apprentice to Pott at St. Bartholomew's. From 1754 to 1756 John was house surgeon at St. George's Hospital, where he received most of his practical training.

William Hunter thought that his younger brother needed to gain sophistication in speech and mannerisms. Accordingly, he sent John to Oxford for lessons in elocution and classical languages. The effort failed: within 2 months John Hunter was back in London, complaining of his unhappiness with being made to understand Latin and Greek when they did not benefit his quest for surgical knowledge.

Hunter was endlessly curious, and for 4 years spent countless hours making thousands of anatomical preparations. He was especially interested in comparative anatomy and dissected animals of every sort to find their differences and note their similarities. In 1761 Hunter became a victim of tuberculosis, which was attributed to the putrid air of dissecting rooms. Realizing his need for rest and using the political connections of his brother, John Hunter secured a commission as an army surgeon. For 2 years he served at Belle Isle, in France, and in Portugal. Although the work was not strenuous, he acquired close familiarity with war wounds and their complications. In his spare time Hunter continued his studies of nature, investigating every change of flora and fauna.

In greatly improved health Hunter returned to London, where he opened his own anatomical school and commenced the private practice of surgery. Although he was well known as an anatomist, the initial growth of his practice was quite slow. To occupy his time, Hunter continued his scientific investigations. At this time he hypothesized that two diseases could not exist simultaneously in the same organ. Therefore syphilis and gonorrhea were believed to be different symptoms of the same sexual illness. To prove the point, he inoculated an individual with gonorrheal pus, not knowing that the pus also harbored syphilis. When the latter disease developed, Hunter believed that his ideas were correct.

Hunter began to receive numerous honors, including election as a fellow of the Royal Society (1767). In 1768 he was appointed surgeon to St. George's Hospital, which provided a needed source of financial stability and made it possible for him to hire hospital pupils to assist with surgery. In the following year he was made a member of the Company of Surgeons but would never hold an officership in the organization.

Like most great surgeons of the past, Hunter stands out because of the volume of his written work and the quality of his research. Considered a dexterous surgeon, he was primarily interested in the pathophysiology of surgical diseases.

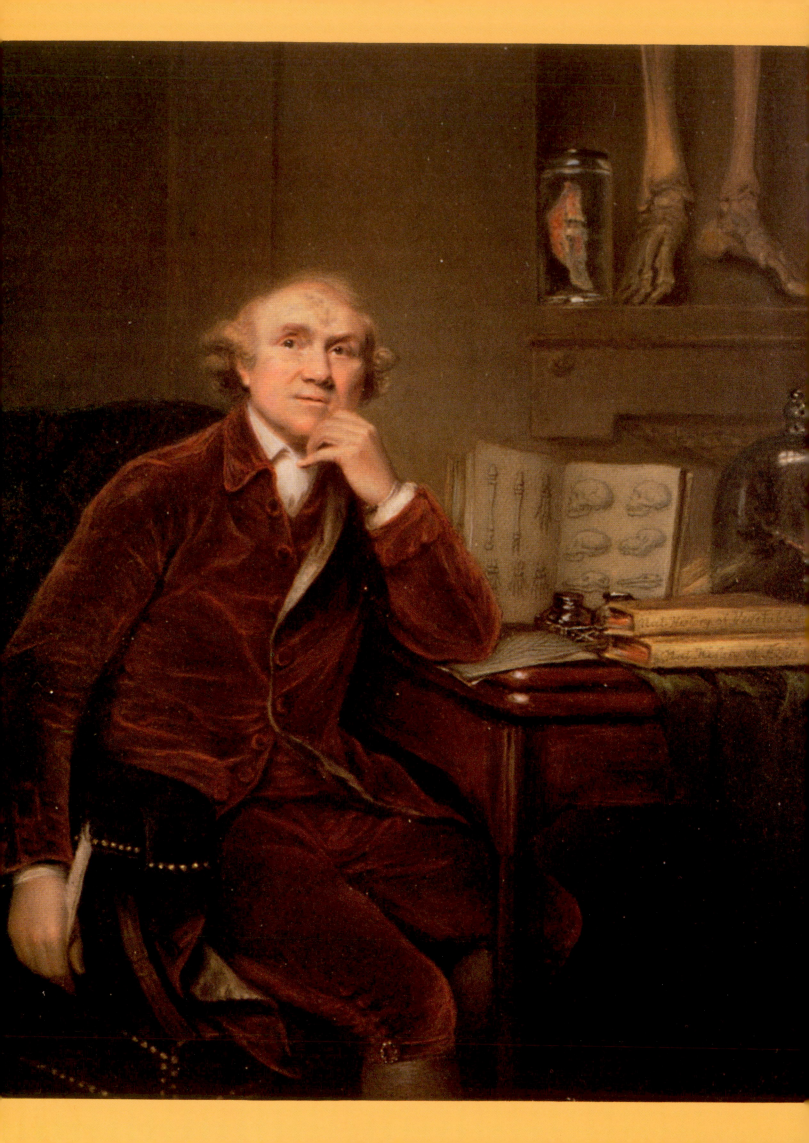

His first book, *The Natural History of the Human Teeth,* was published in 1771. Early in his professional career Hunter had been friends with a number of successful dentists. His observations of these men and their patients, along with studies on the mouths and jaws of cadavers, culminated in the writing of this remarkable text. Hunter's understanding of the growth and development of the jaw and its relation to the muscles of mastication was amazingly precise. He coined the terms *bicuspids, cuspids, incisors,* and *molars.* He correctly disapproved of extracting primary teeth to permit permanent teeth to erupt.

In 1778 Hunter authored his second major book, *A Practical Treatise on the Diseases of the Teeth.* Although not as significant as the 1771 treatise to which it should be considered a supplement, the second work offered excellent clinical pictures of the various stages of inflammation of affected teeth and of decay. Hunter also devised appliances for the correction of malocclusion. Among the most famous of his experiments was the successful implantation of an incompletely formed human tooth into the comb of a cock. The tooth became firmly rooted, and the blood vessels of the comb grew into the tooth. This experiment convinced Hunter of the practicality of transplanting human teeth.

As a surgical pathologist, Hunter studied "the digestion of the stomach after death" (1772) and described shock, phlebitis, pyemia, and intussusception. In *A Treatise on the Venereal Disease* (1786) he differentiated between hard chancre and the chancroid ulcer and made the first suggestion that lymphogranuloma venereum is a distinct disease. Also in 1786, Hunter authored his *Observations on Certain Parts of the Animal Oeconomy.* This unusual work included observations on the secondary sexual characteristics in birds, the descent of the testis, the air sac in birds, and the structure of the placenta, and presented the original description of the olfactory nerves.

In many respects, *Observations on Certain Parts of the Animal Oeconomy* epitomized the amazing achievements of Hunter. His thousands of dissections, both human and animal, formed a unique collection of natural history. He expended large amounts of money for his animal menagerie. Hunter bought a piece of land on the outskirts of London, where he built a house that served as a combined laboratory, museum, and zoo of domesticated and wild beasts. As his assemblage grew, he was forced to purchase an even larger house in Leicester Square, together with a neighboring house and the ground between. Eventually he had on his payroll nearly 50 persons, including servants, stable help, and groundskeepers. It is estimated that Hunter dissected more than 500 different species of living creatures, from insects to whales.

Among Hunter's fundamental pathological studies were those on inflammation, as described in *A Treatise on the Blood, Inflammation, and Gun-shot Wounds* (1794). While serving with the army in Belle Isle, Hunter had begun to collect the material for this epoch-making work. Not having a university education, Hunter relied little on the theories of past authorities but rather on his personal observations. One of his most novel concepts was to treat gunshot injuries just like any other wounds, there being no reason to enlarge them. With the acceptance of his thoughts on these injuries, the old belief that gunpowder was a fatal poison was finally laid to rest:

> It is against all the rules of surgery and against what we know of animal economy to make a wound larger, unless one needs to prepare it to do something more—if it is a complicated wound that must be treated in a special way; it should not be opened simply because it is a wound, but because something must be done which cannot be done without making the wound larger. This is ordinary surgery and it should also be war surgery in regard to shot injuries.

Hunter's research on the surgical pathology of the vascular system remains his most significant work. The most familiar contribution of purely surgical importance was his operation for popliteal aneurysm. Surgeons of the eighteenth century either refused entirely to operate on the artery immediately above the aneurysmal sac or ligated it. The ligature was frequently placed through a diseased portion of the artery, which caused secondary hemorrhage. Hunter's animal

177. *Facing page,* Reproduction by Henry Bone (1755-1834) of the portrait of John Hunter by Sir Joshua Reynolds in the Royal College of Surgeons, London. The original oil painting on canvas has deteriorated, and this reproduction presents the painting nearly as it originally looked. Hunter is shown with some of his books and preserved specimens. In the upper right corner only the feet are visible from the skeleton of Charles Byrne, the Irish Giant. Hunter bought the remains of this "freak" celebrity while Byrne was still alive. When the elderly Byrne felt death approaching, he regretted the sale and tried to flee from London, but Hunter's servants shadowed him and eventually brought back the huge corpse in triumph. *(Reproduced by kind permission of the President and Council of the Royal College of Surgeons of England.)*

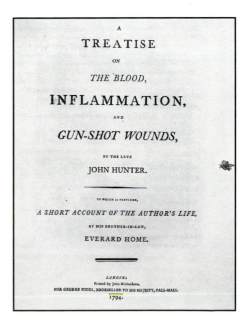

178. Title page of John Hunter's most famous book, published shortly after he died. *(Jeremy Norman & Co., Inc.)*

experimentation convinced him that collateral circulation would support viability of the extremity after ligation of the femoral artery in the thigh.

Two basic principles relating to arterial ligation made Hunter's operations successful where those of other surgeons had failed. First, ligation of the femoral artery at a distance from the diseased aneurysmal sac minimized arterial erosion and postoperative hemorrhage. Second, by placing occluding ligatures in the thigh rather than the popliteal fossa, minimal disturbance to valuable collaterals occurred.

Applying these two basic principles, Hunter first performed his operation for popliteal aneurysm in December 1785 on a 45-year-old coachman. The patient had been symptomatic for 3 years, and the condition of his lower extremity had progressed to severe distal ischemia. Hunter undertook an operation on the patient at St. George's by placing femoral arterial ligatures within the fascial tunnel formed in the anterior thigh, between the femoral triangle and the opening in the adductor magnus muscle. Six weeks later the individual left the hospital fully ambulatory. Hunter's success in this endeavor was first outlined by his brother-in-law, Everard Home (1756-1832), in an article in the *London Medical Journal* (1786):

> . . . making an incision on the anterior and inner part of the thigh, rather below its middle . . . The fascia which covers the artery was then laid bare about three inches in length . . . A double ligature was passed behind it, by means of an eyed probe. The doubling of the ligature . . . was cut so as to form two separate ligatures. The artery was now tied by both these ligatures, but so slightly as to only compress the sides together. A similar application of the ligature was made a little lower. The reason for four ligatures, was to compress such a length of artery as might make up for want of tightness, it being wished to avoid great pressure on the vessel at any one part. The ends of the ligatures were carried directly out of the wound, the sides of which were now brought together.

After the early cases of popliteal artery aneurysm Hunter established primary indications for operative intervention. Certainly, no damage to surrounding structures should be present. Excellent arterial collateralization must always be established for optimal results. Finally, the arterial mass had to be well circumscribed and pulsatile before ligation. He was of the opinion that the operation should be carried out earlier rather than later because an increase in the size of the aneurysm would not always produce a similar increase in the size of collateral vessels, so waiting for the size of the aneurysm to increase was not necessarily effective.

Hunter lived with chronic illness for much of his later life. He was plagued with pulmonary disease and angina pectoris. Despite these problems, his practice grew with his reputation. In 1786 he was appointed deputy surgeon general of the army, and three years later, surgeon general of the army and inspector general of hospitals.

The influence of John Hunter as clinician, researcher, and teacher, was promulgated worldwide by his many pupils, some of whom are listed in the box on p. 277.

The breadth of Hunter's work is evident in an article he published in 1780 concerning a woman with smallpox who had apparently communicated the disease to her fetus. Jenner had been Hunter's house pupil during the preceding decade, and much of Jenner's later work in inoculation can be traced back to experimental protocols inculcated by Hunter. Everard Home related in 1799 that Hunter had first suggested artificial insemination 9 years earlier as a means to relieve infertility. The husband performed the actual insemination by means of a syringe.

Many of the eighteenth-century British surgeons turned their interest in animal research to concern for their humane care and treatment. Hunter became one of the prime supporters of the London Veterinary College. With Hunter's influence a favorite house pupil, Edward Coleman (1765-1839), became the professor and head of this institution. John Wollstein (1765-1839), another pu-

PUPILS OF JOHN HUNTER

ↀ

WILLIAM HEY (1736-1819)

WILLIAM BLIZARD (1743-1835)

EDWARD ALANSON (1747-1823)

BENJAMIN BELL (1749-1806)

EDWARD JENNER (1749-1823)

HENRY CLINE (1750-1827)

WILLIAM LYNN (1753-1857)

EVERARD HOME (1756-1832)

JOHN ABERNETHY (1764-1831)

JOHN THOMSON (1765-1864)

ANTHONY CARLISLE (1768-1840)

ASTLEY COOPER (1768-1841)

JAMES MACARTNEY (1770-1843)

pil, returned to his native Vienna and became director of the Vienna Veterinary Institute and founder of veterinary science in the German-speaking countries.

Ultimately Hunter's voluminous research and clinical work resulted in a collection of more than 13,000 specimens, which became one of his most important legacies to the world of surgery. It represented a unique arrangement of separate organ systems; comparisons of these systems, from the simplest animal or plant to humans, demonstrated the interaction of structure and function. In addition, thousands of clinical pathological specimens were included. For many decades this collection remained the best museum of comparative anatomy and pathology in the world.

After Hunter's death, Home became custodian of his unpublished notes and manuscripts, a source of data numbering in the thousands of pages. Thirty years later Home burned this material. Various reasons have been given for this unreasonable act, but it later became apparent that Home had been plagiarizing Hunter's notes and publishing them as his own research, particularly in the six-volume *Lectures on Comparative Anatomy* (1814-1828). To mask the truth, Home felt compelled to destroy all the evidence.

By the last decade of the century Great Britain, especially London, had displaced Paris as the center for European surgical education and training. Well-known surgeons such as Cheselden, Pott, Hunter, and many others contributed to that success. Among the most prominent of these surgeons were the Scottish physician James Douglas (1675-1742) and his surgeon brother, John. James Douglas mainly practiced midwifery and taught anatomy in London. He is most remembered for his detailed anatomical description of the peritoneum (1730), including the fold, line, and pouch that bear his name, and for his monumental first attempt at writing a systematic medical bibliography (1715).

Claudius Amyand (1680-1740) was sergeant surgeon to George II and principal surgeon to the St. George's and the Westminster hospitals. He was a master of the Company of Barber-Surgeons and is most renowned for his role in introducing inoculation for smallpox in Great Britain. However, his role in surgical history is secured because he performed the first recorded successful appendectomy. Amyand reported the case to the Royal Society and it was published in their *Philosophical Transactions* (1736).

Samuel Sharp (1700-1780) was a pupil of Cheselden and was elected surgeon to Guy's Hospital in 1733. He was reputed to be a conservative surgeon, albeit with great technical ability. In many respects Sharp was the link between the older surgery of Cheselden and Pott and the new surgery of Hunter. Sharp authored two important works, *A Treatise on the Operations of Surgery* (1739) and *A Critical Enquiry into the Present State of Surgery* (1750). The latter was so well received that it was translated into French, German, and Spanish.

Among Sharp's special interests were the anatomy and treatment of hernias. His experiments with instruments led to his suggestion that the barrel of trephines used in craniotomy should be conical. This suggestion became universally adopted. Sharp was elected to the Royal Society of London and its counterpart in Paris in 1749. In his most renowned work he described a method for opening the cornea in cataract extraction. His notion that a special instrument be designed for opening the cornea to extract the "crystaline humor" led to the invention of several forms of cataract knife.

John Pringle (1707-1782) was surgeon general of the British armies from 1742 to 1758. Through his efforts the concepts of modern military medicine were originated, including the neutralization of military hospitals during war. This suggestion was eventually incorporated into the articles of the Geneva Convention (1864). Many of Pringle's principles of military sanitation, such as the ventilation of barracks, were incorporated into his *Observations on the Diseases of the Army* (1752). Pringle did much to improve the daily lives of soldiers, including the distribution of blankets. Besides his pioneer work in military medicine, Pringle helped improve the conditions of sailors at sea in *A Discourse upon Some Late Improvements of the Means for Preserving the Health of Mariners* (1776). He was also a strong advocate of better ventilation in prisons and hospitals as a means of preventing typhoid fever *(Observations on the Nature and Cure of Hospital and Jayl-Fevers* [1750]*)*, which he demonstrated to be the same as "hospital fever."

Joseph Warner (1717-1801) was a pupil of Sharp and a surgeon at Guy's Hospital. Warner held the unique distinction of being a member of all three professional surgical organizations in London during the eighteenth century. He was a barber-surgeon, twice a master of the Company of Surgeons (1755 and 1784), and among the first members of the reconstituted College of Surgeons (1800). His written works included *Cases in Surgery* (1754), *A Description of the Human Eye* (1773), and *An Account of the Testicles* (1774).

William Bromfield (1712-1792) was an authoritative surgical author who worked at St. George's Hospital. Having served as an apprentice to Ranby, he commenced lecturing on anatomy and surgery in 1741. He was also the founder of the well-known Lock Hospital for venereal diseases in London (1746). In 1761 Bromfield was appointed surgeon to George III and Queen Charlotte (1744-1818). Bromfield's most important surgical treatise was the two-volume *Chirurgical Observations and Cases* (1773), which contained many technical hints, including those on the performance of "bilateral lithotomy." He also described the proper procedure for compressing the subclavian artery above the clavicle on the first rib and a special method for ligating this artery after separating it from the brachial plexus. Among his other valuable literary efforts was *Thoughts Arising from Experience, Concerning the Present Method of Treating Persons Inoculated for the Small-Pox* (1767).

OBSERVATIONS

ON THE

Diseases of the Army,

IN

CAMP and GARRISON.

In THREE PARTS.

WITH AN

APPENDIX,

CONTAINING SOME

PAPERS of EXPERIMENTS,

Read at several Meetings of the ROYAL SOCIETY.

BY

JOHN PRINGLE, M.D. F.R.S.

Physician-General to his MAJESTY's Forces employed
abroad during the late War.

LONDON:

Printed for A. MILLAR, and D. WILSON, both in the Strand;
and T. PAYNE, next the Mews-gate, near
St. Martin's Church. MDCCLII.

179. Pringle was the founder of modern military medicine. In the preface of this book he first expressed the idea of the neutrality of military hospitals on the battlefield, a concept that, more than 100 years later, was eventually incorporated into the Geneva Convention's founding of the Red Cross (1864). *(Jeremy Norman & Co., Inc.)*

William Hunter (1718-1783), the elder brother of John Hunter, was born near East Kilbride in Scotland. His early education was unremarkable; he eventually spent 5 years studying liberal arts at the University of Glasgow. Although Hunter had originally intended to enter theology, he was attracted to the medical teachings of William Cullen (1712-1790). Cullen was instrumental in founding the medical school in Glasgow and held the chairs of medicine and chemistry both there and in Edinburgh. For 3 years Hunter served as an apprentice to Cullen. During 1739 Hunter worked in Edinburgh with Monro primus, a man who would later become his bitter rival. Two years later Hunter traveled to London, where he was introduced to William Smellie (1697-1763) and James Douglas. He assisted the latter in his dissecting room and attended lectures at St. George's Hospital. In 1748 Hunter became connected with the Middlesex Hospital and the British Lying-In Hospital. Hunter was long interested in obstetrics, which he had learned from Smellie, and eventually became personal physician to Queen Charlotte, who had 15 children. William Hunter was one of London's leading private teachers in dissection, operative surgery, and bandaging. In 1768 he built the famous anatomical theater and museum in Great Windmill Street, where some of the most renowned British anatomists and surgeons of the mid-eighteenth century were trained.

Hunter's literary efforts were extensive and addressed many medical topics. In 1757 he reported the first known case of arteriovenous aneurysm and said of these aneurysmal varices:

> . . . the vein will be dilated or become varicose, and it will have a pulsatile jarring motion on account of the stream from the artery. It will make a hissing noise, which will be found to correspond with the pulse . . . The artery, I apprehend, will become longer in the arm and smaller at the wrist than it was in the natural state . . . There is a remarkable tremulous motion both in the bag, and in the dilated vein, as if blood was squirted into it through a small hole. It is like what is produced in the mouth by continuing the sound of the letter "R" in a whisper.

William Hunter's first important paper on an obstetrical topic was published in 1762. In it he described a case of osteomalacic pelvis in a patient who had been referred to him by a country practitioner. Ten years later Hunter wrote about retroversion of the uterus. Finally, in 1774 came his most important treatise, *Anatomia Uteri Humani Grabidi Tabulis Illustrata,* which was his best work and one of the finest anatomical atlases ever produced. The 34 life-sized copper plates depicting the gravid uterus are anatomically exact and artistically magnificent. Hunter also wrote important papers on the signs of murder of illegitimate children (1783), and cases of congenital heart disease (1783). Hunter remains eponymically linked with the gubernaculum of the testis, the ligamentum teres of the uterus, the linea alba, and the membrana decidua.

William Blizard (1743-1835) was a student of both Hunters, although he eventually developed a closer friendship with John. Blizard became surgeon to the London Hospital in 1780, and 5 years later was the driving force behind the establishment of the London Hospital Medical School. He served as a member of the court of assistants and as professor of anatomy for the Company of Surgeons and also served a term as president of the College of Surgeons.

Edward Jenner (1749-1823) was the first to test experimentally the folk belief that cowpox conferred immunity to its deadly relative, smallpox, and the first to transmit the cowpox virus from person to person in an attempt to build a population immune to smallpox. Jenner detailed his experiments in his influential *An Inquiry into the Causes and Effects of the Variolae Vaccinae* (1798). Jenner's early medical training was with John Hunter, and Jenner served as one of Hunter's first house pupils. Jenner never truly practiced surgery but lived the life of a quiet country doctor in Berkley, a small dairy town. From 1770, when he became Hunter's pupil, until Hunter's death in 1793, Jenner's scientific work was directed and influenced by Hunter, who bombarded him continually with questions concerning animal life and habits.

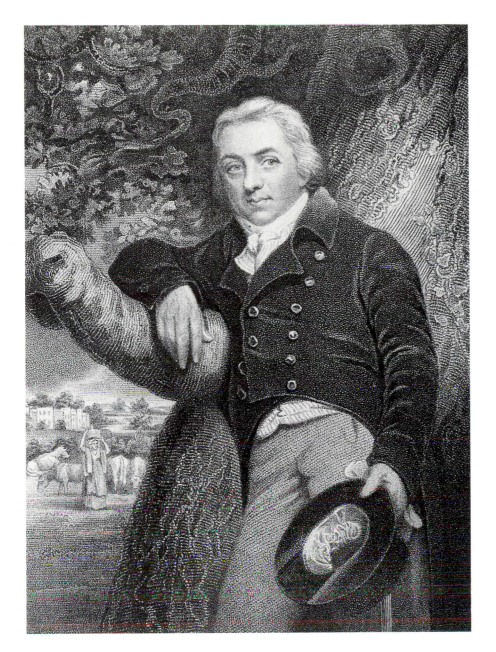

180. Edward Jenner, whose popularization of vaccination for smallpox (1798) was ultimately responsible for eradication of the disease toward the end of the twentieth century. In the lower left corner are Jenner's home, a milkmaid, and cows, source of the conveyance of the disease to humans. Mezzotint by John Raphael Smith and his assistant, William Ward, after 1800. *(Historical Collections, College of Physicians of Philadelphia.)*

Henry Cline (1750-1827) was born in London and received his diploma from the Company of Surgeons. One of John Hunter's most illustrious pupils, Cline became surgeon at St. Thomas's Hospital, where he was instrumental in propagating Hunterian doctrines of surgical pathology. Cline never wrote any lengthy surgical treatises but as president (1823) of the College of Surgeons, he was a major force in its management.

Everard Home (1756-1832) remains one of the most important pupils of John Hunter, even though he is believed to have plagiarized much of his mentor's work. Home had an intimate knowledge of Hunter for 21 years; for 6 of these years he served as house pupil. During the last 8 years of Hunter's life Home lived with him as his brother-in-law, assisted with operations at St. George's Hospital, and took virtually all of Hunter's emergency consultations. Home was a voluminous writer, although it remains uncertain exactly how much of his work might have been taken from Hunter's manuscripts, since he was Hunter's editor. Among Home's most important works were the original description of cornu cutaneum (1791) and a paper containing the first illustrations of microscopic sections of cancerous tissue (1830). He also prepared the six-volume *Lectures on Comparative Anatomy, in Which Are Explained the Preparations in the Hunterian Collection* (1814-1824). Despite the unsavory elements of his character, Home was a skilled technician and was appointed personal surgeon to both George IV (1762-1830) and his brother William IV (1765-1837). Home also served as president of the College of Surgeons for 3 years. He is remembered eponymically for the enlarged middle lobe of the prostate gland.

John Abernethy (1764-1831) was John Hunter's immediate successor in London. He was born in that city and served briefly as assistant to Charles Blicke (1745-1815), a surgeon at St. Bartholomew's Hospital. Abernethy attended the anatomical lectures of Blizard, Hunter, and Pott. In 1787 Abernethy was elected an assistant surgeon at St. Bartholomew's. He became successful in providing private lectures on anatomy in his own house; so the governors at the hospital erected a lecture theater where Abernethy was able to present a series of discussions on anatomy, physiology, and surgery (1791). Thus he became the founder of the medical school associated with St. Bartholomew's.

Abernethy is principally remembered for the first ligation of the external iliac artery for aneurysm (1796). In addition, his name is eponymically linked with a layer of subperitoneal areolar tissue in front of the external iliac artery, and a variety of neoplasm consisting of malignant fat cells (liposarcoma) found on the trunk. Abernethy's *Surgical Observations* was published in 1809.

Charles White (1728-1813) was considered a leader in conservative surgery. He practiced in Manchester, where he performed some of the most impressive surgical procedures in eighteenth-century Great Britain. In 1762 White provided an account of how to reduce the chronically dislocated shoulder by means of placing the heel in the axilla. Seven years later he performed the first recorded excision of the head of the humerus, sparing the periosteum, with consequent complete regeneration of the bone. Among White's important texts was his work on obstetrics, *A Treatise on the Management of Pregnant and Lying-In Women* (1773), in which he pioneered aseptic midwifery. In addition, he provided the first account of phlegmasia alba dolens in *An Inquiry into the Nature and Cause of That Swelling, in One or Both of the Lower Extremities, Which Sometimes Happens to Lying-In Women* (1784). White ascribed the condition to destruction of the lymphatics as a result of pressure from the fetal head.

William Hey (1736-1819) practiced in the General Infirmary in Leeds, which was his native city. He received his surgical education under Bromfield and Donald Monro (1727-1802) at St. George's Hospital. Hey's first important surgical work was his description of congenital hernia in infants (1764), and he is eponymically linked with a bilocular femoral hernia in which one sac is in the femoral canal and the other passes through a defect in the superficial fascia and lies beneath the skin. Eventually his surgical interests focused on orthopedic surgery, and he is remembered for an amputation of the foot in front of the tarsometatarsal joint, dislocation of the semilunar cartilages of the knee joint, and other procedures. In his *Practical Observations in Surgery* (1803) Hey included a description of the falciform ligament of the saphenous opening. Hey is also credited with introducing the once much used but now obsolete term *fungus haematodes* to describe a soft, fungating, easily bleeding, malignant neoplasm.

Henry Park (1744-1831) was a prominent provincial surgeon who studied with Pott and, later, Le Cat in Paris. Park was surgeon at the Royal Infirmary in Liverpool from 1767 to 1798. In 1783 Park authored the 51-page *An Account of a New Method of Treating Disease of the Joints of the Knee and Elbow,* which was originally intended as a letter to Pott. Park became well known for his operation of excision and arthrodesis as a treatment for destructive joint disease. He is also remembered for describing an arteriovenous aneurysm of the bend of the elbow in which the brachial artery communicates with the brachial and median basilic veins.

In 1694 Archibald Pitcairn (1652-1713) attempted to start a medical school in Edinburgh, Scotland. He enlisted the aid of Alexander Menteith to apply to the town council for a grant to obtain an adequate, regular supply of cadavers for dissection. This request was granted, and part of Menteith's promise was that "he would not only lay himself out for the improving of anatomy, but also would serve as chirurgeon to the town's poor gratis, but to be paid for his drogs at prime cost." Menteith was well qualified to undertake these responsibilities; he was one of the leading surgeons in Edinburgh, having been twice elected president of that city's Company of Barber-Surgeons.

For various reasons, primarily because of a lack of cooperation from his peers, Menteith's anatomical venture did not prosper. After 3 years he abandoned the teaching of anatomy to commence a course of instruction on chemistry. Concurrently the Company of Barber-Surgeons had obtained for themselves a further supply of cadavers under the following clause:

> . . . the bodies of foundlings who dye betwixt the tyme that they are weaned and thir being put to schools or trades; also the dead bodies of such as are stiflet in the birth, which are exposed, and have none to owne them; as also the dead bodies of such as are felo de se, and have none to owne them; likewayes the bodies of such as are put to death by sentence of the magistrat, and have none to owne them.

In addition, it was required of the Company that:

> . . . the petitioners shall, befor the terms of Michallmes 1697 years, build, repaire, and have in readiness, ane anatomicale theatre where they shall one a year (a subject offering) have ane public anatomicale dissection as much as can be showen upon one body, and if the failzie thir present to be void and null.

The Company fully complied with the requirement, and because the grant required that the body be buried within 10 days, the surgeons selected 10 of their number, each of whom lectured for 1 day on the 10% of the body that he had dissected. In 1705 this system was altered such that only one surgeon performed the duty, and he became known as the professor of anatomy at the university. This professorship was the formal beginning of the medical school in Edinburgh. However, it was not until 1726, under the influence of John Monro (1670-1738), that the school was completely opened.

John Monro had served with the army of William III in Flanders, and in 1703, after retirement from the military, Monro settled in Edinburgh. There he began to practice surgery and conceived the idea of establishing a "seminary of medical education" in his native country. In 1720 he formulated a plan that was favorably received by the Edinburgh town council. Part of Monro's ambition was to have his son Alexander, known as Monro *primus,* guide the destiny of the new institution.

In Edinburgh the Company of Barber-Surgeons was essentially in the hands of the surgeons by the beginning of the eighteenth century. However, the barbers instituted a legal action in 1718 that proved the original intention that barbers be equal to surgeons in the corporation. The courts ruled that the barbers had the rights to manage their own affairs and to divide equally all existing funds. In effect, this ruling permanently separated the two groups. Because the Company of Barber-Surgeons had already built its new anatomical lecture hall, the surgeons began to form other lectureships and eventually created a formalized extramural school of surgical education.

Alexander Monro *(primus)* (1697-1767) received the most thorough education in preparation for his life's work. After working as his father's assistant, he was sent to London to study with Cheselden, to Paris, and finally, to Leyden to study under Boerhaave. Monro *primus* returned to Edinburgh in 1720 and was nominated to the chair of anatomy in the new Company of Surgeons. With the founding of the medical faculty Monro *primus* was appointed the first professor of anatomy at the University of Edinburgh. For the following 39 years he gave an annual course of lectures from October to May, covering both anatomy and surgery. His most renowned written texts included *The Anatomy of the Humane Bones* (1726), *An Essay on Comparative Anatomy* (1744), and *An Account of the Inoculation of Small Pox in Scotland* (1765). He is eponymically linked with the bursa intratendinea olecrani.

In 1725 a rumor had spread that the graves in the churchyards of Edinburgh were being desecrated to obtain bodies for anatomical dissection, and an angry mob threatened to wreck the private anatomy rooms where Monro *primus* conducted his classes. Because he feared that his numerous preparations would be destroyed, he moved them to more secure quarters in the university. Henceforth he lectured from the new quarters, and the surgeon's theater no longer functioned as the official center of anatomical teaching in Edinburgh. Although Monro *primus* is regarded as the father of the Edinburgh school of medicine and surgery, he actually performed very little surgery.

During the first half of the eighteenth century, while the medical world of Edinburgh was dominated by the teachings of Monro *primus*, surgery was in many respects regarded as an inferior craft. The subject was taught only in perfunctory lectures, usually at the end of the anatomical lecture series. Consequently, few surgeons who practiced during that time are remembered today. However, the reputations of Alexander Wood (1725-1807) and John Bennet (?-1805) endure, although they left little in the way of written reports.

By 1750 almost 200 students a year were attending the anatomical lectures of Monro *primus*. The classes were growing so large that they eventually had to be divided, and none was more qualified to be an anatomical assistant than Monro primus's son, Alexander Monro, known as Monro *secundus* (1733-1817). He had studied anatomy since he was 13 years of age and began his true clinical education as a pupil of William Hunter. Monro *secundus* next studied in Berlin, where, under the tutelage of Johann Meckel, he authored a 59-page thesis on the lymphatics (1759).

The concept of devoting a complete course of lectures to surgery, apart from anatomy, was first broached in Edinburgh in 1764. James Rae, a deacon of the Company of Surgeons, began to conduct a course privately, with considerable success. In 1772 he asked the Company to support its own course of lectures on surgery, and the Company agreed to do so. The course was so successful that 4 years later the Company approached the city council with a view toward establishing a formal professorship of surgery within the university. This proposal was vigorously opposed by Monro *secundus*, who had by that time succeeded his father as professor of anatomy. Monro *secundus*, who was neither a member of the Company of Surgeons nor a practicing surgeon, explained that the teaching of surgery had always been under the purview of his chair. Consequently, the combined political strength of the Monros and the university prevented the city council from granting the petition of the surgeons. In 1777 Monro *secundus* received a new commission as professor of medicine, "particularly of anatomy and surgery."

Monro *secundus* (1733-1817), one of the leading Scottish physicians of his time, was among the world's most celebrated anatomists. Although he is generally acknowledged as the first professor of surgery in the University of Edinburgh, the political shenanigans he instigated delayed the evolution of surgery in the city. His most important written work was *Observations on the Structure and Function of the Nervous System* (1783). In his research he discovered the communication of the lateral ventricles of the human brain with each other and with the third ventricle. He remains eponymically linked with the Monro-Kellie doctrine, which states that the cranial cavity is a closed, rigid box and that a change in the quantity of intracranial blood thus can occur only through the displacement or replacement of cerebrospinal fluid. Other anatomical observations attributed to Monro *secundus* include the hypothalamic sulcus and a line passing from the umbilicus to the left anterior superior spine of the ilium. It has been estimated that from 1720 to 1790, 12,000 students were taught by Monro *primus* and Monro *secundus*.

A definite school of surgery in Edinburgh became evident during the second half of the eighteenth century. Most closely associated with this educational effort has been the surname *Bell*. Two unrelated families and several generations of Bells are involved in this history, and their relationships to one another cause much confusion. Benjamin Bell (1749-1806) was the leading Scottish surgeon of his time and the founder of a surgical dynasty that lasted for more than a century. His two sons, George (1777-1832) and Joseph, were also surgeons in Edinburgh, as were Joseph's son, the second Benjamin (1810-1883), and the latter's son, the second Joseph (?-1911). Bells from a different family included two brothers, John (1763-1820) and Charles (1774-1842).

Benjamin Bell (1749-1806) was born in Dumfries, where he received his early education. He was initially apprenticed to James Hill, a well-known surgeon in that city. In 1766 Bell entered the University of Edinburgh but found the educational opportunities quite limited. After 2 years at the university he went to London to study with the Hunters and also spent a short time in Paris. On his return to Edinburgh (1772) Bell commenced the practice of surgery and in less than a year was appointed surgeon to the Royal Infirmary, a position he held for almost 30 years.

Bell became one of the most active surgeons in Scotland, both in clinical practice and in his writings. His earliest important dissertation was *On the Chirurgical Treatment of Inflammation* (1777). Bell warned against the danger of admitting air to large abscesses and other bodily collections and advised the use of a seton. In 1778 he authored *A Treatise on the Theory and Management of Ulcers* (1778), which contained an important classification of ulcers. His largest and most ambitious work was the six-volume *System of Surgery* (1782-1787), which was written as an attempt to displace some of the systematic surgical texts authored by other European surgeons. Outside of Scotland the demand for *System of Surgery* was greatest in the United States. Bell's most important scientific text was the two-volume *A Treatise on Gonorrhoea Virulenta, and Lues Venerea* (1793). He proved that gonorrhea and syphilis were two separate disease entities, thereby correcting the earlier error made by John Hunter. Among Bell's other accomplishments was the improvement he made in the methods of amputation by introducing the "triple incision of Bell" so that soft tissue could be saved and used to cover the stump.

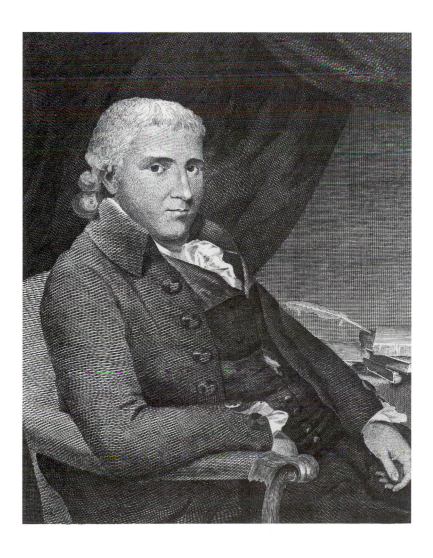

181. Engraving of Benjamin Bell. *(Boston Medical Library.)*

In Ireland a Company of Barber-Surgeons had been in existence since 1446, after receiving a charter from Henry VI (1421-1471). Through the years this manifesto was recast by other English monarchs, but by the beginning of the eighteenth century obvious attempts were being made to separate barbers from surgeons. These efforts were mostly unsuccessful and only propagated the problem that young Irish medical students had in attempting to become surgeons. The only means of self-education was apprenticeship, and no diplomas were available to show that a surgeon was properly qualified. For all practical purposes a young surgeon was forced to leave the country to receive education and training.

In 1765 Sylvester O'Halloran (1728-1807), a successful Limerick surgeon, made recommendations for the advancement of surgical education. O'Halloran had studied in Leyden and Paris and was a founder of and surgeon to the County Limerick Infirmary. His proposals eventually were put into practice when the Royal College of Surgeons of Ireland was created. O'Halloran authored a number of important treatises, including *A New Treatise on the Glaucoma, or Cataract* (1750), *A Complete Treatise on Gangrene and Sphacelus* (1765), and *A New Treatise on the Different Disorders Arising from External Injuries of the Head* (1793).

In late 1765 an act of the Irish Parliament established the first surgical examining body in Ireland, the County Infirmaries' Board, and required that all surgeons appointed to any infirmary in the country pass an examination in anatomy and surgery. A diploma was granted, for which the candidate paid 1 guinea. The examining surgeons received no financial recompense. This board conducted examinations until 1796, when the College of Surgeons was functioning well enough to assume this responsibility.

William Dease (1752-1798), surgeon to the United Hospitals of St. Nicholas and St. Catherine on Francis Street, Dublin, was a pioneer of Irish surgical education. Dease was one of the founders of the Royal College of Surgeons and a prominent lecturer and teacher. In 1776 he authored *Observations on Wounds of the Head* and 6 years later, *Observations on the Radical Cure of the Hydrocele*.

In 1745 the administration of the Company of Barber-Surgeons in Dublin began to disintegrate. By 1784, after the Royal College of Surgeons had been created, the union between the two groups no longer existed. The first president of the Royal College was Samuel Croker-King (1728-1817); the College had a governing body of 6 examiners and 12 assistants. The first students of the College had to pass examinations in Latin and Greek classics, after which they were registered as pupils of the College. Apprenticeships to members of the College followed, and the pupils also attended lectures by the College's professors. After a final examination in anatomy, surgery, and surgical pharmacy was passed, a candidate was awarded the "letters testimonial" and could then apply for election to full membership in the College.

GERMANY AND AUSTRIA

At the end of the Thirty Years' War the emerging kingdom of Prussia was becoming dominant in north central Europe. The Hohenzollerns were a family of German counts; their descendants would become the rulers of Prussia. Frederick I (1657-1713), the son of the Great Elector of Brandenburg, Frederick William (1620-1688), was crowned the first king of Prussia in 1701. Although Frederick I still owed his allegiance to Emperor Leopold I (1640-1705), the antagonism between the two men had become increasingly bitter.

Frederick William I (1688-1740) succeeded his father in 1713 and instituted strict economic controls to fill the Prussian treasury. He also created the most well-disciplined army in Europe. Frederick II (1712-1786), also known as Frederick the Great, started his reign by invading Silesia, one of the wealthiest provinces of Maria Theresa of Austria (1717-1780), the daughter of the Holy Roman emperor, Charles VI of Austria (1685-1740).

In 1756 Maria Theresa organized an alliance of France, Sweden, Russia, Saxony, Austria, and other countries and set out to defeat Frederick II. The Seven Years' War ensued (1756-1763); the result was complete victory for Frederick. In addition, he was able to partition Poland with Russia.

Less skillful rulers followed Frederick the Great, including his nephew Frederick William II (1744-1797), soon to be followed by the nephew's son, Frederick William III (1770-1840). Most of the German-speaking states, including Austria and Prussia, became involved in the wars of the French Revolution after 1792. Napoleon carried the French wars deep into Germany and abolished the Holy Roman Empire in 1806.

When Maria Theresa was married to Francis Stephen, Duke of Lorraine (1708-1765), in 1736, the claim of several German princes that she was no longer the legal ruler of Austria precipitated the war of Austrian succession (1740-1748). Although Maria Theresa lost Silesia to Frederick the Great of Prussia, she was recognized as the ruler of Austria, Hungary, and Bohemia. Her husband was crowned Holy Roman emperor, the last monarch to hold the title. Austria suffered terribly during the wars that followed the French Revolution. Each time Austria went to war with France, Austria lost more territory. In 1797 France took Belgium and Milan but gave Venice to Austria in payment.

In an environment of military and socioeconomic strife, the condition of German surgical practice was also unstable. Formalized surgical education and training were limited. Most individuals obtained surgical treatment from local barbers or itinerant quacks. The populace was overwhelmingly superstitious and ignorant of medical facts. The people believed in charms and relics and relied strictly on the traveling cutters for treatment of bladder calculi and hernia, and on the cataract extractors and the bone setters for other care.

Despite repeated edicts by the kings, nobles, and city authorities to improve conditions for the physicians and surgeons, the unsettled times limited surgical progress. Among the most appalling of situations, public executioners were permitted to compete with surgeons because they were supposed to have special dealing with the power of evil, that is, they understood witchcraft. More important, part of their work as executioners was to dislocate joints with the rack or fracture bones on the wheel. Hence they supposedly had special skills relative to the repair of fractures and dislocations.

Because of the great need for competent surgeons in the Prussian army, the Theatrum Anatomicum, founded in Berlin in 1713 was expanded in 1724 to include the Collegium Medico-Chirurgicum. Three years later the Charité hospital in that city was opened to provide clinical instruction to the students of the new school. In 1748 a military medical and surgical school was opened in Dresden. Still, the Prussian army surgeon of the era was ranked just above a drummer and beneath a chaplain. In most respects the army surgeons remained

Der Pesthof

seuffzet hier mit fast **achthundert Armen**,

Erbarmt diß Hamburg nicht, so wird es GOtt erbarmen.

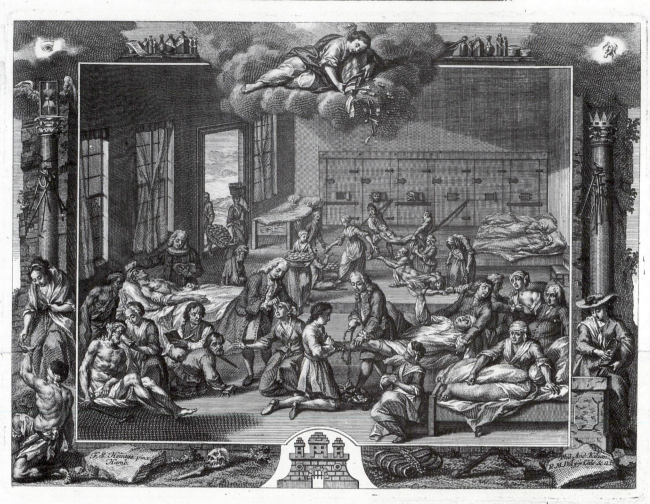

Wann du / O Leser! wilst in einem Bilde sehen /
Wie Jammer-voll der Mensch auf Erden werden kan;
So findest du es hier auf diesem Blate stehen.
Ach! schaue doch die Schaar geplagter Seelen an!
Sie sind von deinem Fleisch; sie sind von deinen Beinen.
Sie rechnen sich mit dir auch zu der Menschen-Zahl.
Kaum aber werden sie dir noch wie Menschen scheinen;
Als bloß nach der Gestalt / und diß auch nicht einmahl.
Ach! möchten sie von Witz und von Vernunft was wissen /
So schätzte man sie noch bey ihrer Noth beglückt.
Ach! aber diese ist dem grösten Theil entrissen.
Ihr Denken ist verkehrt; die Sinnen sind verrückt.
Dort steht ein Greiß und schwärmt / und will dich überreden /
Er sey der wahre GOtt / der Richter aller Welt.
Er droht/ er habe Macht zu straffen und zu tödten /
Ihm sey ein gantzes Heer der Engel zugesellt.
Ein andrer plagt und quält sich mit der Kayser-Crone.
Noch einer denckt ein Prinz und Graf und Fürst zu seyn.
Der dritte spricht voll Muth aus einem Helden-Thone;
Der vierdte bildet sich des Crösus Schätze ein.
Der fünffte rast und meynt/ daß er philosophiret;
Dem sechsten kommt es offt mit der Entzückung an.
Fast jeder hat ein Bild/ womit er phantasiret /
Wovon Vernunfft und Rath ihn nicht ableiten kan.
O Christ! was dünckt dich hier! kanst du wohl dieses lesen/
Daß diese Armen an die Seele gehn /
Ist ihre Noth nicht groß? Ach! lieber nie gewesen/
Als der Verstandes-Krafft sich so beraubet sehn.
Hierdurch vermögen sie nicht nur nicht zu erkennen /
Was dem Gemüthe Trost und Ruh und Hoffnung schenckt.

Nein/ ihre Raserey will ihnen auch nicht gönnen /
Daß ihr elender Leib auf gute Pflegung denckt.
Da die Vernunfft gebricht/ die sonst ein scharffer Zügel
Für den erhitzten Trieb und die Begierden ist;
So öffnen sie alsdenn der Wuth die Thor und Riegel /
So/ daß man Schaam und Scheu und Menschheit gar vergißt.
Der eine schreyt und brüllt mit einem weiten Rachen;
Der andre schäumt und knirscht/ und speyt/ und wirft und schilt.
Der dritte sucht sich selbst das Leben kurtz zu machen;
Der vierdte ist mit Grimm und Blut-Durst angefüllt.
Erfordert nun die Noth/ um Unglück zu verhüten/
Daß man zur Sicherheit sie in Verwahrung bringt/
So stellt auch diese sie nicht mit sich selbst zu frieden.
Sie sind/ als wie ein Thier/ das nur nach Unglück ringt.
Das Haar steht aufgereckt/ der Zorn färbt das Gesichte;
Das starre Auge brennt und strahlet Feur und Gluth.
Der Zahn fällt an den Arm und reist sich selbst zu nichte.
Die Nase raucht und schwillt und schnaubet lauter Wuth.
Die Zung ist nicht geschickt/ geschwind genug zu sprechen;
Der Leib voll Gall und Zorn erzittert und erbebt.
Die Hand will/ was sie faßt/ zerreissen und zerbrechen.
Es kracht/ was nicht mit Macht der Stärcke widerstrebt.
Der Fuß zermalmt den Grund mit fürchterlichem Tritte/
Biß endlich sich der Leib/ mit Kleidern unbedeckt/
Von Kräfften abgematt in seinem Loch und Hütte
Zur Unruh-vollen Ruh auf Wust und Erde streckt.
Ach! bloß die Möglichkeit hievon sich vorzustellen
Entsetzet und betäubt auch ein gesetzt Gemüth.

Was vor ein Urtheil soll der vollends hier nicht fällen/
Der diesen Jammer selbst mit seinen Augen sieht.
Doch/ sich noch mehrere von den geplagten Seelen/
Die aus Erbarmung hier der Pesthof in sich schließt.
Da sind zu Hunderten / die sich mit Kranckheit quälen/
An denen überall fast nichts gesundes ist.
Bey tausend Ach! und Weh! und kläglich harten Schmertzen/
Droht ihnen Krebs und Stein und Gicht und schwere Noth/
Verzehrung/ Wassersucht/ Schlag/ Lähmung/ Angst am Hertzen/
Geschwüre/ Wunden/ Krampf den Jammer-vollen Tod.
So sehnlich mancher da um seine Glieder flehet;
Erfordert doch die Noth die Lösung/ Schnitt und Brand.
Ach! wehe/ denen es also/ wie diesen gehet!
Was die Gesundheit sey/ wird hier bloß recht erkandt.
Noch die Gebrechlichen laß dir/ O Leser! zeigen/
So hast du Elend gnug auf Lebens-Zeit gesehen.
So bist du überzeugt/ wie hoch die Noth kan steigen/
Wenn GOttes Ruthen erst recht an ein straffen geht.
Frag bey dem einen an/ ob er dich sieht und kennet?
Ach! klagt er/ ich bin blind. Der Stab ist mein Gesicht.
Sag jenem/ daß er dich bey deinem Nahmen nennet.
Die Zung ist ihm gelähmt/ er schweigt und kan es nicht.
Sieh dort dem einen Trost/ versprich ihm grosses Glücke.
Er achtet nicht darauf. Ihm fehlet das Gehör.
Ruff ihn zu dir. Er kommt/ allein an einer Krücke.
Und was sind sonst noch hier vor Gebrechen mehr?
Ach! jammert dich denn nicht/ O Leser! diese Armen?
Hast du denn nicht gesehen/ wie sie so elend sind?
Um GOttes willen doch gönn ihnen dein Erbarmen
So viel sich nur dazu in deinen Kräfften findt.

Du weißt es ja noch nicht/ was GOtt vor Unglück schicket/
Daß/ GOtt behüte dich/ auch dich mit treffen kan.
Wer weiß/ wer dich alsdenn auch wiederum erquicket?
GOtt schreibet gantz gewiß sich diese Wohlthat an.
Ach! Stadt/ die du mit Recht die Mitleids-volle heissest/
Durch deine Mildigkeit steht dieses Lazareth.
So manchen hast du hier versorget und gespeiset/
Und dadurch deinen Ruhm bey GOtt und Welt erhöht.
So/ wie der Armen Zahl allmählig zugenommen/
Hat dein mitleidig Hertz sich auch darnach gericht/
Und bist viel reichlicher mit deinen Gaben kommen/
Daß deiner Armuth nichts/ was nöthig ist/ gebricht.
So lange nun bey dir der Armen Elend währet/
So lange zeige auch/ was die Erbarmung ist.
Vornemlich/ da sich jetzt die Zahl der Armen mehret/
Ach! so thu dißmahl auch/ wie du gewohnet bist.
Dein armes Volck steht schon und faltet seine Hände/
Indem du jetzt für sie die Wohlthat giebst.
Es steht aus Danckbarkeit um Heil zum Regimente.
Es steht um Fried und Ruh und alles/ was du liebst.
Wie wird nicht ihr Gebet dir manchen Seegen bringen?
Kirch/ Rathhauß/ Börse wird davon ein Zeuge seyn.
Auch Beck- und Brauerey und Schrangen wirds gelingen.
So fäst du wenig aus/ und erndtest vieles ein.

Philipp Hinrich Stenglin.
1746.

generally ignorant and incompetent. By 1795, because the shortage of army surgeons continued, the Friedrich Wilhelm Institute of Berlin was reorganized into a strictly military medical school and renamed the Pèpiniére.

Beginning with Prussia, the governments of the different German states began to establish examinations for the purpose of determining the qualifications of applicants to practice medicine and surgery. At the same time, the members of the aristocracy began to adopt the practice of taking a surgeon with them on their travels. The desire to be chosen for these privileged positions caused the younger surgeons to obtain greater skill and knowledge.

In Germany the first surgeon of importance in the eighteenth century was Lorenz Heister (1683-1758). He was a native of Frankfurt-am-Main, where he received his early education. Heister was an excellent student and studied at the University of Giessen. He obtained further surgical training in Leyden and Amsterdam; in the latter city he worked as apprentice to the Dutch surgeon-anatomists Frederick Ruysch (1638-1731) and Johann Rau (1668-1719). In 1708 Heister received a doctoral degree in medicine from the University of Hardewyk in Holland. After his formal education and under the sponsorship of Ruysch, he was appointed chief surgeon of the army of the Netherlands.

During the spring of 1710 Heister was invited by the republic of Nuremberg to become professor of anatomy and surgery at the university in Altdorf. He remained in this position for 11 years. During that time he wrote *Chirurgie In Welcher Alles Was Zur Wund-Artzney Gehoret, Nach Der Neuesten Und Besten Art* (1718), which became the most popular surgical text of the eighteenth century and was published in numerous editions and translations into Latin, English, Spanish, French, Italian, and Dutch. The 38 folding copper-plate engravings of instruments and bandages were of considerable value to surgeons who needed more training. As Heister noted in the preface, there were no adequate textbooks to supplement lectures in Germany:

> To our want of such a Compendium I also attributed the general ignorance and insufficiency of the young surgeons and students in this branch of physic, which at that time universally prevailed, through Germany especially. And from the same cause the

182. *Facing page, Der Pesthof.* A surgeon amputates a limb in the midst of a large, busy plaque ward in a Hamburg hospital in 1746. In addition to the surgeon, those attending the patients include nurses and at least one priest. Nurses appear to be handing loaves of bread to some patients. In the background two men carry out a dead body. Heads of two patients peer out of what look like holding cells on the back wall. Many patients have been so weakened by the disease that they require canes or crutches for support. Framing the central image are allegorical representations, including the spirit of pharmacy dispensing medication from a cornucopia in the clouds above, the spirit of charity giving money to a poor crippled patient on the left, and the skeletons of the dead in the foreground. Hanging from the columns on both the left and right sides of the image are more walking sticks and crutches. The hourglass on top of the column on the left has wings attached to it, suggesting the old saying that "time flies" and life is fleeting. Engraving by Phillip Andres Kilian (1714-1759) after a painting by F.S. Heintze. *(Germanisches Nationalmuseum, Nürnberg.)*

183. Eighteenth-century German trephination instrument set finely preserved in its original leather case. *(Germanisches Nationalmuseum, Nürnberg.)*

184. The instruments and technique of cataract extraction, from one of the many editions of Heister's *Chirurgie,* first published in 1718 and widely revised and translated during the eighteenth century. The way Heister combined the instruments and the operative technique for each procedure on a single plate keyed to brief textual commentary made his textbook easy to use and exceptionally popular. *(Jeremy Norman & Co., Inc.)*

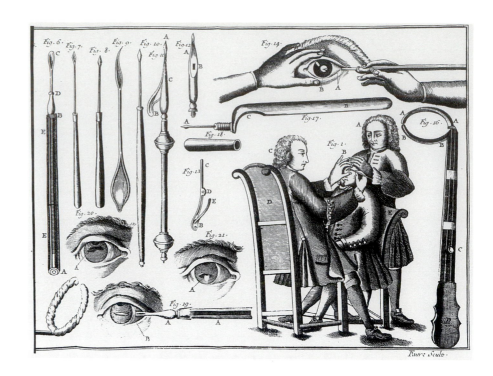

generality of our surgeons, being unequal to the more difficult operations, were content with being able to cure a slight wound, open a vein or abscess, or at most to set a fracture, and reduce a luxation; leaving those disorders and operations, which require the greatest skill, to the management of daring quacks and itinerant operators, with which Germany at that time swarmed.

Shortly after the publication of the surgical text Heister was appointed to the chair of anatomy and surgery at the University of Helmstadt, in the Duchy of Brunswick. Under his leadership the faculty became one of Europe's best, an eminence which lasted only through his tenure.

Among the important works of the prolific Heister was the *Compendium Anatomicum* (1725). It was published in 25 editions in various languages. He is remembered eponymically for diverticulum of the superior jugular vein and for the spiral valves of the cystic duct of the gallbladder. Heister is also acknowledged to be the surgeon who introduced the term "tracheotomy" to the practice of surgery.

During the last half of the eighteenth century the principal German surgeons were Carl Siebold (1736-1807) and August Richter (1742-1812). Siebold studied in Paris under Morand and in London with Pott and Bromfield and was named professor of anatomy, surgery, and obstetrics at Würzburg in 1769. His best-known work was *Chirurgisches Tagebuch* (1792). Siebold is eponymically linked with pubiotomy. He was succeeded by his son Johann (1774-1814), who founded a surgical journal called *Chiron.*

Richter was quite well known and served as professor of surgery in Göttingen. He was considered the best surgical educator in Germany and traveled widely to broaden his experience. Richter's *Abhandlung Von Den Brüchen* (1778) is a classic work on hernia in which he first described partial enterocele. He is also remembered for an interrupted silver suture used for wounds of the intestine. Richter authored a scholarly history of surgery, but the seven-volume *Anfangsgründe Den Wundarznekunst* (1782-1804) is not considered a complete account. He also founded the *Chirurgische Bibliothek* (1771-1796), a journal that did more than any other publication to improve the status of surgery in Germany.

The Meckels were a remarkable family of Prussian anatomists. Johann Meckel the Elder (1724-1774) graduated at Göttingen (1748) and authored a thesis that provided a classic description of the sphenopalatine ganglion and the dural space lodging the Gasserian ganglion. He became professor of anatomy, botany, and obstetrics at Berlin (1751) and was the first teacher of midwifery at the Charité. His son Philipp (1756-1803) served as professor of anatomy and surgery at Halle and was considered a favorite obstetrician at the Russian court. Among the anatomical findings for which he is remembered are a portion of the anterior ligament binding the malleus to the wall of the tympanum, and the receptaculum in the labyrinth of the ear.

In Austria very little of importance to surgery occurred until the end of the eighteenth century. Although Gerard Van Swieten (1700-1772) had introduced clinical instruction in Vienna in 1745, virtually none of the lectures were on surgical topics. The only known surgeon of any repute was Ferdinand Leber (1727-1808), who authored an anatomical text in 1777. Leber is known primarily for his investigations into the use of torture in jurisprudence.

Emperor Joseph II (1741-1790), eldest son of Maria Theresa, traveled widely in Europe and became quite familiar with modern European medical facilities. As a result, in 1784 he transformed the great Vienna Poor-House and Veteran's Hospital into a 2000-bed general hospital. The following year the Academia Medico-Chirurgica, containing more than 1000 beds for members of the military forces and their dependents, was opened adjacent to the general hospital. For more than a century this military medical school, known as the Josephina, provided the Austrian monarchy's forces with well-trained field surgeons.

Giovanni Brambilla (1728-1800), was born in San Zenone al Po, Lombardy, and became the trusted supervisor of all military medical affairs in Austria. An ambitious individual, Brambilla was interested in seeing that surgery was elevated to the same status as medicine. Because he became a favorite of the emperor, his efforts to foster surgery as an academic discipline succeeded. Brambilla's most important works were *Instrumentarium Chirurgicum Viennense Oder Wiennerische Chirurgische Instrumenten Sammlung* (1781), and *Instruktion Fur Die Professoren Der K. K. Chirurgischen Militarakademie* (1784).

185. *The Flayed Man.* Life-sized anatomical wax preparation made in Florence between 1775 and 1786 for the Academia Medico-Chirurgica "Josephina" in Vienna. The end of the eighteenth century was the "golden age" of wax modeling, and this is one of more than 1000 examples preserved in this institution. The increasing availability of cadavers for dissection in the nineteenth century made contemplation of these models more an aesthetic experience than a practical learning experience. Today this art form is confined primarily to museums such as Madame Tussaud's. (*Institute for the History of Medicine, Vienna.*)

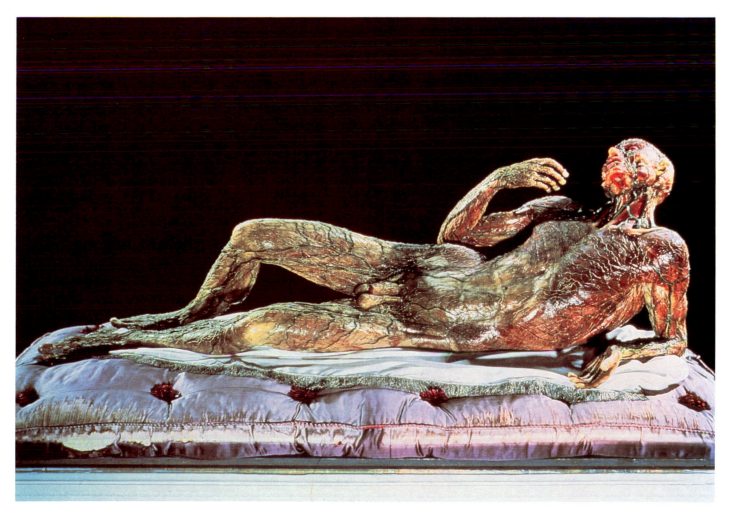

ITALY

After the outbreak of the French Revolution the many Italian states attempted to form a coalition against France. Napoleon subsequently invaded the Italian peninsula and thwarted all such resistance. Under his rule Italy became a French dependency. The Treaty of Campo Formio (1797) gave Venice to Austria and divided the remainder of Italy into five republics with Milan, Genoa, Rome, Bologna, and Naples as their capitals.

Because surgical education and training in eighteenth-century Italy were relatively unorganized, few surgeons gained national reputations. Among those few was Antonio Valsalva (1666–1723), professor of surgery in Bologna and surgeon to the Hospital of the Incurables. In his chief written work (1704) he described and depicted the smallest muscles and nerves of the ear. He divided the ear into external, middle, and internal portions. Valsalva is eponymically remembered for the maneuver that inflates the eustachian tube and tympanum by a forced expiration made with the mouth closed and the nose held by thumb and forefinger.

Gaetano Tacconi (1689–1782) succeeded Valsalva as professor and was surgeon to the Santa Maria hospital. His most important works were *Notizia Della Ferita E Della Cura Chirurgica Seguita* (1738), *De Raris Quibusdam Herniis* (1751), and *De Nonnullis Cranii Ossiumque Fracturis Eorumque Conjunctione* (1751).

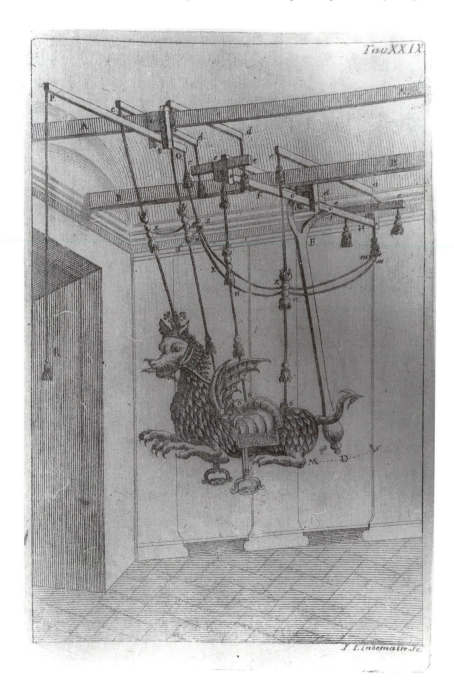

186. Physical therapy by simulation of horseback riding was accomplished by means of this "dragon," a device suspended by an elaborate system of pulleys, displayed at the first museum of medicine and surgery established in Ravenna by Father Ippolito Rondinelli. Used in the era before the invention of the bicycle, this machine might be thought of as the forerunner of the stationary "exercise bike." The engraving by Joh. Lindemain was published in a little-known account of Rondinelli's museum, *Descrizione Degl'Instrumenti . . .* by Mauro Soldo, Faenza, 1766. *(Jeremy Norman & Co., Inc.)*

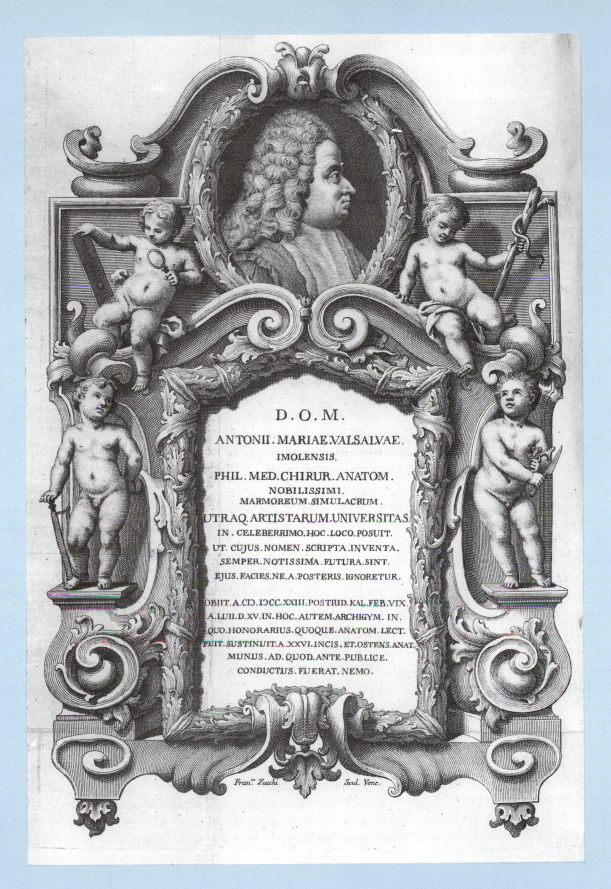

187. Elaborately framed portrait of the otologist, Antonio Maria Valsalva. Engraved by Francesco Zucchi, the portrait graces Valsalva's collected works, edited by Giovanni Baptista Morgagni and published posthumously in 1740. The caption below the cameo details Valsalva's accomplishments. Three putti incorporated in the frame are holding medical and surgical instruments; one is holding the symbol of Aesculapius. *(Jeremy Norman & Co., Inc.)*

293

NETHERLANDS

During the 1700s the Netherlands lost some colonies and much trade. Because of its great wealth from past centuries, however, it was able to continue its dominance over many countries. In 1795 France invaded the Netherlands, and William V, Prince of Orange, the last governor, or *stadthouder,* of the Netherlands, fled to England. The French changed the name of the country to the Batavian Republic and modeled its government after that of France.

The clinical teaching of medicine rather than surgery at Leyden played an important role in early eighteenth-century medicine. Johann Rau (1668-1719) was originally trained as a barber-surgeon. He taught anatomy and surgery in Amsterdam, where he was considered quite skilled as a lithotomist. Although he wrote no significant treatises, he taught many distinguished pupils. Abraham Titsingh (1685-1776) of Amsterdam, less renowned than Rau, was master of the surgeons' guild and authored several lengthy treatises.

The leading Flemish surgeon of the first half of the eighteenth century was Johann Palfyn (1650-1730) of Ghent, who was educated in Paris. After returning to Ghent, he was made master of the barber-surgeons' company in 1698. A decade later Palfyn became professor of anatomy and surgery in that city. He wrote a number of important anatomical works, including the *Nieuwe Osteologie* (1701) and *Anatomie Du Corps Humain* (1726). Palfyn is eponymically remembered for a space within the crista galli of the ethmoid that is described as communicating with the ethmoidal and frontal cells.

188. Abraham Titsingh (1685-1776) lecturing on the art of lithotomy in the presence of other members of the Surgeons' Guild of Amsterdam in 1737. Titsingh was the head of the Surgeons' Guild in Amsterdam. Presumably this is a group portrait of senior members of the guild. One of the surgeons appears to be transcribing Titsingh's words as he speaks. Painting by J.M. Quinkhardt. *(Amsterdams Historisch Museum.)*

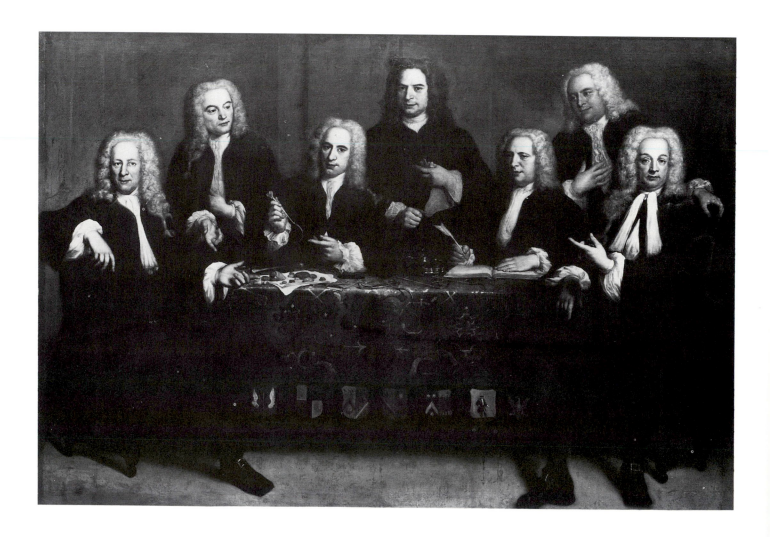

Pieter Camper (1722-1789) played the most important role in promoting the growth of late eighteenth-century Dutch surgery. He was professor of anatomy and surgery at Amsterdam and, later, in Groninge. In Groninge he was the first to open a multispecialty surgical clinic (1764). Camper's works included the three-volume *Sammtliche Kleinere Schriften* (1784-1790), a treatise on physiognomy (1792) that contained descriptions of craniometrical methods and the "facial angle," a classic text on hernia, *Icones Herniarum* (1801), *Observationes Circa Mutationes Quas Subeunt Calculi In Vesica* (1784), and a dissertation on fractures of the patella and the olecranon process (1789). Anatomical structures that bear Camper's name include an angle formed by the intersection of a line drawn from the glabella through the anterior surface of the incisors and a line drawn from the inferior nares point through the porion, a superficial layer of the tela subcutanea of the abdomen, the urogenital diaphragmatic ligament, and a line running from the inferior border of the ala of the nose to the superior border of the tragus of the ear.

189. *The Country Surgeon* by David Teniers the Younger. The surgeon, in fur cap, is on his knees treating a peasant seated on a box-like chair. The peasant's wounded foot is propped on a small block of wood, his discarded shoe and the surgeon's instruments and ointment jars scattered on the ground around it. In the background a boy prepares medicine, and the peasant's wife stands anxiously looking over the surgeon's shoulder. On a ledge beneath an open window high over the patient sits a monkey playing with a ball, a little unlikely, perhaps, but the monkey, something of a trademark for Teniers, is a frequent subject in his paintings. This is an engraved reproduction by Thomas Major (1720-1799) published in Paris by Major in 1747. Major was the first English engraver elected to the Royal Academy. (Jeremy Norman & Co., Inc.)

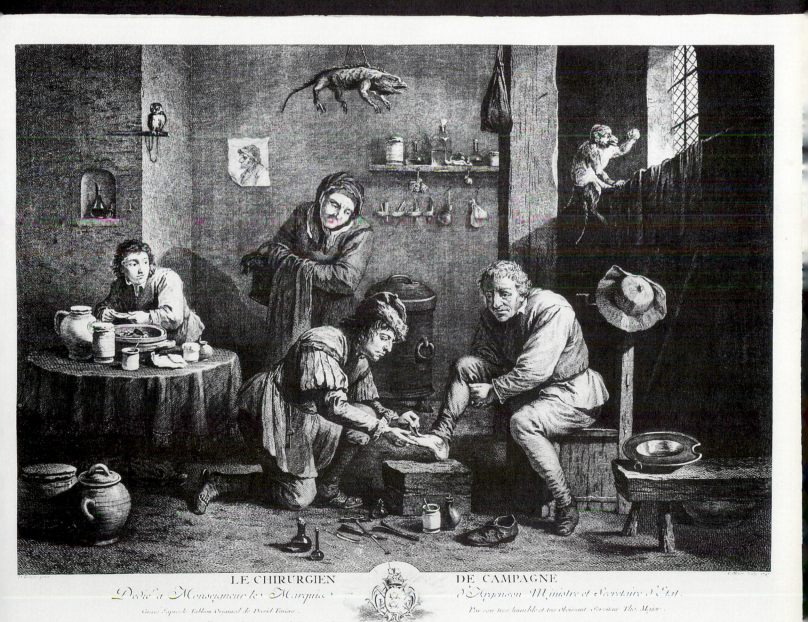

LE CHIRURGIEN DE CAMPAGNE

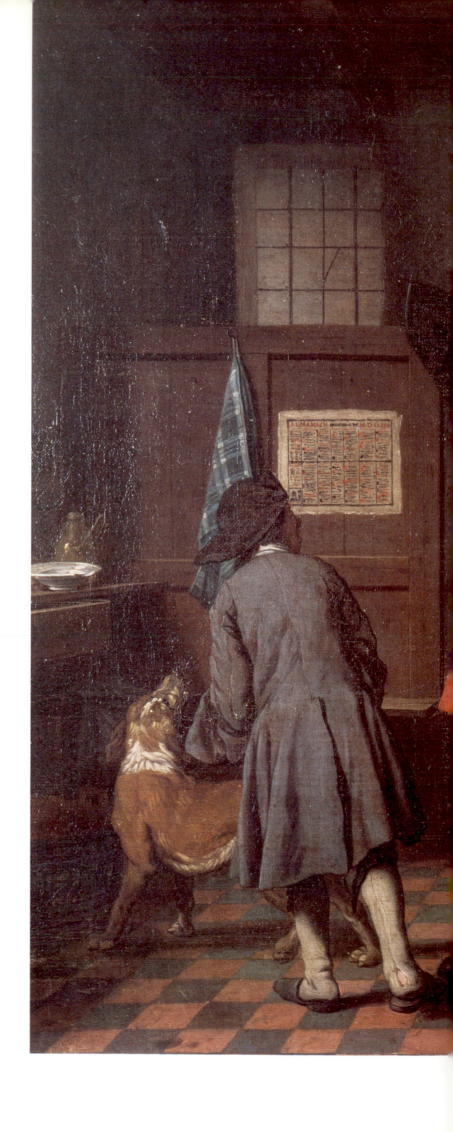

190. Surgical scene attributed to Jan Josef Horemans the Elder (1682-1759). This oil painting, completed circa 1720, is a realistic view of a barber-surgeon at work in his shop. Operations must have been performed rapidly in a noisy and distracting atmosphere. Before aneesthesia, speed was a particularly desirable trait in a surgeon. *(Wellcome Institute Library, London.)*

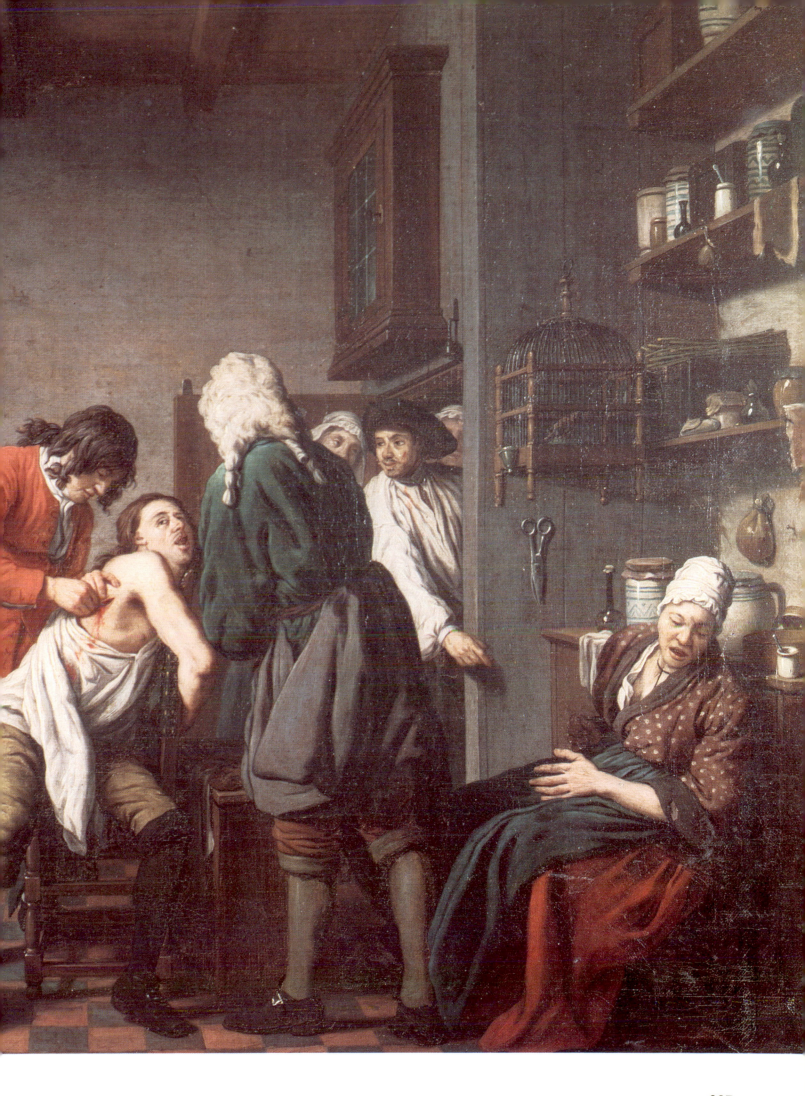

297

DENMARK AND SWEDEN

Scandinavian surgery remained unrefined until near the end of the eighteenth century, when Sweden became an international power. Until that time most medicine and surgery were left in the hands of barber-surgeons. Because physicians were few, most aspiring doctors began their apprenticeships with barber-surgeons. Students with enough ambition and talent could proceed to the universities in Copenhagen, Stockholm, and Uppsala.

In 1736 Simon Krueger (1687-1760), a barber-surgeon in Copenhagen, founded a private school for teaching both anatomy and surgery. It became a successful enterprise for almost 25 years. However, in 1772 the loss of general support from the professional medical community led to its closing. The Academia Chirurgica was founded 10 years later.

Henry Callisen (1740-1824) was one of Krueger's last apprentices and also studied with William Hunter in London. Callisen returned to Copenhagen, where he was nominated as professor of surgery (1773). Among Callisen's most prominent works were *Institutiones Chirurgicae Hodiernae* (1777) and *Systema Chirurgiae Hodiernae* (1778).

The first internationally known Swedish surgeon was Olof Acrel (1717-1806). He studied with Linnaeus and Nils Rosenstein (1706-1773) at Uppsala and received his surgical training from Gerhard Boltenhagen, a military field surgeon. In 1738 Acrel became an assistant to the city surgeon of Stockholm. Two years later he began a tour of major European medical centers: he visited Göttingen with Haller, Paris with Petit, and London with Cheselden. Acrel also found time to travel to Switzerland and Italy. In 1744 he returned to Sweden and passed his final examination before the College of Surgeons.

Through joint effort with the physician Abraham Back (1713-1795), Acrel founded Sweden's first general hospital, the Royal Seraphim Lazarette in Stockholm. Acrel authored many important surgical treatises, including *Utforlig Forklaring Om Friska Sars Egenskaper* (1745), *Chirurgiske Handelser* (1759), and *Heelkundige Waarneemingen* (1771). His name is also linked with a pseudoganglion on the posterior interosseous nerve on the dorsal aspect of the wrist joint and with a cyst on a tendon of an extensor muscle at the level of the wrist.

SPAIN

Much of the progress in eighteenth-century Spain was associated with Don Antonio Gimbernat (1734-1816), who founded and served as the first director of the Royal College of Surgeons of San Carlos (1787). Gimbernat was initially appointed professor of surgery in Barcelona (1762-1774). After his appointment as personal surgeon to the monarch, Gimbernat moved his practice to Madrid. Gimbernat's most important treatise was *Nuevo Método De Operar En La Hernia Crural* (1793), in which he outlined his operation for strangulated femoral hernia. In the same work he described the lacunar ligament.

UNITED STATES

The earliest viable settlement in the New World appeared in 1607 in Jamestown. Within 25 years of the landing of the first English colonists, 40,000 persons lived in what was to become the state of Virginia. In 1620, separatist Puritans fleeing from England because of religious persecution sailed across the Atlantic on the Mayflower and landed at Plymouth. As these Pilgrims prospered, more English people came to establish other northern colonies. Within 12 years almost 20,000 individuals called the future area of New England their home.

Great colonies controlled by individual proprietors were founded in the area between New England and Virginia. The Dutch settled New Netherland in 1624 but were unable to establish a successful government; the English took over in 1664, and the land was renamed New York. New York City grew rapidly and developed a lucrative shipping and trading business with other fledgling colonies. In 1681 William Penn (1644-1718), an English Quaker, founded Pennsylvania. He proclaimed religious and personal freedoms as the most basic tenets of his new society. English, Scotch-Irish, and German settlers soon emigrated to that area.

Life in the colonies was extremely harsh. The winters were bitterly cold, and many of the earliest colonists died before they could provide themselves with shelter or raise crops for food. Disease was rampant: epidemics such as bubonic plague, dysentery, malaria, scarlet fever, smallpox, and yellow fever often swept the land.

Among the most evident of societal problems for the new colonists during the 1600s was a dearth of doctors. Few university-educated physicians or surgeons were willing to permanently settle in the new world, and it was a rare itinerant or barber-surgeon who left his European stronghold. In 1609 John Smith (1580-1631), founder of the colony at Jamestown, was gravely wounded in a gunpowder accident and was obliged to return to England for surgical treatment, since no surgeons were available at the fort.

It is known that Giles Heale (?-1653) was aboard the Mayflower in 1620 and served as surgeon to the 35-man crew. Heale was believed to have undergone an apprenticeship in the Company of Barber-Surgeons of London and to have received a license to practice in 1619. He survived that first New England winter of 1620 and returned to London on the Mayflower in April 1621. Nothing is known of Heale's surgical exploits in Plymouth.

American medicine and surgery made few advances from 1600 to 1750. There were few actual physicians or surgeons of note, and most of the medical needs of the growing populace were served by three classes of health-care providers: governors, clerics, and a wide range of self-educated "physicians," secular preachers, and schoolmasters.

The colonial governors were able to provide for the medical needs of their constituents reasonably well. These governors were among the most educated of the settlers and were familiar with the European medical literature of the day. The most notable, John Winthrop (1588-1649), first governor of the Massachusetts Bay colony, and his son, John Winthrop, Jr. (1606-1676), governor of the Connecticut colony, were particularly well informed. In 1643 the elder Winthrop had written to Edward Stafford (?-1651) of London, an individual known for his scientific interests, requesting medical instructions for treatment of the most common diseases and injuries. Among the offered advice was:

> For a broken bone, or a joynt dislocated, to knit them; take ye barke of elme, or witch-hazle; cutt away the outward part, and cutt ye inward redd barke small, and boyle it in water, till it be thick that it will rope; pound well, and lay of it hott, barke and all upon ye bone or joynt, and tye it on; or with ye mussilage of it, and bole armoniak make a playster and lay it on.
>
> For burning with gunn powder or otherwise—take ye inner green rine of elder, in latine sambucus, sempervive, and mosse that groweth on an old thacht howse top, of each alike; boyle them in stale [lotium] and sallet oyle, so much as may cover them

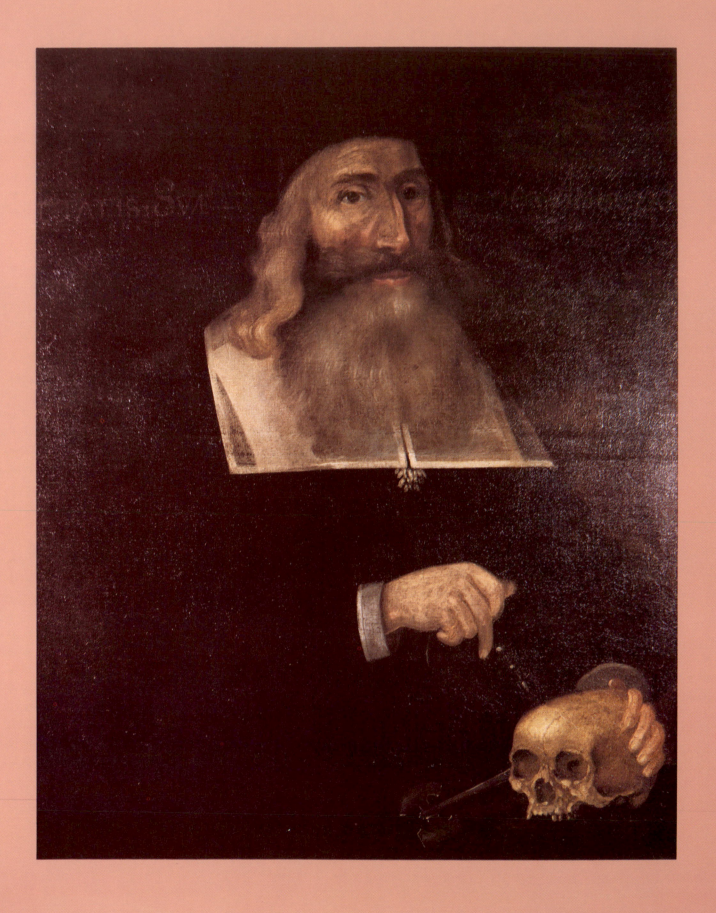

four fingers; let all the [lotium] boyle cleane away, and straine very well; putt new herbes and [lotium] as before, boyle that likewise away, and straine it as before. Then to that oyle adde barrowes grease until it come to be an oyntment, with which an-noynt a paper, and lay it to ye burning anoynting the place also with a feather.

The knowledge received from Stafford's reply was as competent as could be expected at that time. Although the letter consisted entirely of ineffective herbal treatments indicative of the lingering effects of Galen, Paracelsus, and medieval medical thought, it may be assumed that Winthrop's ability to treat patients approached that of the average European physician. In other words, there was little that the seventeenth-century physician could do to thwart most disease processes. Winthrop applied his layman's medical knowledge largely through letter writing and occasionally by seeing patients. Although no information is available concerning his surgical skills, at the time of Winthrop's death an inventory of his estate included "3 sirenges—2 treepans." It can be inferred that the governor thought it wise to have at least a few surgical instruments available as part of his armamentarium.

John Winthrop, Jr. was more famous throughout the New England colonies for his medical skills than his father was. Educated at Trinity College, Dublin, the younger Winthrop was a fellow of the Royal Society of London and counted among his many correspondents the renowned alchemist Kenelm Digby (1603-1665). As governor of the Connecticut colony, Winthrop noted the scarcity of physicians and surgeons and accordingly expressed a willingness to provide medical advice. As such, he was consulted by numerous individuals who wrote lengthy letters explaining their medical problems. Many of these letters remain extant, but there is little in them to indicate that Winthrop performed even the simplest of surgical procedures.

Next to the governors, the clerics were a leading force in early American medicine. Like their political counterparts, the clerics practiced little in the way of actual surgical operations, although some are believed to have been excellent phlebotomists. Among the most notable of this group were Thomas Thacher (1620-1678), Increase Mather (1639-1723), and the latter's son, Cotton Mather (1663-1728).

Thomas Thacher, regarded as the outstanding Puritan preacher of his time and minister of the Old South Church in Boston, became the first American to author a work on a solely medical topic. In 1677 Thacher produced a broadside that described the essential characteristics of smallpox, together with treatment and a recommended diet. Thacher was quite deliberate in informing the reader that he was not a physician and that most of the information was obtained from the writings of the English physician Thomas Sydenham (1624-1689). Since newspapers were not yet printed in the colonies, it is believed that Thacher's papersheet was actually intended for posting or for use as a circular for public instruction during an epidemic of smallpox in the winter of 1677-1678.

There is no evidence that either of the Mathers practiced surgery, although they were closely identified with the earliest attempts to introduce inoculation as preventive treatment against smallpox in the colonies. Increase Mather was born in Dorchester and studied at Harvard College and at Trinity College in Dublin. He was quite conservative in his sociopolitical beliefs and opposed attempts by the British government to reduce the historic independence of the Massachusetts colony. Mather served as pastor of the North Church in Boston from 1664 until his death in 1723. In 1684 Increase Mather authored his *Remarkable Providences Illustrative of the Earlier Days of American Colonisation*. In that work he provided the first written account of a surgical operation to be performed in one of the colonies:

Remarkable was the preservation and restoration which the gracious providence of God vouchsafed to Abigail Eliot. . . of Boston. . that when she was a child under a cart, an iron hinge, being sharp at the lower end, happened to strike her head. . . and pierced into the skull and brain. . . Able chyrurgeons were sent for—in special Mr. Oliver and Mr. Prat. The head being uncovered, there appeared just upon the

191. *Facing page,* Dr. John Clark (1598-1664). Painted in Boston circa 1664 by Augustine Clement or his son Samuel. Clark was the first of a dynasty of Boston physicians and surgeons that spanned seven generations from 1598 to 1800. Physicians in early American communities could hardly specialize; thus it is most probable that Clark practiced the entire range of medicine and surgery. The inclusion in the painting of the skull and trephination instruments clearly indicates that Clark was performing this operation in America; he is the first American surgeon known to have done so. This painting of Clark is the earliest portrait of an American physician or surgeon and is among the earliest portraits painted in North America. The supposed artist, Augustine Clement, is known to have immigrated to America from England in 1635. *(Boston Medical Library.)*

301

place where the iron pierced the skull, a bunch as big as a small egg. A question arose, whether the skin should not be cut and dilated from the orifice of the wound to the swelling. . . This Mr. Prat inclined unto, but Mr. Oliver pleading that then the air would get to the brain, and the child would presently die. Mr. Oliver was desired to undertake the cure; and thus was his operation: He gently drove the soft matter of the bunch into the wound, and pressed so much out as well he could. . . so did he apply a plaister. The skull wasted where it was pierced to the bigness of a half crown piece of silver. The skin was exceeding tender, so that a silver plate, like the skull, was always kept in the place to defend it from any touch or injury. . . This child lived to be the mother of two children, and she was not by this wound made defective in her memory or understanding.

Cotton Mather became known as the leading scholar of early American Puritanism. He is said to have written more than 450 books and pamphlets, many on medical themes. Cotton Mather helped found Yale College and became the first native of America to be elected a fellow of the Royal Society in London. He served as associate pastor in his father's church from 1685 and carried on as pastor after his father's death in 1723.

The two physician-surgeons written about by Increase Mather (Drs. Prat and Oliver) were representative of the final group of important early American health-care providers (that is, inadequately educated or self-taught physicians, lay preachers, and schoolmasters). Most of their work was poorly performed, and as a consequence little is known of their day-to-day medical and surgical activities. Although barber-surgeons were not unheard of in the early colonies, their number was quite small. Barber-Surgeons were known to complete the difficult work of minor surgery, particularly tooth extraction, incision of abscesses, and phlebotomy.

The practice of medicine and surgery in North America assumed characteristics markedly different from those of European medical and surgical practice. The general character of colonial medicine was marked by a low level of sophistication compounded by a scarcity of educated physician-surgeons. Unlike in the European countries, in the colonies there were essentially no dividing lines between physician and surgeon and since apothecaries did not exist, it was necessary for the dispensers of medical advice to act as their own pharmacists. No institutions of higher learning existed to provide for the formal education of individuals interested in studying medicine. An organized profession of surgeons did not exist in colonial America, so an examining body such as London's Company of Barber-Surgeons appeared to be unnecessary.

Early American medicine by its very nature was forced to have a practical tendency. There were no lithotomists, cataract couchers, or herniotomists roaming the frontier. The medical bond between the government officials and clerics and a growing populace was quite strong. By 1700 the apprentice system of medical education was in place, and general practitioners trained in that fashion were overtly pragmatic in their therapeutic decision making. The few physicians who obtained medical degrees in Europe and emigrated to America were regarded by their communities with no more respect than that accorded the government official or cleric who dispensed medical advice. Unlike in European countries, the colonial governments made no attempts to regulate or legislate the practice of seventeenth-century American medicine.

The tenor of American medicine and surgery markedly changed during the eighteenth century. Medicine divorced itself from the influence of the governors and clerics. Apothecary shops came into existence, and attempts to legislate the profession were initiated. In addition, sporadic medical literature indigenous to the American colonies was published. Some of these changes are evident in the controversy surrounding the introduction of inoculation for smallpox into the colonies and in the role played by Zabdiel Boylston (1679-1766) of Boston regarding colonial surgery.

The terrors of smallpox in eighteenth-century colonial America were recurrent and devastating. The epidemics were especially hard on the young and the elderly; death rates ranged from 15% to 50%. Destructive abscesses required surgical drainage, and disfigurement was common. Although the biochemical concept of immunity was not yet appreciated, the scars from a prior attack of smallpox were known to ensure virtual safety from reinfection in those who nursed the sick.

In 1721 the population of Boston was slightly less than 11,000. It had been 20 years since the city had been victim to a smallpox epidemic; during those years the population had doubled, and many children were left unprotected. In April 1721 a maritime fleet that arrived from Barbados brought with it the beginnings of a new epidemic. The disease soon appeared in the city and by autumn had spread into the neighboring towns, especially Roxbury, Charlestown, and Cambridge.

Early in the epidemic Cotton Mather had read in the *Philosophical Transactions* of the Royal Society of London of a method employed in Turkey and neighboring countries to prevent smallpox by inoculating healthy individuals with material taken from a pock of a patient with active smallpox. Mather attempted to interest a number of medical practitioners in Boston in this new process. The physicians, led by William Douglass (1691-1752), a Scottish immigrant who had received his education in Edinburgh, Paris, and Leyden and held the degree of doctor of medicine, ridiculed the idea, treating the concept with outright scorn and equating it with murder.

Despite the setback, Mather decided to visit Zabdiel Boylston, a successful practitioner in Boston and long-time friend of the Mather family. Boylston was educated in medicine by his father, Thomas (1644-?), and was among the busiest physicians in Boston. Zabdiel was considered particularly erudite. He had interests in zoology and botany and carried on an extensive correspondence with the English physician and book collector Hans Sloane (1660-1753). Mather proposed to Boylston the deliberate inoculation of healthy young people. The intent was to produce a mild form of the disease from which the patient would recover and, as a result, be protected against further infection.

Why Mather singled out Boylston, as opposed to other physicians, remains historical conjecture. It is possible that Mather looked upon inoculation as a type of surgical operation and therefore needed the services of a "surgeon." Boylston, although not a surgeon per se, was known to have successfully performed such surgical procedures as removal of bladder stones as part of his general practice. Against vocal and violent opposition Boylston decided to implement Mather's proposal. On June 26, 1721, Mather had his own 6-year-old son, Thomas, and two of the family's black servants inoculated. Shortly thereafter, all three came down with a mild case of smallpox from which they entirely recovered. They began to show resistance to further infections. Nonetheless, the public outcry was horrendous. After a threat of public hanging, Boylston had to go into hiding for 2 weeks.

The results of Boylston's efforts were slowly recognized. By the end of 1721 he had inoculated almost 250 individuals. Other physicians had inoculated another 30 or 40 persons of whom 6 died. In contrast, there were 5759 cases of smallpox in Boston, 844 deaths, and a death rate of almost 15%. The epidemic of 1721-1722 came to an end with a measure of vindication for Boylston and Mather.

Boylston was a true scientific investigator who spent much time analyzing his results. He maintained meticulous records of his patients and their clinical courses. After the epidemic Boylston authored a 22-page pamphlet entitled *Some Account of What Is Said of Inoculating or Transplanting the Small Pox . . . with Some Remarks Thereon.* Two years later Boylston was invited to London by Sloane. As the physician with the largest inoculation experience in the world, Boylston was accorded many honors. He lectured before the Royal College of Physicians and was elected a member of the Royal Society.

Whether Boylston performed any inoculations in Europe remains unknown. There has always been speculation that Boylston was involved in an attempt to inoculate certain members of the royal family, but no written records exist to verify this rumor. At the request of the Royal Society Boylston recounted his

192. *Following pages,* In early eighteenth-century America there were no medical schools. The only options for medical training of the aspiring physician or surgeon were education in Europe or apprenticeship to an American practitioner. These are the original articles of indenture of Joseph Lemmon, Jr., to Dr. Zabdiel Boylston of Boston, on May 18, 1736. The document, signed and receipted by Boylston, provides that Lemmon's father will pay Boylston for his son's instruction "in the Arts Businesses or Mysterys of Physick and Surgery." Boylston is to be responsible for young Lemmon's room and board; Lemmon's father agrees to provide his son "suitable and sufficient apparel and washing." *(Boston Medical Library.)*

Articles of Agreement Indented and made the eighteenth day of May Anno Domini one thousand seven hundred and thirty six Between Zabdiel Boylstone of Boston in the County of Suffolk Practitiöner in Physick & Surgery of the one part, and Joseph Lemmon of Charlestown in the County of Middlesex Esqr on the other part.

Whereas Joseph Lemmon Junr Son of the said Joseph Lemmon Esqr hath lived with the said Zabdiel Boylstone in order to be Instructed by him in the arts Businesses or Mysterys of Physick and Surgery ever since the first of March last, and purposes to continue to live with the said Boylstone until the first day of March one thousand seven hundred and thirty seven if the said Boylstone shall so long live; whereupon It is agreed by and between the said Zabdiel Boylstone and Joseph Lemmon Esqr as follows viz

Imprimis The said Zabdiel Boylstone Doth Covenant and agree for himself to teach and Instruct the said Joseph Lemmon Junr in the arts, Mysterys and Businesses of Physick & Surgery during the term of two years from the first day of March last, provided the said Boylstone should live so long, and if the said Joseph Lemmon Junr shall incline so long to live with and continue in the said Boylstones Employ; and also to find and provide for him good sufficient and suitable Dyet and lodging during the said two years, or so long as the said Lemmon shall see cause to live with the said Boylstone

In

In Consideration whereof the said Joseph Lemmon for himself his Executors and admin.rs doth hereby Covenant and agree to and with the said Zabdiel Boylstone to pay him two hundred pounds in full Satisfaction for his Sons Dyet and Lodging and for the Instruction which the said Boylstone shall give him in the said Mysterys of Physick and Surgery during the term of two years ending in March 1737 vizt. one hundred pounds thereof upon demand; and the remaining sum of one hundred pounds on or before the first day of March next, if the said Boylstone and Joseph Lemmon Jun.r shall be then living. And further the said Joseph Lemmon Esq.r doth hereby Covenant and agree to find and provide for his said Son Suitable and Sufficient apparel and washing during the time he shall be and remain in the Service or Employ of the said Boylstone. In Witness whereof the s.d parties to these presents have hereunto interchangeably Set their hands and Seals the day and year first herein before written.

Signed Sealed & Deliv.d
in presence of us.

Aed: Emerson Jun

Gillam Tailer.

Rec.d of Joseph Lemmon
Consideration

Boston May 18 1736
One Hundred pounds of the within

305

experience with inoculation in a small treatise, *An Historical Account of the Small Pox Inoculated in New England, Upon All Sorts of Persons, Whites, Blacks, and of All Ages and Constitutions* (1726). First published in London, this rare work was dedicated to Caroline, Princess of Wales and daughter of King George I. Boylston was particularly adamant about using statistical tables to analyze patient outcomes, and his treatise was a masterpiece of early scientific investigation.

Boylston soon returned to Boston but was not accorded the celebrity status that he relished in London. In 1730 a second, corrected edition of his treatise was published in Boston. Through unstated means, presumably payment from the British royal family for his professional services, Boylston had acquired great wealth in Europe, which eventually permitted him, in 1752, to retire from active clinical practice. Although the concept of inoculation would not be accepted for some time throughout the North American colonies, Boylston eventually saw his method adopted by many colonial physicians.

By the mid-eighteenth century almost 1.5 million people lived in the thirteen colonies. Although the colonists were British subjects, the British government paid them little attention. The British let the colonies enjoy a certain amount of political freedom but maintained strict economic control over them. Parliament passed laws requiring the colonies to carry goods in British ships. In return, the colonies enjoyed a protected market for their products in Britain. In many instances the British trade restrictions on the American colonists were much less demanding than those that France and Spain imposed on their foreign conquests. Still, the Americans were strong individualists whose resentment of any type of political or economic domination was growing.

The French and Indian War, as the European Seven Years' War was called in America, began in 1754. On North American territory the war was caused mainly by conflicts between the French and British over forts in the Ohio River valley. The war ended with the Treaty of Paris (1763), in which a defeated France ceded to Britain all of Canada and the western part of the American territory as far west as the Mississippi River. Thus Britain and Spain ruled all of the North American continent. Spain, however, was politically and economically the weaker of the two.

Great Britain found the vast administrative responsibilities of its burgeoning empire increasingly difficult to handle. A series of unwise moves were made relative to the American colonies, including the Stamp Tax of 1765. The Stamp Act brought on the rallying cry of "no taxation without representation," and in March 1770 a Boston mob attacked British troops, who fired on the angry crowd and killed several persons in what became known as the Boston Massacre. The First Continental Congress met in September 1774 and resolved that America would resist these increasingly intolerable acts.

Fighting between the colonists and British troops commenced at Lexington and Concord, near Boston, on April 19, 1775. Thus the American Revolution began. It would end in victory at Yorktown in October 1781. As the new nation was being established, a census taken in 1790 estimated that 4 million persons were living in the United States. George Washington (1732-1799) was inaugurated as the first president and remained in office until 1797.

Little original work in science and medicine occurred in America during the eighteenth century. Daily life, even after independence, was quite harsh. Physicians remained few in number, but differences in their educational status and in their acceptance by society were becoming apparent. Governors and clerics were moving away from the dispensing of medical advice. Legislative efforts were being made to control the practice of medicine and surgery. In 1736 the Virginia Assembly passed an act regulating the fees and accounts of physicians. Included in the fee schedule were 2 pounds "for a simple fracture and cure thereof" and 4 pounds "for a compound fracture and cure thereof." In 1792 the New York State legislature promulgated a law that delineated the educational requirements for a physician:

. . . no one should practise physic or surgery . . . before he should have both attended the practice of some reputable physician for two years, if a graduate of a college, or for three years if not a graduate, and been examined, admitted, and approved by the Governor, Chancellor, Judges of the Supreme Court, Attorney-General, Mayor, and Recorder, or any two of them, taking to their aid three respectable physicians with whom the candidate had not lived to acquire medical information . . .

Medical schools were first established in the mid-eighteenth century and included the University of Pennsylvania (1765), King's College, now Columbia University (1767), Harvard University (1782), and Dartmouth College (1797). Concerted activity to organize physicians and surgeons and to meet their educational and clinical needs was minimal. Medical societies were in their infancy: the state medical society of New Jersey (1766) was the first of these, but the Massachusetts Medical Society (1781), the College of Physicians of Philadelphia (1787), and the Medical and Chirurgical Faculty of Maryland (1789) became the most active in physician organization and education. Hospitals of the eighteenth century included the Pennsylvania Hospital of Philadelphia (1756), the Philadelphia Dispensary (1786), the New York Hospital (1791), and the New York Dispensary (1795).

Late eighteenth-century American medicine is distinguished from that of earlier years by the higher regard in which physicians were being held by society and the increasing numbers of Americans who were obtaining their medical degrees in Europe and returning to America with valuable clinical acumen and technical skills. These physicians would serve as a nucleus in providing a more sophisticated level of medical care to the colonists.

193. Holden Chapel in Cambridge, Massachusetts, the original home of Harvard Medical School. The three departments—anatomy and surgery, taught by John Warren; theory and practice, taught by Benjamin Waterhouse; and chemistry and materia medica, taught by Aaron Dexter—each occupied a room in the chapel in 1783. The medical school did not move to enlarged quarters in Boston until 1816. Holden Chapel is now the home of the Harvard Glee Club. (*Harvard Medical Library*.)

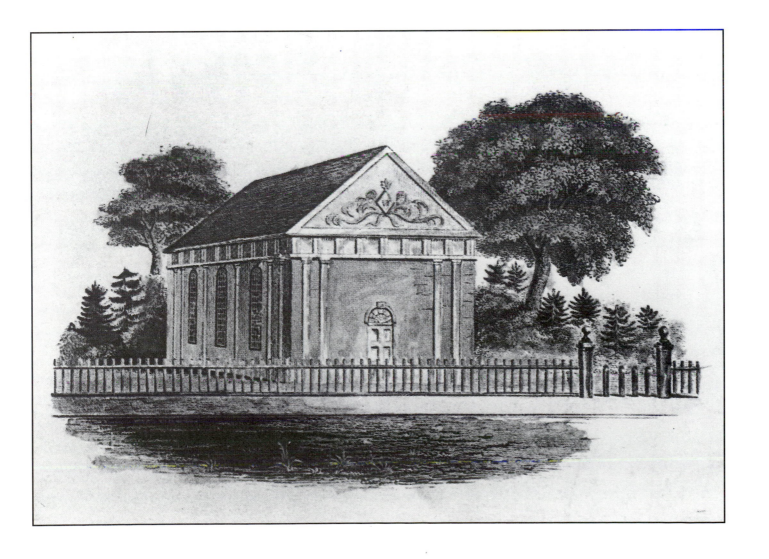

194. *Facing page,* The last page of *The Boston News-Letter* for July 17 to July 24, 1710. The advertisement in the lower right corner of this page represents the first published account of an elective surgical procedure performed in the thirteen colonies. *(Massachusetts Historical Society.)*

It is estimated that there were about 3500 medical practitioners in America at the time of the Revolution. However, less than 10% were doctors of medicine. Because of the severe lack of academic educational facilities, most individuals received their medical training by serving as apprentices to practicing physicians. The duration of apprenticeships varied considerably, as did the degree of formality in the arrangements between preceptor and student. In most instances the apprentice read books recommended by his teacher. No formal study of anatomy was made, and cadaver dissection was limited. The strong prejudice against human dissection was broken only by an occasional case of body snatching. There was little formal instruction in physiology or the new science of pathology. Obstetric cases were usually handled by midwives. The eighteenth century was an age of individualism, with each physician literally practicing his own brand of medicine.

The first printing press in America was established in Cambridge in 1639 under the auspices of Harvard College. However, because so few physicians had anything original to say, no American textbooks of medicine or surgery were published before the Revolution. For those who could afford textbooks, plenty of imported European works were available. Among the favored texts were those by the anatomists Albinus, Cowper, Cheselden, Monro *primus* and *secundus,* and Winslow. Medicine was learned from the works of Boerhaave, van Swieten, and Sydenham; the surgical favorites were treatises by Heister and Pott.

Medical information and important professional announcements were disseminated through newspapers and magazines. From 1704, when the *Boston News-Letter* was first printed, through 1783 almost 200 different newspapers appeared in the colonies. The sheer volume of these periodicals is staggering, considering the size of the populace. It has been estimated that scattered through these quarter-of-a-million pages of newspaper are some 10,000 items of medical interest to the practitioner and the patient. For instance, in the *Boston News-Letter* for the week of July 17, 1710, a small announcement appeared on the back page detailing the events of the first publicly recorded surgical operation in America:

> For the benefit of any that has or may have Occasion, Henry Hill Distiller in the Town of Boston New-England, having had a Child grievously afflicted with the Stone, apply'd himself to mr. Zabdiel Boylstoun [sic] of the said Boston, Practitioner in Physick and Chirurgery; who on the 24th of June last, in presence of sundry Gentlemen, Physicians and Chyrurgeons, Cut the said Child & took out of his Bladder a stone of considerable bigness and with the blessing of God in less than a months time has perfectly Cured him, and holds his Water: This is his third Operation performed in the Stone on Males and Females, and all with good success: He likewise pretends to all other Operations in Surgery. Which Operation the said Hill could not omit to make Publick.

Whether Hill placed the advertisement because he was pleased with the results or at the request of Boylston remains historical conjecture. However, in 1720 a similar piece regarding a mastectomy appeared in the *Boston Gazette,* again with Boylston as surgeon. From the brief notices it may be concluded that major surgical operations were being undertaken, albeit on a modest scale, in early eighteenth-century America. The colonial physician and surgeon used newspapers and magazines as important marketing tools, to further their clinical reputations, and as referral sources. In some instances the misdeeds of the medical profession also were brought to the attention of the unwary public.

By studying colonial medical literature, a clearer determination of the degree of early American cultural dependence on European medical ideas can be made. For example, some European textbooks were highly regarded and were physically reprinted in colonial America, including editions that were translations from foreign languages and abridgements, such as Northcote's *Extracts From the Marine Practice of Physic and Surgery* (London 1771, Boston 1776), Ranby's *The Nature and Treatment of Gun-Shot Wounds* (London 1744, Philadelphia 1776), and van Swieten's *The Diseases Incident to Armies* (Vienna 1758, Philadelphia 1776).

Last year there died in this City and Suburbs 4426 persons, among whom a man of 113 years old, and another 110.

Berlin, Jan. 4. The King of Prussia has been desired by the Regency of Sweden to endeavour an Accommodation between that Kingdom and Denmark, and that the Elector of Hannover has made the like Instances to him: 'Tis said his Majesties Journey to Leipsick is to mediate a Peace between Poland, Sweden and Muscovy, and some seem confident that the Troubles in the North will be composed before the next Campaign, without the least detriment to the cause of the High Allies against *France.*

Moscow, Jan. 4. An Express from Constantinople this day arrived at Court, importing that the Turks have Countermanded their preparations of War.

Deal, Jan. 5. Her Majesty's Ship the Strombulo, Cruising Yesterday to the Westward, brought in hither last Night as Prize a French Snow, with thirty three Men, and four Guns, taken off of Dungeness.

Plimouth, Jan. 6. Yesterday came in the Restoration and Plimouth, with the Bonliver Privateer of St. Malo of 20 Guns and 113 Men. The Plimouth and Salisbury have retaken and sent into Scilly the John and Margate of London from Antego, and the John of Plimouth from Virginia. This day came in the Assurance from Spithead, sailed the Unity Gally of Plimouth, with 300 Prisoners for St. Maloes.

Madrid, Jan. 7. Badajox seems to be threatened again by a Siege from the Portuguise.

Berlin, Jan. 11. They write from Riga of the 30th of the last Month, that the Dome of the great Church in that City had been very much damnified by the Enemies Bombs; and a Magazine of Powder had taken Fire, and blown up a Bastion; by which Accident near one thousand Men were killed. His Czarish Majesty was expected at the Head of his Army the beginning of the next Month. Letters from Warsaw of the 28th of December say, that the Ottoman Port had lately deposed the Hospodar in Walachia, and appointed another to succeed him; and that a French Officer had passed through the Capital of that Country in his Journey to the King of Sweden.

Milan, Jan. 11. N. S. We are advised from Genoa, that a Flushing Privateer had lately brought into that Port a French Vessel laden with Corn, and bound for Marseilles; and that the English Squadron which is Cruising on the Coast of France, had taken fifteen Corn Ships bound for that Kingdom, and sent them to Barcelona; and the Enemy are apprehensive, that a great Fleet laden with that Commodity, which is expected from the Levant, will also be intercepted by the Confederates. These Advices add, that they received an Account from Barcelona of several Advantages which General Staremberg had gained over the Enemy; that he did frequently beat up their Quarters, and had dislodged them from divers considerable Posts on the Frontiers of Arragon. Letters from Naples say, that besides the Loss which the Enemy sustained at the Siege of Orbitello, four hundred of their Men had Deserted since that Expedition, and listed themselves in the Service of his Catholick Majesty.

Vienna, Jan. 11. The Elector of Hannover has resigned the Command of the Imperial Army on the Rhine, because of the disorders of the Empire, that a General cannot Command with Honour, he is also obliged by reason of the troubles in the North rendering his presence necessary in his Dominions.

Falmouth, Jan. 12. This Day came in the Revenge-Galley, a Privateer of Guernsey, of 14 Guns and eighty Men, *Edward du Maresque* Commander, who on the 9th Instant took on the French Coast the St. Antony, of 14 Guns and sixty Men, and the St. Antony de Padua, of ten Guns and thirty five Men both of and from Granville for St. Maloe, with Salt, &c. There are two Vessels in sight, supposed to be the said Prizes, which are plying to the Windward, and endeavour to make his Harbour.

London, Jan. 12. On Tuesday night the Rt. Hon. the Earl of Essex departed this Life.

Paris, Jan. 13. A Declaration is come out, bearing Date the 28th of December, which gives uneasiness to a world of People. The Mint Bills being very troublesome, and the Government taking all possible Measures to suppress them, it was some time ago ordered, that the Farmers of the King's Revenues, and the General Receivers, should give out Notes, or rather exchange them for Mint Bills to the value of 50 Millions of Livres, which they were to pay in a certain time with the Interest; but the King being obliged upon Account of the pressing necessity of his Affairs to make use of the Money designed for the payment of the said Bills, this Declaration imports, that the Payment which the said Farmers were to make the 1st instant, shall be prorogued to the 1st of January 1711. which will prove the ruin of abundance of People, who had given Bonds to pay their Debts about this time, relying on the payment the said Farmers were to make: The Interest due thereupon is to be forthwith paid.

Leghorn, Jan. 13. Yesterday 5 British Men of War and six Dutch arrived here from the Coast of Provence, having been forc'd from their Station by a violent Storm which hindered them from taking a French Fleet laden with Corn from the Levant, except 3 Ships, which they have brought to this Place. Two Zealand Privateers, the Griffin and Grenadier, have taken another Ship out of the same Fleet, and the Dolphin and Tinnepont. 2 other Dutch Privateers have taken a French Ship of 24 Guns, having on Board 110 Lasts of Corn, besides two other Prizes, one a French Ship from the West-Indies, which they have sent to Port Mahon, and another laden with Corn; one of which was formerly an English Ship of 36 Guns. The said Privateers intend suddenly to put again to Sea.

Bristol, Jan. 14. On Thursday arrived here the Union Frigot from Nevis, who left the Island the 12th of December last, and has been in this Channel for 8 days. The Captain says, that the French have taken Statia belonging to the Dutch, and carried off 700 Negroes.

Hague, Jan. 17. N. S. The Allies by shutting the Sluices of Mons, Tournay, and St. Guilain, had drowned all the Territory of Conde, and very much incommoded the Enemy in Valenciennes, Mortagne and St. Amand, so that they will be obliged to withdraw their Troops from those Garrisons, unless the Allies do speedily open their Sluices. We have Advice from Spain, that on the 14th of the last Month, a Body of the Allies, consisting of one hundred Horse, and eight hundred Foot, had burnt down the Bridge of Moncon, & made a Guard of thirty Men, who defended it, Prisoners of War; so that they had entirely cut off all manner of Communication between the Enemy and Lerida, who were also apprehensive that the Allies had a design to attack Tortosa, Balbastro, or Moncon, in order to open a Passage into Arragon, or into the Kingdom of Valencia. These Advices also assure us, that considerable Detachments, of the Allies were filing off towards the Plains of Montblanc and Balaguer, where Count Staremberg had laid in great Stores of Provisions and Ammunition, and had erected Magazines in the Neighbourhood of Fraga, which Place he designs for the general Rendezvous of his Army. Some Advices from Valenciennes import, that they had received an Account from the Court of France of the taking of Farantona by Count Staremberg, which is a Fortified Town on the Frontiers of Arragon, & opens a free Passage into that Kingdom from Catalonia.

South-Carolina, July 4. Edward Tent Esq; our late Governour is Dead, as also Mr. Turvevil, Deputy to His Grace the Duke of Beaufort and Mr. Nathaniel Seales, Receiver to the Lords Proprietors.

Milford, July 12. The Hon. Col. Robert Treat, in the Eighty eighth Year of his Age departed this Life, after he had most diligently and faithfully Served Her Majesties Colony of Connecticut in Quality of an Assistant, Deputy Governour, or Governour and Commander in Chief for the space of about 40 years, whose Piety, Prudence, Fortitude, Temperance, Humility, Integrity recommended him highly Exemplary to all Observers, justly honourable in Life, much lamented in Death; His Funeral accordingly was attended with proper marks of Honour, and a great Concourse of Gentlemen and other People: Several Companies of the Train Bands being under Arms. He was Interr'd the 14th Currant.

New-York, July 17th Just now arriv'd here Roland from Jamaica he left that port the 11th of June with the Fleet for London under Convoy of the Kingston and Portsmouth, he parted with them at the Entring of the Gulph, with a Pink one Frost Master, a Ketch and a Brigt. for Boston.

On Friday last Dirck Adolph and Adolph Degrove arrived here from Boston.

They write from Philadelphia that Privateers have taken several Vessels off the Capes of Virginia, where they still Cruise.

The Kingsayle and Maidstone will not sayle till the 20th Instant, some say the 26th.

His Excellency Col. Hunter designs for Albany about the 25th Instant.

Entered, Out Horton and Gravener for Lisbon, Lawrence for Barbadoes, Ramsey for Madera; Rivers for St. Thomas, Degrove for Boston Elfton for Virginia; and Dowell for Maryland.

Cleared, Out Blackburn for Newfoundland; Nagle for Antigua, Bevis for Lisbon, Aspinall for Philadelphia, and Masse for North-Carolina.

Boston. An Embargo is laid on here on all Vessels Outward bound, excepting Coasters and Wood-boats.

Entered inwards Tho. Miller Ship Paul and Lewis, and Zachary Fowle Ship Unity from London; Joseph Gardner Sloop Content from Pensilvania; Michael Hilman Ship Land of Promise from Isle of May; and William Card Sloop Industry from Virginia.

Cleared Outwards Gross and Perkins for Connecticut; Chase for Rhode-Island; and Blin for Virginia.

Outward Bound Elton and Brown for Connecticut.

Frost from Jamaica arrived here on Saturday night last.

A significant segment of eighteenth-century American medical publications were written and published abroad, generally representing graduation theses of American-born students (listed in the box below) who received European educations and medical diplomas.

If a colonial physician wanted his cases, observations, or opinions to be widely reported within the colonies themselves, he was forced to submit his work to a nonmedical periodical. Among these journals were *The Memoirs of the American Academy of Arts and Sciences*, the *American Museum*, and the *Philadelphia Monthly Magazine*, all of which contained many medical contributions.

In 1790 Thomas Kast (1755-1820) wrote an article entitled "An account of an aneurism in the thigh, perfectly cured by the operation, and the use of the limb preserved" in the *Medical Communications* journal of the Massachusetts Medical Society. Kast was born in Boston and graduated from Harvard College in 1769. He studied medicine as an apprentice to his father and also spent 2 years in London as a wound dresser at Guy's and St. Thomas's hospitals. Kast returned to his native city in 1774, where he soon became a prominent practitioner and one of the founders of the Massachusetts Medical Society. His account of the ligation of a femoral aneurysm is the first article on a surgical topic to appear in the American medical periodical literature. Consequently, it is also the first known femoral ligation to be reported in the United States.

Although not usually recognized as the initial American periodical journal, publication of the first and only volume of the *Medical Communications* preceded the first printing of the more widely known *Medical Repository* by 7 years. The appearance of the *Medical Repository* in July 1797 truly inaugurated the American medical journal. The new journal was edited by three New York physicians, Samuel Mitchill (1764-1831), Edward Miller (1760-1812), and Elihu Smith (1771-1798) and was met with an immediate, gratifying response from the medical profession. It provided American physicians with their first native source of medical news and information and set the example for the many journals that

PROMINENT AMERICAN MEDICAL STUDENTS EDUCATED IN EUROPE

∾

SAMUEL BARD (1742-1821)

THOMAS BOND (1712-1784)

THOMAS BULFINCH (1728-1802)

THOMAS DALE (1700-1750)

ISAAC HALL (1746-?)

ALEXANDER HAMILTON (1712-1756)

BENJAMIN KISSAM (1759-1803)

ADAM KUHN (1741-1817)

JOHN MORGAN (1735-1789)

JOHN REDMAN (1722-1808)

NICHOLAS ROMAYNE (1756-1817)

BENJAMIN RUSH (1745-1813)

WILLIAM SHIPPEN (1736-1808)

JAMES TILTON (1745-1822)

BENJAMIN WATERHOUSE (1754-1846)

would follow in the next century. Within its pages could be found meteorological observations, reviews of foreign medical literature, and numerous clinical articles. It also published some important "firsts," including John Otto's (1774-1844) account of hemophilia (1803).

A most important change in colonial medicine was taking place in the mid- to late eighteenth century. During those years an increasing number of Americans began to study abroad, with the ultimate goal of returning to the colonies and establishing medical practices. In general these young men came from wealthy backgrounds and with their families' support were able to absorb the financial burden of living in London, Edinburgh, or Paris for an extended period. When compared with the number of Americans who obtained their medical knowledge through apprenticeship or self-education, the number of individuals who studied abroad was quite small; nonetheless, these few foreign-educated physicians would have an extraordinary impact on the future direction of medicine and surgery in the United States. Virtually every physician-surgeon of note in late eighteenth-century and early nineteenth-century America was educated abroad.

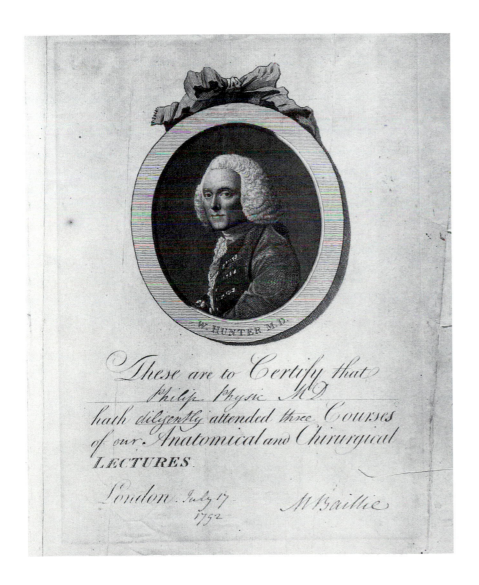

195. The certificate, filled out and signed by Matthew Baillie, nephew, pupil, and successor to William Hunter, stating that Philip Syng Physick attended three courses in anatomy and surgery at Hunter's Great Windmill Street School in July 1792. The certificate unites two of the most famous names in English medicine with Physick, one of the true pioneers of American surgery. The cameo portrait is of William Hunter. (*Historical Collections, College of Physicians of Philadelphia.*)

From the period of the earliest settlement of the colonies to the time of the Revolution the greatest percentage of medical students who studied in Europe went to England and Scotland. For some years after the War of Independence there was a natural tendency to avoid England and to study instead in France. Most of the foreign-educated students came from the central and southern colonies; numbers from New England were smaller. In most instances these students represented their homeland quite well and made quite favorable impressions on the leading teachers of the European countries, especially the Hunter brothers.

The academic achievements of the young Americans abroad were impressive, and they would soon become teachers in the first medical schools established in the United States. Many of them would also have substantive roles in developing the craft of surgery in America. Because surgical activity was limited at best, many of the technical skills needed for performing operations could just as easily be learned in the colonies as in Europe.

John Morgan was the first colonial physician to attempt to separate the practice of internal medicine from surgery. Morgan served a 6-year medical apprenticeship with John Redman (1722-1808) of Philadelphia. On its completion Morgan volunteered to act as surgeon to the provincial troops of Pennsylvania in their campaign during the war between the French and the English. In 1760 Morgan went abroad, studying first in London with William Hunter and, later, traveling to Edinburgh. Letters of introduction from Benjamin Franklin (1706-1790) provided Morgan with entrée to many elite English physicians. In Edinburgh Morgan fulfilled the requirements at its famed medical school and received his doctor of medicine degree (M.D.) in 1763. From Edinburgh, he went to Paris, where he lectured to members of the College of Surgery on suppuration and also presented methods employed by the Hunter brothers to inject and preserve anatomical specimens. To complete his journey, Morgan traveled to Italy, where he made the acquaintance of the 82-year-old Morgagni.

While studying in Europe, Morgan realized the necessity of establishing a school of medicine in his native country. Armed with a letter of endorsement from Thomas Penn (1702-1775), son of William Penn, Morgan introduced the concept to the trustees of the College of Philadelphia. His project met with immediate approval, and in May 1765 Morgan was elected professor of the theory and practice of physick in the new institution, the initial course in what soon became the medical department of the University of Pennsylvania. Later that month Morgan delivered his celebrated *A Discourse upon the Institution of Medical Schools in America,* the first American publication on medical education.

Until Morgan resettled in Philadelphia it had been customary throughout the American colonies for physicians to practice all branches of medicine, including surgery, and to prepare and furnish their own medicines. Morgan began to question that tradition and recommended a separation of pharmacy and surgery from the practice of medicine. In his attempt to improve the level of American surgical skills, Morgan brought David Leighton, an English apothecary and surgeon, to America. Morgan publicly announced that henceforth he would refuse all surgical cases and the furnishing of medicine and that his patients could avail themselves of the services of Leighton or another apothecary or surgeon. No further information is available concerning the surgical career of Leighton and his ultimate impact on the practice of surgery in Philadelphia. What prompted Morgan to make such a momentous decision also remains unknown. He became medical director of the Continental army and was eventually involved in a professional imbroglio surrounding the misappropriation of funds.

Names that recur most commonly in the accounts of surgery in revolutionary times are John Bard, John Jones, William Shippen, Samuel Bard, William Baynham, and John Warren. John Bard (1716-1799) was the first physician in colonial America to perform a human dissection for the purpose of instructing young men engaged in the study of medicine. Bard received his own medical education as an apprentice to a physician in Philadelphia. In 1746, prompted by Benjamin Franklin, Bard moved to New York City to replace a physician who had recently died in an epidemic of yellow fever. Bard became friendly with Peter Middleton (?-1781), founder of the medical department at King's College, and with his assistance completed the first recorded human dissection for instructional purposes in America in 1750. Bard established a lucrative surgical practice but remains best known as the author of the first published scientific paper on a surgical topic to come from the American colonies. In 1759 he wrote a letter to John Fothergill (1712-1780), an English physician, describing a case of ectopic pregnancy: Bard had successfully performed a laparotomy to remove a nonviable fetus from a 28-year-old woman. In 1764 Fothergill had the letter published as a scientific contribution in the Society of Physicians in London's *Medical Observations and Enquiries.*

The most famous eighteenth-century American physician-surgeon was John Jones (1729-1791). He authored the first surgical work written by an American and printed in North America. In 1767 Jones was named professor of surgery and obstetrics in the newly created medical department of King's College in New York City. Jones was also a founder of the New York Hospital and, later, the College of Physicians of Philadelphia. Jones's *Plain Concise Practical Remarks on the Treatment of Wounds and Fractures* (1775) became the accepted guide to

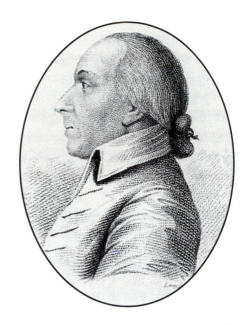

196. John Jones (1729-1791) in profile. Engraving from the *Medical and Philosophical Register. (Historical Collections, College of Physicians of Philadelphia.)*

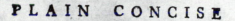

PLAIN CONCISE

PRACTICAL REMARKS

ON THE TREATMENT OF

WOUNDS AND FRACTURES;

TO WHICH IS ADDED, A SHORT

APPENDIX

ON

CAMP AND MILITARY HOSPITALS;

PRINCIPALLY

Designed for the Use of young MILITARY SURGEONS,

in NORTH-AMERICA.

By JOHN JONES, M.D.
Profeſſor of Surgery in King's College, New York.

NEW-YORK:
Printed by JOHN HOLT, in Water-Street, near the Coffee-House.

M,DCC,LXXV.

197. The rare first edition of the first treatise on surgery published in North America. Jones's work was the standard guide for American surgeons during the American Revolutionary War. *(From the author's collection.)*

surgical practice during the revolutionary war. It is among the rarest of American medical texts: fewer than a dozen copies of the 92-page first edition are known to exist. The book provided little more than a condensation of the teachings of Henri LeDran, Percivall Pott, and other European surgeons; Jones had studied with most of them in the early 1750s. As Jones so eloquently noted in the preface:

> The present calamitous situation of this once happy country, in a peculiar manner, demands the aid and assistance of every virtuous citizen; and though few men are possessed of those superior talents, which are requisite, to heal such might evils as now threaten the whole body politic with ruin and desoltion; yet, every man has it in his power to contribute something towards so desireable an end; and if he cannot cure the fatal disease of this unfortunate country, it will, at least, afford him some consoltion, to have poured a little balm into her bleeding wounds. Influenced by these motives, I have endeavoured to select the sentiments of the best modern surgeons upon the treatment of those accidents, which are most likely to attend our present unnatural contest.

William Shippen (1736-1808) studied anatomy in London with John Hunter and midwifery with William Hunter and received his doctor of medicine degree from Edinburgh in 1761. The following year he returned to America and began teaching anatomy at his father's house, using anatomical pictures that Fothergill had given to the Pennsylvania Hospital. In 1765 Shippen was named professor of anatomy and surgery at the College of Philadelphia. He replaced Morgan as chief physician and medical director of the Continental army in 1777 and served until 1781, when he was forced to resign as part of the Morgan scandal associated with financial wrongdoing. Among Shippen's most prominent professional accomplishments was his being the first in America to lecture on midwifery and to establish a hospital for its teaching.

Samuel Bard (1742-1821) was born in Philadelphia and studied for 2 years in London. In 1765 he received his doctor of medicine degree from Edinburgh University. That year, Bard joined the practice of his father in New York City and helped found the school of medicine affiliated with King's College, where he served as professor of the theory and practice of physick. Although known primarily as a physician, Bard did perform an operation on General George Washington for a large abscess of the thigh. Among Bard's prominent written works were *A Discourse upon the Duties of a Physician* (1769), the first American treatise on medical ethics; *An Enquiry into the Nature, Cause and Cure of the Angina Suffocative, or Sore Throat Distemper* (1771), one of the earliest accurate descriptions of diphtheria; and *A Compendium of the Theory and Practice of Midwifery* (1807), the first significant textbook on obstetrics written by an American.

William Baynham (1749-1814) was born in Virginia and initially took a 5-year apprenticeship in his native state. He followed the apprenticeship with several years of study at St. Thomas's Hospital in London, where he gained considerable knowledge of anatomy. From 1772 to 1775 Baynham taught anatomy under the guidance of Charles Collignon (1725-1785), professor of anatomy at Cambridge University. Baynham transferred positions in 1776, returning to St. Thomas's Hospital to instruct students in preparing anatomical specimens and to oversee the anatomical and dissecting rooms. In 1781, after failing to win election by St. Thomas's governors to the professorship of anatomy, Baynham became a member of London's Company of Surgeons. Baynham returned to the United States in 1785 and entered practice in Virginia. Despite the rural background of his patients, Baynham gained a national reputation as a surgeon and frequently traveled to other cities and states to perform surgical operations or provide consultations. He completed operations for ectopic pregnancy in 1791 and 1799 but did not report these procedures until 1809.

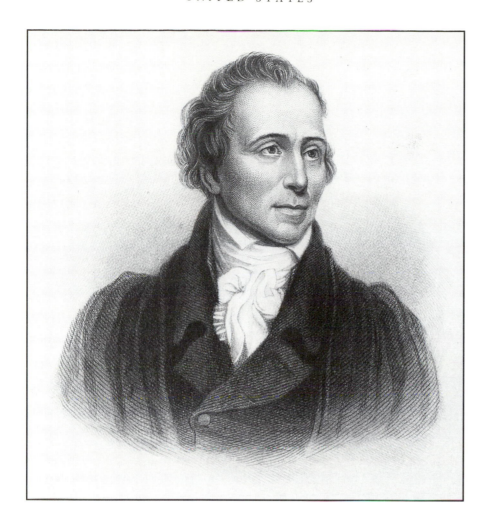

198. John Warren, first professor of anatomy and surgery at Harvard Medical School. Engraving after the painting by Rembrandt Peale (1778-1860). *(Historical Collections, College of Physicians of Philadelphia.)*

John Warren (1753-1815) of Boston studied medicine with his brother Joseph (1741-1775), who later became a hero during the Revolutionary War and was killed at the Battle of Bunker Hill. Unlike most of the prominent physician-surgeons of his era, Warren never studied in Europe. From 1775 until 1782 Warren served in the Continental army as a hospital surgeon. He possessed a lifelong passion for anatomy and was a member of the original faculty of Harvard Medical School, serving as its first professor of anatomy and surgery. Warren, the most influential figure in the early institutionalization of Boston medicine and surgery, is known to have completed an amputation of the shoulder joint on a soldier during the Revolution (1781) and a successful abdominal laparotomy in 1785.

THE NINETEENTH CENTURY

1750	1800	1850	1900	1950

DAILY LIFE

Smithsonian Institution **(1846)**

Neanderthal skull **(1856)**

Public telephones **(1877)**

Electric street lighting **(1878)**

Jack the Ripper **(1888)**

> **POPULATION FIGURES (1800)**
>
> London 864,000
> Paris 547,000
> Vienna 231,000
> Berlin 183,000

SCIENCE AND TECHNOLOGY

Christian Doppler, Austrian physicist **(1803–1853)**

James Joule, English physicist **(1818–1889)**

Gregor Mendel, Austrian geneticist **(1822–1884)**

Thomas Edison, American inventor **(1847–1931)**

Alexander Graham Bell, American inventor **(1847–1922)**

Heinrich Hertz, German physicist **(1857–1894)**

Marie Curie, French physicist **(1867–1934)**

Albert Schweitzer, French missionary **(1875–1965)**

Albert Einstein, German physicist **(1879–1955)**

Niels Bohr, Danish physicist **(1885–1962)**

RELIGION AND PHILOSOPHY

Ralph Waldo Emerson, American philosopher **(1803–1882)**

Charles Darwin, English naturalist **(1809–1882)**

Søren Kierkegaard, Danish philosopher **(1813–1855)**

Karl Marx, German political philosopher **(1818–1883)**

Friedrich Nietzsche, German philosopher **(1844–1924)**

Carl Jung, Swiss philosopher **(1875–1961)**

LITERATURE AND THEATER

Victor Hugo, French poet **(1802–1885**

Hans Christian Andersen, Danish poet **(1805–1875)**

Edgar Allen Poe, American author **(1809–1849)**

Alfred Tennyson, English poet **(1809–1892)**

Charles Dickens, English novelist **(1812–1870)**

Henry David Thoreau, American author **(1817–1862)**

Fyodor Dostoyevsky, Russian novelist **(1821–1881)**

Leo Tolstoy, Russian novelist **(1828–1910)**

Emily Dickinson, American poetess **(1830–1886)**

Lewis Carroll, English author **(1832–1898)**

Mark Twain, American novelist **(1835–1910)**

Oscar Wilde, Irish author **(1856–1900)**

Anton Chekhov, Russian novelist **(1860–1904)**

H.G. Wells, English author **(1866–1946)**

Gertrude Stein, American poetess **(1874–1946)**

Carl Sandburg, American poet **(1878–1967)**

James Joyce, Irish novelist **(1882–1941)**

D.H. Lawrence, English novelist **(1885–1930)**

Ezra Pound, American poet **(1885–1972)**

Sinclair Lewis, American novelist **(1885–1951)**

T.S.Eliot, English poet **(1888–1965)**

Eugene O'Neill, American dramatist **(1888–1953)**

VISUAL ARTS

James Whistler, American painter **(1834–1903)**

Claude Monet, French painter **(1840–1926)**

Pierre Renoir, French painter **(1840–1919)**

Paul Gaugin, French painter **(1848–1903)**

Vincent Van Gogh, Dutch painter **(1853–1890)**

Henri Toulouse-Lautrec, French painter **(1864–1901)**

Henri Matisse, French painter **(1869–1954)**

Frank Lloyd Wright, American architect **(1869–1959)**

Pablo Picasso, Spanish painter **(1881–1973)**

Marc Chagall, Russian painter **(1887–1982)**

MUSIC

Felix Mendelssohn-Bartholdy, German composer **(1809–1847)**

Frederic Chopin, Polish composer **(1810–1849)**

Guiseppe Verdi, Italian operatic composer **(1813–1901)**

Richard Wagner, German composer **(1813–1883)**

Johann Strauss, Austrian composer **(1825–1899)**

Johannes Brahms, German composer **(1833–1897)**

Peter Tchaikovsky, Russian composer **(1840–1893)**

Giacomo Puccini, Italian opera composer **(1858–1924)**

Claude Debussy, French composer **(1862–1918)**

Arturo Toscanini, Italian conductor **(1867–1957)**

Maurice Ravel, French composer **(1875–1937)**

Igor Stravinsky, Russian composer **(1882–1971)**

Irving Berlin, American songwiter **(1888–1990)**

Cole Porter, American songwriter **(1893–1964)**

MEDICINE AND SURGERY

Antonio Scarpa, Italian **(1752–1832)**

Alexis Boyer, French **(1757–1833)**

Franz Hesselbach, German **(1759–1816)**

Vincenz von Kern, German **(1760–1829)**

Nathan Smith, United States **(1762–1829)**

Giovanni Monteggia, Italian **(1762–1815)**

Dominique Larrey, French **(1766–1842)**

Wright Post, United States **(1766–1822)**

Astley Cooper, English **(1768–1841)**

Philip Syng Physick, United States **(1768–1837)**

Ephraim McDowell, United States **(1771–1830)**

Abraham Colles, Irish **(1773–1843)**

Charles Bell, Scottish **(1774–1842)**

Conrad Langenbeck, German **(1776–1851)**

Jacques Delpech, French **(1777–1832)**

Guillaume Dupuytren, French **(1777–1835)**

John Collins Warren, United States **(1778–1856)**

Jean Marjolin, French **(1780–1850)**

Allan Burns, Scottish **(1781–1813)**

Johann Meckel, German **(1781–1833)**

Benjamin Collins Brodie, English **(1783–1862)**

William Lawrence, English **(1783–1867)**

François Magendie, French **(1783–1855)**

Benjamin Travers, English **(1783–1858)**

John Syng Dorsey, United States **(1783–1818)**

William Beaumont, United States **(1785–1853)**

George Guthrie, English **(1785–1856)**

Valentine Mott, United States **(1785–1865)**

John Mettauer, United States **(1787–1875)**

William Gibson, United States **(1788–1868)**

Richard Bright, English **(1789–1858)**

James Blundell, English **(1790–1878)**

Jules Cloquet, French **(1790–1883)**

Jacques Lisfranc, French **(1790–1847)**

Robert Adams, Irish **(1791–1875)**

Jean Cruveilhier, French **(1791–1874)**

George Hayward, United States **(1791–1863)**

Jean Civiale, French **(1792–1867)**

Bransby Blake Cooper, English **(1792–1853)**

Johann Dieffenbach, German **(1792–1847)**

Thomas Addison, English **(1793–1860)**

William Horner, United States **(1793–1853)**

Charles Aston Key, English **(1793–1849)**

Maximilian Chelius, German **(1794–1876)**

Robert Liston, English **(1794–1847)**

John Lizar, English **(1794–1860)**

James Braid, Scottish **(1795–1861)**

Alfred Velpeau, French **(1795–1867)**

Nathan Ryno Smith, United States **(1797–1877)**

John Flint South, English **(1797–1882)**

Thomas Hodgkin, English **(1798–1866)**

James Syme, Scottish **(1799–1870)**

Henry Hickman, English **(1800–1830)**

Willard Parker, United States **(1800–1884)**

Thomas Teale, English **(1801–1868)**

Horace Green, United States **(1802–1866)**

Antoine Lembert, French **(1802–1851)**

John Hilton, English **(1804–1878)**

Carl Rokitansky, German **(1804–1878)**

Matthias Schleiden, German **(1804–1881)**

Georg Stromeyer, German **(1804–1876)**

Samuel David Gross, United States **(1805–1884)**

Charles Jackson, United States **(1805–1880)**

Joseph Pancoast, United States **(1805–1882)**

Joseph Malgaigne, French **(1806–1865)**

MEDICINE AND SURGERY

Gurdon Buck, United States **(1807–1877)**
Auguste Nelaton, French **(1807–1873)**
Washington Atlee, United States **(1808–1878)**
William Bodenhamer, United States **(1808–1905)**
Charles Denonvilliers, French **(1808–1872)**
James Esdaile, English **(1808–1859)**
William Fergusson, English **(1808–1877)**
John Bobbs, United States **(1809–1870)**
Henry Hancock, English **(1809–1880)**
Friedrich Henle, German **(1809–1885)**
Oliver Wendell Holmes, United States **(1809–1894)**
Bernhard von Langenbeck, German **(1810–1887)**
Nikolai Pirogoff, Russian **(1810–1881)**
Theodor Schwann, German **(1810–1882)**
James Young Simpson, Scottish **(1811–1870)**
John Mason Warren, United States **(1811–1867)**
Victor von Bruns, German **(1812–1883)**
James Miller, English **(1812–1864)**
Claude Bernard, French **(1813–1878)**
Frank Hamilton, United States **(1813–1886)**
J. Marion Sims, United States **(1813–1883)**
John Snow, English **(1813–1858)**
James Paget, English **(1814–1899)**
Crawford Long, United States **(1815–1878)**
Horace Wells, United States **(1815–1848)**
William Bowman, English **(1816–1892)**
Charles Brown-Sequard, French **(1817–1894)**
David Hayes Agnew, United States **(1818–1892)**
Henry Bigelow, United States **(1818–1890)**
John Erichsen, English **(1818–1896)**
Ignaz Semmelweis, Hungarian **(1818–1865)**
Thomas Wells, English **(1818–1897)**
William Morton, United States **(1819–1868)**
Florence Nightingale, English **(1820–1910)**
Lewis Sayre, United States **(1820–1900)**
Henry Thompson, English **(1820–1904)**
Hermann Von Helmholtz, German **(1821–1894)**
Rudolf Virchow, German **(1821–1902)**
Louis Pasteur, French **(1822–1895)**
Karl Thiersch, German **(1822–1895)**
Friedrich von Esmarch, German **(1823–1908)**
Stephen Smith, United States **(1823–1922)**
Paul Broca, French **(1824–1880)**
Gustav Simon, German **(1824–1876)**
Nathan Bozeman, United States **(1825–1905)**
Henry Gray, English **(1825–1861)**
Ernst Gurlt, German **(1825–1899)**
Joseph Lister, English **(1827–1912)**
Robert Battey, United States **(1828–1895)**
Thomas Addis Emmet, United States **(1828–1919)**
Albrecht von Graefe, German **(1828–1870)**
Jonathan Hutchinson, English **(1828–1913)**
Theodor Billroth, German **(1829–1894)**
Johann Nussbaum, German **(1829–1890)**
Leopold Ollier, French **(1830–1900)**
Jules Pean, French **(1830–1898)**
Richard von Volkmann, German **(1830–1889)**
Wilhelm His, German **(1831–1904)**
Henry Noyes, United States **(1832–1900)**
Friedrich von Recklinghausen, German **(1833–1910)**
Rudolph Heidenhain, German **(1834–1897)**
Hugh Owen Thomas, English **(1834–1891)**
Ernst von Bergmann, German **(1836–1907)**
William Williams Keen, United States **(1837–1932)**
Morell Mackenzie, English **(1837–1892)**
Henry Marcy, United States **(1837–1924)**

MEDICINE AND SURGERY

Louis Terrier, French (1837–1908)
Jacob DaSilva Solis-Cohen, United States (1838–1927)
Julius Cohnheim, German (1839–1884)
Hugo Kronecker, German (1839–1914)
Eduard Albert, German (1841–1900)
Theodor Kocher, Swiss (1841–1917)
Vincent von Czerny, German (1842–1916)
Carl Gussenbauer, German (1842–1903)
John Collins Warren, United States (1842–1927)
Just Lucas-Championiére, French (1843–1913)
Robert Koch, German (1843–1910)
Eduardo Bassini, Italian (1844–1924)
Robert Gersuny, German (1844–1924)
Lewis Pilcher, United States (1844–1917)
Nicholas Senn, United States (1844–1908)
Friedrich Trendelenburg, German (1844–1924)
Wilhelm Roentgen, German (1845–1923)
Robert Lawson Tait, English (1845–1899)
Charles McBurney, United States (1845–1913)
John Wyeth, United States (1845–1922)
George Fowler, United States (1848–1906)
Arpad Gerster, United States (1848–1923)
William Macewen, Scottish (1848–1924)
Max Nitze, German (1848–1906)
Alexander von Winiwarter, German (1848–1917)
William Osler, United States (1849–1919)
Ivan Pavlov, Russian (1849–1936)
Johannes von Mikulicz-Radecki, German (1850–1905)
Ludwig Rydgier, German (1850–1920)
Anton Wölfler, German (1850–1917)
Paul Kraske, German (1851–1930)
Viktor von Hacker, German (1852–1933)
William Halsted, United States (1852–1922)
Roswell Park, United States (1852–1914)
Arthur Mayo-Robson, English (1853–1933)
Frederick Treves, English (1853–1923)
Adolf Lorenz, German (1854–1946)
John Deaver, United States (1855–1931)
William Arbuthnot Lane, English (1856–1943)
Victor Horsley, English (1857–1916)
Carl Koller, German (1857–1944)
John Benjamin Murphy, United States (1857–1916)
Cesar Roux, Swiss (1857–1926)
Marin-Theodore Tuffier, French (1857–1929)
Robert Jones, English (1858–1933)
Howard Kelly, United States (1858–1943)
Eugene Doyen, French (1859–1916)
Rickman Godlee, English (1859–1925)
Carl Schleich, German (1859–1922)
Joaquin Albarran, Cuban (1860–1912)
Anton von Eiselsberg, German (1860–1939)
Henri Hartmann, French (1860–1952)
Mathieu Jaboulay, French (1860–1913)
Rudolph Matas, United States (1860–1957)
August Bier, German (1861–1949)
William Mayo, United States (1861–1939)
Niels Rovsing, Danish (1862–1927)
Hermann Pfannenstiel, German (1862–1909)
George Crile, United States (1864–1943)
Ernst Wertheim, German (1864–1920)
Berkeley Moynihan, English (1865–1936)
Charles Mayo, United States (1865–1939)
Max Wilms, German (1867–1918)
Fritz De Quervain, Swiss (1868–1940)
Harvey Cushing, United States (1869–1939)
W. Ernest Miles, English (1869–1947)

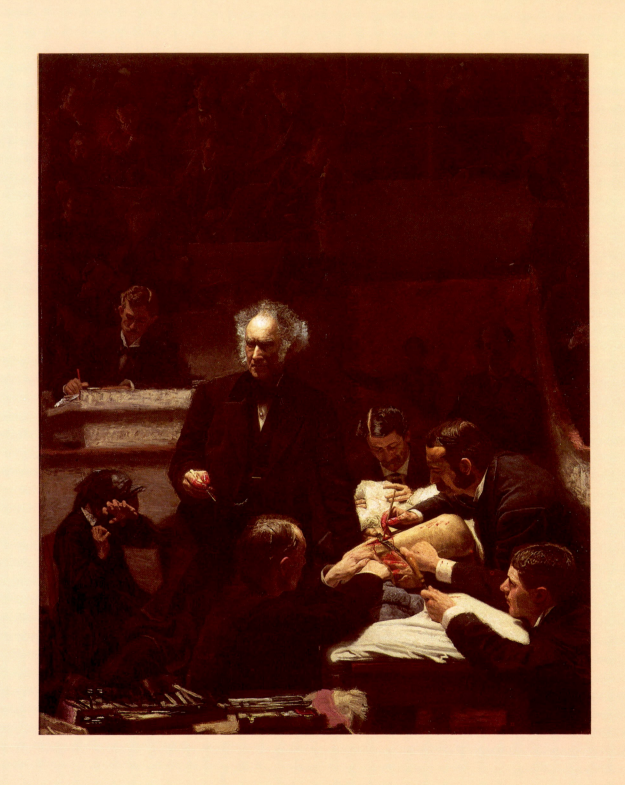

CHAPTER 11

THE NINETEENTH CENTURY

During the nineteenth century the organized advancement of medical sciences began, and the surgeon emerged as a specialist, to become a recognized and respected medical practitioner. Yet, the era began unobtrusively as a direct continuation of the medical and surgical development of the eighteenth century.

Through the first half of the nineteenth century the scope of surgery remained limited. Surgeons, whether university educated or trained in apprenticeships, treated only simple fractures, dislocations, and abscesses and performed amputations with dexterity but high mortality rates. They managed to ligate major arteries for common and accessible aneurysms and made heroic attempts to excise external tumors. Some specialized in the treatment of anal fistulas, hernias, cataracts, and bladder stones. Attempts at reduction of incarcerated and strangulated hernias were made, and an occasional lumbar colostomy was performed for intestinal obstruction. Compound fractures of the limbs with attendant sepsis remained mostly unmanageable, and staggering morbidity and mortality could be anticipated. Although a few bold surgeons endeavored to incise the abdomen, hoping to divide obstructing bands and adhesions, abdominal surgery was virtually unknown.

Within just a few years the practice of surgery would be more abruptly altered than in all of its previous history. Startling new developments rendered the surgery of the 1850s and beyond a scientific profession markedly different from the surgery of the past. Among the most salient of these changes were the discovery and employment of anesthetics; the establishment of antiseptic and aseptic surgery; the improvement on old practices and the advent of radically new operative procedures, especially in the fields of abdominal, gynecologic, intracranial, orthopedic, plastic and reconstructive, and urologic surgery; the use of roentgen rays; the development of more effective methods of hemostasis, aided by the evolution of practical blood transfusion; the total removal of any restrictions on the study of human anatomy and pathology; distinct and far-reaching changes in the methods of educating and training surgeons; the reform of medical care as a result of the rise of nursing as a profession; the formation of national and international surgical societies; and more rapid transfer of information via periodicals and other forms of communication. So great were the innovations and so inclusive was the domain of surgery that the foundation of basic operative procedures to be performed throughout the twentieth century was laid by the time World War I was concluded (1918).

The development of surgery is especially evident in the analysis of operative statistics from the Massachusetts General Hospital. In the decade before the discovery of ether anesthesia (1836 to 1846) only 385 surgical operations were performed in that venerable institution. In the first decade after the employment of ether anesthesia (1847 to 1857) 1893 surgical operations were completed. In the 10 years preceding Lister's visit to the United States (1866 to 1876) 7696 operations were performed. In the next decade (1877 to 1887) the number increased

199. *Facing page, The Gross Clinic, Portrait of Professor Gross* (1875) by Thomas Eakins. Arguably the greatest painting of a medical subject created by an American artist, this large work (96 by 78 inches) is the crowning achievement of Eakins, who studied medicine at Jefferson Medical College under Joseph Pancoast in 1864. Originally Eakins intended to become a surgeon, but his artistic interests won out over a medical career. Several of Eakins's most important portraits are of physicians and surgeons at Jefferson. This painting shows Samuel D. Gross with five other surgeons assisting him as he performs an operation in the amphitheater at Jefferson for the removal of a diseased thigh bone. Apart from the dramatic portrayal of the subject, what is most striking is that the surgeons are operating in their business suits with bare hands and no masks. Although Lister began publishing on the antiseptic principle in surgery as early as 1867, antisepsis was not widely practiced until years later, especially in the United States.

The other surgeons assisting Gross include, in the rear, W. Joseph Hearn, who is administering the anesthetic, and in the front, James M. Barton, Daniel Apple, and Charles S. Briggs. Behind Gross on the left is the clinic clerk, Franklin West. On the right, in the shadow of the entrance to the amphitheater, is Gross's son, Samuel W. Gross. Below the clinic clerk a woman, presumably the patient's mother, shields her eyes in horror. It was a stipulation in charity cases that a member of the patient's family be present; however, wives were specifically discouraged from attending. *(Jefferson Medical College, Thomas Jefferson University, Philadelphia.)*

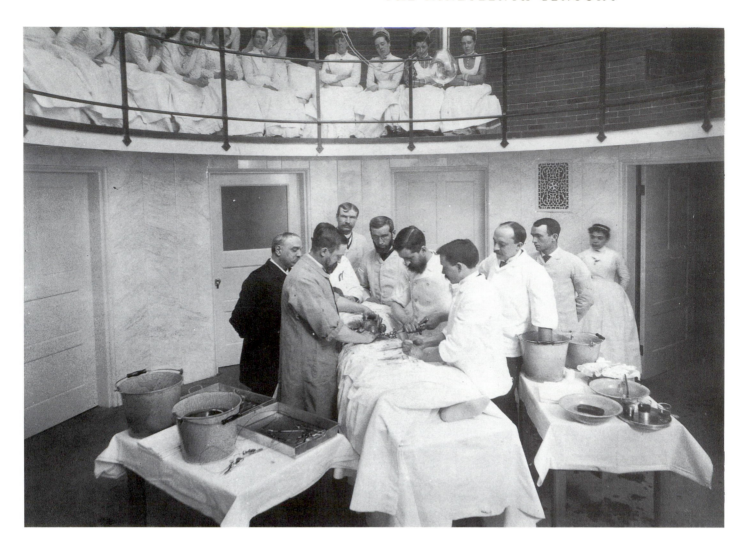

200. One of the first operations performed in the abdominal (Bradley) ward of Massachusetts General Hospital (1889). The large group of nurses watches the operation from the gallery. *(Boston Medical Library.)*

slightly, to 10,119. From 1894 to 1904, however, 24,270 operations were completed, and by the beginning of World War I (1914) more than 4000 surgical procedures a year were being conducted.

The nineteenth century was a time of enormous national growth and development, both in Europe and in the United States. After the defeat of Napoleon the Congresses of Vienna (1814-1815) and Aix-la-Chapelle (1818) brought together all the important European diplomatic communities to redraw the map of that continent. Among the various participants were Robert Castlereagh (1769-1822) and Arthur Wellington (1769-1852) of Great Britain, Alexander I (1777-1825) of Russia, Wilhelm von Humboldt (1767-1835) of Prussia, Klemens Metternich (1773-1859) of Austria, and Charles Talleyrand (1754-1838) of France. The Congresses were instrumental in restoring the rulers of France, some of the German states, Italy, the Netherlands, Portugal, and Spain. Despite all the diplomatic maneuvering, differing alliances and shifting loyalties marked the remainder of this century and culminated in the First World War.

Within medicine a number of fundamental advances were highlighted by profound developments in microscopy, histology, and embryology. The development of the cell theory was furthered by the discovery of the cell nucleus by Robert Brown (1773-1858). Matthias Schleiden (1804-1881) demonstrated that plant tissues are made up of and developed from groups of cells. Theodor Schwann (1810-1882) showed similar findings in animal tissues. By the end of the nineteenth century most of the great accomplishments in topographical and regional anatomy had occurred.

One macabre method used to advance nineteenth-century medical sciences concerned the obtaining of bodies for anatomical studies. In early nineteenth-century Great Britain and the United States no public regulations guided the supply of dissecting materials for teaching purposes. Access to cadavers was an absolute necessity for medical students, and the need was often met by surreptitious methods.

Most bodies were those of executed criminals: professional hangmen, for a small fee, cut them down from the gallows and delivered them to the anatomical schools. If a shortage of bodies occurred, another class of individuals would resort to digging up cadavers during the night, after the funerals. These individuals, usually criminals and ruffians, became known as the "resurrectionists" or the "body snatchers." The most famous corpse suppliers were William Burke and William Hare, called the "sack-'em-up men" of Edinburgh. Quite impatient regarding natural death, they resorted to murder to increase their supply of bodies. Usually the intended victim was first intoxicated, then smothered in an act that became known as "Burking." In 1828 Burke and Hare admitted to killing 16 victims, all for sale to the anatomist Robert Knox. Hare eventually became a witness for the state's prosecution of the body snatchers; Burke was hanged. The magistrate declared that, as an appropriate punishment, Burke's body would be publicly dissected and his skeleton preserved for posterity. A gruesome sequel occurred in November 1831, when two London grave robbers, William and Bishop, were arrested while attempting to sell the body of a 14-year-old boy to King's College Hospital. They eventually confessed to having murdered more than 60 persons. Both were convicted and publicly hanged 1 month later. As a result of the scandal of the black market in human corpses, Parliament passed the Anatomy Act of 1834, which regulated the obtaining of cadavers for anatomical research.

201. The published transcript of the trial (1828) of William Burke and his accomplice, Helen M'Dougal. Burke's other accomplice, William Hare, turned "King's Evidence" to avoid execution. The frontispiece includes portraits of all three notorious criminals, the most famous of the suppliers of illicit dissection material for anatomy courses in the days before the Anatomy Act of 1834 made it possible for medical schools to obtain legally a steady supply of cadavers. *(Jeremy Norman & Co., Inc.)*

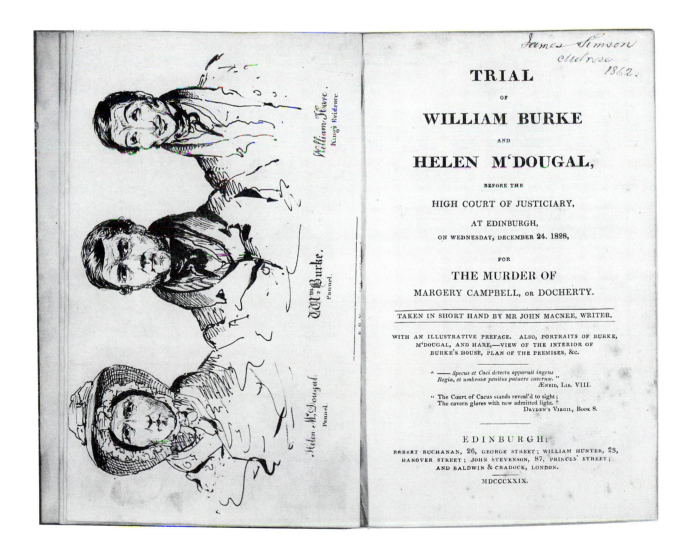

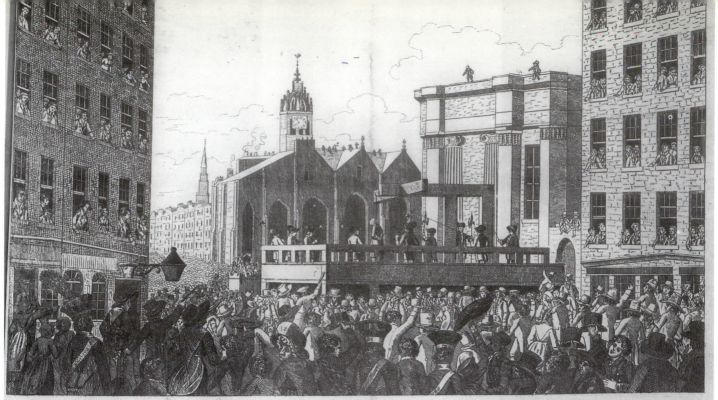

EXECUTION of the notorious WILLIAM BURKE the murderer, who supplied D.ʳ KNOX with subjects.

202. The hanging of William Burke, convicted of murdering people in their sleep so that he could sell their corpses to Robert Knox for his anatomical lectures, was a popular sensation. This original engraving shows the enormous crowd that gathered to witness the event. *(Jeremy Norman & Co., Inc.)*

In America, Valentine Mott (1785-1865), a well-known New York surgeon, described his own travails regarding the procurement of anatomical material in 1810:

Material for dissection was scarce . . . I well remember on one occasion driving, in disguise, a cart containing eleven subjects, from the old Pottersfield Burying ground, sitting on the subjects, and proud enough of my trophies; but we were not always so fortunate, being on many occasions discovered and pursued, and obliged to leave our spoils behind us . . . One little incident of the times occurs to me. A German who had been hung, was "given" for dissection, and with the colored porter, I went in a carriage in the evening, to get the body . . . With great difficulty we exhumed the body, but then my colored associate deserted me, declaring that he could not touch the subject, on account of his having been hung. I had, therefore, to lug the body, attired in its white robes, by my own strength, to the carriage, and partly by menaces, compelled the man to assist me in getting the body into the carriage, and what was still more difficult to get in along with it. So thoroughly was he terrified . . .

During the second half of the nineteenth century the continued advancement of scientific medicine led to the blossoming of such areas of knowledge as cellular pathology, experimental physiology, anesthesia, and bacteriology. The numerous discoveries made in these emerging disciplines in turn stimulated far-reaching advances within surgery. Most important were an understanding and a formal recognition of surgical antisepsis and asepsis. The ability to conduct a surgical operation without fear of the patient succumbing to sepsis would prove a most crucial step in the evolution of the surgical sciences.

CELLULAR PATHOLOGY

Autopsies became one of the major focuses of clinical medicine. Consequently the second half of the nineteenth century was marked by an emphasis on the correlation of the clinical manifestations of illness with specific pathological findings in organs. As surgery became increasingly sophisticated, the importance of pathology became paramount. Each country had its eminent pathologists, who frequently were also practicing clinicians. In many respects the anatomist-surgeon of earlier centuries was replaced by the pathologist-surgeon in the nineteenth century.

The British pathologists were especially brilliant in their descriptions of disease. The earliest of the nineteenth-century British pathologists was Matthew Baillie (1761–1823). His uncle was William Hunter, with whom he had studied at the Windmill Street School. Baillie's *Morbid Anatomy*, published in 1793, was the first systematic textbook of morbid anatomy, which for the first time treated the subject as an independent science. Six years later Baillie produced the first systematic atlas of pathology, *A Series of Engravings, Accompanied with Explanations, Which Are Intended to Illustrate the Morbid Anatomy of Some of the Most Important Parts of the Human Body* (1799–1803). This work was intended to illustrate the preceding *Morbid Anatomy*, but with its extensive descriptive text for each plate the atlas could be appreciated separately. The black-and-white engravings, prepared by John Hunter's artist and amanuensis, William Clift (1775–1849), depicted numerous specimens from Hunter's collection. Within the text were descriptions of the morbid appearances of each organ in systematic succession, accompanied by complete case histories.

Richard Bright (1789–1858), who had studied with Astley Cooper (1768–1841), became a physician at Guy's Hospital, where he worked 6 hours a day in the wards and the postmortem room and lectured on materia medica and clinical medicine. He was considered the leading consultant of his time, and his two-volume *Reports of Medical Cases* (1827–1831) helped solidify his reputation. Bright's name remains associated with his description of chronic nonsuppurative nephritis. His many contributions to medical knowledge included the differentiation of renal from cardiac edema and the correlation of albuminuria with nephritis.

Thomas Addison (1793–1860), like Bright, worked at Guy's Hospital and was considered more brilliant as a lecturer on pathology and as a diagnostician than as a practitioner. He is eponymically remembered for his description of chronic adrenocortical insufficiency caused by destruction of both adrenal glands by tuberculosis or by idiopathic cortical atrophy. Addison's clinical notations were fully detailed in his classic monograph, *On the Constitutional and Local Effects of Disease of the Suprarenal Capsules* (1855).

The pathologist Thomas Hodgkin (1798–1866) strongly stimulated the study of tissue pathology in Great Britain with his two-volume *Lecture on the Morbid Anatomy of the Serous and Mucous Membranes* (1836–1840). An eccentric personality, Hodgkin is best remembered for his description of chronic enlargement of the lymph nodes, often cervical at the onset and then generalized, together with enlargement of the spleen and, sometimes, the liver. He died in Jaffa, Palestine, while on a philanthropic mission.

As in Britain, the principal French studies in pathology were made primarily by clinicians. After the death of Bichat in 1802 his ideas were carried into pathology by Jean Cruveilhier (1791–1874). A pupil of Guillaume Dupuytren (1777–1835), Cruveilhier held the first chair of pathology at the University of Paris. His two-volume *Anatomie Pathologique Du Corps Humain* (1829–1842) was among the most splendidly illustrated works on the subject. Cruveilhier's name is associated with numerous pathological conditions and anatomical entities.

The rise of cellular pathology first became evident in Austria and Germany. Unlike the British and French schools, where the availability of corpses for postmortem examination was often limited, the great medical institutions in the German-speaking countries were the centers where autopsies were most often performed. The prosector and his cadre of eager students completed prodigious numbers of pathological studies.

The first of many great German pathologists was Carl Rokitansky (1804–1878), who ranks with Morgagni among the greatest of all writers on gross pathology. Rokitansky was a Czech who worked in Vienna at the Institute of Pathology. Unlike many of his colleagues in the early nineteenth century, he was a nonpracticing physician. This work arrangement would become commonplace by the end of the century, when pathologists were no longer treating patients. Rokitansky performed an enormous amount of work in pathology: it is estimated that he personally completed more than 30,000 postmortem examinations during his 50-year career. Rokitansky's three-volume *Handbuch Der Pathologischen Anatomie* (1842–1846), his most famous work, appeared when he was 38 years of age.

The rise of modern medicine and surgery is inextricably linked with the career of Rudolf Virchow (1821–1902), one of the greatest figures in the evolution of pathology and a dominant figure in European medicine of the second half of the nineteenth century. Virchow received his doctor of medicine degree from Berlin (1843), became assistant prosector at the Charité in 1845, and 1 year later was promoted to full rank. Virchow was an outspoken personality who often found himself in personal difficulties because of his brash demeanor. In 1856 he was appointed professor of pathology at the university in Berlin and concurrently assumed directorship of that city's Pathologic Institute.

Virchow was an individual of many interests: he served in the Prussian parliament in 1862 and from 1880 until 1893 was a member of the German Reichstag. During the Franco-Prussian War (1870–1871) he organized the Prussian Ambulance Corps and ran an army hospital in Berlin. Among his most lasting contributions to medicine was the founding of the periodical *Archiv Für Pathologische Anatomie,* long known as *Virchow's Archives*.

Virchow's *Die Cellularpathologie In Ihrer Begrundung Auf Physkologische Und Pathologische Gewebelehre* (1858) is one of the most important medical books ever written. Virchow strove to integrate clinical medicine, morbid anatomy, and physiology. As the founder of cellular pathology, Virchow stressed the concepts that all cells come from other cells and that disease is an alteration of the normal structure and function of these cells.

Of Virchow's many students the most prominent was Julius Cohnheim (1839–1884). After having been an assistant in the Pathologic Institute in Berlin, Cohnheim assumed the chairs of pathology in Kiel, Breslau, and Leipzig. He introduced the method of frozen section in microscopic pathology. He was considered an elegant experimental pathologist, as evidenced by the *Neue Untersuchungen Uber Die Entzundung* (1873) and the two-volume *Vorlesungen Uber Allgemeine Pathologie* (1877–1880). The last years of Cohnheim's life were made difficult by severe complications from gout, which caused his early demise.

203. The renowned pathologist Rudolf Virchow attending an operation in Paris in 1900. *(Bildarchiv Preussicher Kulturbesitz, Berlin.)*

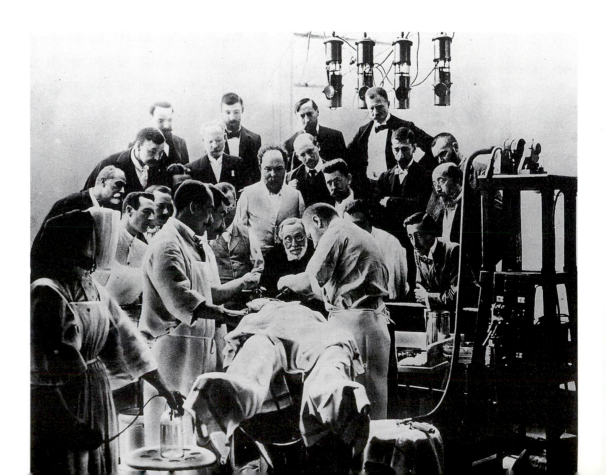

The concept of a surgeon who also acted as a pathologist was most evident in the United States. The country's first extensive and systematic work on the subject, *A Treatise on Pathological Anatomy* (1829), was authored by William Horner (1793-1853). Horner received his degree in medicine from the University of Pennsylvania (1814), and served as prosector to Casper Wistar (1760-1818), the university's first professor of anatomy. Horner later worked with John Syng Dorsey (1785-1818) and Philip Syng Physick (1768-1837). When the latter resigned his position, Horner was named professor of anatomy at his alma mater. Horner in turn was succeeded by Joseph Leidy (1823-1891).

Horner was quite a prolific writer and authored two of the earliest anatomical texts in the United States, *Lessons in Practical Anatomy* (1823) and the two-volume *Treatise on Special and General Anatomy* (1826). Horner's surgical accomplishments included the treatment of ectropion of the lower eyelid (1837) and the first operation to be performed in which the maxilla was excised without an external incision in the cheek (1850). He is eponymically remembered for his description of the tensor tarsi muscle, also known as the pars lacrimalis musculi orbicularis oculi.

The most important pathological text to be written by a bonafide surgeon during the nineteenth century and the first in English was Samuel Gross's (1805-1884) two-volume *Elements of Pathological Anatomy* (1839). Gross was among the most influential surgeons working in the United States. The range of his intellectual work, his prodigious literary output, and his outstanding clinical acumen explain his enormous influence on the practice of medicine, both in his own country and in Europe. Born in Pennsylvania, Gross commenced the study of medicine as an apprentice in 1824. He was a precocious student and within a short time had mastered Wistar's two-volume *System of Anatomy*. Gross desired to increase the breadth of his medical education and matriculated at the Jefferson Medical College in Philadelphia. He graduated in 1828, after writing a thesis on the nature and treatment of cataract.

Early in his professional life Gross's talent as a medical writer first became apparent. In 1828 and 1829 he undertook the translation of four texts authored by French and German physicians. In 1830 he completed his *Anatomy, Physiology, and Diseases of the Bones and Joints*, which represents the first systematic orthopedic text written by a surgeon in the United States.

Gross's clinical practice was minimally successful and in 1833 he was appointed demonstrator of anatomy at the Medical College of Ohio. Two years later, the medical department of Cincinnati College was organized and Gross was offered the chair of pathological anatomy. At that time he delivered the first systematic course of lectures on pathological anatomy ever given in America. His dissections, extensive reading, and numerous visits to the slaughterhouses of Cincinnati constituted the research for his *Elements*.

During the spring of 1840 the chair of surgery at the University of Louisville became vacant. Gross was offered the position, accepted the offer, and spent the next 15 years there. During those years he authored his *Experiments and Critical Inquiry into the Nature and Treatment of Wounds of the Intestines* (1843), the first text on experimental animal surgery to be written in the United States. During the late 1840s he completed *A Practical Treatise on the Diseases, Injuries and Malformation of the Urinary Bladder, the Prostate Gland, and the Urethra* (1851), the first American textbook to provide a systematic approach to genitourinary diseases. In 1854 Gross authored *A Practical Treatise on Foreign Bodies in the Air Passages*.

In 1856 Gross accepted the chair of surgery at his alma mater, where his reputation as the country's most influential surgeon of the nineteenth century would be solidified. In 1859 he authored his massive, two-volume *System of Surgery*. Considered among the most significant surgical treatises of its time, *System of Surgery* went through six editions, the last in 1882.

Among Gross's monographs was *A Manual of Military Surgery* (1861), which was written during the Civil War and was intended to serve as a battlefield surgical manual for the military surgeon. In addition to authoring textbooks, Gross

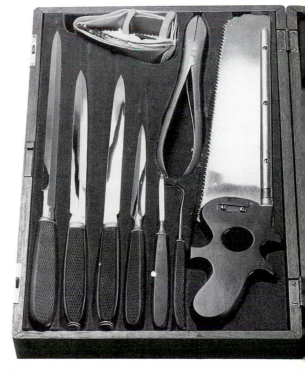

204. An amputation set used by the great American surgeon and medical writer Samuel D. Gross. *(Mütter Museum, College of Physicians of Philadelphia.)*

made numerous contributions to medical journals and founded and edited the *Western Medical Gazette,* the *Louisville Medical Review,* and the *North American Medico-Chirurgical Review.*

Gross was widely acclaimed as a medical historian. In 1861 he found time to complete the 800-page *Lives of Eminent American Physicians and Surgeons of the Nineteenth Century.* Fifteen years later he provided in a lengthy journal article an account of the previous century of American surgery. In addition, he wrote a *History of American Medical Literature from 1776 to the Present Time* (1876).

The most admirable of all Gross's talents was his ability to be organized and supremely efficient. Besides his many clinical responsibilities, he was the twentieth president of the American Medical Association (1868) and founder and first president of the American Surgical Association (1880).

Perhaps Gross's greatest continuing gift to the surgical world has been the famous painting of him by Thomas Eakins (1844-1916). This renowned work depicts Gross in his operative amphitheater before the days of listerian antisepsis. Of underlying significance in this work, Gross was typical of the older American surgeons of that era, who were slow to understand and accept the value of Lister's carbolic acid treatment of surgical wounds.

Among other surgeons in the United States who authored pathology texts was David Gilliam (1844-1923), a gynecologist renowned for his treatment of uterine prolapse. In 1877 Gilliam held the chair of pathology at Columbus Medical College in Ohio. While there, he began writing *The Essentials of Pathology* (1883), the first work devoted solely to pathology and written by an American surgeon. Gilliam is eponymically remembered for an operation for retroversion of the uterus in which the round ligaments are sutured to abdominal wall fascia.

In 1895 John Collins Warren (1842-1927), son of John Mason Warren (1811-1867) and professor of surgery at Harvard Medical School, wrote his *Surgical Pathology and Therapeutics.* Warren, who had taught pathology for many years, intended this work to summarize his lectures and research. He also authored *The Anatomy and Development of Rodent Ulcer* (1872) and *The Healing of Arteries After Ligature in Man and Animals* (1886).

EXPERIMENTAL PHYSIOLOGY

As important as the progress of nineteenth-century pathology was to the overall development of surgery, the rise of experimental physiology was similarly crucial. The masters of physiology in the second half of the century were Hermann von Helmholtz (1821-1894), Claude Bernard (1813-1878), Carl Ludwig (1816-1895), Charles Brown-Sequard (1817-1894), Hugo Kronecker (1839-1914), Henry Bowditch (1840-1911), and Ivan Pavlov (1849-1936). The true pioneer of experimental physiology at the start of the century, however, was Francois Magendie (1783-1855) of France. He was born in Bordeaux and educated in Paris but never held an academic appointment. Like most early nineteenth-century researchers, Magendie combined the dual careers of medical practitioner and laboratory experimentalist. In 1822 he demonstrated that the anterior spinal nerve root is motor and that the dorsal, or posterior, is sensory. Magendie described his momentous experiment:

> . . . section of the dorsal root abolishes sensation, section of ventral root abolishes motor activity, and section of both roots abolishes both sensation and motor activity . . .

Magendie's observations have since been incorrectly attributed to Charles Bell (1774-1842). Magendie was also the founder of the first periodical devoted exclusively to physiology, the *Journal De Physiologie Experimentale* (1821).

Jean-Leonard Poiseuille (1799-1869) of Paris is best remembered for his elaboration of the observation that the quantity of fluid flowing from a narrow tube (comparable in size to that of the small arteries) is directly proportional to the pressure gradient, the viscosity coefficient, and the fourth power of the diameter of the tube.

In the United States little experimental physiologic research was conducted before the Civil War. A paucity of laboratories and the lack of a cadre of scientists able to perform basic research were the major difficulties. One individual, however, did attain worldwide recognition for a series of experiments conducted in an isolated military outpost in northern Michigan and the wilderness of upstate New York. William Beaumont (1785-1853) was the first to study the gastric juice in situ, which was obtained through a permanent fistula. Beaumont received his initial medical education as an apprentice to a general practitioner in St. Albans, Vermont, from 1810 to 1812. In December 1812 he enlisted as a surgeon's mate in the United States Army. After serving for 3 years, Beaumont entered private general practice in Ogdensburg, New York. His experience in practice was unsatisfactory, and in late 1819 Beaumont reentered the army as a post surgeon. He was assigned to Mackinac Island, Territory of Michigan, where he remained through 1825.

On June 6, 1822, a 19-year-old French-Canadian hunter by the name of Alexis St. Martin was wounded in the upper abdomen by an accidental shotgun blast. The incident occurred just outside the fort where Beaumont was stationed, and his treatment of St. Martin's injury was to have a tremendous impact on the evolution of medicine and surgery:

> The charge . . . entered posteriorly, and in an oblique direction, forward and inward, literally blowing off integuments and muscles of the size of a man's hand, fracturing and carrying away the anterior half of the sixth rib, fracturing the fifth, lacerating the lower portion of the left lobe of the lungs, the diaphragm, and perforating the stomach . . .

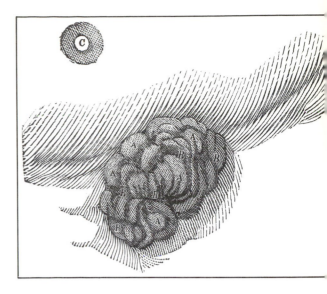

205. The gastric fistula in William Beaumont's patient, Alexis St. Martin, which enabled the army surgeon Beaumont to study the physiology of digestion in vivo. Beaumont was one of the first Americans to conduct medical research of worldwide significance. Remarkably he accomplished this from a rural outpost on the American frontier. *(From the author's collection.)*

206. Portrait of William Beaumont in 1850 by Chester Harding (1792-1866). *(Washington University School of Medicine Library, St. Louis.)*

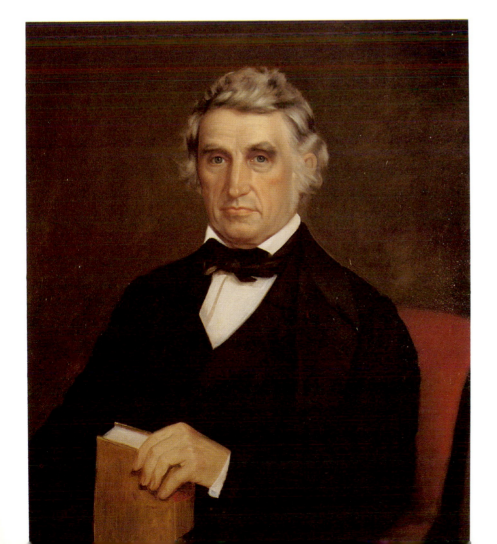

I saw him in twenty-five or thirty minutes after the accident occurred . . . examination proved . . . a portion of the stomach was lacerated through all its coats, and pouring out the food he had taken for his breakfast, through an orifice large enough to admit the fore finger . . .

By the 6th of June, 1823, one year from the time of the accident, the injured parts were all sound, and firmly cicatrized, with the exception of the aperture in the stomach and side . . . The perforation was about two and a half inches in circumference, and the food and drinks constantly exuded, unless prevented by a tent, compress and bandage . . .

In the spring of 1824 he had perfectly recovered his natural health and strength; the aperture remained; and the surrounding wound was firmly cicatrized to its edges. In the month of May, 1825, I commenced my first series of gastric experiments on him . . .

When he lies upon the opposite side, I can look directly into the cavity of the stomach, observe its motion, and almost see the process of digestion—I can pour in water with a funnel, or put in food with a spoon, and draw them out again with a syphon. I have frequently suspended flesh, raw and roasted, and other substances in the hole, to ascertain the length of time required to digest each; and at one time used a plug of raw beef, instead of lint, to stop the orifice, and found that in less than five hours it was completely digested off.

The series of experiments, which continued periodically through 1833, was summarized in Beaumont's classic *Experiments and Observations on the Gastric Juice, and the Physiology of Digestion* (1833). Beaumont's work was the most important research on the physiology of digestion before Pavlov's. The primitive conditions, the lack of laboratory facilities, and the tenacity of Beaumont in completing his tasks made his experiments even more remarkable. The publication of the monograph was treated with indifference in the United States because there were few experimental physiologists to appreciate the importance of his observations. In Europe many of the leading scientists, including Johannes Müller (1801-1858) and Andrew Combe (1797-1847), thought highly of Beaumont's observations.

Henry Bowditch (1840-1911) established the first physiological research laboratory in the United States at Harvard in 1871. His work with nerve conduction was accomplished by paralyzing the motor nerve endings in the muscle with curare. These observations ultimately led to the discovery of local anesthesia (1884), spinal anesthesia (1885), regional nerve blocks (1901), and peridural anesthesia (1921).

In France an early proponent of experimental physiology, Claude Bernard (1813-1878), had abandoned his clinical career for the laboratory. Because his earliest intentions were to become a surgeon, Bernard's first medical textbook, *Precis Iconographique De Médicine Opératoire Et D'Anatomie Chirurgicale* (1848), co-authored with Charles Huette, was on operative surgery. Bernard was a staunch proponent of experimental medicine, and his compulsive attitude toward physiological research resulted in his description of the concept of homeostasis. He was particularly interested in digestive and vasomotor systems and clarified the multiple functions of the liver, the association of the pancreas and diabetes, and the ability of the nervous system to dilate and constrict the smaller arteries.

Under the direction of Ivan Pavlov (1849-1936), a pupil of Rudolph Heidenhain (1834-1897) and Carl Ludwig, great advances were made in late nineteenth-century Russian physiology. Pavlov was director of the Institute for Experimental Medicine in St. Petersburg (1890) and in 1904 received the Nobel Prize for Medicine. Although he is rarely recognized as a surgeon, much of his success can be traced to his technical skills in operating on laboratory animals. He was known by his assistants as an outstanding ambidextrous surgeon who could construct gastric and pancreatic fistulas with great ease. Pavlov clearly learned his operative skills from Heidenhain, who is remembered primarily for his operative creation of a small sac or pouch of the stomach totally separated and closed off from the main cavity but with an opening through the abdominal wall, fashioned for the purpose of obtaining gastric juice and for studying gastric secretions. Pavlov improvised on his mentor's surgical creation by fashioning a

Профессоръ И. П. Павловъ.

ЛЕКЦIИ
о
РАБОТѢ ГЛАВНЫХЪ
ПИЩЕВАРИТЕЛЬНЫХЪ ЖЕЛЕЗЪ

С.-ПЕТЕРБУРГЪ.
1897.

207. First edition of Pavlov's classic work on the physiology of digestion, published in St. Petersburg in 1897, which led to the concept of conditioned reflexes. *(Jeremy Norman & Co., Inc.)*

miniature stomach in which a section of the stomach of a dog was physically shut off from all communication with the main part of the organ and was connected to the outside by a fistula. Through the use of the "Pavlov stomach" Pavlov's most influential work on the conditioned reflex was able to proceed.

ANESTHESIA

Numerous efforts have been made throughout history to relieve the discomfort of surgical operations by various measures, and the epoch of ultimate conquest of pain is one of the most important in the evolution of surgery. Soporific, narcotic, and analgesic agents such as hashish, mandrake, and opium had been put to use for thousands of years. Alcoholic beverages, too, had been used to render a patient oblivious enough to pain to permit the performance of surgical procedures on the surface of the body or on the bones. However, the systematic operative invasion of body cavities and the inevitable progression of surgical history could not occur until an effective means of rendering a patient insensitive to pain was developed.

In the late eighteenth century Franz Mesmer (1734-1815) of France began to promote a system of medical treatment based on his confused doctrine of a universal magnetic fluid that influences tides and humans alike. Mesmer was a great showman and self-promoter, and his treatment became such a popular health care sensation that it was as much a social movement as a medical practice. Mesmer proposed the concept of animal magnetism, in which certain individuals possessed the power of transmitting what he termed "the harnessed powers of the cosmic energies." These cosmic energies were supposedly remarkable in their abilities to alleviate pain and suffering. Although Mesmer was a blatant charlatan, his *Mémoire Sur La Découverte Du Magnétisme Animal* (1779) served as a basis for the scientific development of hypnosis and suggestion in psychiatry, which has been termed, after him, "mesmerism."

After the publication of Mesmer's book, the use of hypnotism and its offshoot, somnambulism, emerged as a method of pain relief for surgical operations. William Topham (1810-1895) authored an account of the first major operation performed in England with the use of hypnosis as a form of anesthesia (1842). The hip amputation was performed by Squire Ward, a surgeon, and the hypnotic state was induced by Topham. Controversy caused by this operation led to the publication of several additional texts about mesmerism.

James Braid (1795-1861) of Fifeshire, Scotland, was a surgeon who settled in Manchester and became interested in the subject of animal magnetism (1841). He proved that a self-induced sleep could be brought about by a fixed stare at a bright, inanimate object. Braid also showed that the mesmeric influence is entirely subjective, and he could find no evidence to suggest that a fluid or other "energy matter" passes from the operator to the patient. He termed this subjective trance hypnosis and authored a monograph on the subject, *Neurypnology, or the Rationale of Nervous Sleep* (1843).

John Elliotson (1791-1868) was president of the Royal Medical and Chirurgical Society in London. In 1843 he authored *Numerous Cases of Surgical Operation Without Pain in the Mesmeric State*. Disputes about his views of hypnotism were quite bitter and led to his eventual resignation.

The most impressive record regarding hypnosis was compiled by James Esdaile (1808-1859), a British surgeon who practiced in India. He performed more than a hundred operations after induction of a mesmeric state in Hindu convicts. Esdaile described these stunning successes in *Mesmerism in India, and Its Practical Application in Surgery and Medicine* (1846). On returning to Scotland, Esdaile found that self-reliant Europeans differed from the more impressionable Hindus in not being particularly susceptible to the hypnotic state.

As anatomical knowledge and surgical techniques improved, the search for safer methods to prevent pain became more pressing. In 1784 James Moore (1763-1834) revived the concept of nerve compression as a means of achieving

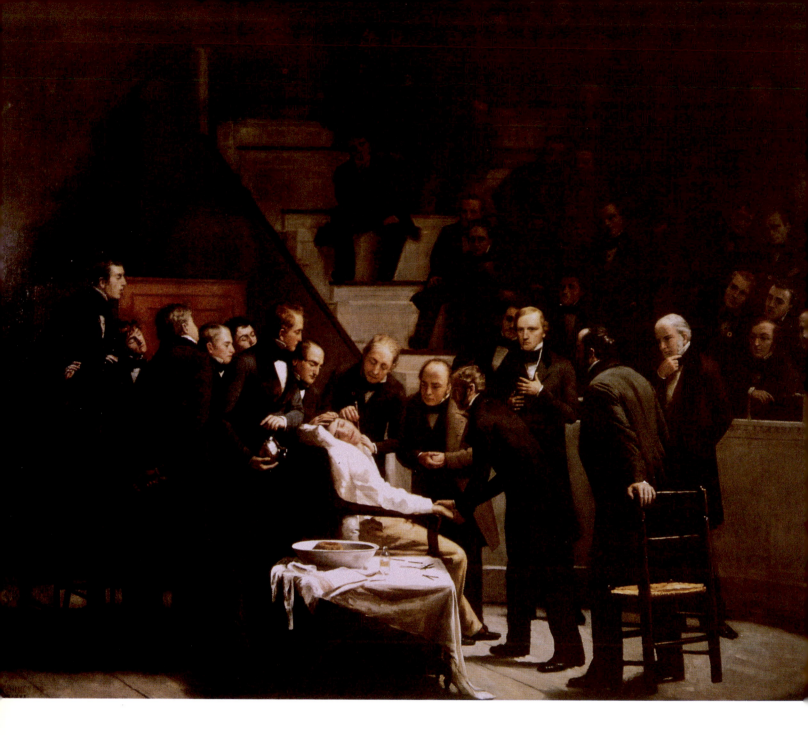

208. *Ether Day* by Robert Hinckley (1853–1941). This huge canvas (96 by 115 inches) was a somewhat romanticized reconstruction of the world's first surgical operation conducted with the use of chemical anesthesia at Massachusetts General Hospital on October 16, 1846. Hinckley, an American artist who had studied in Paris, is believed to have begun the painting in 1882 and to have spent more than 10 years researching the historic event that it records before finishing the painting in 1893. In the center, rear, is John Collins Warren, who performed the surgery. *(Boston Medical Library.)*

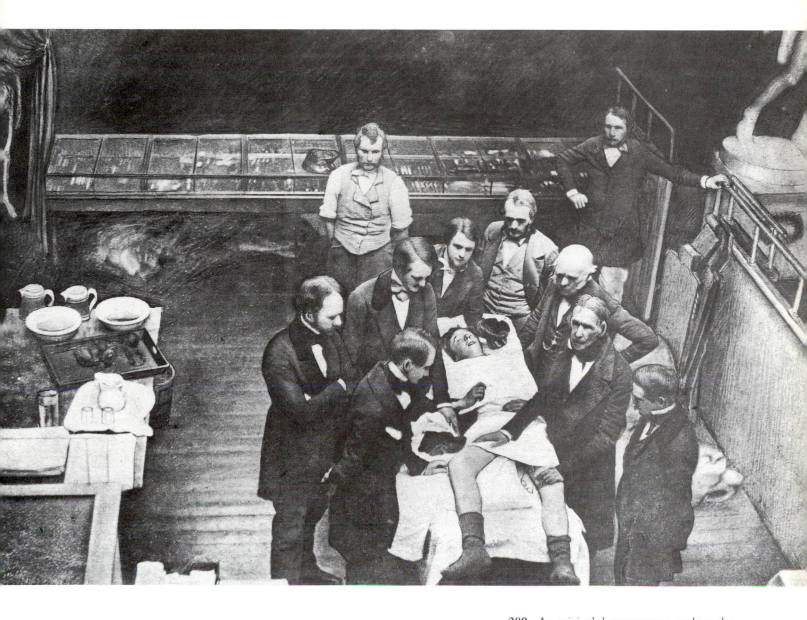

209. An original daguerreotype made at the second operation performed with the use of ether anesthesia on October 17, 1846. During the first operation on the previous day the photographer, Josiah Hawes of the daguerreotype studio of Southworth and Hawes in Boston, was so unnerved at the sight of blood that he did not take any photographs. Presumably he or his assistant had a less delicate stomach on the following day. Compare this actual photograph of the ether dome at Massachusetts General Hospital with Hinckley's painting. The chair in which the patient sat during the demonstration on the previous day is on the right. The surgeon, John Collins Warren, who is said to have appreciated the value of surgical anesthesia with the remark, "Gentlemen, this is no humbug," stands in the right foreground. At the head of the operating table, in the center rear of the photograph, wearing a checked vest, is the anesthesiologist, the dentist William T. C. Morton. In the left foreground facing Warren is the orthopedic surgeon, Jacob Henry Bigelow, who announced the discovery of ether anesthesia to the world in his scientific paper published in the *Boston Medical & Surgical Journal. (Boston Medical Library.)*

333

analgesia. In his *A Method of Preventing or Diminishing Pain in Several Operations of Surgery* he described a special clamp to be used in extremity amputation.

By the early 1830s ether, nitrous oxide, and chloroform had been discovered. Humphry Davy (1778-1829), who early in his career had been a surgeon's assistant, revealed the anesthetic properties of nitrous oxide and suggested its use during surgical operations (1800). Henry Hickman (1800-1830) was only 20 years of age when he was made a member of the Royal College of Surgeons of London. In 1824 he carried out a series of experiments by operating, without causing pain, on animals after the administration of carbon dioxide gas. His work, the first true research regarding inhalation anesthesia during surgery, was received with little interest, and no clinical applications were ever made of it.

Concurrent with the research being conducted in Europe, interest in nitrous oxide and ether was developing in the United States. "Laughing gas" parties and "ether frolics" were in vogue. Young people were amusing themselves with the pleasant side effects of these compounds. Throughout the 1830s and 1840s itinerant "professors" of chemistry would travel to villages, towns, and cities to lecture on these new gases and demonstrate their exhilarating effects. Often the most important part of such presentations consisted of having young members of the audience inhale ether vapor or nitrous oxide. These individuals lost the sense of equilibrium, felt little pain, and acted with an apparent loss of inhibition.

It became evident to various American physicians and dentists that the pain-relieving qualities of ether and nitrous oxide could be applicable to surgical operations and tooth extraction. By December 1844 a dentist from Hartford, Horace Wells (1815-1848), had grasped the concept of inhalation anesthesia. To publicize his discovery, Wells asked John Collins Warren (1778-1856), professor of surgery at the Massachusetts General Hospital, for permission to demonstrate his claims. In January 1845, in front of a class at Harvard Medical School, Wells administered nitrous oxide to a schoolboy as an anesthetic for tooth extraction. The level of anesthesia was too light, however, and the boy screamed out. Wells was labeled a fake, and his career never recovered from the embarrassing episode.

Wells had ventured into a brief dental partnership with another dentist, William Morton (1819-1868), during the mid-1840s. He shared his findings with Morton, but little of consequence came from this initial briefing. Shortly thereafter Morton resettled in Boston, where he became acquainted with Charles Jackson (1805-1880), one of the most eccentric and bizarre of all personalities connected with the discovery of surgical anesthesia. Jackson, an 1829 graduate of Harvard Medical School, was more a mineralogist and geologist than a physician. In September 1846 Jackson suggested to Morton that sulfuric ether mixed with air would make a more suitable anesthetic agent than nitrous oxide. Morton proceeded to experiment with this new concept. He in turn asked John Collins Warren to let him administer the substance to another surgical patient. On October 16, 1846, Morton gave his first public demonstration of the effects of the then "anonymous" liquid in a patient from whom Warren removed a small, congenital vascular tumor of the neck. After the operation Warren, greatly impressed with the new discovery, uttered his famous words: "Gentlemen, this is no humbug." Morton repeated his successful demonstration the following day in another patient, and the second operation, for a small lipoma of the arm, was performed by George Hayward (1791-1863). Although both demonstrations were successful, Morton initially was unwilling to disclose the nature of his new agent because of his desire to patent it, so he permitted no more public trials for 3 weeks.

In early November of 1846 Henry Bigelow (1818-1890) began to "force the issue" of further demonstrations by telling Morton that his demonstration would have no meaning unless the agent were used during the performance of a "capital," or major, operation. Bigelow also suspected that the preparation was sulfuric ether, and he so advised Morton. Subsequently, on November 6, Morton again called on George Hayward, the surgeon from Massachusetts General Hospital, and asked if he might use his preparation on a patient for whom Haywood

THE

BOSTON MEDICAL AND SURGICAL JOURNAL.

VOL. XXXV.   WEDNESDAY, NOVEMBER 18, 1846.   No. 16.

INSENSIBILITY DURING SURGICAL OPERATIONS PRODUCED BY
INHALATION.

Read before the Boston Society of Medical Improvement, Nov. 9th, 1846, an abstract having been
previously read before the American Academy of Arts and Sciences, Nov. 3d, 1846.

By Henry Jacob Bigelow, M.D., one of the Surgeons of the Massachusetts General Hospital.

[Communicated for the Boston Medical and Surgical Journal.]

It has long been an important problem in medical science to devise some method of mitigating the pain of surgical operations. An efficient agent for this purpose has at length been discovered. A patient has been rendered completely insensible during an amputation of the thigh, regaining consciousness after a short interval. Other severe operations have been performed without the knowledge of the patients. So remarkable an occurrence will, it is believed, render the following details relating to the history and character of the process, not uninteresting.

On the 16th of Oct., 1846, an operation was performed at the hospital, upon a patient who had inhaled a preparation administered by Dr. Morton, a dentist of this city, with the alleged intention of producing insensibility to pain. Dr. Morton was understood to have extracted teeth under similar circumstances, without the knowledge of the patient. The present operation was performed by Dr. Warren, and though comparatively slight, involved an incision near the lower jaw of some inches in extent. During the operation the patient muttered, as in a semi-conscious state, and afterwards stated that the pain was considerable, though mitigated; in his own words, as though the skin had been scratched with a hoe. There was, probably, in this instance, some defect in the process of inhalation, for on the following day the vapor was administered to another patient with complete success. A fatty tumor of considerable size was removed, by Dr. Hayward, from the arm of a woman near the deltoid muscle. The operation lasted four or five minutes, during which time the patient betrayed occasional marks of uneasiness; but upon subsequently regaining her consciousness, professed not only to have felt no pain, but to have been insensible to surrounding objects, to have known nothing of the operation, being only uneasy about a child left at home. No doubt, I think, existed, in the minds of those who saw this operation, that the unconsciousness was real; nor could the imagination be accused of any share in the production of these remarkable phenomena.

I subsequently undertook a number of experiments, with the view of ascertaining the nature of this new agent, and shall briefly state them,

16

210. The first page of Henry Jacob Bigelow's paper, which announced to the world the discovery of ether as an anesthetic in surgery, as published in the *Boston Medical & Surgical Journal* (1846) vol 35, pp 309–317 and 379–382. *(Jeremy Norman & Co., Inc.)*

was preparing to perform an amputation. Hayward agreed but with the stipulation that Morton must tell the surgeons what the vapors were. Morton acquiesced, and the following day, after Morton had rendered the patient unconscious and insensitive to pain, Hayward successfully performed the amputation. Morton then authorized Bigelow to make a detailed public announcement, and the discovery of surgical anesthesia was formally announced in the *Boston Medical and Surgical Journal* on November 18. News of the momentous event spread rapidly throughout the United States and Europe: a new epoch in the history of surgery had begun.

The lives of many of the principles involved in the initial discovery of surgical anesthesia ended in tragedy. Morton and Jackson became involved in a dispute concerning priority in the discovery of surgical anesthesia. Multiple lawsuits were filed and culminated in Morton's retirement from dental practice. Morton then became involved in one failed business venture after another; he died in abject poverty after having a stroke while on the way to his lawyer to institute another set of lawsuits against Jackson. Late in life Morton was somewhat vindicated by the United States Congress, when members of Congress investigated his claims and a committee composed of physicians reported, after

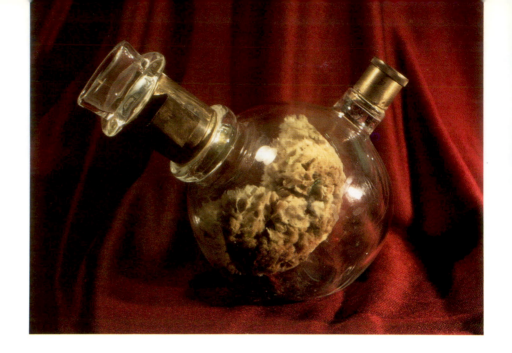

211. Morton's ether inhaler. *(Warren Museum, Harvard Medical School.)*

hearing the evidence on both sides, that he was entitled to the merit of the discovery. Bills appropriating $100,000 for the discovery of practical anesthesia were introduced into Congress during three separate sessions of that body but were never passed. Jackson continued his lifelong struggle to proclaim himself the inventor of surgical anesthesia. His efforts culminated in mental instability, and he spent the last 15 years of his life in the McLean Asylum for the Insane in Massachusetts. After Bigelow's announcement about inhalational anesthesia, Wells attempted to establish his priority in both the United States and France. In late 1847 he moved to New York, where in January 1848 he was arrested and incarcerated for throwing sulfuric acid on a prostitute. That night Wells, who had become mentally deranged, committed suicide by severing a vein in his arm.

The American surgeon Crawford Long (1815-1878) also played an important role in the early history of anesthesia. Long practiced surgery in Georgia, where in January 1842 a group of his friends induced him to have an "ether frolic" in his home. His friends proceeded to inhale the ether and during their antics received various bruises and cuts. None of these had been felt, and Long concluded that ether must abolish pain. He promptly attempted to prove the value of his observation and in March 1842 successfully removed a small cyst from the neck of a patient who had been etherized. The gentleman underwent a second such procedure that June. By September 1846 Long had performed eight various surgical operations after the administration of ether. Only after he had become aware of the controversy that had surrounded the claims of Jackson, Morton, and Wells did Long publish his results (1849). Consequently, although Long's use of sulfuric ether for surgical anesthesia antedates Morton's by more than 4 years, he never received credit for this discovery.

Oliver Wendell Holmes (1809-1894) supplied the term *anesthesia* for the new discovery, which would become firmly established in the surgeon's repertoire by the end of 1847. In that year Marie Flourens (1794-1867) of Paris authored a paper announcing that chloroform had an anesthetic effect analogous to that of ether. Little notice was taken of this report until later in the year, when James Young Simpson (1811-1870) of Edinburgh independently demonstrated the value of chloroform as an anesthetic agent.

Simpson studied surgery under Robert Liston and at the age of 19 years obtained his license to practice medicine. He obtained additional training under John Thomson (1765-1846) and in 1840 was elected professor of obstetrics at the University of Edinburgh. Simpson had used ether as early as January 1847. In an attempt to find an anesthetic agent less irritating to the eyes and nose than ether he discovered the advantages of chloroform, or, as it was first called, chloric ether. On November 15, 1847, the first public demonstration of this new anesthetic occurred when Simpson, acting as anesthesiologist, placed a 4-year-old boy under the influence of chloroform. James Miller (1812-1864), who was professor of surgery, proceeded to remove one of the bones in the youngster's forearm. Simpson advanced the thesis of chloroform's superiority over ether in a paper presented before the Medico-Chirurgical Society of Edinburgh (1847). He advocated the use of chloroform not only in operative surgery but also in childbirth.

In 1853 and 1857 John Snow (1813-1858), the royal accoucheur, delivered Queen Victoria's child with the aid of chloroform. The Boston-based physician Walter Channing (1786-1876) was an early advocate of anesthesia in obstetrics. He authored *A Treatise on Etherization in Childbirth* (1848), which brought the importance of this branch of anesthetics into the foreground of attention for the American physician. By the 1850s chloroform was being used more frequently than ether in Europe, whereas the converse was true in the United States.

Although anesthesiology would eventually develop as its own specialty within medicine, virtually all of the early work in the field was completed by surgeons. Snow became the first physician to specialize in anesthesiology. In his *On the Inhalation of the Vapour of Ether in Surgical Operations* (1847) he included an account of a regulating inhaler, which controlled the amount of ether vapor administered to the patient. A year later he described a chloroform inhaler. His most important text, *On Chloroform and Other Anaesthetics: Their Action and Administration* (1858), established a sound scientific basis for the administration of chloroform and ether. Other nineteenth-century discoveries in anesthesiology are listed in the box on p. 338.

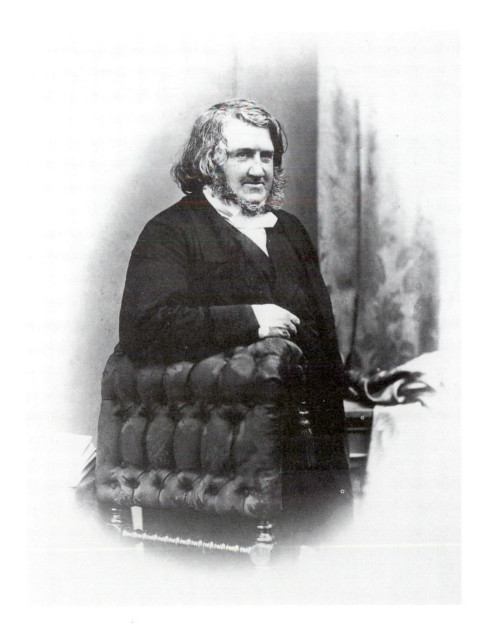

212. Photograph of James Young Simpson, who introduced the use of chloroform as an anesthetic. *(Historical Collections, College of Physicians of Philadelphia.)*

NINETEENTH-CENTURY DISCOVERIES IN ANESTHESIOLOGY

JOHANN HEYFELDER (1798-1869)
Ethyl chloride (1848)
Trichloroethylene (1864)

AUGUST FREUND (1835-1892)
Cyclopropane (1882)

ALFRED EINHORN (1856-1917)
Procaine (1899)

EDMUND ANDREWS (1824-1904)
Oxygen-nitrous mixture (1868)

LÉON LABBE (1832-1916)
Preanesthetic medication (1872)

PIERRE ORÉ (1828-1889)
Human intravenous anesthesia (1874)

Local anesthesia was introduced in 1884. Most of the credit for the discovery of the local anesthetic property of cocaine belongs to Carl Koller (1857-1944), a German ophthalmological resident. However, some research indicates that a suggestion made by Sigmund Freud (1856-1939) in a paper describing his observations on the effects of cocaine (1884) and Freud's recognition of the drug's anesthetizing qualities may actually have given Koller the idea to revolutionize eye surgery by using cocaine as the first local anesthetic. Koller used a 2% solution of cocaine and described its potent local anesthetic action on the conjunctiva and cornea. After conducting experiments in animals, he self-administered cocaine and, later, administered cocaine to patients while performing various types of ophthalmological operations. In September 1884 Koller reported the results in his important paper, *Vorläufige Mitteilung Uber Locale Anästhesirung Am Auge*. His discovery aroused enormous interest, and his methods were soon adopted for various otolaryngological procedures.

Koller's discovery was reported back to American physicians by Henry Noyes (1832-1900) in a short letter published in the New York *Medical Record*. Publication excited great interest in the New York City medical community, and demand for the alkaloid derivative of the coca leaf skyrocketed. William Halsted and several of his associates at Roosevelt Hospital, including Richard Hall (1856-1897) and James Corning (1855-1923), began performing experiments with the drug and demonstrated that it could be used to anesthetize deeper structures via injection into all parts of the body. Such conduction anesthesia gained rapid popularity, since it was simple and required minimal amounts of cocaine. Hall wrote in the first article of this research group in December 1884:

> I made some experiments on myself, to determine the best mode of using it. The preparation was a four-per-cent solution . . . Injecting subcutaneously six minims on the dorsal surface of the forearm . . . caused complete loss of sensation over an area extending downward . . . obviously following the distribution of a cutaneous branch of the ulnar nerve . . . Thus, in a number of experiments made by Dr. Halsted and myself, we have found that, injected subcutaneously into the leg or forearm . . . it will cause anaesthesia for a distance of two or three inches below the point of injection . . . it is obvious that, when the limits of safety have been determined, it may find very wide application.

In 1885 Halsted wrote his *Practical Comments on the Use and Abuse of Cocaine.* It is a poignant irony of surgical progress that after repeated self-experimentation both Hall and Halsted suffered the ravages of cocaine addiction for the remainders of their adult lives. Hall died of a ruptured appendix after having moved to Santa Barbara, California, to seek improvement in his health. Halsted, one of America's greatest surgeons, kept the secret of his addiction from all but his closest associates.

Corning demonstrated that cocaine exerted a prolonged anesthetic effect when the circulation in the anesthesized area was decreased. Thus longer operations could be performed without repeated injections of cocaine and possible problems with overdosage. More important, Corning performed spinal block within a year after the demonstration of the anesthetic property of cocaine, only 10 months after the discovery of conduction anesthesia. He also authored *Local Anesthesia in General Medicine and Surgery* (1886), the first textbook on local anesthesia.

Carl Schleich (1859-1922), a German surgeon, introduced the method of infiltration anesthesia (1892). He showed that local anesthesia can be induced by the injection of a local anesthetic solution directly into the tissues to be anesthetized. Both infiltration and conduction anesthesia were further improved by the work of Karl Bier (1861-1949) at his surgical clinic in 1899.

BACTERIOLOGY AND SURGICAL ANTISEPSIS AND ASEPSIS

Although the introduction of general anesthesia had occurred by the mid-nineteenth century, the evolution of surgery could not proceed smoothly until the grave problem of postoperative and hospital-acquired infection was resolved. Hospital diseases such as erysipelas, septicemias and fulminating gas gangrene were of paramount concern in the health of a postoperative patient. Without a clear understanding of bacteriology and the sources of infection, however, most surgeons could do little more than provide high standards of surgical cleanliness, adequate hemostasis, and open-wound management.

Historically most of the deadly diseases had been viewed as the result of some form of "contagion." It was incorrectly believed, however, that these various infections were generated spontaneously in wounds and, alternatively, that air itself was the etiological agent for suppuration. Accordingly, since the time of Paré, increasingly sophisticated attempts had been made to exclude air from wounds by means of elaborate dressings. The spurious notion that suppuration in a wound favored healing, expressed by the term "laudable pus," would plague surgeons until the pathogenic character of bacteria was completely understood and accepted.

Despite prophetic work by many individuals, most physicians and surgeons were slow to accept the theory of infection caused by microorganisms. For the surgeon the most frightening scourge, especially after traumatic injuries, was hospital-acquired gangrene. Thus it was the military surgeons who toward the end of the eighteenth century and in the early nineteenth century sounded warnings that went largely unheeded regarding the nature and origin of wound infection.

In 1753 John Pringle (1707-1782) had shown that putrescence in dead flesh could be prevented and suspended by submersion in acid solutions. Still, any recognition of the nature of the contagion responsible for wound infection and any thought of implementing chemical means to render surgical instruments and other operative material reasonably safe were a century away.

"Hospital gangrene" was first given its name by Claude Pouteau (1724-1775), a surgeon from Lyon, France. In 1744, when Pouteau was a young medical student, he pricked his finger while working on a cadaver. He continued to care for the infected, gangrenous wounds of many patients. At the same time, his finger became inflamed and gangrenous. Pouteau was able to recover but not before he realized that wound infection was contagious. Throughout his professional career Pouteau maintained an active interest in the problem of wound infection and authored several treatises on the subject. In 1760 he recognized the similarity between surgical wound infections and puerperal fever. In his *Mélanges De Chirurgie* (1760) he wrote about an outbreak of puerperal fever in Lyon and noted that the bodies of women who had died of puerperal fever revealed an erysipelas-like inflammation. In 1775 Pouteau emphasized the importance of clean hands for wound dressers, calling the neglect of this observance detrimental to any patient. He exhorted hospital administrators to enforce the measure. Pouteau's three-volume *Oeuvres Posthumes* (1783) provided an exacting description of hospital-acquired gangrene and provided its name, *pourriture d'hôpital*.

During the American Civil War the evils of hospital gangrene were most evident. For a wounded or sick soldier no surgical disease was more horrible than what began as a small black spot on an extremity and soon spread throughout the limb, causing a rotten, evil-smelling mass of dead flesh. The condition occurred chiefly in hospitals and temporary shelters, where sick and wounded soldiers were crowded together, ventilation was poor, and the supply of utensils, bandages, lint, and clean instruments was insufficient.

The overwhelming majority of cases of hospital gangrene seem to have been bacterial in origin, but because hospital gangrene is an extinct pathologic entity, whether it was a *Streptococcus* species, a mixed infection, or a *Clostridium* organism remains historical conjecture. Contemporary descriptions of various cases suggest that virtually all the acute and chronic gangrenous infections and progressive ulcerative lesions were labeled as hospital gangrene, such as gas gangrene, acute hemolytic gangrene *(S. pyogenes),* progressive bacterial synergistic gangrene, and chronic undermining burrowing ulcer.

During the Civil War Joseph Jones (1833-1896), a surgeon-major in the Confederate army who extensively studied hospital gangrene and in 1869 authored a 60-page account of the surgical difficulties encountered by the wounded soldier, stated:

Whether we regard the local affection as a poisoned wound, in which contagious poisonous matters are continually generated, and from which the surrounding living tissues are contaminated; or look upon the destruction of the tissues as the result of deficient and perverted inflammatory reaction, the principles of the local treatment would in either view be much the same. These indications are best fulfilled by the liberal and thorough application of concentrated nitric acid to the gangrenous parts.

213. Hospital gangrene of the upper extremity secondary to a gunshot wound. Chromolithograph after the painting by Edward Stauch. From the *Medical & Surgical History of the War of the Rebellion,* vol 2, part 2, p. 739, 1877. *(From the author's collection.)*

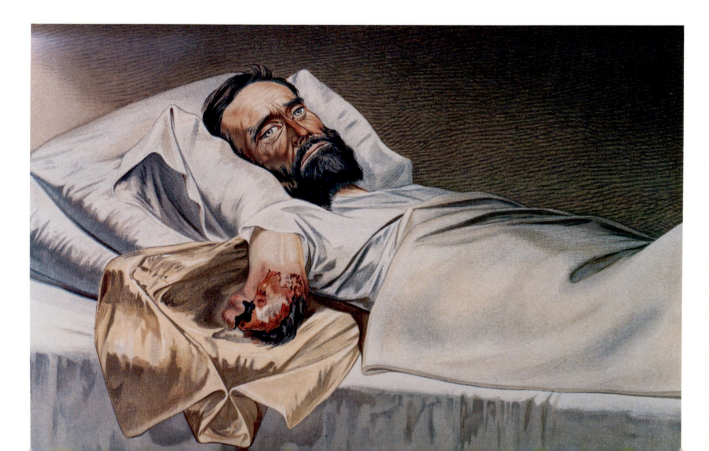

As this is a painful procedure, the patient as a general rule should be placed under the influence of chloroform and sulfuric ether. During the insensibility of the patient, the surgeon should carefully examine the wound, and first remove all the gangrenous tissues, using the scalpel and scissors, and causing the part beneath to bleed quite freely. All sinuses formed under the skin, or between the muscles, or in the cellular or areolar tissue, must be freely laid open, and the dead tissues removed. The entire wound is then to be carefully wiped out with a sponge or dry lint, and the concentrated acid applied with a brush or mop to the entire surface; and care should be taken that the acid penetrate into all the sinuses and cavities. If any diseased part be untouched or undestroyed by the acid, the disease will recommence and spread from that point.

Although the death of young mothers as a result of childbed (puerperal) fever had been known for centuries, few satisfactory attempts were made to correct the situation. Besides Pouteau, other individuals who had sharply reduced the occurrence of postpartum infection by regimens of personal and environmental cleanliness, limited vaginal examinations during labor, and active cleansing of beds and linens were Charles White (1728-1813), Alexander Gordon (1752-1799), Joseph Clarke (1758-1834), and Robert Collins (1801-1868).

In 1843 Oliver Wendell Holmes (1809-1894) read a paper, *On the Contagiousness of Puerperal Fever,* to the Boston Society for Medical Improvement. He had learned that a New England physician had been able to halt an epidemic of puerperal fever in his obstetrical practice in the summer of 1835 by washing his hands in calcium chloride after attending women in childbirth who were affected by the disorder. In a strongly worded presentation Holmes argued that women in childbirth should never be treated by physicians who had been conducting postmortem sections or treating patients with puerperal fever. He felt that the disease could be conveyed in that manner from patient to patient.

Holmes was a graduate of both the Harvard medical school and the Harvard law school. He became known as a poet and a physician and served his alma mater as professor of anatomy and physiology (1847-1882). Holmes was also dean of the medical school from 1847 to 1853. His writings, including an 1855 monograph entitled *Puerperal Fever as a Private Pestilence,* were vigorously attacked and were not accepted for many years by the medical establishment.

Holmes's views predated the findings of Ignaz Semmelweis (1818-1865), one of the most tragic figures in the history of medicine. Semmelweis, a Hungarian pupil of Rokitansky, became an assistant to Johann Klein in the first obstetrical department of the Allgemeines Krankenhaus in Vienna, where the maternity clinic was divided into two sections. The first, ward 1, was run by Klein and the second, ward 2, by midwives. Ward 1, in which 10% of the women died, had acquired a particularly bad reputation concerning puerperal fever. Ward 2 had a 3% death rate.

Semmelweis noticed that the two wards differed in that students came directly into ward 1 from the postmortem room. They would immediately undertake vaginal examinations with unclean hands. In ward 2 the midwives devoted much attention to personal cleanliness, particularly the washing of hands before any examinations.

In March 1847, at approximately the same time that Semmelweis had made the preceding observation, a professional acquaintance of his died of sepsis after sustaining a prick of the finger while performing an autopsy. Semmelweis was present at this man's autopsy, and when he examined the body of his colleague, he was struck by its pathological appearances, which were the same as those in the women of ward 1 who had died of puerperal fever. Semmelweis believed that his observations were proof of the infectious nature of puerperal sepsis. To bolster his belief, Semmelweis demonstrated transmission of fatal puerperal fever to parturient rabbits directly after delivery by introducing pus that had been recovered from the vaginal tract of women dying of the disease into the rabbits' vaginas. Sepsis did not occur when chlorinated lime also was introduced.

By mid-May Semmelweis, with the approval of Klein, instituted a vigorous program of obligatory handwashing with chlorinated water before the performance of any vaginal examinations. Almost immediately the death rate in ward 2 dropped to the same level as that in ward 1. Like those of most innovators, Semmelweis's viewpoints were met by vigorous opposition. The most vocal of his newfound critics was his own chief, Klein, who recommended Semmelweis's dismissal to the minister of education, over the strenuous objections of several prominent members of the Vienna medical faculty, especially Rokitansky, Josef Skoda (1805-1881), and Ferdinand von Hebra (1816-1880).

Semmelweis became bitterly discouraged and disgusted with his treatment in Vienna. He returned to Budapest, where he eventually became professor of obstetrics at the University of Pest. While there, he published his important monograph *Die Aetiologie, Der Begriff Und Die Prophylaxis Des Kindbettfiebers* in 1861. By that time the world of medicine had essentially forgotten about Semmelweis, and his unstable, brooding personality disintegrated into mental instability. He was committed to a mental institution in July 1865 and within 1 month was found dead, supposedly as a result of sepsis.

As important as the work of the early obstetricians and gynecologists was, it had no immediate repercussions in surgical practice. Although simple, routine methods of cleanliness were quite effective in reducing sepsis, an understanding of bacteria and antisepsis lacked a scientific basis, which remained to be elucidated by the research of Louis Pasteur.

Pasteur (1822-1895) graduated from the Ecole Normale in Paris in 1847, eventually to serve as professor of chemistry at the Sorbonne (1867-1889) and director of the Institut de Pasteur (1889-1895). Pasteur was not a physician, but his research into fermentation and microorganisms probably had as great an influence on medicine's progress as that of any individual in history.

Pasteur's earliest research concerned the fermentation of wine, which had long been thought to be caused by the spontaneous generation of some noxious agents or by purely chemical means. He showed conclusively (1856-1859) that the conversion of sugar to lactic acid in fermentation was due to "small corpuscles." By 1861 the success of his experiments led to the downfall of the theory of spontaneous generation. Pasteur further confirmed that putrefaction was a biological process and that meat and fluid, like tissue and blood, did not putrefy if they were kept in such a way that all air was excluded from them. He next showed that putrefaction was caused by the presence of bacteria and that this cause applied to putrefaction in wounds. Pasteur differentiated between aerobic and anaerobic organisms and discovered that the spoiling of wine by microorganisms could be prevented by partial heat sterilization (pasteurization) at a suitably high temperature (55° to 60° centigrade).

Around 1875 Pasteur focused his attention on microorganisms that cause disease in humans. He discovered *Clostridum septicum,* the first pathogenic anaerobe to be identified. By 1880 Pasteur had begun work on the attenuation of infective organisms. Noting that fowls inoculated with an attenuated form of the chicken cholera bacterium acquired immunity, he developed the concept of a protective inoculation with attenuated living cultures. Pasteur's principles laid the foundations of the science of immunology; he was able to develop vaccines against anthrax, rabies, and swine erysipelas.

In 1878 Pasteur presented a paper on the theory of germs and its application to surgery before the Academy of Medicine in Paris. On that occasion he stated:

> If I had the honor of being a surgeon, impressed as I am with the dangers of exposure to the germs and microbes scattered on the surface of all objects, particularly in hospitals, not only would I use only perfectly clean instruments, but after washing my hands with the greatest care and submitting them to a rapid flaming, which would cause no more discomfort than a smoker feels in passing a burning coal from one hand to the other, I would use charpie, bandages, sponges previously exposed in air at 130 to 150 [C] degree temperature; I would never use water which had not been submitted to a temperature of 110 to 120 [C] degrees. All this is practical. In this way I would have to fear only the germs in suspension in the air around the patient's bed; but observation shows us each day that the number of such germs is insignificant compared to those scattered in the dust on the surface of objects or in the clearest of ordinary water.

The burgeoning of bacteriology was ably continued by Robert Koch (1843-1910). Unlike Pasteur, Koch was a physician; he received his degree in medicine from Gottingen (1866). He was profoundly influenced by the teachings of the histologist Friedrich Henle (1809-1885), the pathologist Wilhelm Krause (1833-1910), and the physiologist George Meissner (1829-1905). After serving as a military physician in the Franco-Prussian War, Koch was appointed a district physician at Wollstein, where he began his studies in microbiology by curtaining off a corner of his office for a laboratory.

By 1876 Koch had worked out the life cycle of the anthrax bacillus *(Bacillus anthracis)*. Although this work was met by initial skepticism, he persisted and in the following year described techniques for staining and photographing bacteria. In 1878 appeared Koch's famous monograph, *Untersuchungen Uber Die Aetiologie Der Wundinfektionskrankheiten*. This work on the origins of wound infection provided convincing evidence, for the first time, of the pathogenicity of pyogenic organisms. The bacteria of six different kinds of surgical infections were described, along with pathological findings and methods for culturing the microorganisms through successive generations.

Koch was soon recognized as the world's most innovative microbiologist; he moved to Berlin, where he became a member of the Imperial Board of Health and professor of hygiene and bacteriology at the university. There he discovered (in 1882) the tubercle bacillus *(Mycobacterium tuberculosis)* and in the accompanying paper characterized the steps necessary to establish the specific causative role of a microorganism in disease. Koch's postulates included (1) that the organism must be present in all cases of the disease, (2) that it is capable of cultivation in pure culture, (3) that animal inoculation from the culture reproduces the disease, and (4) that the organism can be recovered from inoculated animals and again be grown in pure culture.

Among Koch's many experimental observations was that certain kinds of bacteria were killed by aqueous dilutions of mercuric chloride. In addition, he noted that for purposes of disinfection chlorine, bromine, and iodine were reliable and quick acting. These facts complemented Koch's demonstration of the superiority of heat over chemicals in destroying and inhibiting bacterial action and became important to the progress of surgery.

In the long evolution of surgery the contributions of few individuals are preeminent. Joseph Lister (1827-1912) can be placed in such an elite list because of his monumental efforts to introduce systematic, scientifically based antisepsis in the treatment of wounds and the performance of surgical operations. Lister pragmatically applied Pasteur's findings to disease. Since infection was now known to be caused by a microscopic living body carried in the air, Lister devised a means of prevention and secured its adoption by a skeptical profession.

Lister was born into a well-to-do Quaker family from Upton in Greater London. His father, Joseph Jackson Lister (1786-1869), was a wine merchant who devoted his leisure time to microscopy and optics. Lister's father is considered one of the founders of modern microscopy because of his important improvements in achromatic lenses. Father and son were strongly devoted to one another; there is little doubt that the father's "hobby" and pursuit of scientific knowledge strongly influenced the son's approach to experimental research.

Young Lister, not a member of the Church of England, could not attend Oxford or Cambridge college. Instead, he entered the arts faculty of University College in London in 1844, graduated with a bachelor of arts degree in 1847, and commenced his medical course at University College in October 1848. There he came under the influence of the physiologist William Sharpey (1802-1880), the chemist Thomas Graham (1805-1869), and the ophthalmologist Thomas Wharton Jones (1808-1891). On completion of his medical studies (1851), Lister served for 9 months as house physician under Walter Walshe (1812-1892) and house surgeon under John Erichsen (1818-1896). By 1852 Lister was a fellow of the Royal College of Surgeons.

Guided by the advice of Sharpey, Lister proposed making a tour of various surgical centers, starting with Edinburgh. He intended to stay 1 month in Scotland but

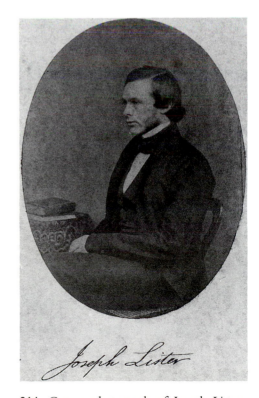

214. Cameo photograph of Joseph Lister, beneath which he inscribed his signature. This photograph was taken about 1865, near the time when Lister made his revolutionary discoveries concerning the value of antisepsis in surgery. *(Jeremy Norman & Co., Inc.)*

343

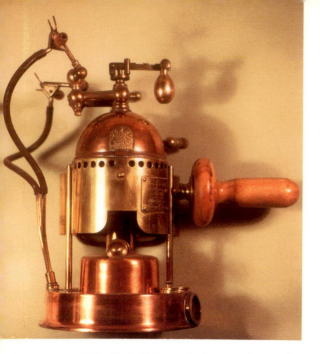

215. Carbolizer used for spraying a fine mist of disinfectant carbolic acid over the operative field and the operative team during surgery, according to Lister's antiseptic principles. *(Warren Museum, Harvard Medical School.)*

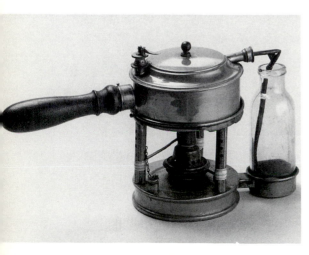

216. Carbolic acid diffuser presented by Joseph Lister to the American surgeon, William Williams Keen. *(Mütter Museum, College of Physicians of Philadelphia.)*

remained for 24 years. In Edinburgh Lister became assistant to James Syme (1799-1870), who made Lister his house surgeon at the Royal Infirmary (1854). It is said that Lister was the only individual with whom Syme never quarreled. The relationship was further strengthened when Lister married Syme's daughter Agnes in April 1856. In the autumn of that year Lister was appointed assistant surgeon to the Edinburgh Royal Infirmary and remained on the staff for just over 3 years. During that time he began his initial studies of the early stages of inflammation and authored a paper (1858) on that subject and on wound healing.

At the urging of Syme, Lister applied for the position of professor of surgery in Glasgow. Although elected to that position, he had to wait almost 2 years before he was appointed surgeon to that city's Royal Infirmary. The 9 years that Lister spent in Glasgow are the most important period in his career as a surgeon-scientist. In his Croonian Lecture (1862) Lister dismissed the idea that coagulation of the blood is due to the liberation of ammonia and showed instead that the blood coagulates when the vessels are injured. More important, he demonstrated that by carrying out strict precautions, he could keep blood free from putrefaction indefinitely, thus supporting his theory that bacteria were the cause of wound suppuration. That Lister was a technically adept surgeon was evident in his classic paper on excision of the wrist for tuberculous caries (1865). Still, he noted that amputations and joint excisions he performed continued to carry a death rate of almost 50%.

In the early spring of 1865 a member of the chemistry faculty at Glasgow told Lister about Pasteur's work on putrefaction. Lister was one of the few practicing surgeons of his day who, because of his familiarity with the microscope, possessed the education to accept Pasteur's findings without question. Although he had not heard of Pasteur, these findings were of extreme importance to Lister because they were consistent with his own theories and with his scanty knowledge of wound infections. To Lister it was obvious that an injury inflicted by a traumatic accident was already full of bacteria before the patient arrived at the hospital. Therefore the concept of a hospital-acquired infection was not necessarily correct, since at the moment of injury bacteria were introduced into the wound. Lister conceived that a method must be found to prevent the ingress of germs into the wound deliberately inflicted at operation and that germs must also be destroyed in wounds created outside the hospital.

It was evident to Lister that Pasteur's method of destroying bacteria by excessive heat could not be applied to a patient. He turned to chemical antisepsis, however, and after experimenting with zinc chloride and the sulfites, decided on carbolic acid. Lister was prompted to use the latter substance because it had just been successfully employed to combat the odor of sewage in Carlisle. By April 1865 Lister was instilling pure carbolic acid into wounds, although he would later decrease the concentration. On August 12, 1865, he successfully employed it in a case of compound fracture of the tibia in 11-year-old James Greenlees. In 1867 Lister authored two monumental papers in which he reported on his 2 years of experience with carbolic acid and described its use as an antiseptic principle in the practice of surgery. Lister gave his own account of the epoch-making first case:

My house surgeon, Dr. Macfee, acting under my instructions, laid a piece of lint dipped in liquid carbolic acid upon the wound, and applied lateral pasteboard splints padded with cotton wool, the limb resting on its outer side, with the knee bent. It was left undisturbed for four days, when, the boy complaining of some uneasiness, I removed the inner splint and examined the wound. It showed no signs of suppuration, but the skin in its immediate vicinity had a slight blush of redness. I now dressed the sore with lint soaked with water having a small proportion of carbolic acid diffused through it, and this was continued for five days, during which the uneasiness and the redness of the skin disappeared, the sore meanwhile furnishing no pus . . . But the epidermis being excoriated by this dressing, I substituted for it a solution of one part of carbolic acid in from ten to twenty parts of olive oil, which was used for four days . . . It was clear that there was no longer any danger of deep-seated suppuration, and simple water dressing was employed. Cicatrization proceeded just as in an ordinary granulating sore. At the expiration of six weeks I examined the condition of the bones, and, finding them firmly united, discarded the splints; and two days later the sore was entirely healed . . .

The remarkable retardation of suppuration, and the immediate conversion of the compound fracture into a simple fracture with a superficial sore, were more encouraging facts.

Lister made numerous modifications in the technique of the dressings, the manner of applying and retaining them, and the choice of antiseptic solutions of varying concentrations. Although the use of a carbolic acid spray remains the best-remembered detail, it was eventually abandoned in favor of other substances. Lister not only used the carbolic acid in the wound but also sprayed the atmosphere around the operative field and table. Lister did not emphasize hand scrubbing but merely dipped his fingers into a solution of phenol and corrosive sublimate. He deliberately avoided scrubbing because he was convinced that such action created crevices in the palms of the hands in which bacteria would grow.

A second important contribution that Lister made to surgical technique was the development of sterile absorbable sutures. He was convinced that much of the deep suppuration found in wounds was created by previously contaminated silk ligatures. Lister evolved a carbolized catgut ligature, which was better than any previously produced (1869). He was able to cut short the ends of his suture, thereby closing the wound tightly and eliminating the necessity of bringing the ends of the suture out through the wound.

217. The correct setup for aseptic surgery according to listerian principles:

> The spray is very important in many cases, for it provides an atmosphere in which instruments, & C., may be kept without danger of contamination. In order to have a wide and large antiseptic area in which to work, the spray ought not to be too near, about six or eight feet or more being a suitable distance for a good spray. Care must be taken that the spray is not blown off the part by draughts or by people moving about. The spray is most necessary in opening abscesses or in stitching up wounds, for, to take the latter case, as the wound is not syringed out after the stitches are inserted, septic air may be inclosed in the cavity of the wound, and may give rise to putrefaction if the spray has not been playing over the wound while the stitches were being introduced.

Quotation is from the first treatise on antiseptic and aseptic surgery, W. Watson Cheyne's, (1852-1932) *Antiseptic Surgery, its Principles, Practice, History and Results* (London, 1882). *(Jeremy Norman & Co., Inc.)*

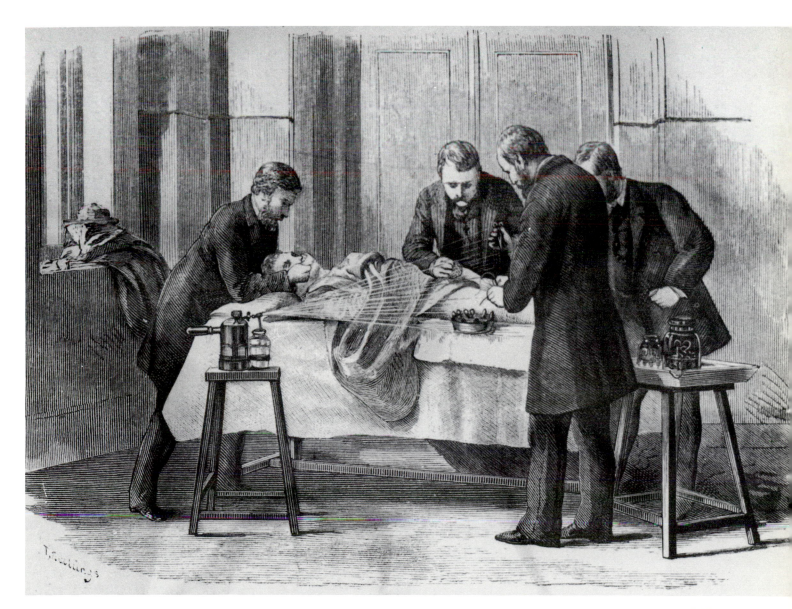

Lister apparently was not happy at Glasgow because he felt overburdened with routine work and lecturing. Twice he applied for other academic appointments but without success. In April 1869 his father-in-law suffered a debilitating stroke, which forced Lister to relinquish his chair of surgery. Syme wanted Lister to succeed him at the hospital, and the governing body agreed. In October Lister left Glasgow to return to Edinburgh.

The next 7 years would be among the happiest of his professional life; nonetheless, Lister's methods were not met with unanimous approval. In 1870 he presented one paper on the salubrious effects of the antiseptic system of treatment on a surgical hospital and another on a method of antiseptic treatment applicable to wounded soldiers. In the latter report Lister described the simplest method he could devise for the use of carbolic acid as an antiseptic on the battlefield, and that year French and German army surgeons implemented the procedure for the first time. In addition, Lister continued his pure scientific research, and in 1873 he isolated *Bacterium lactis* and gave it its name. Four years later he became the first person to obtain a pure culture of a bacterium. Despite his scientific prowess in most cases, his clinical methods were being met with indifference and occasionally with violent opposition.

Like those of Semmelweis and Holmes, neither of whom Lister knew, Lister's theories were most strongly opposed in his own country, particularly by the renowned gynecologist Lawson Tait (1845-1899). Continental surgeons, however, especially those in Germany, quickly adopted the treatment and enthusiastically confirmed the excellent results reported by Lister. The practice gained considerable momentum when Matthias Saxtorph (1822-1900) of Copenhagen (1870), Richard von Volkmann (1830-1889) of Halle (1874), and Johann Nussbaum (1829-1890) of Munich (1875) commented favorably on their treatment of compound fracture with the listerian methods. The latter two surgeons also noted the disappearance of hospital gangrene and pyemia from their respective institutions. In France, Just Lucas-Championière (1843-1913) became Lister's greatest champion and pioneered antiseptic measures in that country.

In 1876 Lister traveled to the United States, where he spoke on his antiseptic dressings at the International Medical Congress being held in Philadelphia in honor of the country's centennial. It was a memorable presentation, lasting more than 3 hours, but American surgeons remained unconvinced of the method's efficacy. As late as 1883, at the first official meeting of the American Surgical Association, more speakers opposed listerian practices than supported them.

In 1877 Lister was invited to accept the chair of surgery at the Anglican King's College Hospital in London. The appointment could not have been offered to a Quaker, so Lister's marriage to Syme's daughter and consequent conversion to the Anglican faith proved important to the latter part of his career. Many of the surgeons of that institution and the general medical profession of London neither openly encouraged nor warmly endorsed the appointment.

It had long been Lister's ambition to return to London, and the opportunity at King's was not to be denied. His initial reception was disheartening. Whereas in Edinburgh he had lectured to throngs of eager, devoted students, in London he gave presentations to apathetic and disinterested young men. His peers generally ignored him, although he was always being sought out by a constant stream of visitors from foreign lands. However, by the time of his retirement in 1893 the number of students in attendance at his biweekly lectures had grown considerably. By patient and persistent effort Lister was able to overcome the resistance of well-known London surgeons to his techniques and saw his doctrines accepted worldwide.

Great achievement and much personal gratification marked Lister's professional life. In 1885 the Royal College of Surgeons invited him to accept the presidency, but Lister, immersed in research and uninterested in medical politics, declined the honor of holding England's premier surgical office. He received a baronetcy in 1883 and became the first medical personage in Great Britain to be raised to the peerage in 1897. His marriage to Agnes Syme was satisfying and serene. Although they never had children, she shared all his work and accompanied him on virtually every trip he made. She was stricken with a fulminating pneumonia while on vacation in Italy and died in April 1893. Without her guidance and support Lister remained a lonely and depressed individual until he died.

Over the years Lister's principles of antisepsis gave way to those of asepsis, or the complete elimination of bacteria. Asepsis was especially promulgated by Ernst von Bergmann (1836–1907), who merged the corrosive sublimate method into steam sterilization (1886) and eventually into the elaborate method of general asepsis (1891). Any lingering doubts about the validity and significance of the momentous concepts Lister had put forth were eliminated on the battlefields of World War I. There the importance of plain antisepsis became an invaluable lesson for surgeons around the world.

218. Surgical instrument set made in London by S. Maw, Son and Thompson, sometime between 1870 and 1900. This set is unusual in that it was made to fit into a doctor's bag for easy transportation. Because these instruments were intended for sterilization, they were made entirely of plated steel. Thus the set can be dated after Lister's exposition of his antiseptic and aseptic principles in 1867. During the last three decades of the nineteenth century Lister's principles were gradually accepted by the surgical community. *(Reproduced by permission of the Trustees of the Science Museum, London; 1188/82.)*

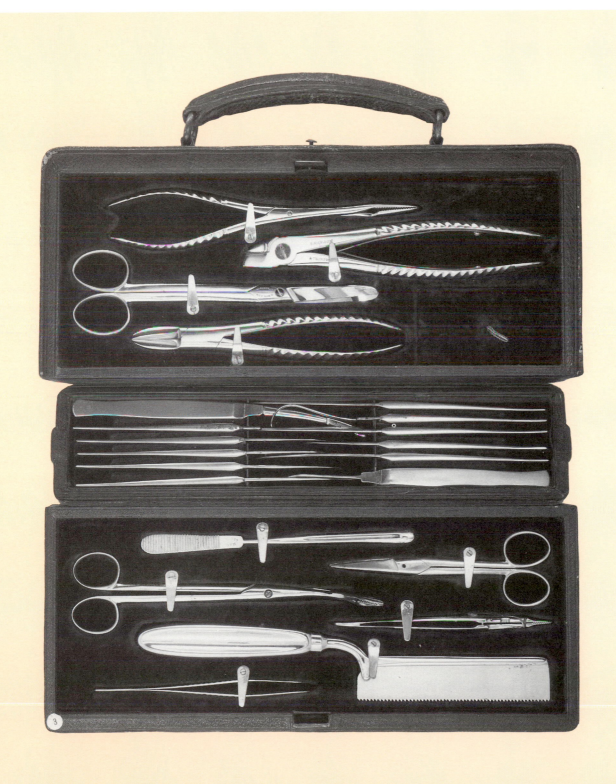

347

Once antiseptic and aseptic techniques had been finally accepted as part of routine surgical practice, it was inevitable that other elaborate antiseptic rituals would similarly take hold. The use of gloves, face masks, operating gowns, and hats naturally evolved. Semmelweis had given significant emphasis to strict hand care, but he had never advocated the use of gloves to protect the patient from the physician or vice versa. There is some indication that a fingernail brush was in vogue by the middle of the nineteenth century, but its use was far from widespread. Johann Walbaum (1724-1799) had first broached the subject of surgical gloves when he described an obstetrical glove that he had devised and used for version (1758). It was made of the cecum of a sheep and was soaked in lukewarm water to make it pliable. When in place, it covered the third, fourth, and fifth fingers and the dorsum of the hand. The thumb and second finger were left bare. In his *Die Beschwerlichkeiten Der Geburtshulfe* (1769) Walbaum noted that the glove and the exposed portions of the hand were smeared with animal fat before introduction into the vaginal canal. Thus the glove was designed primarily as a mechanical contrivance to prevent the hand from sticking to the vaginal walls or the uterus. Secondarily it covered the fingernails so that painful scratches would not occur. This device was not intended to serve any purpose of antisepsis, since the concept did not exist at that time.

The Viennese dermatologist Joseph Plenk (1739-1807) first suggested that a glove could be used for prophylactic purposes. He wrote that a midwife should be careful about introducing an ungloved hand into the vagina of a venereally diseased patient. During the first half of the nineteenth century, gloves had been used or suggested by various physicians. In most instances such gloves were particularly clumsy and interfered with the performance of all types of surgical operations.

In 1843, along with other developments in rubber processing, the process of vulcanization was patented and the use of rubber gloves became a possibility. Five years later William Acton presented a report to the Royal Medical and Chirurgical Society on the advantages of caoutchouc and gutta percha in protecting skin from infection. However, his report dealt strictly with dissections and postmortem examinations, not surgical operations.

Surgeons were generally reluctant to use gloves, primarily because until the 1870s no truly flexible, functional glove had been designed. This situation changed in 1878, when Thomas Forster, an employee of the India-Rubber Works in Surrey, England, was granted both British and United States patents for the "manufacture of gloves for surgical operations." Rubber gloves and surgical operations had finally been brought together.

As physicians and surgeons began to understand the work of Pasteur, Koch, and Lister, it was inevitable that hand coverings would be introduced. Even with the advent of antisepsis, however, surgical garb remained decidedly unsanitary. Berkeley Moynihan (1865-1936), a well-known surgeon from Leeds, wrote of his house-surgeon days (1888) as an assistant to Arthur Mayo-Robson (1853-1933):

> The surgeon arrived, doffed his coat lest he should soil it with blood or pus, rolled up his shirt-sleeves and took down from a cupboard in the passage leading to the theatre an old coat, as a rule a frock coat of antique design which bore many marks of usage, and was stiff here, there, and everywhere with blood. One at least of the coats was worn with special pride, indeed with a certain jauntiness, for it had been inherited from a retiring member of the staff. The cuffs were rolled back a little, just above the wrists, and the hands were washed in a basin. The hands, when clean in a social sense, were soaked in a solution of carbolic acid. The instruments were taken from the cupboard, whose shelves were lined with green baize, and placed in a tray of 1 in 20 carbolic acid, about half an hour before the operation. When all was ready the spray was turned on, and a fine mist of steam, odorous with carbolic acid, soon bathed all engaged in the operation.

The identity of the first surgeon who required that flexible rubber gloves be routinely worn for every surgical operation remains uncertain. William Stewart Halsted (1852-1922), professor of surgery at the Johns Hopkins Hospital in Baltimore, is commonly regarded as the individual who popularized their use. His interest in them, as he described it in his 1913 account of the introduction of gloves in his clinic, was accidental:

> Rubber gloves must, of course be worn by all concerned in the operation . . . In the winter of 1889 and 1890 . . . the nurse in charge of my operating-room complained that the solutions of mercuric chloride produced a dermatitis of her arms and hands. As she was an unusually efficient woman, I gave the matter my consideration and one day in New York requested the Goodyear Rubber Company to make as an experiment two pair of thin rubber gloves with gauntlets. On trial these proved to be so satisfactory that additional gloves were ordered . . . I think it was Dr. Bloodgood, my house surgeon, who . . . was the first to wear them, invariably, when operating . . .
>
> In the report which I made of the first year's work at the hospital, written in November and December, 1890 . . . I stated that the assistant who passed the instruments wore rubber gloves. This assistant was given the gloves to protect his hands from the solution of phenol (carbolic acid) in which the instruments were submerged rather than to eliminate him as a source of infection . . . Dr. Hunter Robb in 1894, in his book on aseptic technic recommended that the operator wear rubber gloves . . . Thus the operating in gloves was an evolution rather than an inspiration or happy thought, and it is remarkable that during the four or five years when as operator I wore them only occasionally, we could have been so blind as not to have perceived the necessity for wearing them invariably at the operating-table.

An element of romance concludes the story of Halsted and the rubber gloves: the operating-room nurse for whom he had ordered the gloves later became his wife.

By the mid-1890s surgeons were becoming satisfied with their antiseptic methods and the attendant results. Wound infection was becoming less of a concern, although difficulties still existed. Rubber gloves remained a curiosity, however, and were not yet considered a part of surgical operative routine. This attitude changed, at least in Germany, when Bernard Krönig (1863-1917) presented results of his research (*Versuche Uber Spiritusdesinfektion Der Hände,* 1894) before his fellow obstetricians of Leipzig. He thoroughly examined the time-honored methods of hand washing, which consisted of a dip in water and a dip in mercury chloride or carbolic acid. Krönig spread gas gangrene spores on the arms of cadavers of children. He then applied various disinfecting agents. Scrapings from the skin were cultured and mice injected. As he expected, most of the animals died of gas gangrene. It is not difficult to imagine the stunned silence of the surgical community as Krönig told them that mechanical cleansing alone, even if carried out for half an hour, is not sufficient to make their skin surfaces bacteria free. Despite Krönig's presentation, the international acceptance of rubber gloves as a necessary adjunct to any surgical operation would not occur until after World War I.

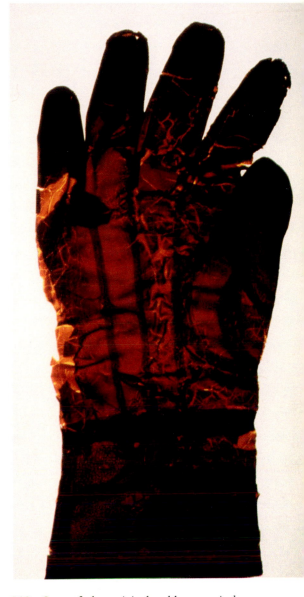

219. One of the original rubber surgical gloves designed by William Stewart Halsted and preserved in lucite. Although Halsted neither invented rubber gloves nor originated their use in surgery, he was the first to promote their widespread application in the surgical community and he is consequently credited with the discovery of rubber surgical gloves. Halsted became interested in the use of rubber gloves as a way of protecting the hands of his favorite operating-room nurse, in whom a dermatitis caused by mercuric chloride developed about 1889. This favorite nurse later became his wife. *(The Alan Mason Chesney Medical Archives of The Johns Hopkins Medical Institutions.)*

X RAYS

Especially prominent among the nineteenth-century discoveries that had an enormous impact on the evolution of surgery were the research conducted by Wilhelm Roentgen (1845-1923) and his elucidation of X rays. Roentgen was professor of physics at Würzburg when, on December 28, 1895, he presented to that city's Physical Medical Society a paper on his most recent work. Having grown interested in the phosphorescence from metallic salts that are exposed to lights, Roentgen made a chance observation in November 1895. When passing a current through a vacuum tube, he noticed a greenish glow coming from a screen on a shelf 9 feet away. This strange glow continued after the current was turned off. Roentgen found that the screen had been painted with a phosphorescent substance (barium platinocyanide). Proceeding with full experimental vigor, he found these invisible rays to be capable of passing through solid objects made of wood, metal, and other materials. Most significant, these rays also passed through the soft parts of the body in such a manner that the bones of his hand were revealed on a photographic plate that he had set up. Within weeks Roentgen presented his findings, and 6 years later, in 1901, he was awarded the first Nobel prize for physics.

Few medical discoveries have been accepted as quickly as X rays were. With amazing rapidity numerous applications were developed, particularly for surgeons. However, because the dangers of X rays were not immediately realized, numerous "martyrs" to the new science learned too late of the seriousness of their X ray–induced injuries.

Surgeons immediately applied the new discovery to the diagnosis and location of fractures, dislocations, and removal of foreign bodies. By March 1896 William Keen (1837-1932), professor of surgery at Jefferson Medical College in Philadelphia, had written America's first article on X rays for the *American Journal of the Medical Sciences*. It included five photographic plates of actual radiographs. During late March, April, and May other published articles discussed further experiments with X rays and their contribution to surgical diagnosis. The most detailed information on roentgenography and surgery was provided by Keen in a chapter in Frederick Dennis's (1850-1934) four-volume *System of Surgery*. Dennis, professor of the principles and practice of surgery at Bellevue Hospital Medical College, had at the last minute asked Keen to contribute a chapter on the newly discovered X ray and its use in surgery. The volume itself was published in July 1896 and represents the first American medical textbook to contain an account of X rays that included actual roentgenograms. Keen was particularly interested in the semantics of roentgenography and wrote that:

> . . . the nomenclature of this subject is a matter of some importance. The popular use of the terms "shadowgraph," "radiography," "rayograph," etc. is greatly to be deplored. Such philological abominations, hybrids of Greek and English are of course wholly inadmissible. The word shadowgraph can only plead its evident meaning as a possible justification. The word skiagraph . . . is far the best, being derived from the Greek word meaning shadow . . . a somewhat similar instrument devised by Mr. Edison is called the fluoroscope.

During the late spring of 1896 the most active American proselytizer for X rays was the Philadelphia surgeon De Forest Willard (1846-1910), professor of orthopedic surgery at the University of Pennsylvania. Willard provided fellows of both the American Surgical Association and the American Orthopedic Association with their first demonstrations of roentgenograms. He showed a series of "roentgen-ray skiagraphs" that included images of talipes equinovarus, tubercular knees, knock-knees, and congenital absence of the fingers, all of which had been made by Arthur Goodspeed (1860-1943), an assistant professor of physics at the University of Pennsylvania.

James White (1850-1916), professor of clinical surgery at the University of Pennsylvania, during a presentation before the American Surgical Association in May 1897, said about X rays:

I must confess that, as with every new discovery, my thoughts turn to its possible application to a subject which has an invincible attraction for me—the cure of cancer . . . I have no results to report . . . I intend to continue my own experiments until I am convinced that they are useless . . . I feel reasonably sure, as in the cancer cases, of doing my patients no harm, if the experiment is an entire failure.

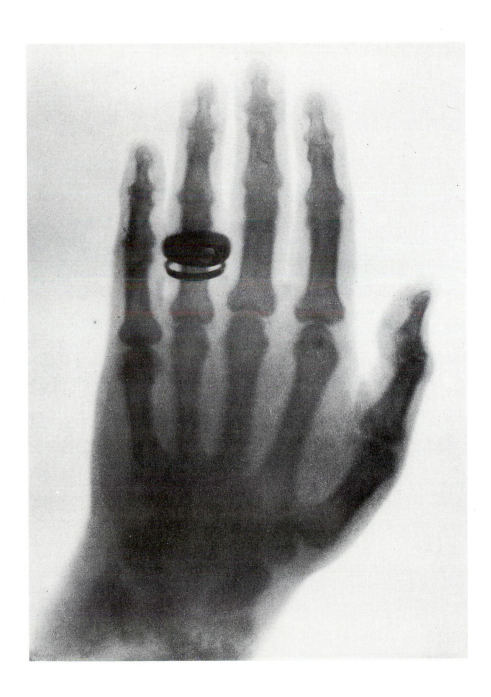

220. Roentgenogram of the hand of the anatomist Rudolph von Kölliker (1817-1905) made in the first and only public demonstration of radiographs (X-rays) by Wilhelm Conrad Roentgen. Roentgen's first paper on radiographs was published and distributed during the first days of January in 1896. The discovery of this imaging method filled such a widely perceived need that the process was almost immediately accepted by the scientific community. By January 23 there was such a clamor for a demonstration that Roentgen appeared before a large audience at the University of Würzburg and radiographed the hand of his colleague, von Kölliker. Copies of this small poster reproducing the radiograph he made were offered for sale. Having no taste for publicity, Roentgen never made another public demonstration of X-rays. (*Jeremy Norman & Co., Inc.*)

BLOOD TRANSFUSION

In 1818 James Blundell (1790-1878), professor of physiology and obstetrics at St. Thomas's and Guy's Hospitals, invented a syringe by means of which he was able to perform transfusions in dogs. In the same year, Blundell recorded the first human-to-human transfusion: a man received 12 to 14 ounces of blood from several donors by means of Blundell's funnel and syringe. The patient died 56 hours after the transfusion. In 1828 Blundell announced the first human-to-human transfusion that did not result in the death of the patient. Blundell established the fundamentals of transfusion, including the incompatibility of interspecies transfusion and the method of indirect transfusion. Blundell, by describing approximately ten cases in a 10-year period, revived interest in blood transfusion after a century-long hiatus.

Among other surgical pioneers in blood transfusion was William Halsted, who in 1881 successfully performed a transfusion in his sister for postpartum hemorrhage with blood drawn into a syringe from one of his own veins. In 1869 the English gynecologist John Braxton Hicks (1823-1897) described the use of sodium phosphate as an anticoagulant in blood transfusion. Further progress in this field was made in 1900, when Karl Landsteiner (1868-1943), who was to win the Nobel prize for medicine in 1930, demonstrated the immunological importance of blood-group antigens and isoantibodies. In 1915 Richard Lewisohn (1875-1962), a New York surgeon, introduced the citrate method of blood transfusion.

SURGICAL EDUCATION AND TRAINING

Far-reaching changes in the manner and methods of educating and training surgeons were among the most important organizational advances in surgery. The haphazard education of surgeons that had held sway for more than 2000 years became a well-defined system, as first promulgated in Germany, Austria, and the United States. By the mid-nineteenth century Germany and Austria had supplanted England and France as the centers of European surgical knowledge, a success due in large measure to the German system of surgical training.

Among the outstanding features of German surgical training were a highly successful integration of the basic sciences with practical clinical teaching by full-time teachers and an unending competitive spirit among the young surgeons in training, with rewards accruing only to the brightest and most strong-willed. The talented German student would choose his area of specialization in his third or fourth year of medical school. If the choice was surgery, for instance, he would petition for a position as demonstrator or voluntary technician in the basic science laboratory. The student would perform simple research assignments and hope to establish a reputation with the head of the institute for the specialty in which he wished to obtain his assistantship. On graduation and at the end of internship, which was considered an integral part of the general medical curriculum, the young doctor would, if fortunate, be asked to become an assistant. The new assistant doctor was then thrust into the thick of an intense competition to become the first assistant. The first assistant, known as the house surgeon or, in modern terms, the chief resident, was selected after several years from a number of well-tried and exhausted assistants. There was no regular advancement of the assistant resident from the bottom to the top of the staff, and only a few assistants ventured to entertain the hope of becoming the first assistant. The first assistant would hold his position until called to a chair of surgery in a small university or until he tired of waiting and went into private practice.

The German plan was adopted by Halsted in his program at the Johns Hopkins Hospital. Although Halsted has long been recognized for his original contributions to the science of surgery, the most far-reaching of his concepts lay in the education, training, and inspiration of a school of surgeons who were imbued with his principles of thought and action. The "Halsted tradition" remains the *sine qua non* of modern surgical residencies.

The resident system of training for surgeons, which Halsted inaugurated in 1889, was unique in its primary purpose. Halsted wished to establish a school of surgery that would eventually disseminate throughout the surgical world the principles and attributes he considered sound and proper. Halsted's aim was to train teachers, not merely competent operating surgeons. His system, however, was not an exact duplicate of the German approach. He insisted on a more clearly defined pattern of organization and division of duties. A larger volume of operative material was at the disposal of the residents, who had a more intimate contact with practical clinical problems and less preoccupation with the pure basic sciences, and responsibility and authority were more concentrated in the resident than in the teacher. In Halsted's classic paper on the training of a surgeon (1904) he described his philosophy and his system:

> We need a system, and we shall surely have it, which will produce not only surgeons but surgeons of the highest type, men who will stimulate the first youths of our country to study surgery and to devote their energies and their lives to raising the standard of surgical science . . .
>
> The surgical staff consists of nine men, eight interns and one extern. The extern is an assistant in surgical pathology . . . four of the interns serve for one year, only the honor men of each class at graduation being entitled to these positions; but the permanent, so-called, consists of four men, the house surgeon and three in line of preferment . . . Great care is exercised in the filling of the vacancy on the permanent staff, which occurs once in two or three years, and advancement is not guaranteed to the appointee. The house surgeon's term of service is still optional. He receives a salary: the other assistants are not paid. The assistants are expected in addition to their ward and operating duties, to prosecute original investigations and to keep in close touch with the work in surgical pathology, bacteriology and, so far as possible physiology.

SURGICAL NURSING

Among the most important principles derived during the evolution of surgery in the nineteenth-century were the need for excellent postoperative care and the awareness that a professionally trained individual would be required to provide such care. Accordingly, the nursing of sick patients by properly trained personnel became a nineteenth-century institution.

During the seventeenth and eighteenth centuries the status and competence of female attendants in hospitals had become quite poor. Theodor Fliedner (1800-1864), pastor at Kaiserwerth on the Rhine, revived the concept of a training program for women, who could then perform social service and take care of the sick. Florence Nightingale (1820-1910), his most famous student, devoted her life to nursing.

The Crimean War (1854-1856) concerned the domination of southwestern Europe, with the allied armies of England, France, Turkey, and Sardinia defeating Russia. The English hospital at Scutari was known to have horrible conditions for its patients. War correspondents vividly described problems at this institution to the English public. National indignation was aroused, and the minister of war asked Nightingale to take charge of the barracks hospital at Scutari.

Nightingale reformed the entire hospital so that within 3 months she was feeding nearly 10,000 men from her diet kitchen and providing them with basic necessities. The death rate among soldiers quickly fell from 42% to 2%. The extent of Nightingale's success was remarkable, and when she returned to England, she was able to raise enough funds to establish the Nightingale Training School for Nurses in 1860, the first organized program of training for nurses and an entirely independent educational institution. Her *Notes on Hospitals* (1859)

221. *Following pages, Florence Nightingale Receiving the Wounded at Scutari. The figure of Florence Nightingale, certainly the most famous nurse of all time, is highlighted in the left center of the painting. Through the doorway on the right the city of Istanbul (Constantinople), Turkey, is visible. Oil painting by Jerry Barratt, late nineteenth century. (Courtesy National Portrait Gallery, London.)*

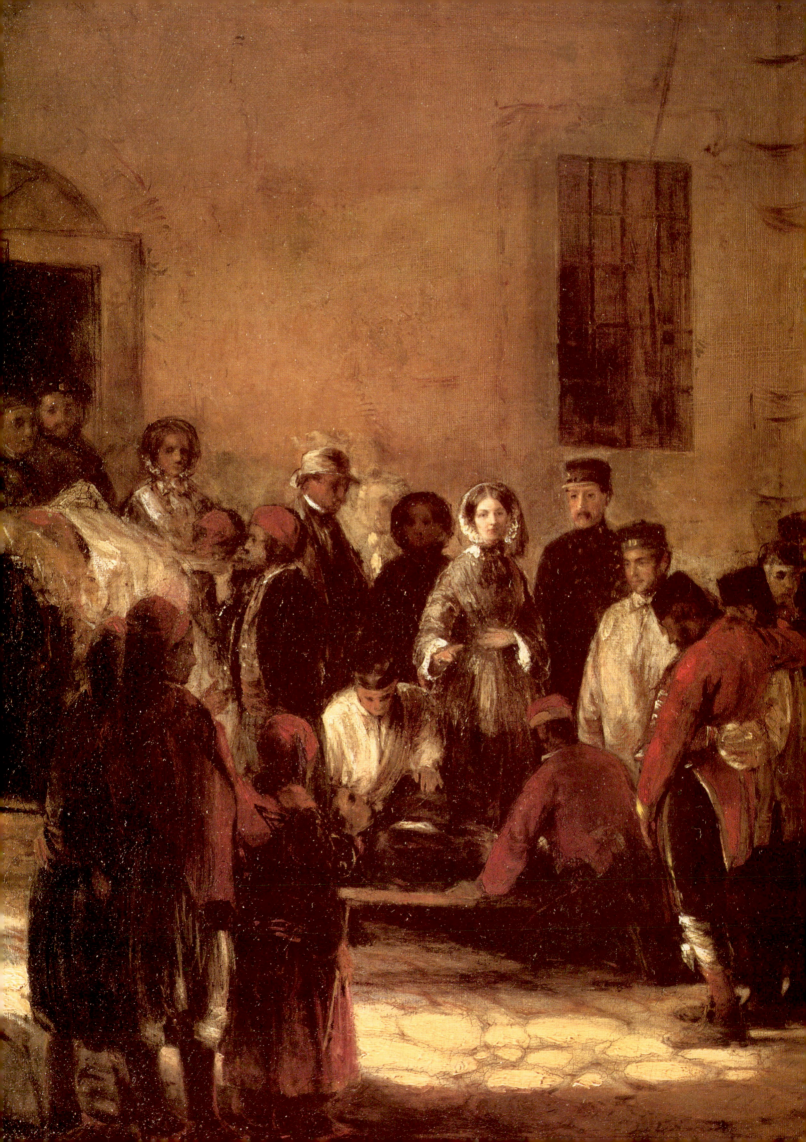

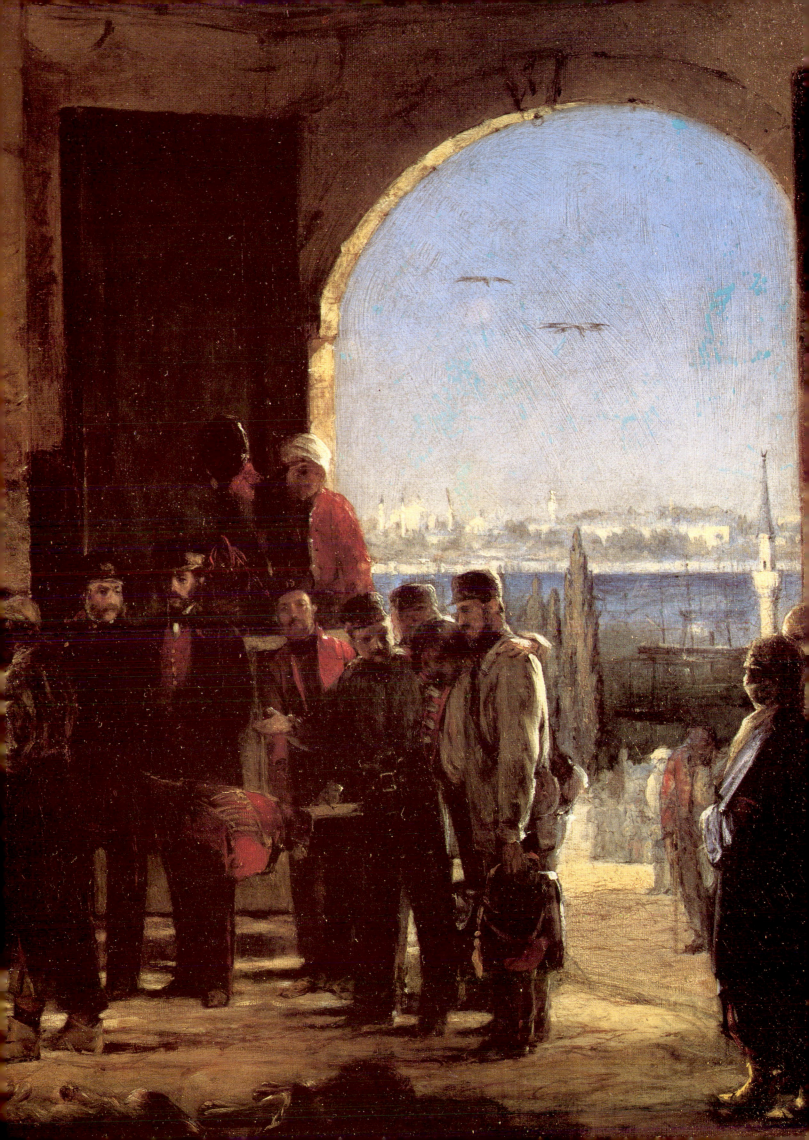

and *Notes on Nursing* (1860) became medical classics and served as the basic texts for the many other nursing schools that were established throughout the world. "Nightingale nurses" were sought everywhere, and the nursing movement quickly made its way to the United States, where Clara Barton (1821-1912) founded the Bellevue Hospital School for Nurses in 1873.

Henri Dunant (1828-1910), a Swiss philanthropist, authored his account of the great suffering endured by those wounded in the Crimean war at Solférino. His *Un Souvenir De Solférino* (1862) led to the International Conference of Red Cross Societies in 1863 and to the signing of the Geneva Convention in 1864.

SURGICAL SOCIETIES AND JOURNALS

The inevitable formation of national and international surgical societies and the emergence and development of medical periodicals were important adjuncts to the evolution of surgery. For the most part the professional associations began as a method of providing mutual improvement via personal interaction with surgical peers and publication of presented papers. Unlike surgeons of earlier centuries, who were known to closely guard "trade secrets," members of these new organizations were emphatic about publishing transactions of their meetings.

The first of these surgical societies was the Academie Royale De Chirurgie in France. Its transactions appeared sporadically from 1743 through 1838. Of the journals of nineteenth-century associations the most prominent are the *Memoires* and *Bulletins* of the Societé De Chirurgie De Paris (1847), the *Verhandlungen* of the Deutsche Gesellschaft Für Chirurgie (1872), the *Transactions of the American Surgical Association* (1883), and the *Proces-Verbaux, Mémoires, Etc.* of the Congres Français De Chirurgie. No surgical association that published professional reports existed in nineteenth-century Great Britain, and the Royal Colleges of Surgeons of Edinburgh, England, and Ireland never undertook such projects.

One of the most striking features of late nineteenth-century medicine and surgery was its internationalism. International medical congresses were held in Florence (1869), Vienna (1873), Brussels (1875), Philadelphia (1876), Geneva (1877), Amsterdam (1879), London (1881), Copenhagen (1884), Washington (1887), Berlin (1890), Rome (1894), Moscow (1897), Paris (1900), Madrid (1903), Lisbon (1906), Budapest (1909), and London (1913). The onset of World War I interrupted the scheduling of such gatherings.

Although textbooks, monographs, and treatises had always been the foundation of medical writing, the introduction of journals to the surgeon's written armamentarium had a tremendous impact on the development of surgery in the nineteenth century (see the box on p. 357).

As surgery became increasingly internationalized, much interest came to be focused on the individuals who participated in its progress. Accordingly, surgical history can also be seen as the biography of great men and women. Similarly, national differences existed within the profession, and progress made in one country did not necessarily correspond with gains made in other countries.

GENERAL SURGERY PERIODICALS

AUGUST RICHTER (1742-1812)
Chirurgische Bibliothek (1771)

CONRAD LANGENBECK (1776-1851)
Bibliothek Für Die Chirurgie (1805)
Neue Bibliothek Für Die Chirurgie Und Ophthalmologie (1815)

ALBRECHT VON GRAEFE (1828-1870)
Journal Der Chirurgie Und Augen-Heilkunde (1820)

JOSEPH MALGAIGNE (1806-1865)
Journal De Chirurgie (1843)

BERNARD LANGENBECK (1810-1887)
Archiv Für Klinische Chirurgie (1860)

KARL HEUTER (1838-1882) AND GEORGE LÜCKE (1829-1924)
Deutsche Zeitschrift Für Chirurgie (1872)

LOUIS TERRIER (1837-1908) AND LEOPOLD OLLIER (1830-1900)
Revue De Chirurgie (1881)

LEWIS PILCHER (1844-1917)
Annals of Surgery (1885)

JONATHAN HUTCHINSON (1828-1913)
Archives of Surgery (1889)

GREAT BRITAIN AND IRELAND

At the beginning of the nineteenth century Great Britain was in socioeconomic and political decline. After 13 months of peace with France, war broke out (1802-1803). Admiral Horatio Nelson (1758-1805) won a brilliant victory over the French fleet at Trafalgar (1805). Great Britain and its allies, including Prussia and Russia, did not defeat the French on land until almost a decade later. Napoleon was sent into exile but escaped within a year and started war again. An allied army under the command of the future Duke of Wellington (1769-1852) permanently defeated Napoleon at Waterloo (1815).

The first 40 years of the century proved to be an era of political reform. The Whigs, who looked at reform as a way to break the power of the Tories, prepared a bill that gave the property-owning middle class the right to vote. The House of Commons passed the bill in 1832, but the House of Lords planned to reject it. Under pressure from the Whigs William IV (1765-1837), who had succeeded his brother George IV (1762-1830), threatened to name enough new lords to ensure the bill's passage, and in response to his threat the House of Lords finally passed it. The new parliament of reform elected under this bill immediately made slavery illegal in Great Britain's colonies, improved child labor laws, and established safety standards for factories.

Queen Victoria (1819-1901) began a 65-year reign in 1837. The British empire exercised great power during her rule, which was marked by the able leadership of several outstanding prime ministers, including Robert Peel (1788-1850), Henry Temple, also known as Lord Palmerston (1784-1865), Benjamin Disraeli (1804-1881), and William Gladstone (1809-1898).

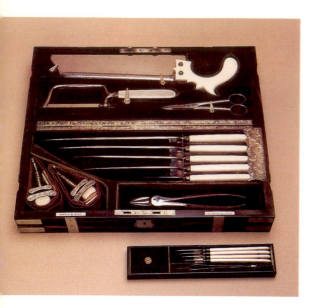

222. Amputation set, steel with ivory handles, made by the London firm of Arnold and Son in 1871. An example of the finest and most expensive instruments available at the time, this set was a prizewinner at the London International Exhibition of 1871. Whatever the set might have cost, the joints where the ivory handles are attached would have harbored bacteria. From 1875 to 1895, as listerian antiseptic principles were gradually adopted throughout the world, surgical sets of this type gave way to all-steel instruments that could be completely sterilized. *(Reproduced by permission of the Trustees of the Science Museum, London; MS575.)*

Life in Great Britain changed greatly during Victoria's reign. Roads and railroads spread across the land, and telephone and telegraph lines linked major cities. Although the population doubled, the middle class prospered and the poor were more comfortable than they had ever been.

Daniel O'Connell (1775-1847) became the first Irish leader in Parliament. He pressed for Irish political independence and for the right of Roman Catholics to hold office, a right that was finally granted in 1829. The potato famine of the 1840s caused widespread misery in the country and resulted in the emigration of hundreds of thousands of individuals.

By the end of the eighteenth century, London had displaced Paris as the center of international surgical excellence, partially because of the manner in which surgical practice and the education of surgeons had been organized. Hunter's teachings had also influenced the practice of British surgery. By 1797, the old Company of Surgeons had ceased to be an effective managerial body and plans were under way to organize a more responsive institution. Accordingly the Royal College of Surgeons received a new charter in March 1800 and would soon be led by men imbued with the hunterian tradition.

While the new charter was being obtained, a momentous negotiation was taking place that would have an enormous influence on the future of the new Royal College of Surgeons. In April 1799 the trustees of John Hunter's museum of comparative anatomy and pathology were petitioning the soon-to-be-reorganized College to take over custody of the museum. Parliament eventually purchased the Hunter Museum for 15,000 pounds, and the College was made permanent custodian. The museum was officially opened in 1813 and grew rapidly; a library was soon added. A decided indirect benefit accrued to the College in its association with the Hunter Museum. Many of the trustees, who were to continue inspecting the museum and to whom the College was responsible, were among the country's foremost scientists and politicians, including the lord chancellor, first lord of the treasury, chancellor of the exchequer, first lord of the admiralty, speaker of the House of Commons, and secretary of war. Their continued and constant social mingling with the surgeons of the College gave the College increased visibility.

In 1800 the Royal College of Physicians, the Royal College of Surgeons, and the Society of Apothecaries controlled the three types of practice, which officially remained mutually exclusive. The members of the Royal College of Physicians were few and had minimal influence outside London. The larger membership of the Royal College of Surgeons included about 400 to 500 individuals who were trained to practice only surgery. The apothecaries, theoretically under the control of the Royal College of Physicians, were permitted to advise on medical cases but were not allowed to charge for that advice unless they prescribed a medicine. When a surgeon was called in to operate, an apothecary frequently was required to attend the patient afterward or to dress the wound, but he could receive no fee unless he induced the patient to take potions and dressings.

As a result of the changing socioeconomic climate in England the people were able to pay for more medical care. Because there were so few physicians, the requirement for more personnel fell to the apothecaries and members of the Royal College of Surgeons. To better care for patients, the apothecaries, who knew little surgery, joined the College to learn surgery. The typical surgeon, conversely, knew little about pharmaceutical medicine and was forced to obtain an apothecary's license. It became apparent that this new class of "general practitioner," or "surgeon-apothecary," needed a comprehensive, regulated form of training.

In 1815 the apothecaries obtained an Act of Parliament that enabled them to hold an examination for all who practiced in England and to prosecute unqualified practitioners, the first statute in Great Britain to impose penalties on unlicensed practitioners. Within a few years of the passage of the Act of 1815 the Royal College of Surgeons began to more clearly define its educational requirements and made them complementary to those required by the Society of

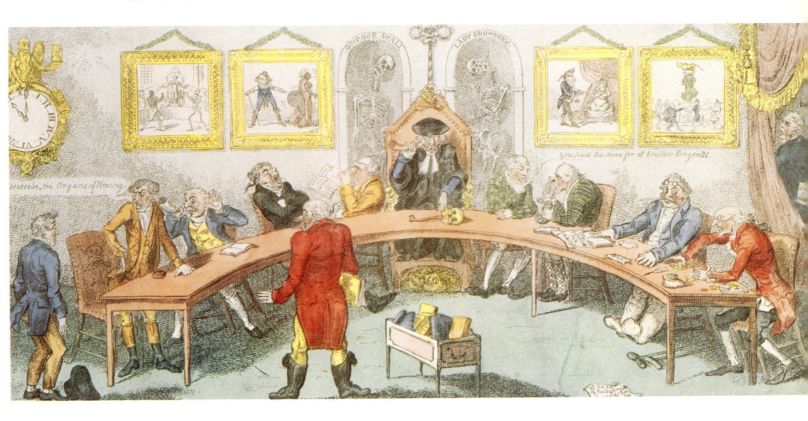

Apothecaries. Thus candidates who intended to enter general practice usually obtained both licenses, and a Master of the Royal College of Surgeons, Licentiate of the Society of Apothecaries (M.R.C.S., L.S.A.) became the common qualification.

The College of Surgeons became a licensing body and over the course of the nineteenth century gradually assumed increasing responsibility for the education of surgeons. Its license, however, was purely optional, and anyone could practice without restriction. In 1843 the College charter was again reformed: the name was legally changed to the Royal College of Surgeons of England, and the Fellowship of Surgeons was created. The Fellows were given the authority to elect the council, whose members had previously been tenured for life. In addition, the Court of Examiners was to be chosen from the Fellows. Not unexpectedly, quarrels arose as to the particular schools that should be recognized as preparing candidates for examination. Eventually standards were established and accords were reached.

The Medical Act of 1858 had the most far-reaching consequences for the College. This opportunity for medical and surgical reform was instigated by the unsettled conditions that had surrounded medical practice for some time. A general medical council for the registration and control of education and practice was instituted. No unregistered individual was allowed to hold a public office or sign medical certificates unless he had been properly examined by one of the royal colleges and placed on an official register.

During the first half of the nineteenth century many medical societies were started throughout Great Britain and Ireland. Many of the societies formed ethical committees, which settled disputes and ejected members guilty of serious breaches. The societies' powers were aided by the formation of the General Medical Council and its revival of penal powers.

The private schools of anatomical and surgical education gradually disappeared by the third decade of the century. Such important institutions as the Great Windmill Street and Aldersgate Street Schools in London and The Webb Street School in Birmingham were no longer needed, since the hospital-based schools were becoming better organized. Thus in England surgical education became entirely associated with these special hospital-based schools apart from any universities and received little recognition from the state. The converse occurred in Scotland and Ireland, where the older universities took a leading role

223. *The Examination of a Young Surgeon* (1811) by George Cruikshank. The process of taking the surgical boards has always been stressful. Here Cruikshank caricatures the elderly surgeons quizzing the young candidate. While one old surgeon asks the young recruit to describe the organs of hearing, several old men on the examining board hold up their ear trumpets. *(National Library of Medicine, Bethesda, Md.)*

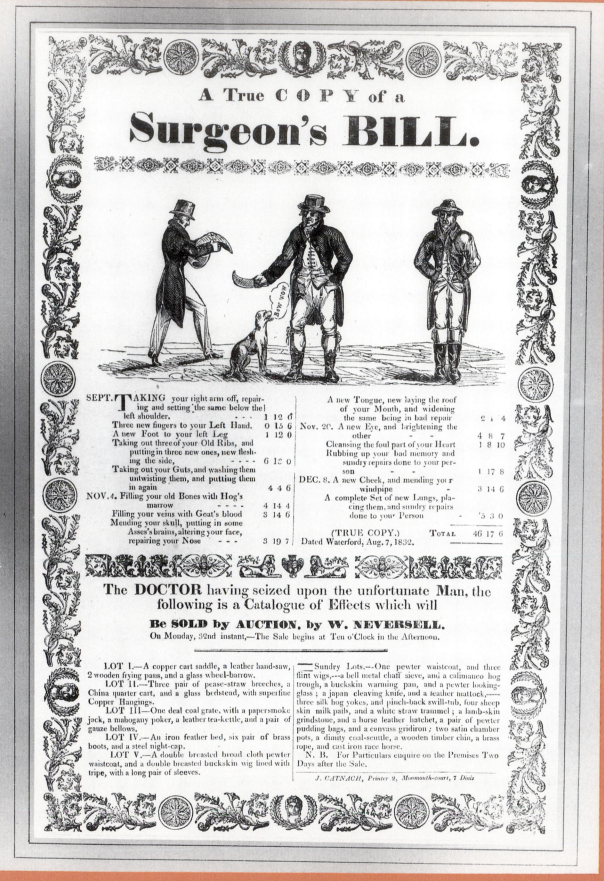

224. Surgeons' fees have always been a controversial aspect of medicine. This broadside, circa 1830, is an indelicate satire on surgeons' practices as well as their fees. Published in London by a prolific printer of children's books, ballads, and broadsides, James Catnach of the Seven Dials. *(Jeremy Norman & Co., Inc.)*

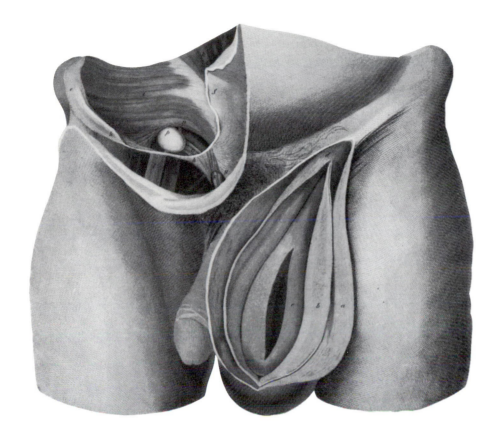

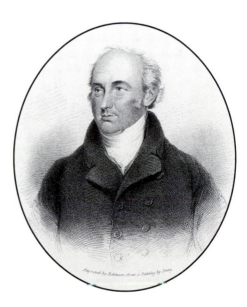

225. Two inguinal hernias. "That on the left side, having existed many years, has descended into the scrotum, and become of great magnitude. That on the right side, is in an incipient state, and shows the distance from the abdominal ring, at which it first protrudes from the abdomen." Plate 3, much reduced, from the life-sized engraving in Astley Cooper's *The Anatomy and Surgical Treatment of Inguinal and Congenital Hernia* (London, 1804). *(Jeremy Norman & Co., Inc.)*

and the medical schools formed by them at an earlier period continued to flourish. Therefore two systems of medical and surgical education existed in the British Isles, which both taught and licensed all who chose to obtain their diplomas.

Astley Cooper (1768-1841) contributed more than any other London surgeon to the brilliance of early nineteenth-century London surgery. He was the son of a clergyman, and both his paternal grandfather and his uncle were prominent surgeons. The latter, William Cooper, was on staff at Guy's Hospital, and under his tutelage Astley first began to study medicine. Astley Cooper soon transferred his apprenticeship to the auspices of Henry Cline, and Cline eventually convinced the younger Cooper to attend the lectures of John Hunter. Cooper did this for 2 years and in the winter of 1787 also spent a few months studying anatomy at the University of Edinburgh.

The zeal with which Cooper took to his studies was extraordinary. In 1789 he became demonstrator in anatomy at St. Thomas's Hospital. Two years later he completed his apprenticeship and was invited by Cline to become his assistant in practice. This meant that Cooper would share the private lectureship in anatomy and surgery that Cline had started in London. In 1793 Cooper was also chosen to give the lectures on anatomy for the Company of Surgeons.

226. Sir Astley Cooper, engraved by John Henry Robinson after the painting by Penny. *(Historical Collections, College of Physicians of Philadelphia.)*

In 1800 William Cooper relinquished his position at Guy's Hospital. Astley Cooper was asked to assume the post, which he did without hesitation. A bit of politics entered into this decision because during his early education Astley Cooper had embraced the democratic ideals of the French Revolution. The excesses of terror and brutality brought upon the monarchist victims were all looked upon quite unfavorably by the British establishment. To secure his position at Guy's, Cooper had to convince the authorities that he would withdraw from any political action and devote his time solely to surgery.

Cooper's contributions to surgery and anatomy were varied and numerous. He was known as a bold and innovative surgeon who completed work in a number of fields. In 1800 Cooper presented to the Royal Society three cases of eustachian-obstruction deafness. In each instance he performed a myringotomy to relieve the symptoms and was also able to demonstrate air and bone conduction by watch (precursor of Rinne's test, which uses a tuning fork). For this work he received the Copley Medal.

Cooper's monumental two-part *The Anatomy and Surgical Treatment of Inguinal and Congenital Hernia* was published in 1804 and 1807. The result of an enormous amount of work on both patients and cadavers, the book is regarded as one of the seminal works in the field. In the text Cooper first described the cremasteric fascia; a femoral hernia with two sacs, the second passing through a defect in the superficial fascia and appearing immediately beneath the skin and the first being in the femoral canal; the pectineal ligament of the pelvis; and the transversalis fascia, a thin, semilunar expansion of the anterior aponeurosis of the transversus abdominis muscle, sometimes prolonged beyond the conjoined tendon to be attached to the deep crural arch. Cooper also discussed the use of a slender bistoury with a short cutting edge for dividing the constricting tissues at the neck of a hernial sac.

In the management of aneurysms and arterial surgery Cooper performed some of his most heroic feats. In 1805 he unsuccessfully ligated the common carotid artery for aneurysm. Three years later he performed the same operation but with a successful result. That same year he successfully ligated the external iliac artery in a case of femoral aneurysm. In 1817 Cooper tied off the abdominal aorta for aneurysm, but the patient died the next day. In 1820 Cooper was asked to perform an operation on George IV for an infected sebaceous cyst of the scalp. He was assisted by Cline and described the surgery for which he was later made a baron:

> I made an incision into the tumour and emptied it of its contents. Then I found it adhered strongly to the scalp . . . I with great difficulty detached it from the skin without cutting the skin itself. On that side on which Cline stood I begged him to detach it which he did but it took up a great deal of time on the whole. The edges of the wound were brought together and lint and plaster applied. The King bore the operation well, requested there might be no hurry and when it was finished said, "What do you call the tumour?" I said, "A steatoma, Sire." "Then," said he, "I hope it will stay at home and not annoy me anymore."

Cooper always remained actively involved in organized surgery. In 1813 he was appointed professor of comparative anatomy and received the professorship in surgery at the Royal College of Surgeons. Within a few years it was evident that he was overworked and in danger of becoming ill. Toward the end of 1824 his syncopal attacks were becoming worse, and dyspnea was evident on exertion. Cooper was forced to give up his lecturing and resigned from St. Thomas's. He had hoped that his pupil Charles Aston Key (1793-1849) and his nephew Bransby Blake Cooper (1792-1853) would receive the surgical and anatomical lectureships, respectively. When they did not, Cooper induced the trustees of Guy's Hospital to secede from their union with St. Thomas's Hospital and form a separate medical school.

Cooper's two-volume collection, *Surgical Essays,* jointly written with Benjamin Travers (1783-1848), appeared in 1818 and 1819. In 1822 Cooper published his *Treatise on Dislocations and on Fractures of the Joints,* and from 1824 to

1827 he authored his three-volume *Lectures on the Principles and Practice of Surgery*. Cooper's final three monographs were among his best-known works. *Illustrations of the Diseases of the Breast* (1829) included the earliest description of chronic inflammation of the breast with the formation of cysts and the first detailing of that gland's suspensory ligaments. In 1830 he published *Observations on the Structure and Diseases of the Testis* and 2 years later, *The Anatomy of the Thymus Gland*.

In the last few years of his life Cooper traveled extensively. He was made sergeant surgeon to George IV and, subsequently, to William IV and Queen Victoria. In addition, he was elected a fellow of the Royal College of Surgeons in both London and Edinburgh. Twice he assumed the presidency of the Royal College. Cooper was a magnetic personality, distinguished by his handsome looks and personal charm. His reputation at the height of his career was enormous, and he was able to amass a personal fortune. Historically he remains known more as a great surgical technician than as a creative contributor to the advancement of surgery.

In the first half of the nineteenth century many great surgeons practiced in London. Charles Bell (1774-1842) was the younger brother of John Bell of Edinburgh, with whom he initially studied medicine. Charles Bell assisted his brother in the anatomical school that the latter ran, and he also attended lectures in his native city. He was a precocious anatomist and by the age of 28 years had authored his important two-volume *A System of Dissections* (1799-1801), which became the most used anatomical manual in the British Isles after the turn of the century. Bell's career was distinguished by his magnificent artistic abilities, which were highlighted in the illustrations he himself made for his many textbooks. Medical politics forced him to leave Edinburgh in 1804, and he permanently resettled in London. He soon began to teach anatomy from his own house and eventually became associated with the Great Windmill Street School. Although Bell's early years in London were filled with loneliness, frustration, and discouragement, he also had triumphs. In 1806 he authored his *Essays on the Anatomy of Expression in Painting*. This beautiful work earned him high praise in artistic circles but brought little recognition from surgeons. In response, during the following year he began to publish his two-volume *A System of Operative Surgery*. In 1811 Bell married and used his wife's modest dowry to purchase the Great Windmill Street School. His reputation was soon established, and in 1813 he was elected surgeon to the Middlesex Hospital. His *Illustrations of the Great Operations on Surgery,* considered a classic technical atlas, was published in 1821. "To the Reader," Bell's preface to this book, is one of the best expressions of the surgeon's credo (see the box on p. 364). In 1836 Bell accepted the chair of systematic surgery at Edinburgh, which he retained until his death. Bell's true fame rests with his many contributions to the study of the nervous system. His *Idea of a New Anatomy of the Brain* (1811) contained the first reference to experimental work on the motor functions of the ventral spinal nerve roots. He did not, however, establish the sensory functions of the dorsal roots. In a series of papers written in 1821 he described the long thoracic nerve and the facial paralysis caused by certain lesions of the motor nerve of the face. In 1830 Bell authored the second edition of his monumental *The Nervous System of the Body,* in which he recorded that the fifth cranial nerve has a sensory-motor function and also included the first description of myotonia. He aptly described a patient with peripheral facial paralysis who could not close the eyelids of the affected side without at the same time moving the eyeball upward and outward, and he also discussed facial tics. Among his other important monographs were *Letters Concerning the Diseases of the Urethra* (1810), *A Dissertation on Gun-Shot Wounds* (1814), and *The Hand: Its Mechanism and Vital Endowments as Evincing Design* (1833).

James Wardrop (1782-1869), a native of Scotland, received his medical degree from the University of Edinburgh and permanently moved to London in 1809. In 1808 he had authored the first of two volumes of his *Essay on the Morbid Anatomy of the Human Eye* (1808-1818). Wardrop was the first to classify the various inflammations of the eye according to the structures involved. He also

TO THE READER

The reader will forgive me, if I now address him with the same freedom I would a pupil who had sat beside me for successive winters.

Before entering on the subject of this work, in which there will be few opportunities of discussion, in which the demonstration only is to be made, I take the occasion to impress upon him the necessity of his prescribing strict rules for himself, in the performance of operations.

The Public, who are so ready to determine on the merits of our Profession, and even the patients who are to suffer, are surprisingly ignorant both of the Surgeon's motives for what he does, and the propriety of the methods he puts in practice. He is continually operating in secret as a matter of necessity; the most sensible give the decision up to him; so that he is answerable to his own conscience, and to that alone. Nor is the Public aware of the temptations which men of our Profession withstand. Credit for great abilities, gratitude for services performed, and high emoluments, are ready to be bestowed for a little deception, and that obliquity of conduct, which does not amount to actual crime. This is precisely the situation in which a man requires a thorough devotion to the principles of honour and right conduct, to preserve him from the commission of error. These are the considerations which should make it the interest of Society to hold the Profession in respect, and which make the duty of every member of it to keep it pure.

I shall place the matter before you in another light. If we go into a court of law, we see the bench occupied by the learned judges; before them are counsel, skilled in the law, and a jury of twelve honest men, to hold the balance betwixt the severity of the law and the weakness of human nature. What are they met to decide? Perhaps a matter of money or of succession. Even if it should be a criminal court, what a contrast have we with the situation of the Surgeon, on whose single decision the life of a fellow-creature depends; one, perhaps, bearing all the relationships of society; having all the ties which bind a man to existence, and the virtues which make his life dear. The Surgeon cannot lean upon the judgment of others, nor say, for this the wisdom of the legislature has provided. He has to examine an evidence, often strangely perverted; he must judge, unaided by friendly counsel; and, to determine upon what is right to be done, when the life of a friend hangs on the issue, and where the execution depends on his own dexterity, is a thing of the greatest difficulty.

When we consider the weight of responsibility, it is not surprising, that so many shrink from the performance of the duties which belong to our Profession; the more especially that success in it draws no sympathy. If there be some eminent men who esteem our Art, and express themselves differently, yet it must be acknowledged, that the Public consider him, who deserves the first honors of the Profession as only more eminently divested of common feeling.

That the surgeon, in order to do his duty, must be divested of the common feelings of Humanity, is a vulgar error. Let my lady's maid still suppose, that he must be a brute whose occupation soils his hands with blood. It is not supposed that she can have very accurate notions of the difference of his service who inflicts the wound, and of his who closes it; but for a reasonable man, and most of all, for one educated to Surgery, it is very ridiculous to assign as a reason for not doing his duty, that his feelings prevent him. These feelings are not for his patient! Instead of having a true compassion for the wounded or for the diseased, instead of neglecting his first painful impressions, and being happy to render assistance, he stands, like the foolish maid, who holds her apron betwixt her pretty eyes and the object of her horror. Let no man boast of feelings, until they are of that genuine kind, and amount to that degree, that he can forget himself, in the desire to give aid to another.

In performing the operations of Surgery, this neglect of yourself is very necessary. Why simplicity should be so rare a virtue in Operators, is very remarkable; since it requires but this one rule—think only of your patient. Any thing like a flourish on such an occasion, does not merely betray vanity, but a lamentable want of just feeling. It is as if a man said—Look at me now—see how unconcerned I am, while the patient is suffering under my hand! Simplicity is always becoming; often a great excellence; but, in regard to operations performed on a fellow-creature, it is a moral obligation.

In truth, the anxiety of a Surgeon, before an important operation, is the greatest any man can suffer, where there is not a consciousness of crime; and do not suppose that this belongs to a Surgeon in his early practice only, or to such feeble spirits as cannot summon resolution to do their duty. The greatest Surgeon this country has produced, the celebrated Cheselden, was, even in his later days, anxious to sickness, before the performance of a severe operation.

These are the considerations which incline me to believe, that our Profession has not been sufficiently honored; and that men are esteemed, only in proportion to the emoluments they have drawn from it. It depends on the conduct of those who are now entering their Profession, whether Surgery will continue to be confounded with the meaner arts, or rise to be the very first in estimation; as requiring great abilities and long study to attain the knowledge of it, and purity and the strictest honor in the practice of it.

Preface to
Illustrations of the Great Operations of Surgery
Charles Bell (1821)

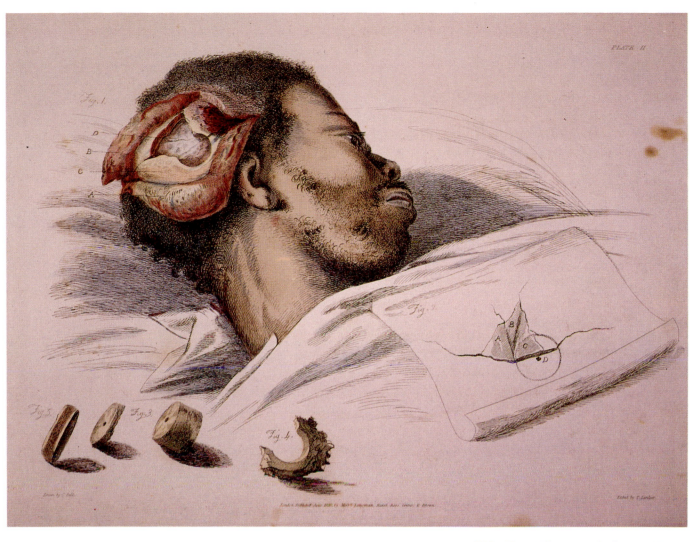

PLATE II

227. *Above,* The wound after trephination, with a sketch of the fractured bone, and the portions of the cranium cut out by the trephine, as drawn by Charles Bell and engraved by Thomas Landseer. Charles Bell remains one of the greatest of all surgeon-artists. Starting in medical school, he prepared virtually all the illustrations for his publications. This hand-colored plate from Bell's *Illustrations of the Great Operations of Surgery* (1820-1821) reflects an unusual level of artistic sensitivity for a surgical treatise. (*Jeremy Norman & Co., Inc.*)

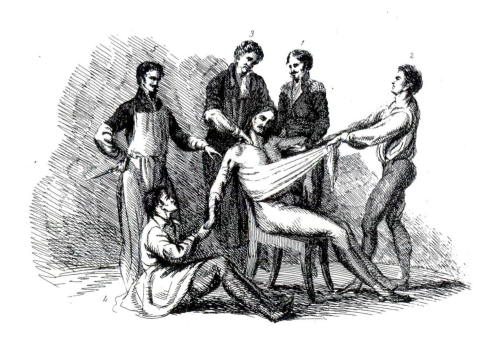

228. The surgeon and his assistants prepared to perform the operation of amputation at the shoulder joint, as drawn by Charles Bell and engraved by Thomas Landseer in Bell's *Illustrations of the Great Operations of Surgery* (1820-1821). (*Jeremy Norman & Co., Inc.*)

used the term *keratitis* for the first time. In 1826 Wardrop founded the West London Hospital of Surgery and began to lecture at the Aldersgate Street Medical School. Two years later he was appointed surgeon to George IV. Wardrop is remembered for successfully treating aneurysms of the carotid artery (1809) and innominate artery (1827) by placing a single distal ligature in a manner originally proposed by Brasdor. He was an extremely ill-tempered, unpleasant individual who heaped abuse on many of his peers in articles published in the *Lancet* (founded 1823). Wardrop is also remembered eponymically for an acute onychia occurring spontaneously in debilitated patients or in response to slight trauma.

Benjamin Collins Brodie (1783-1862) was the son of a Wiltshire clergyman. In 1801 Brodie moved to London and registered for the private anatomical lectures given by Abernethy, while also attending sessions at the Great Windmill Street School. In 1803 he was enrolled in St. George's Hospital as an apprentice to Home. Two years later Brodie was appointed house surgeon and demonstrator in anatomy at the Windmill Street institution. In time, Brodie became personal assistant to Home, and in 1808 he was appointed to the surgical staff at St. George's. His reputation grew immensely, and by 1822 Brodie was full surgeon, from which position he retired in 1840. The contributions Brodie made to surgery span several different fields. From 1810 to 1814 he authored a number of papers on various topics in physiology. Among the most important were those regarding the effect of the brain on the action of the heart (1810) and the influence of the pneumogastric nerve on gastric secretion (1814). At around the same time, Brodie began to operate on varicose veins and eventually devised a test to determine the insufficiency of venous valves. Brodie believed strongly in conservative surgery, especially as applied to bones and joints. His most important textbook is the 1818 *Pathological and Surgical Observations on the Diseases of the Joints,* in which he provided descriptions of a bursa beneath the medial head of the gastrocnemius; hysterical arthralgia and hysterical spinal neuralgia, simulating Pott's disease, after trauma; chronic hypertrophic synovitis of the knee; and, for the first time, ankylosing spondylitis. In 1828 Brodie described a chronic, inactive abscess of the bone marrow surrounded by dense fibrous tissue and sclerotic bone. His *Lectures on the Diseases of the Urinary Organs* first appeared in 1832, a report on rectal disease involving spasm of the anal sphincter was written in 1835, and a paper on serocystic tumors of the breast was published in 1840. In 1846 his 352-page *Clinical Lectures on Surgery* and the important *Lectures Illustrative of Various Subjects in Pathology and Surgery* were published simultaneously. The latter work contained the first clinical description of intermittent claudication in humans. Brodie was always involved in organized medicine, serving as president of the Royal College of Surgeons (1844), the Royal Society (1858), and the General Medical Council (1858).

William Lawrence (1783-1867) was the son of a surgeon and a surgical apprentice of Abernethy. The latter was especially fond of his young student and appointed him demonstrator in anatomy at St. Bartholomew's Hospital, where he served for 12 years. In 1813 Lawrence was made assistant surgeon at that institution and was also elected a Fellow of the Royal Society. In the following year Lawrence was appointed Benjamin Travers's associate at the London Infirmary for Diseases of the Eye. In 1815 Lawrence was named professor of anatomy and physiology at the Royal College of Surgeons. Lawrence succeeded Abernethy as lecturer on surgery at St. Bartholmew's in 1823 and within 2 years was elevated to professor of surgery. He authored a number of outstanding texts, including *Treatise on Hernia* (1807) and *A Practical Treatise on Diseases of the Eye* (1830). The latter included a classical description of the symptoms of glaucoma and was probably the first work to draw attention to the increase of intraocular pressure as a characteristic of the condition. He introduced the term *asthenopia* and was the first to describe sympathetic ophthalmia as a distinct disease. Lawrence's last major text was *Lectures on Surgery* (1863).

Benjamin Travers (1783-1858) served as an apprentice to Astley Cooper for 6 years. He eventually became prosector of anatomy at Guy's Hospital and surgeon at St. Thomas's. Travers's most important early work was in vascular surgery and included the ligature of the common carotid artery to cure an aneurysm (1811). In 1812 Travers authored *An Inquiry into the Process of Nature in Repairing Injuries of the Intestines,* which recorded the first accurate information on the subject. As mentioned earlier, Travers and Cooper coauthored a two-volume text, *Surgical Essays* (1818). Early in his career Travers became interested in ophthalmology. Before his appointment to St. Thomas's he also served at the London Infirmary for Diseases of the Eye. In 1820 Travers authored his *Synopsis of the Diseases of the Eye,* which was the earliest systematic treatise in English on that subject. Travers wrote a number of monographs on physiopathology, including *Constitutional Irritation* (1824), *A Further Inquiry Concerning Constitutional Irritation and the Pathology of the Nervous System* (1834), and *The Physiology of Inflammation* (1844). He was twice president (1847 and 1856) of the Royal College of Surgeons. In 1857 Travers served for 1 year as sergeant surgeon to Queen Victoria.

George Guthrie (1785-1856) was England's greatest military surgeon of the nineteenth century. He served a surgical apprenticeship in London and by the age of 16 years had already qualified for the Royal College of Surgeons. Deciding on a military career, he joined the army and became an assistant surgeon (1801). Five years later he accompanied his regiment to North America; later he served under Wellington during the War of the Peninsula in Spain. Guthrie was active during the Napoleonic Wars and saw action at Waterloo. In 1806 he authored an important text, *On Gun-Shot Wounds of the Extremities, Requiring the Different Operations of Amputation, With Their After Treatment.* He urged prompt amputation, and the book remains among the most important in the history of military surgery. At Waterloo Guthrie successfully ligated the peroneal artery of a German soldier who had been wounded. In the second edition of his *Treatise on Gun-Shot Wounds* (1820), Guthrie described a successful amputation at the hip joint that he had performed on a French soldier. After the slaughter at Waterloo, Guthrie remained at York Hospital, taking charge of wounded British soldiers for 2 years. He became lecturer on surgery at the Westminster Hospital in London in 1816, assistant surgeon 7 years later, and surgeon to the same institution in 1827. In 1828 Guthrie was named professor of anatomy at the Royal College of Surgeons. Among his many accomplishments were the founding of the Royal Westminster Ophthalmic Hospital in London (1816) and the writing of an important text, *Lectures on the Operative Surgery of the Eye* (1823), which contained interesting research on artificial pupils. In 1834 Guthrie wrote *On the Anatomy and Diseases of the Neck of the Bladder and of the Urethra,* the first urological text to describe nonprostatic obstruction of the bladder neck and to provide a description of his prostatic catheter for use in transurethral prostatectomy. Guthrie remains eponymically linked with the urethral sphincter muscle. During the 1840s he wrote a series of four books on injuries of the head, arteries, abdomen and pelvis, and chest. Guthrie had the honor of being elected president of the Royal College of Surgeons in 1833, 1841, and 1854.

Joseph Green (1791-1863) was a nephew and pupil of Henry Cline. He qualified for the Royal College of Surgeons in 1815 and soon began the private practice of surgery in London. Green became surgeon at St. Thomas's Hospital in 1820 and professor of surgery in King's College a decade later. From 1823 to 1828 he held the office of professor of anatomy, physiology, and surgery at the Royal College of Surgeons. His most prominent written work is the lengthy *Dissector's Manual* (1820). Green has been credited with performing the first recorded thyroidectomy in 1828; the patient died of sepsis 15 days after the operation. Green was twice president of the Royal College (1849 and 1858). Green was a close friend of the writer Samuel Taylor Coleridge (1772-1834), and in 1865 a two-volume work by Green entitled *Spiritual Philosophy, Founded on the Technique of S. T. Coleridge* was published posthumously.

Edward Stanley (1791-1862) studied at St. Bartholomew's Hospital, where he became assistant surgeon in 1816 and surgeon in 1838. He twice served as president of the Royal College of Surgeons. In 1833 Stanley wrote about liver puncture as a means to diagnose an abscess of that organ. His most important

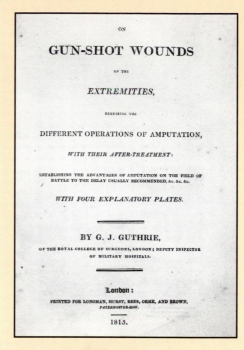

229. George Guthrie's classic of military surgery. *(Jeremy Norman & Co., Inc.)*

work was in orthopedic surgery: he was the first to describe disease of the posterior columns of the spinal cord (1839). In 1849 he authored his principal text, *A Treatise on the Diseases of the Bones*. Stanley is remembered for his description of ligamentous fibers of the capsule of the hip joint that reflect onto the neck of the femur.

Charles Key (1793-1849) was a pupil of Astley Cooper and married Cooper's niece. Key became demonstrator of anatomy at St. Thomas's Hospital in 1820, assistant surgeon at Guy's Hospital in the following year, surgeon in 1824, and professor of surgery at its medical school in 1825. He qualified for the Royal College of Surgeons in 1821 and eventually became a member of its council. His gruff personality, however, prevented him from receiving the honor of its presidency. Key was quite innovative in vascular operations and in 1823 successfully ligated the subclavian artery for an aneurysm at the axilla. In 1836 he reported the successful ligation of the external iliac artery for a femoral aneurysm. Key's other major clinical accomplishment was his introduction of the principle of dividing a stricture outside the sac in cases of strangulated hernia, which was first recorded in his *Memoir on the Advantages and Practicability of Dividing the Stricture in Strangulated Hernia on the Outside of the Sac* (1833).

Robert Liston (1794-1847) was a native of Scotland but spent most of his professional life in London. At the age of 16 years he began an apprenticeship under John Barclay (1758-1826), a renowned anatomist who had written *A New Anatomical Nomenclature* (1803). After completing studies with Barclay, Liston moved to London, where he attended lectures by Abernethy and Blizard. Having passed the qualifying examination of the Royal College of Surgeons of both London and Edinburgh (1818), Liston returned to Edinburgh to become assistant in surgery to Barclay. A misunderstanding between the two men led to Liston's opening his own private school of anatomy and surgery, where James Syme was his chief associate. Most of the cadavers in Edinburgh ended up with the Monros or with Barclay, so both Liston and Syme were forced to do some grave robbing to supply their new school with adequate dissection material. Edinburgh surgery before Lister reached its zenith through the efforts of Syme and Liston. For 5 years both men conducted their anatomy school with ever-increasing success; however, they were more interested in the practice of surgery. Liston became a surgeon's clerk under George Bell (?- 1862) in the Royal Infirmary, and Syme clerked with William Newbigging. Not unexpectedly, these two men, especially Liston, were soon viewed with suspicion by their older rivals. Together, Liston and Syme performed many operations that have since been shown to have historical precedent. Professional jealousies began to plague their daily activities, and the managers of the infirmary finally expelled Liston from the institution. Liston appealed for help from the Royal College of Surgeons, but his pleas went unheard. For 5 years Liston was forced to perform surgical operations in patients' houses and other private institutions, and he was not reappointed to the Royal Infirmary until 1827. By the mid-1820s various differences were driving Liston and Syme apart. Their personal relationship had become so acrimonious that when Syme applied for the surgeonship of the Royal Infirmary, the managers declined to appoint him for fear that his feud with Liston would be carried into the classroom. The conflict came to a resounding end when Syme defeated Liston in a bitter contest for the chair of clinical surgery in the University of Edinburgh. Liston then spent much time preparing his three-volume *Elements of Surgery* (1831). Liston was considered among the most dexterous of all British surgeons in his day, and his dexterity is evident in many of his remarkable surgical achievements. In 1820 he maintained that a fracture of the neck of the femur should not be neglected, as was the common practice. Liston argued that such fractures should be reduced and treated with splints, as would any other fracture, and he described a long splint extending from the axilla to the sole of the foot for use in femoral fractures. He also developed a strong shear for cutting plaster-of-paris bandages. Liston himself designed bone forceps, which remain an indispensable implement in bone surgery, and also described long-bladed knives of various sizes for use in amputations. In 1835 Liston decided to leave Edinburgh and accepted the professorship of surgery at University College in London. Five years later a reconciliation between the two men occurred, which lasted until Liston's premature death. In London Liston had so many professional duties that he had little time left for his clinical practice or his writings. However, in 1837 he did manage to author *Practical Surgery,* in which he suggested the use of a mirror for viewing edematous tumors of the larynx. In 1846 he became the first surgeon in England to use ether as an anesthetic for a lower extremity amputation.

John Flint South (1797-1882) served an apprenticeship with Cline and was admitted as a member of the Royal College of Surgeons in 1819. He took additional studies in Germany and returned to become demonstrator of surgery at St. Thomas's Hospital, then lecturer, and ultimately surgeon. While studying in Germany he became friendly with Max Josef von Chelius (1794-1876) and translated the latter's *Handbuch Der Chirurgie* (1821) into English, adding a great number of notes. South is remembered by surgical historians because he gathered together a large collection of reference materials, which were edited by D'Arcy Power (1855-1941) and published as *Memorials of the Craft of Surgery in England* (1886).

John Hilton (1804-1878) studied at Guy's Hospital and was eventually appointed demonstrator of anatomy (1828) at his alma mater. In 1845 he was named assistant surgeon, and 4 years later, surgeon at Guy's. Hilton was reputed to be the best anatomist in London and in 1833 described *Trichinella spiralis* in human muscle and suggested its parasitic nature. An 1847 paper recorded the first operation for internal strangulation of the small intestine by Hilton at Guy's Hospital; no anesthetic was used, and the patient died 9 hours later. Hilton's most important written work is the monograph *On the Influence of Mechanical and Physiological Rest in the Treatment of Accidents and Surgical Diseases, and the Diagnos-*

230. The old operating theater and herb garret of Guy's and St. Thomas's Hospitals, London, the only operating theater in England that has remained intact since the nineteenth century. (*St. Thomas's Hospital, London.*)

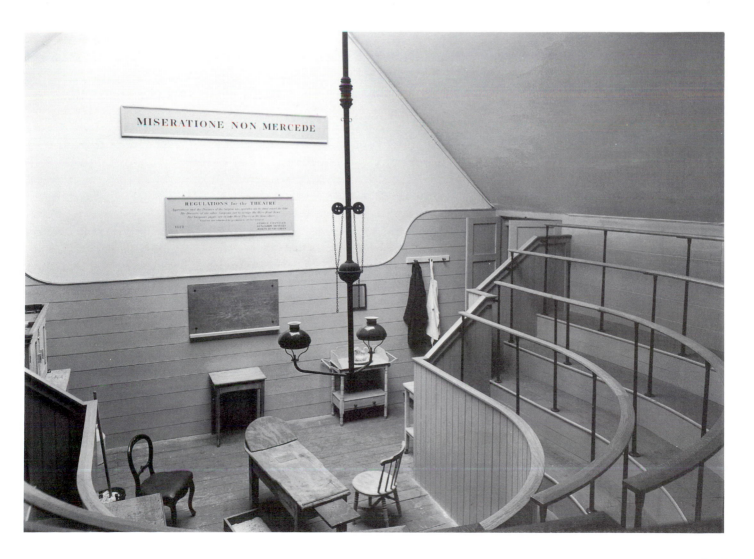

tic Value of Pain (1863). He suggested that symptoms are disordered reflexes and advocated complete rest in the treatment of surgical disorders of all parts of the body. This book has long been considered a surgical classic; later editions are entitled *On Rest and Pain*. Hilton's name is eponymically linked with a law stating that the nerve supplying a joint also supplies the muscles that move the joint and the skin covering the articular insertion of those muscles; a method that employs division of the nerves supplying a superficial ulcer to aid in relief of pain; and a laryngeal sac.

Edward Cock (1805-1892), a nephew and pupil of Astley Cooper, was appointed demonstrator of anatomy at Guy's Hospital Medical School when it first opened (1825). In 1838 Cock was named assistant surgeon to the hospital and in 1848, surgeon. His most memorable paper concerned the first case of pharyngotomy in England (1856). Cock's major written work was his *Practical Anatomy of the Nerves and Vessels Supplying the Head, Neck and Chest* (1835). His name is remembered for a fungating mass of inflamed granulation tissue that may develop in adjacent tissue after the rupture of a suppurative sebaceous cyst.

William Fergusson (1808-1877), a native of Scotland, was educated in Edinburgh as an apprentice under Knox. Knox recognized Fergusson's capabilities and encouraged him in his anatomical studies. In 1829 Fergusson was admitted as a fellow to the Royal College of Surgeons of Edinburgh. Two years later, after serving as lecturer on anatomy, he became surgeon to the Edinburgh Royal Dispensary. In 1839 Fergusson was appointed surgeon to the Royal Infirmary as successor to Liston. In the following year a vacancy occurred in the chair of surgery at King's College in London, and on the recommendation of Astley Cooper, Fergusson was invited to take the position. Within a few years of his arrival in London most of the older, well-known surgeons had retired, and Fergusson rapidly became the most respected surgeon in that city. He received many honors, among them a barony and in 1867, service as sergeant surgeon to Queen Victoria. Fergusson has been called the originator of conservative surgery in England because of his horror of amputation. Quite a prolific writer, his most important paper described an operation for partial excision of the scapula (1842). His *System of Practical Surgery* was also published in 1842, a text that would go through numerous editions. Fergusson's *Lectures on the Progress of Anatomy and Surgery During the Present Century* (1867) remains a classic text in the history of surgery. His name is eponymically linked with an incision for excision of the maxilla and with a cylindrical vaginal speculum of silvered glass with a coating of caoutchouc.

Many distinguished provincial English surgeons practiced during the first half of the nineteenth century. Joseph Hodgson (1788-1869) of Birmingham is best known for his *Treatise on the Diseases of Arteries and Veins, Containing the Pathology and Treatment of Aneurisms and Wounded Arteries* (1815). His work included some of the best illustrations of aneurysms and of aortic valvular endocarditis yet published. Hodgson's name is eponymically linked with a nonsacculated dilation of the aortic arch associated with insufficiency of the aortic valve.

Thomas Teale (1801-1868) founded the Leeds School of Medicine. He remains best known for his important text, *A Practical Treatise on Abdominal Hernia* (1846). Teale's name is associated with an amputation of the forearm in its lower half, or of the thigh, with a long posterior rectangular flap and a short anterior one as well as an amputation of the leg, with a long anterior rectangular flap and a short posterior one (1858).

Through the 1830s most surgical teaching in London was still provided in private schools, which remained without connection to the larger hospitals. However, as more surgeons with excellent reputations began to perform their operative cases in the hospitals and expanded their lecture series within them, it was inevitable that the private schools would gradually disappear. This change was especially evident after Robert Liston and William Fergusson moved to London. Through the middle of the nineteenth century, London and Paris remained surgical meccas, but their reputations were being rapidly displaced by those of the German-speaking countries. From 1850 to the end of the 1880s, London's hospitals and medical schools were guided by a group of able but less renowned men than had previously been in control.

Henry Hancock (1809-1880) was an apprentice of Guthrie and became demonstrator of anatomy at the Westminster Hospital School in 1835. Four years later he was named assistant surgeon at the Charing Cross Hospital and succeeded to its professorship of surgery on the death of John Howship (1781-1841). In 1848 Hancock recorded the first successful operation for peritonitis caused by abscess in the appendix. He authored the monograph *On the Operation for Strangulated Hernia* in 1850. Hancock's name is eponymically linked with an amputation of the foot through the astragalus, which was described in his *Operative Surgery of the Foot and Ankle-Joint* (1873).

William John Little (1810-1894) was the first eminent orthopedic surgeon in the British Isles; because of him orthopedics emerged as a specialty in that country. Little studied in London and qualified as a surgeon in 1832. After having been passed over for a staff post at the London Hospital, Little went to Berlin to work in the anatomical institute of Johannes Müller (1801-1858). Little had contracted poliomyelitis at 2 years of age and was left with a deformity of one foot. No treatment or appliances had been successful in his native country. Muller advised him to consult George Stromeyer (1804-1876), and in June 1836 Stromeyer performed a tenotomy with complete success. Little, always grateful to Stromeyer for transforming his life, remained with him for a few months to study orthopedic techniques. Stromeyer suggested that Little found a hospital in England to perform tenotomies on the poor. Little's Infirmary opened in 1840; it was later named the Orthopaedic Institution and then, in 1845, the Royal Orthopaedic Hospital. Little wrote much of orthopedic interest, including *On the Nature of Club-Foot and Analogous Distortions* (1839) and *On the Nature and Treatment of the Deformities of the Human Frame* (1853). Little's most important student was William Adams (1810-1900), who succeeded Little and became the preeminent London orthopedic surgeon of the mid-Victorian era.

James Paget (1814-1899) of Great Yarmouth was a graduate of St. Bartholomew's Hospital and was affiliated with that institution for his entire professional life. Paget's career was distinguished by his masterful abilities as a surgical pathologist. In many respects he was a direct descendant of the hunterian tradition of linking pathological changes in the body with surgical operations. He was a close associate of Virchow and received numerous honors throughout his life. Paget served as sergeant surgeon to Queen Victoria, became a baron in 1871, and was president of the Royal College of Surgeons in 1875. His best written works are his *Lectures on Tumours* (1851), *Surgical Pathology* (1863), and *Clinical Lectures and Essays* (1875). Among his original clinical observations were venous obstruction in the upper extremity (1866); an 1874 description of an eczema of the nipple with underlying breast cancer; and a classic description of osteitis deformans (1877). Paget is eponymically linked with numerous medical items, including large, neoplastic epithelial carcinoma cells with hyperchromatic nuclei and palely staining cytoplasm found in neoplastic eptithelium of the ducts and in the epidermis of the nipple, areola, and adjacent skin; and pagetoid osteitis or osteitis fibrosa cystica with marked deformity of the bones.

John Erichsen (1818-1896) served his apprenticeship with Liston at the University College Hospital. By the age of 32 years he had been elected professor of surgery and full attending surgeon at his alma mater. Erichsen became known as one of the ablest surgical teachers of his time; his skill is evident in the popularity of his text, *The Science and Art of Surgery* (1853). Lister and many other well-known British physicians served as his house surgeon. Erichsen's name is associated with a clinical sign that, when sudden pressure is placed approximate to the iliac bones, pain is caused in the presence of sacroiliac disease but not in that of hip disease. He was quite influential in the affairs of the Royal College of Surgeons and served as its president in 1880. Queen Victoria made him a baronet in 1895.

John Marshall (1818-1891) was a student of Liston and became professor of surgery at University College Hospital. Most of his experimental work was related to physiology and pathology, and his name is associated with a vestigial fold of the left vena cava and a small oblique vein on the posterior wall of the left atrium, which is a tributary of the coronary sinus. Marshall was president of the General Medical Council; his principal textbook was the two-volume *Outline of Physiology* (1867).

Thomas Wells (1818-1897) studied at Leeds under Hey and Teale and in London with Travers and Green. Initially Wells worked as a naval surgeon, but he settled permanently in London in 1853, where he began to specialize in gynecological surgery with an emphasis on ovariotomy. Wells achieved spectacular results for his time: women came great distances to have him perform surgery on them. He was president of the Royal College of Surgeons and was made a baronet in 1883. Wells's most renowned text is the two-volume *Diseases of the Ovaries* (1865 and 1872). He is eponymically remembered for his invention of a hemostatic forceps and the description of facies ovarica.

Henry Thompson (1820-1904), the son of a lay preacher, was born in Framingham. He entered University College Hospital as a student in 1846. He qualified 3 years later and became house surgeon to Erichsen. After his training Thompson decided to specialize in urological surgery and was awarded two Jacksonian prizes for essays on urethral stricture and prostatic enlargement. He eventually became professor of clinical surgery at his alma mater. Thompson's two most important texts were *Clinical Lectures on Diseases of the Urinary Organs* (1868) and *On Tumours of the Bladder* (1884). His name is associated with the two-glass test, in which the urine from a patient with gonorrhea is passed into two glasses; if the gonococci and gonorrheal threads are found only in the first glass, the probability is that the process is limited to the anterior urethra.

In Edinburgh during the early years of the nineteenth century, after the expulsion of John Bell (1763-1820) from the Royal Infirmary, no surgeons of special note were engaged in teaching. As with many others in surgical history, the life of Bell was full of political intrigue. He was an apprentice to Alexander Wood and also attended lectures at the University of Edinburgh, his native city. He became a member of the Royal College of Surgeons in 1786. His fellowship entitled him to the privilege of acting in rotation as one of the surgeons to the Royal Infirmary. In so doing, his clinical abilities and manual dexterity became readily apparent to all members of the staff. Besides his clinical responsibilities, Bell lectured on anatomy and surgery (1786-1796) in the extramural school at Surgeon's Square. Bell's success was extraordinary and was greatly helped by the publication of his *Anatomy of the Bones, Muscles, and Joints* (1793) and an accompanying self-illustrated atlas. In 1800 a change was made in the manner in which surgeons were selected to the Infirmary. James Gregory (1753-1821), professor of medicine, attempted to exclude the younger surgeons while retaining his older, less reactionary peers. Bell vigorously protested the events, but to no avail. The controversy became quite bitter: Bell authored several pamphlets attacking Gregory with tremendous acrimony, including *Letters on Professional Character and Manners* (1810). The Edinburgh medical community was split asunder by the feud; Bell was forced out of the hospital and discontinued his lectures. For the next 20 years he devoted himself to the private practice of surgery. Bell's success was evident in both the size of his practice and the extent of his writings. Among his most popular texts was the 1795 *Discourses on the Nature and Cure of Wounds*. His continued interest in military surgery was reflected in the *Memorial Concerning the Present State of Military and Naval Surgery* (1803). Bell's most influential textbook was his three-volume *The Principles of Surgery* (1801-1808). He was the first to ligate the gluteal artery for aneurysm. Bell's name is associated with a band of muscular fibers that forms a slight fold in the wall of the bladder, running from the uvula to the opening of the ureter on either side, bounding the trigonum. Like his brother Charles, John Bell was a noted artist who illustrated his books with his own paintings and drawings. Bell's last book, *Observations on Italy,* was issued posthumously (1825).

Because of the adamant opposition of Monro *(secundus)*, a separate chair of systematic surgery was not established at the University of Edinburgh until 1831. In reaction to this lack of progress the Royal College of Surgeons of Edinburgh decided to institute their own professorship. John Thomson (1765-1846) assumed their chair in 1804 and held the position until 1821, when he was succeeded by his assistant, John Turner (1790-1836). When Turner resigned 10 years later to become professor of systematic surgery at the university, he was succeeded by John Lizars (1783-1860). Since the university had established a surgical professorship within its academic walls, when Lizar retired (1839) from the chair of the Royal College of Surgeons, no successor was appointed and this extramural teaching position was discontinued.

Part of the university's decision to finally acquiesce regarding a professorship of systematic surgery was a result of the lessening influence of Monro *(secundus)*. He retired from his position at the university in 1798, only to be succeeded by his son, Monro *(tertius)*. The latter was said to be the worst lecturer at the university, a speaker with little originality who made no attempt to render his subject more interesting. Thus after the Monros had monopolized the university teaching of surgery for 110 years, the separate chair of systematic surgery was finally established at the University of Edinburgh.

The last of the prelisterian surgeons to hold the chair of systematic surgery was James Miller (1812-1864). He was an apprentice to Liston and was his assistant in practice before Liston resettled in London. At 30 years of age Miller succeeded Charles Bell and spent 22 years in the post. His most important published work is the two-volume *Principles and Practice of Surgery* (1850).

Clinical surgery was the premier surgical chair in Edinburgh. It was established by George III and thus antedated the founding of a separate chair of systematic surgery by almost 30 years. The first incumbent of the clinical chair was James Russell (1755-1836), who had been a leading member of the Company of Surgeons for many years and its president in 1796. Russell had been one of the first surgeons on staff of the Royal Infirmary and was among the most popular of individuals who practiced in Edinburgh. Russell's most important text was *A Practical Essay on a Certain Disease of the Bones Termed Necrosis* (1794), which was one of the first attempts to provide a complete, detailed description of this pathological process. The last of his monographs was *Observations on the Testicles* (1833). Russell was a cagey personality; after acting as professor for 30 years he had fully established the teaching of clinical surgery at the university. He made it a condition of his retirement at 81 years of age that his successor should pay him the sum of 300 pounds a year for life. James Syme (1799-1870) and Liston were initially involved in the negotiations to be the next professor of clinical surgery, but Liston refused to pay this retirement allowance, so Syme was eventually elected Russell's successor.

Syme was born in Edinburgh and began his medical studies under Barclay at the extramural school at Surgeon's Square. Before he studied medicine, Syme was a chemistry student at the university, where he discovered a method by which rubber (caoutchouc) could be dissolved and thus made suitable for painting onto cloth, rendering the cloth waterproof. Syme submitted his discovery to the editor of the *Annals of Philosophy,* but for various reasons publication was delayed. During that interim, Charles Mackintosh (1766-1843), a Scottish inventor, learned of the method, elaborated on it, developed it further, and patented it for commercial purposes. As a result, the Mackintosh raincoat was born and Syme lost out on an inestimable fortune. Inspired by Barclay and under the direction of his chief assistant, Liston, Syme quickly became a master anatomist. Both Liston and Syme left Barclay to open their own school of anatomical instruction in 1818. By 1823 the once close friends had become bitter enemies, which caused professional repercussions throughout the remainder of their lives. Within 2 years Syme had started giving private lessons in surgery, and because of ongoing political difficulties with Liston and other individuals, he was not able to receive an appointment to the surgical staff of the Royal Infirmary. For the next few years Syme's principal goal was to further his reputation as a teacher of

231. James Syme, leader of the Edinburgh school of surgery and father-in-law of Joseph Lister. *(Historical Collections, College of Physicians of Philadelphia.)*

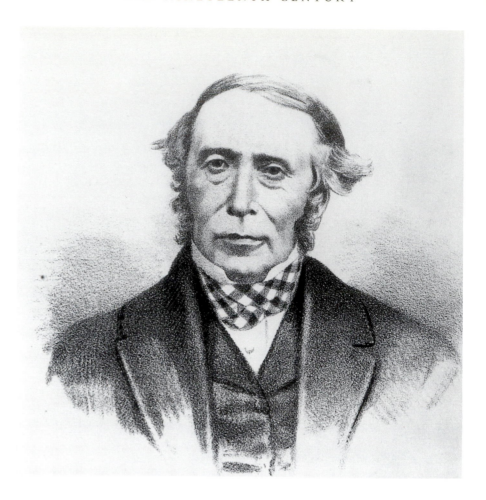

surgery. During that time he began to make his numerous contributions to surgery of the bones and joints. In 1828 he reported his remarkable excision of the lower jaw for osteosarcoma. It is important to keep in mind that most of the difficult, dangerous operations carried out during the early nineteenth century were performed in the humble homes of poor patients. The surroundings were unfavorable; modern conveniences were few. Desperately in need of a private hospital, Syme started his own facility in 1829. His growing reputation was enhanced by the publication in quick order of another important paper on excision of elbow joints (1829) and his monumental *Treatise on the Excision of Diseased Joints* (1831). The latter work demonstrated that excision of joints is usually preferable to amputation, a principle that was soon generally adopted. Syme's *Principles of Surgery* was also published in 1831. By the early 1830s Syme and his rival Liston had become the most well-known surgeons in Edinburgh. In 1833 Russell resigned his position as professor of clinical surgery at the university. After lengthy negotiations Syme was offered the professorship when Liston refused to pay Russell a retirement allowance. In a more than symbolic way, Syme had won his lifelong battle. He had established himself in the premier surgical chair in Edinburgh, he had been placed on the staff of the Royal Infirmary, and his surgical and academic reputations were secure. The teaching of clinical surgery in Edinburgh took on a new meaning with Syme's accession to the professorship. Bedside teaching and student access to the patients were considered integral to his method:

> To bring the cases one by one into a room, where the students are comfortably seated, and if the patients have not been seen by the surgeon beforehand, so much the better; then ascertaining the seat and nature of their complaints, he points out their distinctive characters.
>
> Having done this so that everyone present knows the case under consideration, the teacher, either in the presence or absence of the patient, according to circumstance, proceeds to explain the principles of treatment, with his reasons for choosing the method preferred; and, lastly, does what is requisite in the presence of the pupils.

The great advantage of this system is that it makes an impression at the same time on the eye and ear, which is known by experience to be more indelible than any other, and thus conveys instruction of the most lasting character.

As a teacher, Syme was the undisputed leader in Edinburgh, but Liston continued to rival him as a surgical operator and had a larger consulting practice in Scotland. In 1835, however, Liston assumed a professorship in London and Syme was left in undisputed possession of Edinburgh and Scottish surgery.

In 1847, after the unexpected death of Liston, Syme was offered and accepted the professorship of clinical surgery at University College Hospital in London. He moved in February 1848 but was unhappy with his new life and returned to Edinburgh by July to reclaim his still vacant former position.

Syme made many of his most memorable contributions to surgery during the 1840s, such as his amputation of the foot at the ankle joint, the malleoli being sawed off, and a flap being made with the soft parts of the heel (1842). Syme was the first important European surgeon to generally adopt the use of ether anesthesia in surgical operations (1847). In 1848 he authored *Contributions to the Pathology and Practice of Surgery,* which summarized his professional contributions up to that time. Syme had many prominent students; the most famous of these, Joseph Lister, became his son-in-law. Syme's name is also associated with operations for the excision of the tongue and an external urethrotomy. He resigned his position in 1868 and died 2 years later.

The professorship of military surgery, begun in 1806, was an important surgical chair in prelisterian nineteenth-century Edinburgh. Founded within the University of Edinburgh, its first incumbent was John Thomson (1765-1846), who concurrently served as professor of surgery in the Royal College of Surgeons. He held the chair for 16 years, but his only written work relating to military surgery was *Report of Observations Made in the British Military Hospitals in Belgium after the Battle of Waterloo* (1816). Thomson resigned in 1822 and thereafter mainly studied pathological anatomy. In 1831 a chair of pathology was begun at the university, and Thomson was nominated as the first recipient. This was the third professorship in Edinburgh that Thomson was the first to hold. In many respects his earliest written work, *Lectures on Inflammation, Exhibiting a View of the General Doctrines, Pathological and Practical, of Medical Surgery* (1813), was a prelude to his life's later work.

When Thomson retired from the chair of military surgery, George Ballingall (1786-1855) was appointed his successor (1823). Ballingall had extensive military experience, having entered the army in 1806, and had written *Practical Observations on Fever, Dysentery, and Liver Complaints, as They Occur Among the European Troops in India* (1822). Ballingall remained as professor for more than 30 years, during which time he wrote *Outlines of the Course of Lectures on Military Surgery* (1833). After Ballingall's death the chair of military surgery was abolished.

In tracing the growth of surgical education and training in Edinburgh, the influence of the extramural school must be taken into account. The individual private schools that made up the extramural school functioned as classrooms outside the formal academic activities of the university. In many respects the various private schools (such as Surgeons' Square, Argyll Square, Brown Square, Minto House, Park Place, and New School) acted as catalysts for the future direction of the university in medical and surgical education. In many instances the most famous of Edinburgh's professors of surgery initially taught at the extramural school. The fame of the University of Edinburgh medical school was at its zenith during the first half of the nineteenth century, largely because of the surgeons of the extramural school.

John Lizar (1794-1860) was among the most prominent of the surgeons of the extramural school. A pupil of John Bell, Lizar began teaching at the extramural school in 1815. In 1831 he succeeded Turner as professor of surgery in the Royal College of Surgeons. In the process of his appointment to the position much political animosity developed between Lizar and Syme. In one instance Syme sued Lizar and forced him to pay damages for supposedly false statements. Lizar resigned his appointment in 1839, at which time the professorship was abolished. He was the first in England to perform ovariotomy, which was duly noted in his *Observations on Extraction of Diseased Ovaria* (1825). In addition to publishing a series of anatomical plates (1822-1826), Lizar authored a *System of Practical Surgery* (1842).

Richard Mackenzie (1821-1854) studied under Syme at the Royal Infirmary and then traveled throughout Europe to complete his surgical education. In 1844 he returned to Edinburgh, where he was made a fellow of the Royal College of Surgeons. During 1849 he lectured at the extramural school and in the following year was appointed surgeon to the Royal Infirmary. Mackenzie's most important surgical contribution was his modification of Syme's method of amputation of the ankle, in which the skin flap was taken from the inner side (1849). In 1854 the army needed medical volunteers to serve in Crimea. Mackenzie entered the army as a military surgeon and died of cholera within 4 months.

In Glasgow at the beginning of the nineteenth century the leading surgeon was John Burns (1775-1850). Initially he gave private lessons in anatomy, but in 1815 he was appointed Regius professor of surgery at the University of Glasgow. Burns was an uninspiring teacher but was quite a prolific writer. His most important work was *The Principles of Midwifery* (1809), which went through 10 editions. His other texts included *Anatomy of the Gravid Uterus* (1799), the two-volume *Dissertations on Inflammation* (1800), *Observations on Abortion* (1806), *Practical Observations on the Uterine Hemorrhage* (1807), and *Popular Directions for the Treatment of the Diseases of Women and Children* (1811).

Alan Burns (1781-1813) became more famous than his older brother, John Burns. He developed an interest in anatomical research during his initial studies with his brother. In 1811 Alan Burns authored *Observations on the Surgical Anatomy of the Head and Neck,* in which he described the fascial space at the suprasternal notch. He also suggested for the first time the feasibility of ligating the innominate artery and provided a description of the first recorded case of chloroma. Burns's name is associated with the superior horn of the saphenous opening, which is the upper part of the falciform margin of the opening of the fascia lata, through which the greater saphenous vein passes. In addition, the falciform process, a continuation of the inner border of the sacrotuberous ligament upward and forward on the inner aspect of the ramus of the ischium, is eponymically linked with him. His *Observations on Some of the Most Frequent and Important Diseases of the Heart* (1809) contained an early description of endocarditis and reported three cases of mitral stenosis. Burns recognized the thrill present in mitral stenosis and appears to have understood the mechanism of the cardiac murmur. He also described unilateral paralysis of the diaphragm resulting from pressure placed on the phrenic nerve by a thoracic aneurysm. Burns was among the first to suggest that angina pectoris is a consequence of coronary artery insufficiency.

In Dublin, surgical practice was quite limited when the Royal College of Surgeons of Ireland was founded. However, the College assumed the task of educating and training surgeons by naming its first professor of surgery in 1785. William Dease (1752-1798), who had written *Observations on Wounds of the Head* (1776), was named as the first incumbent. His tenure lasted 10 years before he suddenly died with a ruptured aneurysm.

The Royal College of Surgeons of Ireland at first granted several varieties of diploma, including those for military surgeons and midwives. The examination for licensure was quite rigorous, frequently lasting 2 days. Until 1828 the College could not legally insist that candidates for the license produce evidence of having attended College-sponsored lectures; the only requirement was an apprenticeship of 5 years to a recognized surgeon. During the first half of the century the College prospered both organizationally and financially. A museum of anatomy and pathology was opened, for which John Houston (1802-1845) served as curator. Houston is eponymically linked with the transverse rectal folds or valves. By 1835 the College's school of medicine was flourishing, as were other private medical institutions throughout Dublin. The increasing respectability of surgery led in 1849 to the creation of a chair of surgery at the University of Dublin. Although the establishment of this chair was looked upon unfavorably by the College, little could be done to prevent it.

The influence of the Royal College of Surgeons of Ireland was evident not only in surgery but also in the strengthening of general medical practice in Dublin. Among the more prominent practitioners were John Cheyne (1777-1836), Robert Graves (1796-1853), Dominic Corrigan (1802-1880), and William Stokes (1804-1878). Abraham Colles (1773-1843) was the most prominent Irish surgeon of his day and a leader of the Royal College of Surgeons. He was born near Kilkenny and matriculated at the University of Dublin in 1790. At the same time, he was apprenticed to a surgeon at Steevens' Hospital. Five years later Colles earned a diploma from the Royal College of Surgeons. Wishing to pursue his studies, he spent 2 years at the University of Edinburgh, from which he received a degree in medicine. Colles then spent a short time assisting Astley Cooper in London with his anatomical studies. In 1797 Colles returned to Dublin and was appointed resident surgeon at Steevens' Hospital. He remained in that position from 1799 to 1813, when he was elected visiting surgeon to that institution. Colles was an excellent clinical surgeon who became most famous for his technical skills. From 1804 to 1836 Colles also served as professor of anatomy and surgery at the Royal College of Surgeons of Ireland. In 1814 he authored his most famous paper, which described a fracture of the lower end of the radius with displacement of the hand backward and outward. One year later he reported two cases in which he ligated the subclavian artery. Among his textbooks the earliest was the partially completed *Treatise on Surgical Anatomy* (1811). In 1837 he wrote *Practical Observations on the Venereal Disease, and on the Use of Mercury,* in which he introduced the hypothesis of immunity in the mother of a syphilitic infant when the mother has never had any symptoms of the disease. Colles's principal textbook was the two-volume *Lectures on the Theory and Practice of Surgery* (1744-1745). His name is also eponymically associated with the superficial perineal fascia; the triangular fascia, a fibrous band extending from the aponeurosis of the external oblique to the pubic tubercle of the opposite side; and the superficial compartment of the perineum. Colles served as president of the Royal College of Surgeons of Ireland in 1802 and 1830.

There were several other prominent prelisterian Irish surgeons. Philip Crampton (1777-1858) was appointed surgeon to the Meath Hospital when he was only 21 years old. He was one of the founders of the first private schools for anatomy and surgery in Dublin. His name is associated with a line from the apex of the cartilage of the last rib downward and forward nearly to the crest of the ilium, then forward and parallel with it to a little below the anterior superior spine, which acts as a guide to the common iliac artery. He is also known for the radiating fibers of the ciliary muscle of the eye.

William Porter (1790-1861) was a pupil of Crampton and was elected surgeon to Meath Hospital in 1819. He succeeded Colles as professor of surgery in the Royal College of Surgeons (1836). Porter's most prominent work was *Observations on the Surgical Pathology of the Larynx and Trachea* (1826). In it he included a description of tracheal tugging in aortic aneurysm and of the pretracheal fascia.

Robert Adams (1791-1875) was surgeon to the Jervis Street and Richmond Hospitals. In 1861 he was appointed Regius professor of surgery at the University of Dublin. Although a surgeon, Adams remains best known for his work with cardiac disease. In 1827 he reported a classic account of heart block with syncopal attacks. Adams also recognized a thrill in mitral regurgitation and understood tricuspid incompetence. His most important textbook was *A Treatise on Rheumatic Gout, or Chronic Rheumatic Arthritis, of All the Joints* (1857). It included an excellent description of chronic rheumatic arthritis.

Robert Smith (1807-1873), a native of Dublin, apprenticed with Richard Carmichael (1779-1849). Smith was appointed first professor of surgery in the School of Physic of the University of Dublin (1849). The chairs of anatomy and surgery had been united before that time. His principal written work was *A Treatise on the Pathology, Diagnosis, and Treatment of Neuroma* (1849). It included a full description of generalized neurofibromatosis. Smith's name is eponymically associated with a fracture of the radius near its lower articular surface with displacement of the fragment toward the palmar aspect.

William Wilde (1815-1876), father of the dramatist Oscar Wilde (1854-1900), was born in Castlereagh and worked in Dublin as an oculist and otologist. His most important work was *Practical Observations on Aural Surgery and the Nature and Treatment of Diseases of the Ear* (1853). This text did more to place British otology on a firm scientific basis than anything previously published. Wilde showed that the middle ear was the site of origin of most of the diseases of the ear. He is remembered for his method of treating acute mastoiditis, in which an incision parallel to the pinna of the ear and about half an inch behind it is used to relieve tension in mastoid periostitis. Wilde is also eponymically linked with transverse markings on the corpus callosum.

Thomas Tufnell (1819-1875) studied in London under Brodie and Hawkins and entered the army medical service in 1841. After the Crimean War he retired from active service and permanently settled in Dublin. He was surgeon to the City of Dublin Hospital and professor of military surgery at the school of the Royal College of Surgeons. He authored *Practical Remarks on the Treatment of Aneurism by Compression* (1851) and *The Successful Treatment of Internal Aneurism* (1864). Tufnell's name is associated with a permanent bandage consisting of a cheesecloth roller impregnated with a mixture of flour and egg white.

Joseph Gamgee (1828-1886), the son of a veterinary surgeon, studied at University College in London. Most of Gamgee's professional life was spent in Birmingham, where he was surgeon to the Queen's Hospital. He advocated the dry, infrequent dressing of wounds and is eponymically linked with a material consisting of a thick layer of absorbent cotton between two layers of absorbent gauze, which was used in surgical dressings. His major monographs were *On the Advantage of the Starched Apparatus in the Treatment of Fractures and Diseases of Joints* (1853) and *On the Treatment of Wounds* (1878).

Jonathan Hutchinson (1828-1913) studied at St. Bartholomew's Hospital, served as surgeon to the London Hospital, and was professor of surgery at the Royal College of Surgeons of England (1879-1883). He also was editor of the *Archives of Surgery* (1889-1899), one of earliest periodicals related to surgery. Hutchinson was an excellent surgeon and pathologist. His many writings included an 1858 article describing notched incisors in congenital syphilis. His name is also associated with the clinical triad of interstitial keratitis, notched incisors, and labyrinthine disease in congenital syphilis. In 1871 he was the first surgeon to successfully operate on an infant for intussusception. Among his many clinical observations were summer prurigo (1878), dyshidrosis, sarcoidosis, hydradenitis destruens suppurativa, and varicella gangrenosa (1882), Hilliard's lupus (1889), and angioma serpiginosum (1891). Hutchinson's name is associated with senile guttate choroidopathy; progeria; the peculiar facial expression produced by the drooping lids and motionless eyeballs of ophthalmoplegia; the sensation in tabes dorsalis that makes the face feel as if it were covered with a mask or with cobwebs; and an immobile dilation of the pupil on the side of the lesion, with contraction of the other pupil, that occurs when meningeal hemorrhage compresses the third nerve at the base of the brain. Among Hutchinson's textbooks were *Illustrations of Clinical Surgery* (1875) and *Lectures on Clinical Surgery* (1879).

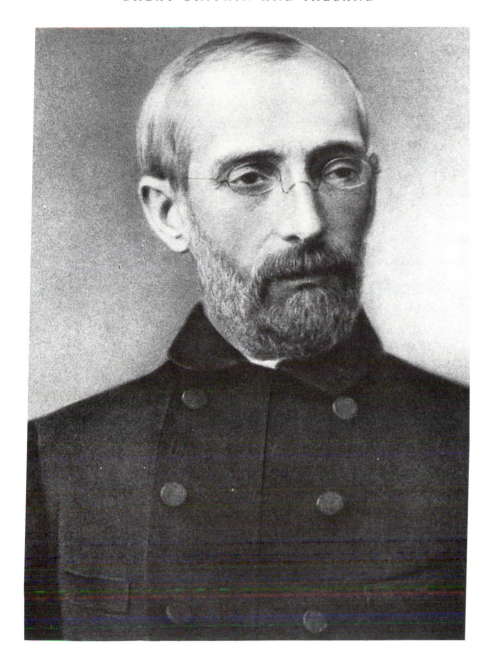

232. Hugh Owen Thomas of the "Thomas Splint" and the "Thomas Heel." Descended from a line of bonesetters, Thomas benefitted from an excellent medical education and proved to be a profound innovator in orthopedic surgery. Although Thomas achieved results superior to those of his traditional-minded colleagues, his lack of tact and diplomacy antagonized them. It fell upon Robert Jones, Thomas's nephew, to convey Thomas's innovations to the surgical community and by so doing to revolutionize orthopedics throughout the world. *(Jeremy Norman & Co., Inc.)*

Hugh Owen Thomas (1834-1891) was trained in both Edinburgh and London and received his M.R.C.S. degree in 1858. He practiced in Liverpool, where he specialized in orthopedic surgery and became a founder of modern British orthopedics. Thomas never served an apprenticeship with any university lecturer, nor had he even been a surgical tutor or a house surgeon. Yet, he was able to develop ideas that he could put to practical clinical use, especially concerning fractures. In his *Diseases of the Hip, Knee and Ankle Joints, with Their Deformities, Treated by a New and Efficient Method* (1875), Thomas introduced a rigid splint made of steel bars curved to the shape of the limb and retained by plaster-of-paris bandages. He is also remembered eponymically for a rigid metal splint extending from a ring at the hip to beyond the foot, which allows traction to a fractured leg and is used for emergencies and during transportation.

Morell Mackenzie (1837-1892) is considered the founder of modern British laryngology. In 1863 he founded the Golden Square Throat Hospital in London, the first hospital in the world devoted solely to diseases of the throat. Mackenzie also started the *Journal of Laryngology*. His most important works included *The Use of the Laryngoscope in Diseases of the Throat; with an Appendix on Rhinoscopy* (1865), *Essay on Growth in the Larynx* (1871), and the two-volume *A Manual of Diseases of the Throat and Nose* (1880-1884).

Robert Lawson Tait (1845-1899) was a native of Edinburgh, where he was educated under James Young Simpson (1811-1870). Tait moved to Birmingham in 1871 and remained there for the rest of his professional life. He was the first British surgeon to diagnose acute appendicitis and to treat it by removal of the appendix (1880), and he performed many other surgical feats. His greatest clinical contributions are found in gynecological surgery, especially ovariotomy. In 1879 Tait reported the removal of normal ovaries. Two years later he removed the uterine appendages. His *General Summary of Conclusions from One Thousand Cases of Abdominal Section* (1884) reveals him to be probably the greatest of all nineteenth-century ovariotomists. In the late 1880s Tait devised a flap-splitting operation for rectocele, also called a perineoplasty. He was also apparently the first to describe ovarian fibroma combined with pleural effusion (1892). Much of Tait's clinical attention centered on obstetrics, and in 1884 he performed the first successful operation for ruptured ectopic pregnancy. Four years later he detailed his wide experience in *Lectures on Ectopic Pregnancy and Pelvic Haematocele*. In 1890 he reported the performance of cesarean section in cases of placenta previa. Tait is eponymically associated with a double ligature passed through the substance of the pedicle of an ovarian tumor, the loop then being reversed over the end of the pedicle and placed between the two free ends of the ligature that are tied over it; and a "law" stating that an exploratory laparotomy should be performed in every case of obscure pelvic or abdominal disease that threatens health or life. In 1884 Tait helped organize the British Gynecological Society, and he served as its second president. Tait was a vociferous, often demeaning critic of Lister and his experimental research. Tait was never convinced of the pathogenic nature of bacteria, yet his insistence on absolute cleanliness proved to be remarkably close to aseptic techniques.

William Macewen (1848-1924) studied at the Royal Infirmary in Glasgow and in 1869 became house surgeon to George Macleod of that city. By 1875 Macewen was appointed assistant surgeon at the Royal Infirmary and 2 years later, full surgeon. In 1892 he succeeded Macleod as Regius professor of surgery and transferred his clinical work from the Royal Infirmary to the Western Infirmary. After Lister's death Macewen was recognized as one of the preeminent living British surgeons. Among his most important texts was *The Growth of Bone* (1912), which contained his research on osteogenesis. Macewen's most prominent papers discussed the first allograft transplantation of bone in humans (1881); a method for the radical cure of inguinal hernia, in which the sac was folded into a pad and used as a plug at the internal ring, the ring being closed in layers (1886); and a removal of a section of the left lung for tuberculosis (1906). He performed his greatest clinical work in neurosurgery, as most graphically detailed in his *Pyogenic Infective Diseases of the Brain and Spinal Cord* (1893) and its accompanying *Atlas of Head Sections* (1893). In the text he included extensive case reports of 65 patients under his care, with details of operative procedures. Along with Fedor Krause (1856-1937) and Harvey Cushing (1869-1939), Macewen pioneered the development of neurosurgery as a specialty. Macewen was also the first physician to administer an anesthetic (chloroform) through a metal tracheal tube introduced into the mouth (endotracheal anesthesia). He is eponymically remembered for a supracondyloid osteotomy of the femur for knock-knee; percussion of the skull giving a cracked-pot sound in cases of hydrocephalus; and the suprameatal triangle. In 1889, overtures had been made to Macewen to become surgeon-in-chief at the Johns Hopkins Hospital in Baltimore. He declined the post, however, and William Halsted was eventually appointed. If Macewen had accepted the position, the history of surgery would have been markedly different in that (1) the achievements of Halsted at Johns Hopkins would never have occurred, (2) Harvey Cushing's neurosurgical career would have been partially eclipsed, and (3) the development and professionalization of nursing in the United States would have been affected, since Macewen limited nurses to secondary, supportive roles. MacEwen served as president of the British Medical Association in 1922.

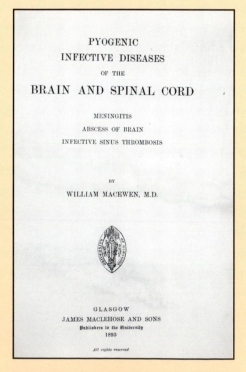

233. Macewen's classic work on neurological surgery. *(Jeremy Norman & Co., Inc.)*

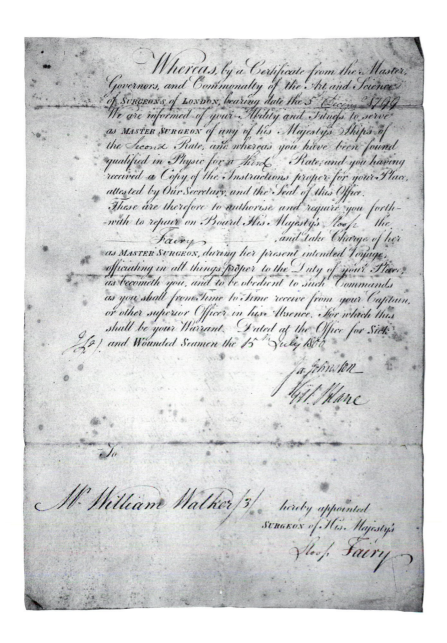

Arthur Mayo-Robson (1853-1933) received his medical training at the Leeds School of Medicine. From 1890 to 1904 he was professor of surgery at his alma mater while also serving as surgeon to the Leeds General Infirmary. After 1904 Mayo-Robson moved to London, where he maintained a busy clinical practice. In 1901 Mayo-Robson jointly authored, with his pupil Moynihan, *Diseases of the Stomach and Their Surgical Treatment*. Mayo-Robson's name is associated with a point just above and to the right of the umbilicus, where tenderness exists in disease of the pancreas; and a position in which the patient lies on the back with a thick pad under the lumbosacral region, causing a marked lordosis in this region, which is used in operations on the gallbladder. In 1897 he served as president of the British Gynecological Society.

Frederick Treves (1853-1923) entered London Hospital as a student in 1867 and spent his entire professional life at that institution. Treves was sergeant surgeon to the monarchy and performed an appendectomy on Edward VII (1841-1910) in 1902, for which he was made a baronet. Treves is best remembered for his fascinating stories about and treatment of John Merrick, the young man with neurofibromatosis who became known as the elephant man. Treves's major written work was *Intestinal Obstruction* (1884), an essay for which he was awarded the Jacksonian prize. He is eponymically associated with the ileocecal fold.

235. Frederick Treves, sergeant surgeon to the king of England, and his most famous patient, John Merrick, "The Elephant Man," whom he rescued and maintained in a room in the London Hospital from 1886 until Merrick's death in 1890. Neither the play nor the film adapted from Treves's own account of this case could depict the true scope of Merrick's deformities, which were caused by a terrible case of neurofibromatosis, but both dramatizations were able to contrast Merrick's noble, romantic spirit with his unspeakably repulsive appearance. *(The Trustees of The Wellcome Trust, London.)*

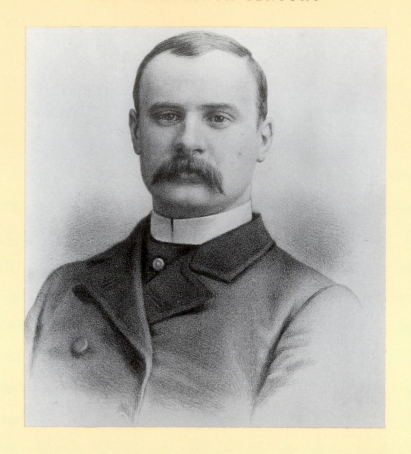

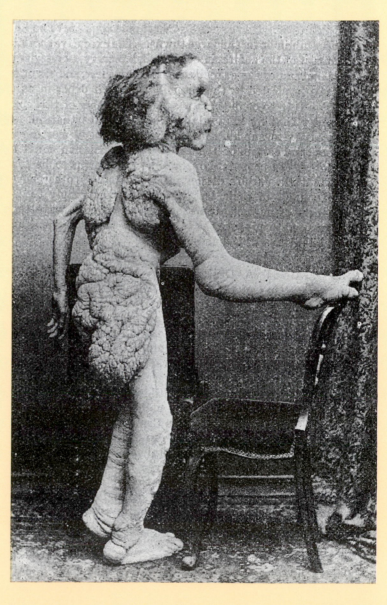

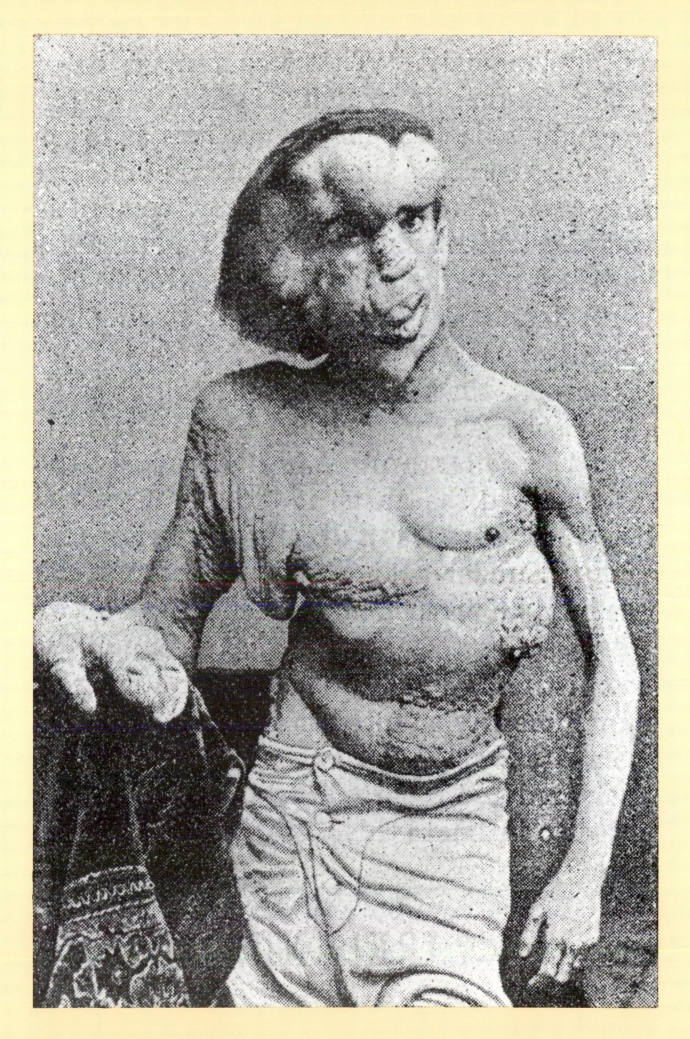

William Battle (1855-1936) practiced in London, where he described a vertical incision of the abdominal wall with retraction of the rectus muscle medially (1895). In 1901 he detailed his operation for femoral hernia. Battle's name is associated with a postauricular ecchymosis in cases of fracture of the base of the skull.

William Arbuthnot Lane (1856-1943) was a native of Scotland and studied at Guy's Hospital. He was eventually appointed chief surgeon at both his alma mater and the Ormond Street Hospital. His most important surgical work was his treatment of chronic intestinal stasis by "short-circuiting" the intestine as described in *The Operative Treatment of Chronic Constipation* (1909). It is unlikely that any other surgeon before or after him ever completed as many colectomies as Lane did. He was also quite well known for his research into orthopedic surgery, which included the treatment of fractures by the perfect reapposition of the affected parts by means of operative intervention (1894) and the use of plates and screws for union of fractures (1907). Lane also wrote an important paper on mastoidectomy for the efficient drainage of middle-ear suppuration (1892). His name is associated with a congenital band on the distal ileum that supposedly causes intestinal stasis; hereditary palmar erythema; a decompression operation that consists of removing segments of bone from the roof of the skull; and flattened, narrow metal plates of various shapes and sizes, perforated for screws, that are used to hold the fragments of a fractured bone in apposition.

Victor Horsley (1857-1916) was one of England's earliest neurosurgeons. He received his medical education at the University College Hospital in London. Most of his professional life was spent on the surgical staff of his alma mater. His early interest in neurology brought him an appointment to the National Hospital for the Paralyzed and Epileptic. He made numerous lasting contributions to surgery, including evidence to support the view that myxedema, cretinism, and operative cachexia strumpriva are all caused by thyroid deficiency (1884); he also performed the first successful experimental hypophysectomy (1886). His neurological experiments included investigations into the localization of cerebral function (1887), demonstration that electrical currents are produced in the mammalian brain (1891), and the development of a stereotactic apparatus for the accurate location of electrodes in the brain (1908). In 1888 Horsley performed the first successful operation for the removal of an extramedullary tumor of the spinal cord. He devised an operation for the treatment of trigeminal neuralgia in which the gasserian ganglion is removed by a temporal approach (1891) and showed that the removal of the precentral cortex in humans abolishes athetosis (1909). Horsley is eponymically associated with a test for sugar in the urine, the presence of which is indicated when a green color is produced by boiling urine with potassic hydrate and potassium chromate, and bone wax. At 50 years of age Horsley resigned his position as surgeon at the University College Hospital and began to devote himself largely to political matters. He advocated such politically unpopular causes as women's suffrage and temperance. At the outbreak of World War I, Horsley enlisted as a surgical consultant. He died of heatstroke in the Mesopotamian desert.

Robert Jones (1858-1933) was lecturer on orthopedic surgery at Liverpool University, orthopedic surgeon at the Royal Infirmary there, and later, director of orthopedics at St. Thomas's Hospital in London. His uncle was Hugh Owen Thomas, from whom he obtained his early orthopedic knowledge. Jones communicated the revolutionary ideas of Thomas to the world, thereby helping to establish his uncle's reputation and orthopedic surgery as a specialty. Jones's own reputation was solidified when he was named director of orthopedics of the British army during the First World War. In 1896 Jones authored the first published report of the clinical use of an X ray to locate a bullet in the wrist. His most important text was *Orthopaedic Surgery,* jointly written with Robert Lovett (1859-1924). Other works included *Injuries of Joints* (1915) and *Notes on Military Orthopedics* (1917). Jones was a forceful advocate of tendon transplantation, bone grafting, and other conservative, restorative procedures.

Rickman Godlee (1859-1925) studied medicine at University College Hospital in London, where he later became professor of clinical surgery and attending surgeon. His mother was Lister's sister: Godlee was one of the major adherents to listerian principles in late nineteenth-century London. Godlee served as president of the Royal College of Surgeons of England (1911-1913) and surgeon to Queen Victoria's household. His most important surgical case was the first known instance of the diagnosis, accurate clinical localization, and operative removal of a tumor of the brain (1884).

Berkeley Moynihan (1865-1936) was born on the island of Malta and pursued his medical studies at Leeds School of Medicine. He later received his degrees of Bachelor of Medicine and Bachelor of Surgery (M.B. and B.S.). from London University. Moynihan was initially an associate of Thomas Jessop (1837-1903), a surgeon at Leeds who later became his father-in-law. From 1907 to 1927 Moynihan was surgeon at the Leeds General Infirmary and later held the chair of clinical surgery at London University. During World War I he was chief surgeon of the British army in France. Moynihan was an outstanding abdominal surgeon who wrote several authoritative texts, in particular, *Diseases of the Stomach and Their Surgical Treatment* (1901), jointly written with his mentor Mayo-Robson, and *Duodenal Ulcer* (1910), in which he presented the so-called ulcer sequence: pain-food-ease. Moynihan stressed the well-ordered sequence of symptoms. He more than any other surgeon established the surgical treatment of duodenal ulcer disease. Additional treatises included *Diseases of the Pancreas* (1902) and *Gall Stones and Their Surgical Treatment* (1904). Much of his later professional life was spent in London, where he was actively involved with the organization and management of the Royal College of Surgeons of England. He also served on the editorial boards of the *British Journal of Surgery* and the American College of Surgeons's journal, *Surgery, Gynecology and Obstetrics*.

W. Ernest Miles (1869-1947) received his surgical training at St. Bartholomew's Hospital, where he first became interested in colon and rectal surgery, and later was appointed surgeon at both the Cancer Hospital at Brompton and the Gordon Hospital for Diseases of the Rectum. In 1908, Miles authored a report that described the one-stage operation of abdominoperineal resection for cancer of the rectum.

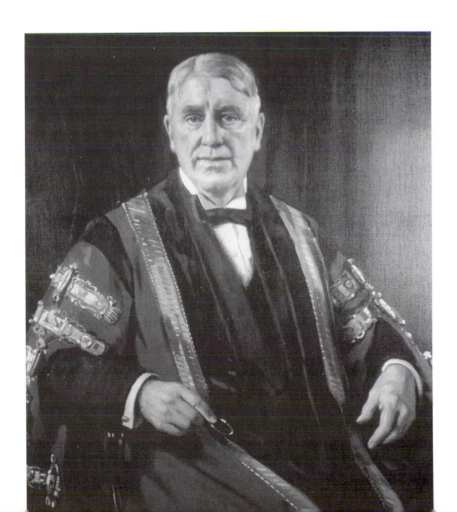

236. Moynihan established the so-called ulcer sequence: pain-food-ease. *(Jeremy Norman & Co., Inc.)*

385

GERMANY, AUSTRIA-HUNGARY, AND SWITZERLAND

After the defeat of Napoleon a peace conference was held in Vienna (1814-1815). Austria, however, would not join with the numerous independent German states to form a national union of Germany, fearing that it would lose its power if it became a member of such a coalition. As a result of the conference, Prussia took part of Saxony and certain lands along the Rhine and Austria received Venice and portions of northern Italy. The more than 300 independent states of the old Holy Roman Empire were reduced to 38. A German Bund was established in place of the empire.

A new movement to unify Germany occurred during the 1850s and 1860s. Prussia was well suited to assume the leadership of the splintered German states. In 1861 Wilhelm I (1797-1888) was proclaimed king of Prussia and immediately became a strong advocate of his prime minister Otto von Bismarck's (1815-1898) goals to unify the confederation. Bismarck fought three wars in the process of unification, including those against Denmark, Austria, and France.

The German Empire, or Second Reich, grew out of the victories of a newly awakened German nationalism. Wilhelm I took the title of German emperor, or kaiser (1871), and appointed Bismarck as chancellor to look after the details of government.

The growth of Germany's industries further empowered the nation. Wilhelm I was succeeded by his son Frederick III (1831-1888), who died of a laryngeal cancer within 100 days of his coronation. Frederick had married a daughter of Queen Victoria. Because of this English connection, Morell MacKenzie had been brought in to treat the illness of the future king but in the process had misdiagnosed the tumor. Against the advice of various German surgeons, including Theodor Billroth, to undergo laryngectomy, the crown prince, heavily influenced by his wife, had decided to continue under the care of MacKenzie.

MacKenzie's surgical misjudgment would have serious future political repercussions, since Frederick's son Wilhelm II (1859-1941) dismissed Bismarck and insisted on a massive reorganization and buildup of the German army and navy. He alarmed the British with his military policy, lost the friendship of Russia, and made enemies on every side. Wilhelm II's miscalculations, perhaps caused by his having to assume the emperorship at a relatively early age as a result of his father's premature death, were among the many reasons for the outbreak of World War I. Wilhelm II was ultimately forced to flee Germany (1918). He was the last emperor, and the Hohenzollern dynasty ended with his departure.

From 1815 to 1848 the leading figure in Austrian affairs was Klemens von Metternich (1773-1859). He was minister of foreign affairs for the Hapsburg emperors and worked diligently to put down all liberal or nationalist movements in the Hapsburg empire. After the forced resignation of Metternich in 1848, Francis Joseph I (1830-1916) was named emperor of Austria and eventually, king of Hungary (1867). In the new Austria-Hungary, often called the Dual Monarchy, the Austrian empire and the kingdom of Hungary were united under one ruler. Foreign affairs, war, and the treasury were combined for both countries, but each had a separate national government.

In 1803 Napoleon gave Switzerland a new constitution, establishing a federal republic of 19 cantons. The Congress of Vienna guaranteed the neutrality of Switzerland, which remained unbroken throughout the century.

The ascendancy of German medicine and surgery did not occur until the latter half of the nineteenth century. Surgical education and training persisted in an undeveloped state in the German-speaking countries longer than in most other regions in western Europe. Undoubtedly, a major reason for the delay was that at the beginning of the century Germany was a conglomeration of divided, independent political units, with no one central city representing the focus of governmental organization. There is no better example of the effect of politics on the delivery of health care and physician education and training than that of the German-speaking countries at the end of the eighteenth century and the beginning of the nineteenth century.

The nineteenth-century German unification process under Prussia presented unlimited opportunities for surgery. As the new Germany began to present itself to the international markets, it looked to its universities for image building. In Prussia a system of medical study had been arranged in 1825. It provided both for physicians who studied at the universities and for surgeons, who were delineated into first and second classes. The surgeons of the first class were required to study at either a university or a "medico-chirurgical school" for 3 years. Unlike the physicians, however, they were not required to know Latin, an indication, perhaps, that surgery was thought of as the more practical craft. Surgeons of the second class were educated only through an apprenticeship with a practicing second-class surgeon. In most instances the second-class surgeons served for a short time in a military hospital or attended a few lectures at a "medico-chirurgical school." At mid-century the Prussian government decreed that there should be but a single class of doctors and that more than a medical degree was necessary before doctors could obtain the right to practice.

As early as 1810 the government in Austria began to require a 5-year course in medicine or surgery, whereas only 2 years were required of country doctors. In 1822 the curriculum at the Military Medico-Chirugical Academy, better known as the Josephina in Vienna, was extended to 5 years, and the college was granted the right to award its own degrees. By 1850 much more power had been given to the professors in the various universities regarding the design of their courses. However, a complete separation between the university faculties and the various medical associations was not made until 1873. It was only in 1872 that separate diplomas for surgery were abolished.

237. Elaborate orthopedic apparatus from Arnold Leopold Richter's (1798-1876) *40 Lithographirte Tafeln,* Berlin, 1828. Richter's book illustrated virtually every type of surgical instrument then available. *(Boston Medical Library.)*

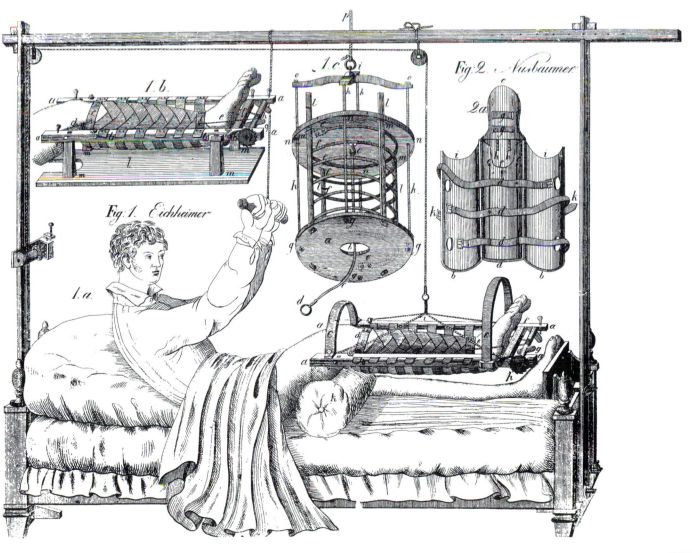

As the German-speaking empire grew, a great scholastic achievement was coming to fruition in the form of the richly endowed state university—highly organized, academically free, crowded with laboratories, and ever growing. The German university system was marked by the following distinctive features: freedom in what was taught; absence of any compulsion in the order, choice, and duration of studies other than those imposed by examinations; release from division of students into classes according to fixed annual courses; academic wandering of students from one university to another; the outside-lecturer system; and academic competition between teachers of similar subjects in the same and different institutions.

The national achievements of Germany soon became international, and from the 1860s through 1914 its educational system attracted aspiring students, including physicians and surgeons, from all over the world. In a mighty academic upsurge of less than 40 years, German surgeons wrenched the world surgical stage away from England and asserted their own dominance. In 1872 the Deutsche Gesellschaft für Chirurgie was formed. This national organization soon began to hold annual meetings, during which papers were read and criticized. In effect it acted as a gathering place for the free interchange of new German surgical ideas.

The reasons for the rapid development of surgery in Germany are not easily defined, but it was undoubtedly related to political and economic changes, as well as to the general cultural and scientific climate. The multiplication in the number of chairs of surgery at the universities, the unification of the disparate branches of the healing art, and the organization of learned societies with journals to publicize their proceedings can be counted among the most important factors. William Halsted cogently commented on Germany's stunning educational achievement in his paper *The Training of the Surgeon* (1904):

> What are the inducements which make it worth while for the young men in Germany to devote so many years to preparation for the practice of surgery, what are the careers to which they aspire, and what manner of men are they who furnish by their example and by their achievements the great stimulus?
>
> Not only the first assistants but all the members of the surgical staff of one of the great university clinics in Germany enjoy almost ideal facilities for learning surgery and for prosecuting researches. The amount of clinical material is great. The operative work begins early in the morning and often does not cease till late in the afternoon. The outpatient department is controlled by the chief surgeon and is conducted by his assistants; a patient when discharged is consequently not referred to some dispensary or other and lost sight of. The pathological material obtained at operation is carefully worked up in the special laboratories for surgery and, if need be, is preserved in the museum, which should always be an important feature of the surgical department of a university. Every facility and the greatest encouragement is given each member of the staff to do work of research . . . the real life of a German surgeon begins when he is invited to fill a professorial chair. He now longs to prove himself worthy of the new position, he has the incentive to inspire others to achieve, he measures himself by a new standard, and there is born in him the desire to rise higher, to sow the seed which will produce a bloom worthy of the greatest universities. In European countries no effort, no amount of time, few sacrifices would be considered too great if thereby the chair of surgery in a university might be secured. In Germany the prestige of the position is something that we in the United States . . . cannot truly comprehend. In each university the chair has its imperishable traditions, its long line of famous surgeons, whose names are cherished and revered for their services to science, to their universities, to their country and to their fellows.

During the first 15 years of the nineteenth century the Napoleonic Wars produced an urgent demand for army surgeons, especially in Austria, the site of numerous conflicts. Vienna had the leading surgical schools of the German-speaking countries at that time, in particular, those founded by Ferdinand Leber (1727-1808) and Giovanni Brambilla (1728-1800).

Few surgeons of distinction practiced in Germany during the early part of the nineteenth century. Franz Hesselbach (1759-1816) studied with Siebold at

Würzburg and also acted as Siebold's assistant in anatomical demonstrations. Hesselbach is principally remembered for his monograph on hernia, *Anatomisch-Chirurgische Abhandlung Uber Den Ursprung Der Leistenbruche* (1806). In it he described the cribriform fascia over the femoral canal; the interfoveolar ligament; a hernia with diverticulae through the cribriform fascia, presenting a lobular outline; and an anatomical triangle bounded by the inguinal ligament, the edge of the rectus abdominis muscle, and the deep or inferior epigastric artery.

Vincenz von Kern (1760-1829) was born in Graz and studied surgery at the Universities of Salzburg, Trieste, and Venice. He was appointed professor of surgery at Laibach in 1797. Kern gained the most important Austrian surgical position in 1805, when he was elected professor of practical and clinical surgery at the University of Vienna. He developed a large surgical practice and was the leader of surgical education and training in Germany and northern Italy until his resignation in 1824. In joining the faculty in Vienna, Kern became a member of what has been named the "first Vienna school" to distinguish it from future faculties. He founded an institute for surgeons in experimental surgery on the cadaver that was among the earliest of such schools in Europe. Kern is best remembered for simplifying the prevailing treatment of wounds by using bandages moistened with plain water as a substitute for various salves and plasters.

By the fourth and fifth decades of the nineteenth century a growing number of German surgeons were achieving prominence. Although their influence would be the catalyst that later propelled Germany toward world prominence, most of them did not live to see the heights to which German surgery rose.

Johann Rust (1775-1840) received his surgical education and training in Prague and Vienna. He was named professor of surgery at Kracow in 1803 and 7 years later became one of the surgeons of the General Hospital in Vienna. In 1816 Rust succeeded Mursinna in the army medical school at Berlin; subsequently he became professor of surgery at the University of Berlin (1824). Rust's most important paper described tuberculous spondylitis of the cervical vertebrae (1834). His name is associated with the phenomenon that in cancer or caries of the upper cervical vertebrae the patient always supports the head with the hands when changing from the recumbent to the sitting posture or the reverse.

Conrad Langenbeck (1776-1851) was born in Horneburg and studied at Jena, Vienna, and Würzburg. In 1802 he settled in Göttingen, where he began lecturing on anatomy and surgery. During the Napoleonic Wars Langenbeck served as a military surgeon, and in 1814 he became surgeon general of the Hanoverian army. In that same year Langenbeck was elected professor of anatomy and surgery at the University of Göttingen, where he founded a renowned anatomical amphitheater and established both surgical and ophthalmological clinics in the university. In 1802 Langenbeck authored a monograph on lithotomy, and 4 years later the first volume of his *Bibliothek Für Die Chirurgie* was published. This eight-volume set was completed in 1828. Among his other written works were *Commentarius De Structura Peritonaei, Yesticulorum Tunicis, Eorumque Ex Abdomine In Scrotum Descensu Ad Illustrandam Herniarum Indolem* (1817), the five-volume *Nosologie Und Therapie Der Chirurgischen Krankheiten* (1822-1850), and the two-volume *Icones Anatomicae* (1826-1841) along with its accompanying four-volume *Handbuch Der Anatomie Mit Hinweisung Auf Die Icones Anatomicae* (1831-1847). In Langenbeck's most important monograph, *Prüfung Der Keratonyxis* (1811), he described the operation of iridencleisis for construction of an artificial pupil. He is eponymically linked with the lateral supraclavicular nerve.

Johann Meckel (the younger) (1781-1833) came from a lengthy line of distinguished anatomists and surgeons. He studied at the University of Halle and after spending some time in Göttingen, received his medical degree (1802). The sudden death of his father Philipp Meckel (1756-1803) caused him to return to Halle, where in 1808 he was named professor of anatomy, surgery, and obstetrics. Meckel was an irascible personality but one who spent much time on and obtained delight from his massive anatomical collection. He received an invitation to the chair of comparative and morbid anatomy at University College in London, but the Prussian minister of education increased his salary and appointed him Royal Privy Counsellor in Medicine. Satisfied with his increased responsibilities, Meckel stayed in Halle for the remainder of his professional life. He was quite a prolific writer and authored the two-volume *Beitrage Zur Vergleichenden Anatomie* (1808-1811), the five-volume *System Der Vergleichenden Anatomie* (1821-1831), the four-volume *Handbuch Der Menschlichen Anatomie* (1815-1820), and the four-part *Tabulae Anatomico-Pathologicae* (1817-1826). The latter was the first systematic work on human abnormalities and brought about a greater understanding of congenital malformations. In 1809 Meckel wrote an important paper describing a diverticular remnant of the omphaloenteric duct located on the ileum, a short distance from the cecum. His name is also associated with the mandibular cartilage and a craniometric plane cutting the alveolar and the auricular points.

Philipp von Walther (1782-1849) was born in Bavaria and received his surgical education at Heidelberg and Vienna. At the age of 21 years he was made surgeon to the Bamberg Hospital; 1 year later he was elevated to a similar position at Landshut. After the Napoleonic Wars, when the University of Bonn was founded, Walther was named first professor of surgery. He remained there until 1830, when he was called to Munich; in Munich he established the first surgical clinics in Bavaria while serving as surgeon-in-ordinary to the Bavarian monarchy. Walther began writing his six-volume *System Der Chirurgie* in 1843 and the two-volume *Lehrbuch Der Augenkrankheiten* in 1849. He remains best known for his description of corneal opacity (1845). Walther was also coeditor with Carl von Graefe (1787-1840) of the important *Journal Der Chirurgie Und Augen-Heilkunde* (1820-1850).

Carl von Graefe was born in Warsaw and received his medical education at Dresden, Halle, and Leipzig. He began the practice of surgery in Berlin (1810), where he was named professor and director of the surgical clinic in the newly founded university of that city. From 1813 to 1815 Graefe served as surgeon general of the Prussian army. He remained at Berlin for more than 30 years. Graefe is regarded as one of the founders of modern plastic and reconstructive surgery. In 1818 he authored *Rhinoplastik, Oder Die Kunst Den Verlust Der Nase Organisch Zu Ersetzen,* the first formal book devoted to rhinoplasty, and revived the operation in Germany with his survey of what he called the three methods: the Italian and Indian methods and the German method, his own variation on the Italian method. Graefe also described the first truly successful performance of blepharoplasty in 1809. In 1820 Graefe wrote a paper in which he described an operation for the treatment of congenital cleft palate.

Johann Fricke (1790-1841) studied at Göttingen (1810) and under Graefe in Berlin (1812). In 1814 he settled in Hamburg, where he became surgeon to the General Hospital. He described his clinical work in two volumes of archives of the hospital (1828-1833). Fricke's name is eponymically linked with a bandage that envelops the scrotum with adhesive plaster strips and is used in inflammation of the testicles and epididymis.

Wilhelm von Ludwig (1790-1865) was born near Stuttgart, where his father was a minister. In 1807 Ludwig matriculated at the University of Tubingen, where, 4 years later, he obtained his medical degree. After military service Ludwig became professor of surgery and obstetrics at his alma mater. Shortly thereafter, he was appointed personal physician to the Bavarian monarchy. In 1836 Ludwig authored a paper in which he described a severe inflammatory condition with suppuration in the region of the submaxillary gland and floor of the mouth, usually originating from a dental infection.

Johann Friedrich Dieffenbach (1792-1847) was born in Königsberg, where he studied medicine from 1816 to 1820. He then went to Bonn, where he worked with Walther. In 1821 Dieffenbach traveled to Paris and Montpellier, attending the clinics of Guillaume Dupuytren (1777-1835) and Jacques Delpech (1777-1832), respectively. Dieffenbach received his medical degree from Würzburg (1822), where he wrote a thesis entitled *Nonnulla De Regeneratione Et Transplantatione.* After graduation Dieffenbach moved to Berlin and began to concentrate on plastic and reconstructive surgery. In 1829 he became surgeon to the Charité and 3 years later, professor extraordinary in that city's university. In 1840, when Graefe died, Dieffenbach was named his successor and became professor of surgery and director of the surgical clinic in Berlin. By that time he was recognized as one of Germany's greatest surgeons and among its most prolific medical writers. In 1829 he authored the first of three volumes of his classic plastic surgical text, *Chirurgische Erfahrungen, Besonders Uber Die Wiederherstellung Zerstörter Theile Des Menschlichen Körpers Nach Neuen Methoden.* In 1841 came *Ueber Die Durchschneidung Der Sehnen Und Muskeln,* outlining 140 cases of treatment for clubfoot. In the following year Dieffenbach described the first successful attempt at treating strabismus by means of myotomy in his classic monograph *Ueber Das Schielen Und Die Heilung Desselben Durch Eine Operation.* Most of his contributions to clinical surgery were summarized in the two-volume *Operative Chirurgie* (1845–1848). In an 1832 paper Dieffenbach described the first known example of cardiac catheterization, which was performed during an unsuccessful attempt to obtain blood from a patient with cholera. In 1836 he attempted a resection of the human intestine in which the sutures described by Antoine Lembert (1802–1851) were first used. Dieffenbach also authored a text on the history of blood transfusion in 1828. His name is associated with a circular amputation at the hip joint with temporary elastic ligature and a plastic operation for covering a tissue defect by sliding a flap with a broad pedicle.

Maximilian Chelius (1794–1876) was born at Mannheim and educated in surgery at Landshut with Walther. When only 25 years of age, he was named professor of surgery at the University of Heidelberg, where he founded a surgical and ophthalmological clinic and also authored his renowned two-volume *Handbuch Der Chirurgie* (1822). Although this text contained little that was original, it may be regarded as the most influential German surgical book of the first half of the nineteenth century, since it was translated into Danish, Dutch, English, French, and Italian. Chelius's interests in ophthalmology were summarized in his *Handbuch Der Augenheilkunde* (1839).

238. Nasal deformities before rhinoplasty, from Dieffenbach's *Surgical Observations on the Restoration of the Nose . . .* [Translated with notes and additional cases, by John Stevenson Bushnan] (London, 1833). *(Jeremy Norman & Co., Inc.)*

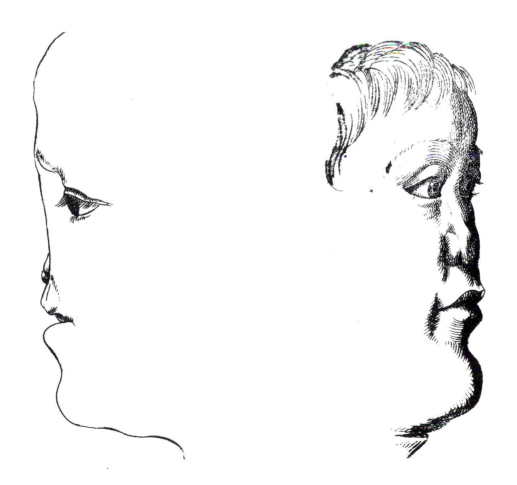

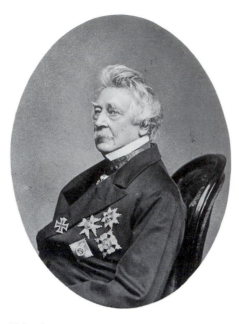

239. Georg Stromeyer in old age, wearing his many decorations. Photograph by F. Wunder Sohn, Hanover. *(Historical Collections, College of Physicians of Philadelphia.)*

Friedrich von Ammon (1799-1861) studied in Göttingen and Leipzig and received his medical degree in 1821. He soon settled in Dresden, where he became professor in the surgical school from 1828 to 1837. Among his most important writings were the two-volume *Die Angeborenen Chirurgischen Krankheiten Des Menschen In Abbildungen Dargestellt* (1842) and *Die Plastische Chirurgie* (1842). Much of Ammon's clinical interest was in ophthalmology, and between 1838 and 1847 he authored a classic four-part atlas, *Klinische Darstellungen Der Krankheiten Und Bildungsfehler Des Menschlichen Auges, Der Augenlider Und Der Thranenwerkzeuge Nach Eigenen Beobachtungen Und Untersuchungen*. He is eponymically associated with blepharoplasty by transplantation from the cheek and with dacryocystotomy.

Jacob von Heine (1800-1879) came from a family with a long tradition of bonesetting. He studied at Würzburg (1827) and soon established an orthopedic hospital in Cannstatt. His most important monograph was *Beobachtungen Uber Lahmungszustande Der Untern Extremitaten Und Deren Behandlung* (1840). In it he provided the first description of acute anterior poliomyelitis, which Heine separated from other forms of paralysis. Heine outlined the deformities arising from the disease and called attention to congenital spastic paraplegia. His other texts included *Uber Spontane Und Congenitale Luxationen* (1842) and *Spinale Kinderlahmung* (1860).

Georg Stromeyer (1804-1876) was the son of a surgeon who was physician to the king of Hanover. Stromeyer obtained his medical education at Berlin, Hanover, and Göttingen and received his degree in 1826. From 1829 to 1838 he taught at the surgical school in Hanover. He was appointed successor to Jaeger at Erlange and in 1842 accepted the professorship of surgery in Freiburg. His final career move was to Kiel (1847), where he succeeded Bernard Langenbeck (1810-1887). Stromeyer played an active role in military surgery and was surgeon general of the Schleswig-Holstein army (1849) and the Hanoverian army (1854). His *Maximen Der Kriegsheilkunst* (1855) was a landmark in military surgical writing. Stromeyer remains best known as the founder of modern surgery of the locomotor system. In 1833 he reported a successful tenotomy for clubfoot. Five years later he authored *Beitrage Zur Operativen Orthopadik,* in which he advocated subcutaneous tenotomy for all deformities of the body arising from muscular defects. Among his other important texts was the two-volume *Handbuch Der Chirurgie* (1844-1848). Stromeyer is eponymically linked with an operation for abscess of the liver, the pus being found by a cannula and the abscess being then opened by a knife running along the cannula as a guide; and for a hinged splint for the knee, which can be set at any angle.

Edward Zeis (1807-1868) was born in Dresden and studied at Bonn, Leipzig, and Munich. After receiving his medical degree (1832), Zeis returned to his native city. From 1844 to 1850 he served as professor of surgery at Marburg, but he resigned to become surgeon to the city hospital back in Dresden. Zeis was quite active in ophthalmology, and his name is associated with the sebaceous glands that open into the follicles of the eyelashes and with a sty that develops when one of the glands becomes inflamed. Zeis's most important clinical work was in plastic surgery: in his *Handbuch Der Plastischen Chirurgie* (1838) he introduced the term "plastic surgery." He is also important to the written history of plastic and reconstructive surgery because of his authoritative *Die Literatur Und Geschichte Der Plastischen Chirurgie* (1863). The main bibliography of this work had 2008 references and was the most extensive annotated bibliography of plastic surgical literature available before 1860.

August Burow (1809-1874) studied in Königsberg and was a student of Dieffenbach. Burow was best known for his work in ophthalmology. His name is associated with a blepharoplasty in which triangles of skin adjacent to the sides of the prepared sliding flap are excised to facilitate mobility. His name is also connected with a flap operation for closing a defect in the lip; a solution of aluminum acetate; and an occasional vein that passes from the inferior epigastric vein, sometimes receiving a tributary from the bladder, which empties into the portal vein.

During the 1860s German surgery began its rapid climb toward world prominence. In most instances it fell to the surgeons who were born during and after the second decade to help showcase the astounding medical and surgical advances and superb technical achievements of the German-speaking countries.

Bernard von Langenbeck (1810-1887), the nephew of Conrad von Langenbeck, received his medical degree from Göttingen (1835). He studied further with Brodie, Lawrence, and Green in London. Langenbeck returned to Göttingen as a private practitioner and in 1842 was appointed professor of surgery at Kiel. He was also director of the Friedrich Hospital, and during the Holstein Wars he left his professorship for a short time to serve as an army surgeon. Langenbeck, who was extremely successful in all that he did regarding surgery, was invited to succeed Dieffenbach in the chair of surgery at Berlin (1847). A firm believer in conducting animal experimentation before undertaking new surgical operations in his clinic, Langenbeck is considered the founder of German scientific surgery. He was made baron in appreciation of his military services against Denmark (1864), Austria (1866), and France (1870). His most prominent textbook, *Chirurgische Beobachtungen Aus Dem Kriege* (1874), is considered a classic text in the military sciences. He performed many important surgical operations, including the complete excision of the scapula (1850) and repair for cleft palate (1862). Langenbeck also discovered *Candida albicans* (1839). His name is associated with a method of amputating the foot; a surgical incision through the linea semilunaris made to expose the spleen or tail of the pancreas; and an anatomical triangle formed by lines drawn from the anterior superior spine of the ilium to the outer surface of the great trochanter and to the surgical neck of the femur, indicating that in this area a penetrating wound probably involves the joint. Among Langenbeck's other achievements was the founding, in conjunction with his pupils Theodor Billroth and Ernst Gurlt (1825-1899), of the *Archiv Für Klinische Chirurgie*, long known as *Langenbeck's Archiv*. In addition he started the Deutsche Gesellschaft für Chirurgie (1872). Langenbeck was most attracted to the education and training of surgeons, and his greatest contribution to surgery is found in that area. His school of surgery produced such luminaries as Friedrich von Esmarch (1823-1908), Ernst Gurlt, Theodor Billroth, Friedrich Trendelenburg (1844-1924), and Rudolf Kronlein (1847-1910).

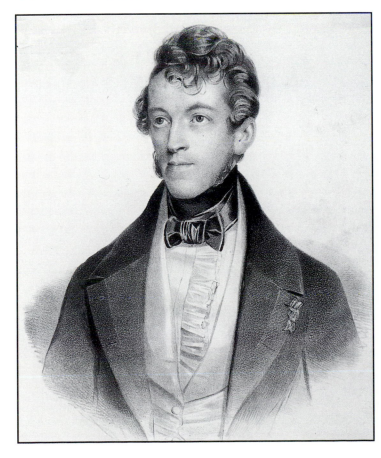

240. Bernard von Langenbeck. *(Historical Collections, College of Physicians of Philadelphia.)*

393

Victor von Bruns (1812-1883) was born in Helmstadt and studied at the Universities of Berlin, Brunswick, Halle, and Tübingen. He gained his degree from the last school (1836) and became professor of surgery there in 1843, a position he held until 1882. Bruns is considered one of the founders of modern laryngology. His work in this area included the first enucleation of a laryngeal polyp by the bloodless method (1862) and his *Die Laryngoskopie Und Die Laryngoskopische Chirurgie* (1865). In the latter treatise Bruns claimed to have been the first to remove a laryngeal tumor with the aid of the laryngoscope. He was also an early pioneer of listerian techniques in Germany.

Karl Thiersch (1822-1895) was a native of Munich and studied with Stromeyer. He became professor of surgery at Erlangen and Leipzig. Among his important written works was *De Maxillarum Necrosi Phosphorica* (1867), a classic description of phosphoric necrosis of the jaw. In 1865 he authored *Der Epithelialkrebs Namentlich Der Haut*, in which he disproved Virchow's theory of the connective tissue origin of cancer and promulgated evidence of its epithelial cell origin. Thiersch also wrote the first paper on transplantation of skin (1874). His name is associated with minute canaliculi in newly formed reparative tissue, which permit the circulation of nutritive fluids and are the precursors of new

241. Esmarch's bandage was printed with a battle scene showing how it could be applied to different wounds. *(Blocker History of Medicine Collections, Moody Medical Library, University of Texas Medical Branch at Galveston.)*

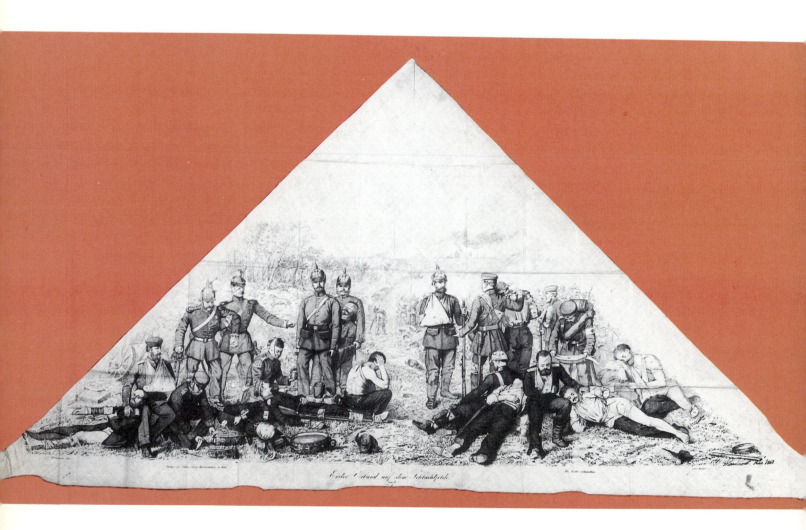

vascularization; a method of skin grafting with films of epidermis and a portion of the dermis shaved off in strips and applied to the surface after shaving down the granulations; and a broad, hollow-ground knife used for cutting sections of skin in such dermoepidermic grafting.

Friedrich von Esmarch (1823-1908) was born in Schleswig-Holstein and matriculated at the University of Kiel. He completed his medical education at Göttingen and then enlisted as a military surgeon. Esmarch served through the campaigns of 1848-1850, 1864-1866, and 1870-1871 and made invaluable contributions to military medicine. In 1869 he authored *Der Erste Verband Auf Dem Schlachtfelde,* in which the first-aid bandage on the battlefield was introduced. Esmarch also described his bandage for surgical hemostasis in an 1873 paper. From 1857 to 1899 he served as professor of surgery at Kiel. Esmarch's name is linked with a mask with a metal frame with strips of gauze stretched across the center and a rubber cover on the outside, which was used for giving chloroform or ether by inhalation. Esmarch was married twice, first to the daughter of Bernard Langenbeck and, later, to a royal princess; the second marriage made him an uncle to Wilhelm II.

242. Friedrich Esmarch amputating with the use of anesthesia and with antisepsis. Although complete listerian methods were impractical for emergency surgery on the battlefield, they worked in military hospitals like that illustrated here. Nevertheless, the principles of antisepsis and aseptic surgery were slow to gain acceptance. Woodcut from Esmarch's *Handbuch Der Kriegschirurgischen Technik* (1877). *(Jeremy Norman & Co., Inc.)*

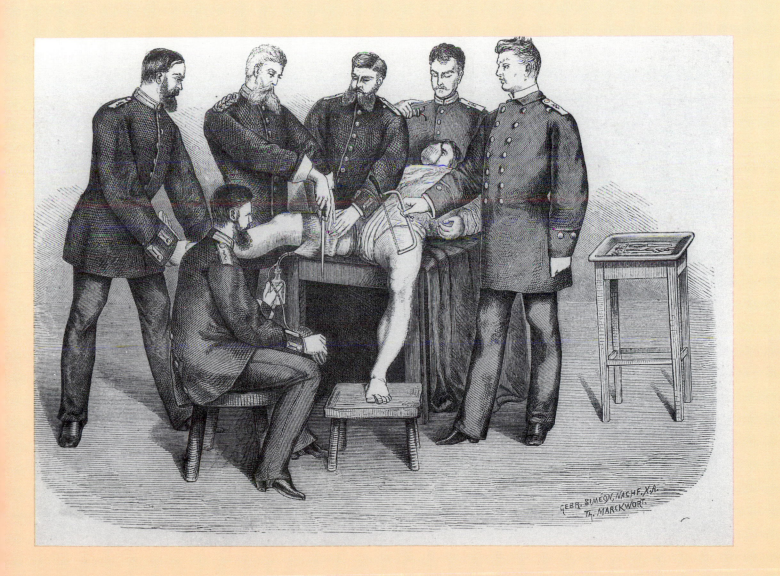

Gustav Simon (1824-1876), born in Darmstadt, was a medical student at Giessen and Heidelberg. After graduating in 1848, he immediately entered the Hessian army, to which he became medical director (1861). From 1861 to 1865 Simon served in the surgical chair at Rostock, and in 1867 he accepted the position in Heidelberg. During the Franco-Prussian War (1870-1871), he was surgeon general of the German reserves. Simon was regarded as a bold, daring surgical technician who made a number of important contributions to clinical surgery, especially urology. In 1870 he reported the first successful planned nephrectomy for urinary tract fistula and also wrote a detailed two-volume text on renal surgery, *Chirurgie Der Nieren* (1871-1876). Simon also authored treatises on vesicovaginal fistula (*Ueber Die Heilung Der Blasen-Scheidenfisteln,* 1854), the spleen (*Die Exstirpation Der Milz Am Menschen,* 1857), and plastic surgery (*Beitrage Zur Plastischen Chirurgie,* 1868). His name is associated with an operation for the repair of a ruptured perineum by suturing, first, the vaginal mucous membrane and then the cutaneous surface; and a position used for vaginal examination, in which the woman is lying on the back with hips elevated, thighs and legs flexed, and thighs widely separated.

Ernst Gurlt (1825-1899) was born in Berlin and received his medical degree from the university of that city. From 1852 to 1856 he was an assistant in Bernard Lagenbeck's clinic, and in 1862 he was nominated as professor of surgery at his alma mater. Gurlt was actively involved in the Prussian military and was one of the organizers of the German Red Cross. His greatest gift to the world of surgery has been his unsurpassed, incredibly detailed three-volume *Geschichte Der Chirurgie Und Ihrer Ausubung* (1898). This history of surgery remains the most exhaustive treatise on the subject and stands as a monument to German thoroughness in the late nineteenth century.

Albrecht von Graefe (1828-1870), the son of Carl von Graefe, is considered one of the outstanding ophthalmological surgeons of the nineteenth century. Graefe studied in Berlin, where he received his medical degree (1847). Most of his years in training were spent studying ophthalmology with the leading physicians in Europe. In 1857 Graefe was appointed professor of ophthalmology at his alma mater. He was an exceptionally prolific writer, and among his important texts was *Symptomenlehre Der Augenmuskellahmungen* (1867), which discussed the symptoms of ocular paralyses. During the 1850s he introduced iridectomy in the treatment of iritis, iridochoroiditis, and glaucoma. He perfected an operation for strabismus (1857) and 2 years later showed how an embolism of the retinal artery could cause sudden blindness. In the 1860s he improved on cataract surgery by using a modified linear extraction and authored classic contributions concerning sympathetic ophthalmia (1866) and keratoconus (1868). During the same decade, Graefe wrote papers showing that most cases of blindness and impaired vision associated with cerebral disorders could be traced to optic neuritis rather than to paralysis of the optic nerve (1860) and described the failure of the eyelid to follow the eye when it is rolled downward as a diagnostic sign of exophthalmic goiter (1864). In 1854 Graefe founded the *Archiv für Ophthalmologie,* universally known as *Graefe's Archiv,* which became the foremost international journal of ophthalmology. The true importance of Graefe lies beyond his own clinical work and his journal. In his short, incredibly brilliant career, Graefe trained an entire school of ophthalmologists who in turn advanced the field immensely. Graefe's name is eponymically associated with a narrow-bladed knife used in making a section of the cornea; the removal of a cataract by a limbal incision with capsulotomy and iridectomy; small areas over the vertebrae or near the supraorbital foramen, pressure on which causes relaxation of blepharofacial spasm; and a test for heterophoria. Graefe succumbed to tuberculosis at the early age of 42 years.

Theodor Billroth (1829-1894) was a native of Bergen, on the island of Rugen; he studied at Berlin, Göttingen, and Greifswald. He received his medical degree in 1852 and immediately became an assistant to Langenbeck. Billroth was made privatdocent in 1856, professor of clinical surgery at Zurich in 1860, and professor of surgery at the University of Vienna in 1867. Billroth embodied the tremendous achievements of German surgery and became that country's most celebrated surgeon. An outstanding surgical technician, he was able to bring his experimental successes to the practical side of clinical medicine. Billroth's views on surgical training were unique for the time in which he lived. Billroth thought that the student would be ready to start surgical training only after he had completed his medical studies and had preliminary experience working in a hospital. Performing operations on cadavers and experimental animals, 2 or 3 years of assistantship in a surgical department, studies of the surgical literature, writing patient histories, and acquiring advanced practical experience in a hospital were necessary to prepare the surgeon for independent work. Billroth firmly believed that anything that concerned a patient, including nursing duties, had to be experienced by the surgeon in training. These viewpoints were promulgated to an attentive surgical world via the graduates of his own training program (see the box below).

In understanding Billroth's success, it is essential to appreciate the evolution of the Viennese surgical school and its relationship with the Allgemeine Krankenhaus, or general hospital, of that city. The hospital was founded in 1784 with Ferdinand von Leber (1729-1808) as its first head of surgery. He in turn was succeeded by Kern and, later, by Joseph von Wattman (1779-1866). During Wattman's professorship (1830-1847) the surgical service was split into first and second surgical divisions (1842). Johann Dumreicher (1815-1880) became head of the first division, to be succeeded by Eduard Albert (1841-1900). The latter was professor of surgery from 1881 to 1900, and his overlapping service with Billroth caused a great rivalry. Franz Schuh (1804-1865) became head of the second division in 1842 and was succeeded by Billroth, who remained in the position until his death in 1894. Anton von Eiselsberg (1860-1939), one of Billroth's most brilliant protégés, succeeded Albert. Eiselsberg was professor of surgery of the first division from 1901 to 1938. Billroth was succeeded by Carl Gussenbauer (1842-1903), who served as professor of surgery of the second division from 1894 to 1903. When Gussenbauer died prematurely in 1903, he was

GRADUATES OF THEODOR BILLROTH'S TRAINING PROGRAM

VINCENT VON CZERNY (1842-1916)

CARL GUSSENBAUER (1842-1903)

ROBERT GERSUNY (1844-1924)

ALEXANDER VON WINIWARTER (1848-1917)

JOHANNE VON MIKULICZ-RADECKI (1850-1905)

ANTON WÖLFLER (1850-1917)

VICTOR VON HACKER (1852-1933)

ALBERT FRANKEL (1857-1929)

ANTON VON EISELSBERG (1860-1939)

ALBERT NARATH (1864-1924)

243. *Facing page, Theodor Billroth Operating in the Auditorium of the Allgemeine Krankenhaus, Vienna (1889).* This painting by Anton F. Seligmann shows Billroth, pale of complexion and with a white beard, at the peak of fame at 60 years of age. The painting, recently cleaned and restored, seems to glow with the brilliance of the white surgical gowns and the like. However, it appears that although Billroth operated with sterilized instruments, he may have allowed the public to come extremely close to the operating field, contrary to aseptic operating conditions. According to notes made by the painter, the patient was an old man on whom Billroth was performing a neurotomy for trigeminal neuralgia. Many of the figures in the painting have been identified. Most interesting are the portraits of the Duke of Bavaria, who commonly attended Billroth's lectures for entertainment, and the self-portrait of the artist. The Duke is sitting at the far left in the first row of seats; Seligmann is at the far right. *(Österreichische Galerie, Vienna.)*

succeeded by Julius von Hochenegg (1859-1940), one of Albert's most famous pupils. Hochenegg served as head of the second division from 1904 to 1930. By such curious crossings of paths, justice was done to both Billroth and Albert and to the rival branches of the Vienna surgical school. Billroth authored a number of prominent texts, including a study of the history of military and naval hygiene (1859), his great *Die Allgemeine Chirurgische Pathologie Und Therapie* (1863), and a treatise on breast surgery, *Die Krankheiten Der Brustdrusen* (1880). In 1872 he reported the first resection of the esophagus; the initial resection of the pylorus for cancer was completed a decade later. He is eponymically linked with a mixture of one part alcohol, two parts chloroform, and three parts ether (ACE) for anesthesia; splenic cords; excision of the pylorus with end-to-end anastomosis of stomach and duodenum (Billroth I); and resection of the pylorus with the greater part of the lesser curvature of the stomach, closure of the cut ends of the duodenum and stomach, and a posterior gastrojejunostomy (Billroth II). Billroth was a man of immense charm with a genial personality. His strong artistic bent was evident in his lifelong friendship and correspondence with the composer Johannes Brahms (1833-1897).

Richard von Volkmann (1830-1889) was the son of Alfred Volkmann (1800-1877), the well-known German physiologist. Volkmann was educated at Berlin, Giessen, and Halle and received his degree in 1854. Within the year he was named assistant at the surgical clinic of Blasius in Halle, in 1857, instructor in surgery, and a decade later, professor. He was instrumental in introducing antiseptic techniques to German surgeons after the Franco-Prussian War. Volkmann was a founder of the Deutsche Gesellschaft für Chirurgie and was elected president in 1876. Two years later he assumed the position of president of the University of Halle. Volkmann's written contributions to surgery were numerous and included the first description of industrial tar- and paraffin-induced cancer (1875) and the first excision of the rectum for cancer (1878). His name is associated with glandular cheilitis; tissue degeneration produced by ischemia leading to a late contracture involving muscles, tendons, fascia, and other soft tissues, usually caused by interference with blood flow as a result of direct vessel compression, prolonged spasm, or trauma; a congenital luxation of the tibiotarsal joint; a splint for fractures of the lower extremity consisting of a guttered splint with a footpiece and two lateral supports to prevent turning; a sharp spoon for scraping away carious bone or other diseased tissue; and a subluxation of the knee usually caused by tuberculous arthritis. Volkmann was a man of varied interests and wrote poetry under the pseudonym of Richard Leander.

Franz Koenig (1832-1910) was professor of surgery at Rostock and Göttingen. He was primarily interested in orthopedic surgery and in 1888 was the first to use the term *osteochondritis dissecans.* Two years later he provided a complete description of joint involvement in hemophilia. His name is associated with a shelving operation for congenital dislocation of the hip, in which reduction of the dislocation and formation of a lip to the upper edge of the acetabulum by an osteoperiosteal strip cut from the surface of the ilium are performed; and a syndrome consisting of alternating attacks of constipation and diarrhea, with colic, meteorism, and gurgling in the right iliac fossa, said to be symptomatic of cecal tuberculosis.

Ernst von Bergmann (1836-1907) was born in Riga and received his medical degree from the university in Dorpat (1860). He was quite active as a military surgeon, serving with the Prussian army in 1866 and 1870 and with the Russian army in the Turko-Russian campaign of 1877. In recognition of his many surgical accomplishments Bergmann was named professor of surgery at his alma mater, was given the chair in Würzburg (1877), and succeeded Langenbeck at Berlin (1882). He was considered a pioneer in the evolution of asepsis (1887) because of his corrosive sublimate method of antisepsis, which gradually merged into steam sterilization. In 1888 Bergmann reported a radical mastoidectomy. His best-known monograph, *Die Chirurgische Behandlung Von Hirnkrankheiten* (1888), described the surgical treatment of diseases of the brain. His name is linked with a surgical incision in the flank for exposing the kidney.

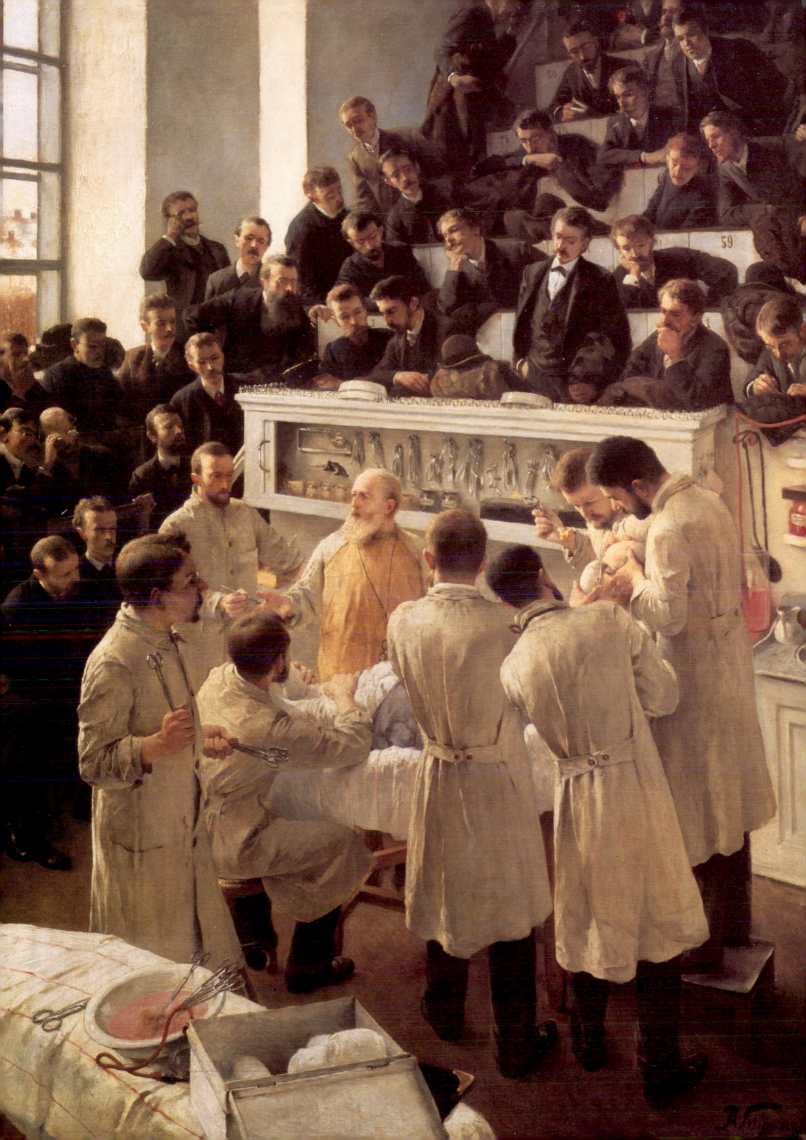

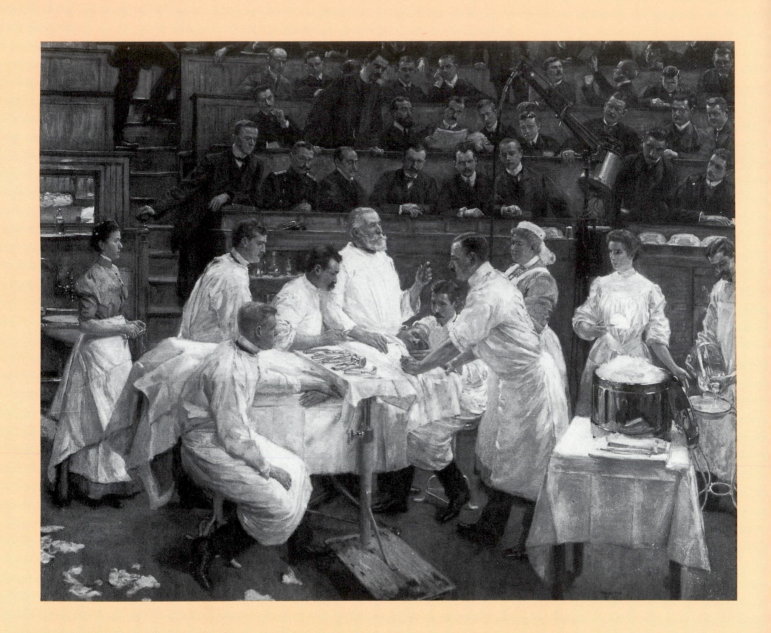

244. Ernst von Bergmann ready to perform a neurosurgical operation, perhaps a craniotomy, as recorded by artist Franz Skarbina in Berlin in 1906. None of the operating team is wearing gloves, although antiseptic technique is being strictly followed. From a 1907 black-and-white collotype reproduction of the painting. *(Jeremy Norman & Co., Inc.)*

Carl Heuter (1838-1882) graduated from Marburg in 1859. He later studied in London, Paris, and Vienna and became an instructor and assistant to Langenbeck. In 1868 Heuter succeeded Simon as professor of surgery at Rostock and within 12 months had accepted the chair at Greifswald. His principal texts were *Klinik Der Gelenkkrankheiten* (1870), *Die Allgemeine Chirurgie* (1873), and *Grundriss Der Chirurgie* (1880). Heuter's name is linked with a maneuver used in passing a stomach tube, whereby one presses the patient's tongue downward and forward with the left forefinger; a point for the application of a trephine in case of hemorrhage from the middle meningeal artery; and a sign that when the soft parts intervene in a case of fracture, the vibration, on tapping the bone, is not transmitted.

Theodor Kocher (1841-1917), a pioneer in thyroid surgery, is commonly regarded as one of the greatest Swiss surgeons of all time. This winner of the Nobel prize in medicine (1909) was born into a well-to-do family in Bern. He matriculated at the university in his native city, from which he received his medical degree. After graduation Kocher traveled for a year, visiting the famed surgical clinics of Europe. He returned to Bern in 1865 and within 7 years was awarded the professorship of surgery at his alma mater. Kocher's adult life was dedicated solely to surgery, and little time was available to spend with his family or on other outside activities. He traveled sparingly: except for a single trip to England, he was never out of continental Europe. His greatest achievements were related to his success in attacking the problem of hyperthyroidism and its alleviation through surgery. Year after year, Kocher issued successive reports of his studies. These traced the refinement of his surgical methods from those described in his first important written paper on thyroidectomy (1878) and disclosed a reduction in mortality from high initial figures to 13% (1883), and eventually, to less than 1%. Among Kocher's most important clinical observations was his use of the term *cachexia strumipriva* to describe the myxedema that follows total thyroidectomy (1883). He was active in many different fields of surgery, as revealed in his papers, which recorded a method of reduction of subluxation of the shoulder joint (1870), a radical extirpation of the tongue for carcinoma (1880), and an operation for hernia (1892). In 1888 Kocher introduced silk sutures as part of aseptic surgical technique. His name is associated with a clamp for grasping tissues in a surgical operation or for providing compression of bleeding structures; a surgical incision parallel with the right costal margin for exposing the gallbladder; a resection of the wrist by means of an incision on the ulnar side of the dorsum; and a clinical test in toxic hyperthyroidism such that when the examiner's hand is placed on a level with the patient's eyes and then suddenly raised higher, the upper lids move upward more rapidly than the eyeballs, giving the appearance of globe lag.

Vincenz Czerny (1842-1916) received his medical degree from the University of Vienna in 1866. Two years later he was appointed assistant in Billroth's clinic and in time became one of his most important pupils. In 1871 Czerny received an official appointment as instructor in surgery at his alma mater. His abilities were quite apparent because within 6 months he was appointed professor of surgery at the University of Freiberg. While there, he married the daughter of Adolph Kussmaul (1822-1902). Czerny was an outstanding teacher and in 1877 was appointed professor of surgery at Heidelberg, succeeding Simon. He was quite adept technically and in that year authored a series of papers on a new, radical operation for inguinal hernia. In 1879 he performed the first total hysterectomy by the vaginal route, and two years later he introduced the operation of enucleation of subperitoneal uterine fibroids by the vaginal route. Czerny served as president of the Deutsche Gesellschaft für Chirurgie (1901) and the International Surgical Congress (1908). His name is associated with a method of intestinal suturing whereby the needle enters the serosa, passes out through the submucosa or muscularis, and then enters the submucosa or muscularis of the opposite side and emerges from the serosa.

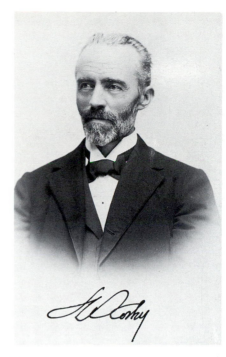

245. Theodor Kocher. Photograph by E. Mauvillier, Besançon, France, 1900. *(Historical Collections, College of Physicians of Philadelphia.)*

Carl Gussenbauer (1842-1903) was one of Billroth's earliest house surgeons and would succeed his mentor as head of Vienna's famous second surgical clinic. On the last day of 1873 Billroth performed the first complete excision of the larynx for cancer. Gussenbauer assisted at the operation and reported the case in 1874. Gussenbauer also assisted Billroth in the first abdominal resection of a tumor of the bladder and later reported it (1875). In 1876 Gussenbauer described a practical method for the excision of the pylorus in a dog, which led to Billroth's famous operations for gastric resection. Seven years later Gussenbauer became the first surgeon to treat a pancreatic cyst surgically by marsupialization. His name is linked with a figure-of-eight intestinal suture.

Jacques Reverdin (1842-1929) was born in Geneva but studied medicine in Paris. He became an *interne des hôpitaux* in 1865 and 4 years later, an assistant to Felix Guyon (1831-1920). At the Hôpital Necker with Guyon, Reverdin began his work on the transplantation of free skin, which contrasted with the previous method of pedunculated flaps (1869). After the 1870 war between France and Germany Reverdin returned to Geneva, where he became chief surgeon of its city hospital and professor of pathology at the University of Geneva. During the next 30 years he remained in his native city, where he authored numerous important papers concerning the experimental production of myxedema by removal of the thyroid gland.

Friedrich Trendelenburg (1844-1924) was a native of Berlin and received his degree from that city's university (1866). His doctoral thesis, *De Veterum Indorum Chirurgiais,* discussed surgery in ancient India. Trendelenburg initially served in the German army and after 2 years was appointed assistant in Langenbeck's clinic in Berlin. In 1874 Trendelenburg was made a director of the surgical ward at the Friedrichshain Hospital in his native city. In the following year he went to Rostock, succeeding Koenig as professor of surgery. From 1882 to 1895 Trendelenburg served as professor in Bonn. His last chair was at Leipzig, where he was successor to Thiersch. Trendelenburg performed many remarkable surgical feats, including the provision of endotracheal anesthesia for a patient with a tracheostomy (1871). In 1890 he reported his operation for the ligation of the great saphenous vein as treatment for varicose veins in the leg and also described his clinical test to determine insufficiency of the venous valves. In that same year he attempted to cure hydronephrosis via operative intervention in the first recorded surgical procedure for the relief of this condition. Also in 1890 Trendelenburg first described a supine position on the operating table or the bed, with the patient inclined at an angle of 45 degrees so that the pelvis is higher than the head. He proposed a clinical test to determine congenital dislocation of the hip joint (1895). Trendelenburg first attempted pulmonary embolectomy, albeit unsuccessfully, in 1908. Trendelenburg's name is linked with a cannula covered with a dilatable rubber bag that occludes the trachea, which is applied during operations on the mouth or larynx, and with a waddling gait in paresis of the gluteal muscles, as in progressive muscular dystrophy.

Carl Langenbuch (1846-1901) was a native of Berlin and director of that city's Lazarus Hospital. Although he held no formal academic positions, Langenbuch accomplished several notable feats in surgery. In 1877 he performed the first nephrectomy for malignant disease, and 5 years later he completed the first successful removal of a gallbladder.

Rudolf Krönlein (1847-1910), a surgeon in Zurich, performed one of the first resections of a portion of a pulmonary lobe that had been invaded by sarcoma of the rib. His name is linked with an operation consisting of a resection of the anterior portion of the lateral wall of the orbit and with a properitoneal inguinal hernia.

Max Nitze (1848-1906) is considered one of the founders of modern urology. He studied medicine at Heidelberg, Leipzig, and Würzburg and received his medical degree in 1874. In that year he received a staff appointment to the state hospital in Dresden, where he remained for 4 years. After spending further research time in Vienna, Nitze came to the University of Berlin, where he was a privatdocent. In 1890 he was appointed professor of urology. In 1877 Nitze had devised an electrically lighted cystoscope, which made possible great improvements in the surgery of the bladder. Almost a decade later he authored his important monograph on cystoscopy, *Lehrbuch Der Kystoskopie*. During the late 1890s Nitze's operative cystoscope made it possible to excise bladder tumors in situ.

Alexander von Winiwarter (1848–1917) obtained his medical degree in Vienna and after 6 years as assistant to Billroth became docent (1876). Earlier, Winiwarter had demonstrated a practical method for excision of the pylorus in dogs, and that work led to Billroth's research in gastric resection. During Winiwarter's time as docent his younger brother Felix (1852–1931), also working in Billroth's clinic, gave a description of thromboangiitis obliterans. In 1878 the elder Winiwarter accepted the surgical professorship in Liege, where he remained for the rest of his life.

246. Illustration of the first electrically lighted cystoscope (1879), which enabled great advances in surgery of the bladder. Developed by Max Nitze in 1877, this is the forerunner of arthroscopic and laparoscopic surgery, which is currently being applied to so many different operations. (*National Library of Medicine, Bethesda, Md.*)

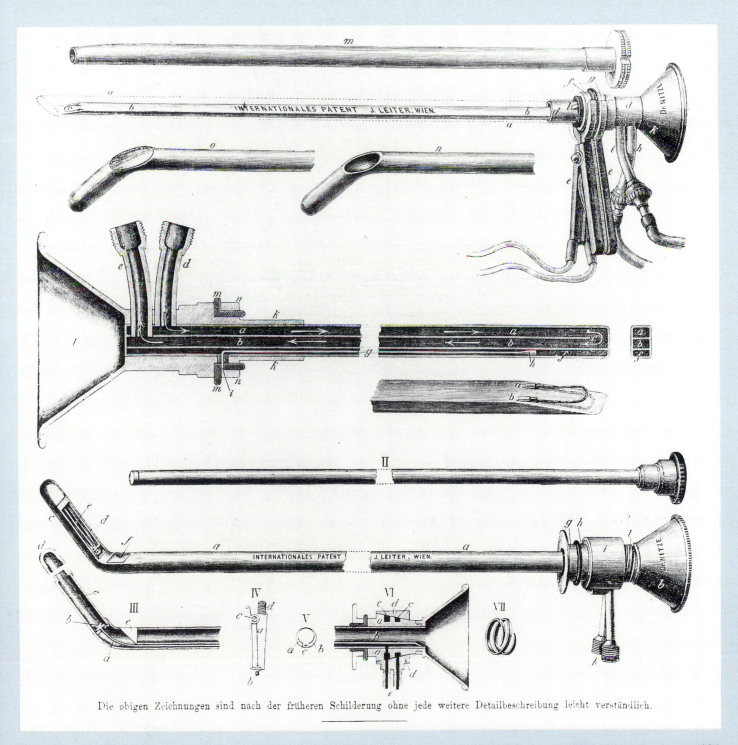

Die obigen Zeichnungen sind nach der früheren Schilderung ohne jede weitere Detailbeschreibung leicht verständlich.

Johann von Mikulicz-Radecki (1850-1905) received his medical degree in Vienna (1875) and became an assistant in Billroth's clinic. Mikulicz-Radecki remained with Billroth until 1882, when he accepted the professorship of surgery at the University of Kracow. Five years later he transferred to Königsburg; he ended his career in Breslau, where he died of gastric cancer. Mikulicz-Radecki was a voluminous contributor to the surgical literature and introduced many new surgical techniques. He described an operation for the treatment of disease of the accessory nasal sinuses (1887), proposed a procedure for complete prolapse of the rectum (1888), completed the first enterocystoplasty (1889), and eventually perfected a two-stage operation for resection of tumors of the rectum (1903). In 1881 Mikulicz-Radecki first used an electric esophagoscope, and 5 years later he completed a reconstruction of the esophagus after resecting the cervical portion for cancer. His name is linked with an osteoplastic resection of the foot; foamy macrophages containing *Klebsiella rhinoscleromatis* that are found in the mucosal nodules in rhinoscleroma; a drain made of several strings of gauze held together by a single layer of the same material; a method for increasing the infection resistance of an individual before abdominal operations by injecting a solution of nucleinate of sodium; an exsection of the sternocleidomastoid muscles in torticollis; a type of pyloroplasty in which a short longitudinal incision is made over the pylorus and then closed transversely, usually with one layer of nonabsorbable sutures; and a pad made from several layers of guaze folded into a rectangular shape, which is used as a sponge for packing off the viscera in abdominal operations. In 1892 Mikulicz-Radecki gave the first description of the syndrome of symmetrical inflammation of the lacrimal and salivary glands caused by the replacement of the normal gland structure with lymphoid tissue. He is also credited with being the first surgeon to require that a face mask be used during all operations.

Ludwig Rydygier (1850-1920) was born in Grudziadz and completed his medical education at Berlin, Greifswald, and Strassburg. In 1879 he returned to his family's home in Chelmno and began a private practice in his own clinic. In November 1880 Rydygier performed an unsuccessful excision of a carcinomatous pylorus. Within the year he refined his techniques, and a successful procedure was soon completed. Rydygier succeeded Mikulicz-Radecki in the chair of surgery at Kracow in 1887. Ten years later he became chairman of surgery and dean of the faculty of the University of Lvor.

Anton Wölfler (1850-1917) obtained his medical degree in 1874 (Vienna) and then worked under Billroth. In 1881 Wölfler perfected the operation of gastroenterostomy and achieved considerable acclaim. By 1886 his surgical triumphs led to his nomination as professor of surgery at Graz. A decade later he transferred to a similar position in Prague. Wölfler's name is associated with an accessory thyroid gland and an intestinal suture by which broad layers of the serosa are united and the knots are tied on the inner surface of the bowel.

Paul Kraske (1851-1930) studied in Halle and Leipzig and became an assistant under Volkmann. His surgical skills were clearly evident, and in 1883 he was appointed professor of surgery at Freiburg. There he perfected the sacral method of resection of the rectum for carcinoma (1887).

Victor von Hacker (1852-1933) was born in Vienna, where he received his medical degree in 1878. After an assistantship under Billroth, Hacker became director of the Sophien-Spital in his native city. He was appointed professor of surgery at Innsbruck (1895) and later, at Graz (1903). When Billroth performed his first resection of the pylorus followed by a posterior gastrojejunostomy, Hacker assisted at the operation and later authored the first account of the procedure (1885). In 1886 Hacker's method of gastrostomy was presented in the periodical literature.

Adolf Lorenz (1854-1946) was born in Weidenau and became professor of surgery in Vienna. His primary interest was orthopedic surgery, and he suggested a bloodless method for closed reduction of congenital dislocation of the hip joint (1894). He is eponymically linked with a bifurcation operation for congenital dislocation of the hip that involves an oblique osteotomy of the upper femur with placement of the distal end in the acetabulum and with stiffness of the thoracic spine in early pulmonary tuberculosis.

Cesar Roux (1857-1926) of Mont-La-Ville received his medical education in Bern. He became an assistant to Kocher and eventually settled in Lausanne, where he was appointed professor of surgery at the newly established university in that city. He is best known for the operation in which the distal end of the divided jejunum is anastomosed to the stomach and the proximal end is implanted into the side of the jejunum, about 3 inches below the first anastomosis.

Fedor Krause (1857-1927) was born in Silesia and studied with Volkmann in Halle and Langenbeck in Berlin. In 1889 Krause was appointed professor and placed in charge of the city hospital in Altona. There he reported his extradural operation for the removal of the gasserian ganglion for the treatment of trigeminal neuralgia (1892), popularized the use of whole-thickness skin grafts (1893), and performed a total cystectomy and bilateral ureterosigmoidostomy (1903). In 1909 Krause was appointed surgical director of the Augusta Hospital in Berlin. There he acquired an international reputation for his work in neurosurgery, especially for his successful removal of a pineal tumor (1913). With William Macewen and Harvey Cushing, Krause pioneered the development of neurosurgery as a specialty. Among Krause's textbooks were *Lehrbuch Der Chirurgischen Operationen* (1912), which was translated into English, Spanish, and Russian, and the comprehensive two-volume *Chirurgie Des Gehirns Und Ruckenmarks Nach Eigenen Erfahrungen* (1908-1911).

Anton von Eiselsberg (1860-1939) was born in Steinhaus and after studying in many of Europe's leading universities, obtained his medical degree from Vienna (1884). He became Billroth's assistant in 1887 and 6 years later was appointed professor of surgery in Utrecht. In 1896 Eiselsberg accepted the post of professor of surgery at the University of Königsberg, and in 1901 he was chosen professor of surgery to the first surgical division in Vienna. His most important research was conducted early in his career, when he was able to demonstrate experimental production of tetany by excision of the thyroid of a cat, which had previously been successfully transplanted into the abdomen (1892).

August Bier (1861-1949) was born in Waldeck and studied at Berlin, Kiel, and Leipzig. He was a protégé of Esmarch and shortly after his graduation (1888) was named professor at Greifswald and Bonn and, in 1907, successor to Bergmann in Berlin. While at Greifswald, Bier engaged in research on spinal anesthesia and introduced the use of cocaine as a spinal anesthetic (1899). His work in active and passive hyperemia as adjuncts to surgical therapy was aptly described in *Hyperaemie Als Heilmittel* (1903). He is eponymically linked with an osteoplastic amputation of the tibia and fibula and with intravenous local anesthesia.

Hans Kehr (1862-1916) of Thüringia studied at Berlin, Freiburg, Halle, and Jena. In Berlin he was appointed professor of surgery and became prominent in the field of biliary tract and liver surgery. In 1903 he published a report detailing the successful ligation of the hepatic artery. Kehr's name is associated with a surgical incision from the xyphoid process to the pubis and with a clinical sign of violent pain in the left shoulder that indicates splenic rupture.

Hermann Pfannenstiel (1862-1909) was professor of gynecology in Breslau. Among his most important texts was *Uber Die Pseudomucine Der Cystischen Ovariengeschwulste* (1890). In 1908 he provided the first detailed description of familial icterus gravis neonatorum. Pfannenstiel is best remembered for his description of a surgical incision made transversely down to and including the external sheath of the rectus muscles, about an inch above the pubes, the muscles being split or separated in the direction of their fibers (1900).

Carl Schlatter (1864-1934) was educated in Heidelberg and Zurich and later served as an assistant to Albert in Vienna. Schlatter subsequently became professor of surgery at the University of Zurich. In 1897 he performed the first successful total gastrectomy. He is also remembered for his description of a painful affliction consisting of osteochondritis in the tibial tuberosity of children.

Ernst Wertheim (1864-1920) was born in Graz and educated in Vienna, where he later became professor of surgery. His interest was mostly in gynecological surgery. In 1895 Wertheim emphasized the importance of latent uterine gonorrhea, and in the following year he demonstrated the gonococcal organisms in acute cystitis. His most important technical contribution was a radical operation for cancer of the uterus (1902). Wertheim's name is associated with a reconstructive operation for prolapse of the uterus consisting of amputation of the cervix, vaginofixation, and posterior colporrhaphy.

Max Wilms (1867-1918) described an embryoma of the kidney in young children in 1899. He was also the first to carry out full excision of burnt tissue and sometimes grafted excised areas (1901). His name is associated with a perineal prostatectomy through a lateral incision and a resection of the ribs anteriorly and posteriorly so that the chest may be flattened and the lungs compressed by the sinking in of the chest wall, which is used in the treatment of certain cases of pulmonary tuberculosis.

Fritz De Quervain (1868-1940) studied at Bern with Kocher and participated in his mentor's thyroid studies. After working at La Chaux-de-Fonds (1894), De Quervain became professor of surgery at Basel. He succeeded Kocher as professor of surgery at the Inselspital in 1918. He is eponymically remembered for a radial styloid tenosynovitis that causes fibrosis of the sheath of a tendon of the thumb, a fracture of the navicular bone with dislocation of the lunar bone, and a subacute granulomatous thyroiditis.

George Perthes (1869-1927) studied at Berlin, Bonn, and Freiburg. He received his medical degree in 1891 and immediately became an assistant in Trendelenburg's clinic. When the latter moved to Leipzig, Perthes joined him. Shortly thereafter, Perthes was appointed Bruns's successor at Tübingen. In 1910 Perthes described epiphyseal aseptic necrosis of the upper end of the femur. He was among the first surgeons to study the inhibitory effect of X rays on carcinoma (1903) and became a pioneer in radiotherapy. He is eponymically linked with a surgical incision for exposure of organs in the right upper abdominal quadrant, with a method of continuous aspiration of a pleuritic exudate in which the drainage tube passes into an airtight receiving vessel that is connected with a water-powered exhaust, and with a clinical test for assessing the patency of the deep femoral vein.

FRANCE

In 1799 Napoleon I seized power in France and within 5 years crowned himself emperor of the French. For most of the next decade his armies crushed one European foe after another. However, his own pride and stubbornness forced him to go ahead with doubtful military plans that ended with a disastrous defeat in Russia (1812). By 1814 his friends and political allies had deserted him, and in April he abdicated. Napoleon I was sent to supposedly permanent exile on the tiny island of Elba, off the coast of Italy. In less than a year he managed to escape, and in March 1815 he landed in southern France with a handful of followers and marched toward Paris.

During Napoleon I's brief exile the Bourbons had returned to power under Louis XVIII (1755-1824). When Napoleon I approached Paris with his growing military force, the king fled and Napoleon I once again ruled. Allied armies took to battle against Napoleon I, and he was decisively defeated on June 18 at Waterloo. He was taken prisoner of war and exiled to the barren island of Saint Helena, off the west coast of Africa. He died of gastric cancer on May 5, 1821, and was buried on the island. Napoleon's body was later reentombed at the Hôtel des Invalides, which once served as a hospital for sick, needy soldiers.

Louis XVIII returned to power and was soon succeeded by his brother Charles X (1757-1836), who attempted to increase the political strength of the aristocracy by compensating them for property lost during the Revolution. His endeavors at absolutism ended in a popular revolt. Charles X fled, and the mod-

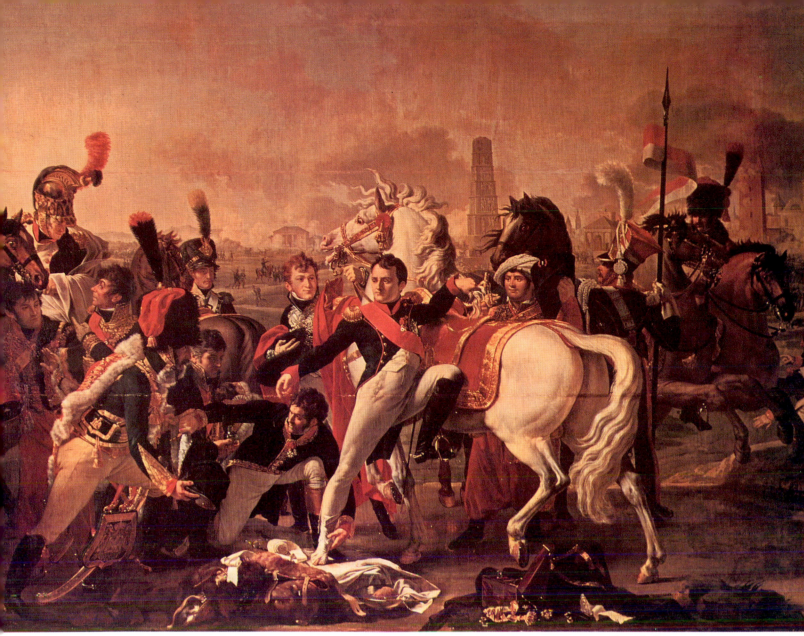

erates selected Louis Philippe (1873-1850) of the House of Orléans to become the "citizen king." His interests, however, were not truly with the people, and he was exiled in 1848.

The Second Republic was proclaimed by the French Parliament, who elected Napoleon III (1808-1873), nephew of Napoleon I, to be president. Within 3 years he had managed to concentrate all power in his hands and proclaimed himself emperor (1852). Napoleon III led France into a long series of unfortunate adventures in other countries. His political blunders led to the Franco-Prussian War (1870), which ultimately helped establish the German Empire. Napoleon III surrendered his troops at Sedan in September 1870, and his empire immediately ceased.

A provisional government was established in France in 1871, to be followed by the Third Republic (1875). Jules Grévy (1807-1891) was elected president and was succeeded by Sadi Carnot (1837-1894), whose term was ended by assassination. A series of presidents was elected, and then Emile Loubet (1838-1929) began his administration in 1899. During the late 1890s the French people were absorbed in the infamous case involving Alfred Dreyfus (1859-1935), who was convicted of treason but was later found to be a victim of virulent anti-Semitism and outright conspiracy.

247. *Napoleon Wounded at Ratisbon* by Claude Gautherot (1765-1825). Napoleon's wound could not have been severe, but the detail preserved in this idolatrous painting indicates that the surgeon has washed and bandaged the wound to Napoleon's foot and ankle. The surgeon is about to replace Napoleon's boot to enable the commander to remount his proud steed and return to his troops. From the medals the surgeon is wearing it appears that the surgeon treating Napoleon is Dominique Jean Larrey. *(Versailles Museum.)*

407

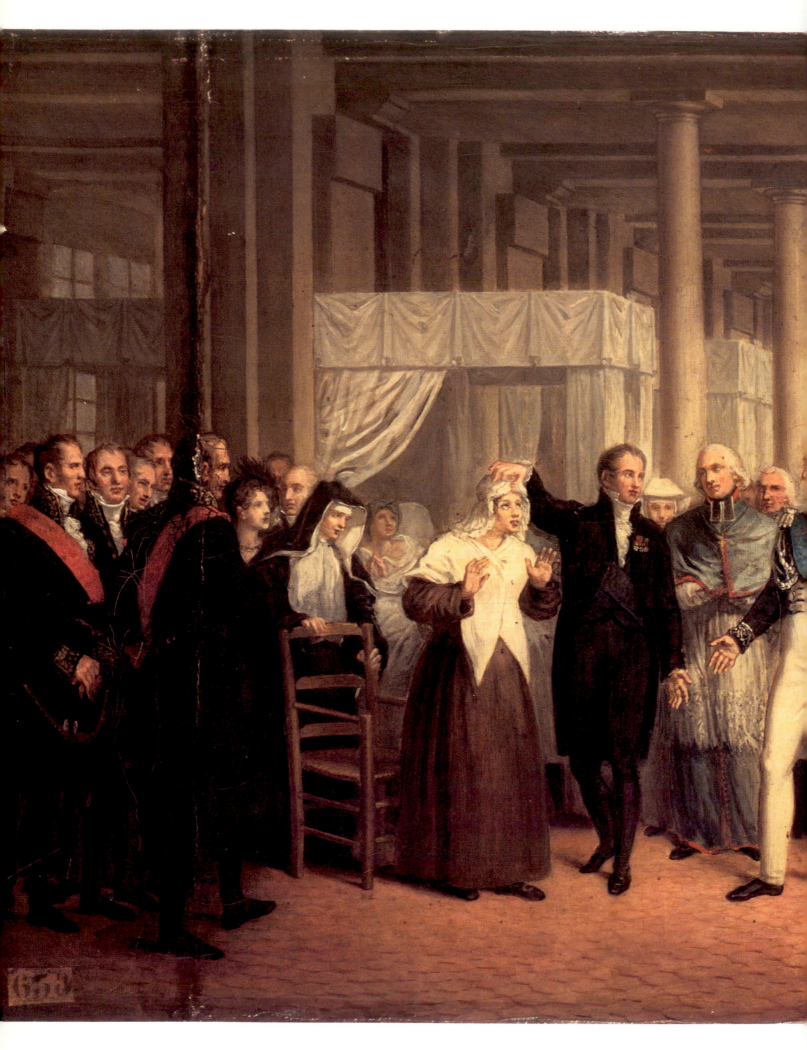

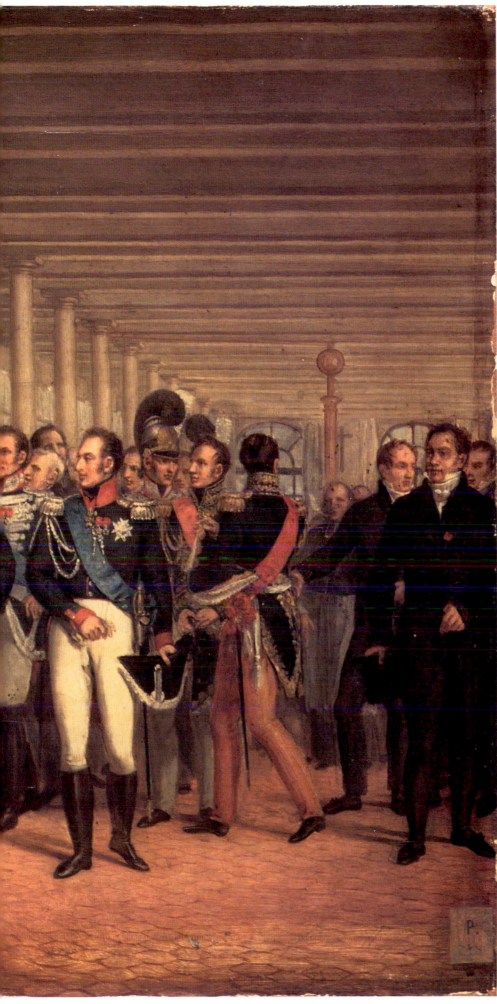

248. *Opération De La Cataracte Par Dupuytren En Présence De Charles X à l' Hôtel Dieu.* Guillaume Dupuytren presents a patient on whom he had successfully operated for cataract to King Charles X during a royal visit to the Hôtel Dieu in Paris in 1824. Dupuytren was the King's Chief Surgeon. He made such a great fortune from surgery that when Charles was deposed and needed money, Dupuytren offered to give him a million francs, stating that he was saving another million for his daughter and a third for his old age. *(Musée Carnavalet, Paris.)*

Paris surgery had achieved European preeminence during the eighteenth century, whereas French medicine tended to be held in low esteem. However, medicine underwent radical changes during the Revolution, and during the first few decades of the nineteenth century, Paris again became the world center for medical science and education. In many respects this new Paris medicine had a decidedly surgical character because the transformation of French medicine depended on the assimilation of surgical concepts and educational patterns that had helped produce the brilliant surgical results of the previous century.

The new Paris medical school was basically the old College of Surgery with the addition of a few physicians. Although surgeons did not literally replace physicians, most physicians of the revolutionary era and the early nineteenth century had strong surgical backgrounds. In a matter of great symbolism, the new Paris medical school was provided a home within the spacious facilities of the former College of Surgery.

The reform of hospital training for young doctors also indicated the strength of Parisian surgeons. In the nineteenth century, hospital service became an integral aspect of overall medical training. Consequently such features as the competitive examinations, known as *concours,* and the division of nonresident students (externs) and resident students (interns) were throwbacks to earlier surgical precedents. Many chores that had previously been assigned to young surgeons (wound dressing, phlebotomy, minor surgery, and the like) were now undertaken by medical students. Thus French physicians had a strong surgical inclination, even if they were not going to actually specialize in surgery. By uniting with medicine (1794), French surgery had ceased being a separate, autonomous profession and had become specialty within medicine. Nonetheless, the new Parisian medicine of the nineteenth century came to be dominated by the surgical forces of the eighteenth century.

In 1804 a revamped Paris Faculty of Medicine was organized; Napoleon I desired it to be not only a center of clinical instruction, but also an institute of medical science capable of acting as a governmental scientific body. This governmental advisory institute was disbanded when the Academy of Medicine was established in 1821. The Faculty of Medicine experienced additional managerial changes during the first three decades of the century but achieved a measure of stability by the 1830s.

Prelisterian nineteenth-century French surgery falls into four natural periods: the first, or Napoleonic, era (1800-1814); the second era, from 1815 to 1835, which closely parallels developments in the career of Guillaume Dupuytren (1778-1835); a preanesthetic period, from Dupuytren's death until 1847; and a fourth period, which lasted until the mid-1870s, when listerian techniques were finally accepted by most French surgeons. In many respects French surgery of the nineteenth century, like the surgery that evolved in other countries, is a record of magnificent personalities and individual clinical achievements.

Pierre François Percy (1754-1825) was one of Napoleon's leading surgeons. In his *Manuel Du Chirurgien-D'Armée* of 1792, Percy laid down his principles of the practice of military surgery. In that same year he was appointed medical consultant to the army of the north. Percy devised his own instrument for bullet extraction, the tribulcon. He was responsible, with Larrey, for the invention of special ambulances and squads of litter bearers, including a "super ambulance" capable of carrying 8 surgeons, 8 attendants, and dressings for 1200 men.

Joseph Souberbielle (1754-1846) apprenticed with Desault and became a military surgeon. In 1813 he received his formal medical degree and began a clinical practice in Paris. Souberbielle was a relative of Frère Côme and his nephew Baseilhac and inherited their instruments and professional reputations. Consequently most of Souberbielle's later professional life was devoted to lithotomy, in particular, to the suprapubic method of extracting bladder calculi.

Alexis Boyer (1757-1833) was born in Uzeriches, the son of poor parents. Through the efforts of an uncle, Boyer eventually obtained his medical education in Paris, where he studied with Desault. He was a studious, hardworking surgeon who became known for his teaching abilities. In 1804 Boyer was appointed to the surgical staff of the Hôtel Dieu and shortly thereafter became professor of surgery at the Ecole de Santé, where he would also hold the chair of clinical surgery. Boyer's reputation was gained primarily through his close association with Napoleon I. In 1805 Boyer was named surgeon to the imperial family, and in the following year he received the Legion of Honor, and the title "Baron of the Empire" was bestowed on him. During the same period he personally accompanied Napoleon to Prussia (1806) and Spain (1807). Most of Boyer's early reputation was gained in anatomy and was enhanced by his authoring of the four-volume *Traité Complet D'Anatomie* (1797-1799). His largest work was the eleven-volume *Traité Des Maladies Chirurgicales* (1814-1826). The practical system of surgery therein described remained the most complete surgical authority in France for many years and was later edited by his son Phillippe (1801-1858). After the fall of Napoleon, Boyer remained in favor with the succeeding monarchs and served as court surgeon. In 1825 he was appointed surgeon-in-chief to the Charité. Boyer's name is linked with the retrohyoid bursa and with a subhyoid cyst.

Dominique Jean Larrey (1766-1842) was the outstanding French surgeon during the Napoleonic era, serving as Napoleon I's chief military surgeon. Larrey was born in the village of Baudean in the Hautes Pyrenées and orphaned at the age of 13 years. Under the supervision of an uncle, who served as chief surgeon to a hospital in Toulouse, Larrey studied for 6 years to become a surgeon. In 1786 he went to Paris with the intention of completing his studies under Desault. Larrey learned, however, that a competitive examination was being held for the posts of assistant surgeons in the French navy. He took the examination and won one of the coveted appointments. Larrey was considered so well prepared as a surgeon that he was given the then-unprecedented commission of chief surgeon on the frigate *Vigilanté*. This vessel made a long and dangerous journey to North America, which Larrey vividly described in his later writings. After his return to Paris, Larrey decided to complete his training and for a period of 3 years served as an assistant to Desault and Sabatier. When war broke out in 1792, Larrey became an assistant surgeon and was assigned to the French army stationed on the Rhine. He shortly realized the need for better transport of the wounded, which led to his important proposal of constructing an ambulance sufficiently mobile to follow the advance guard into combat. These so-called "flying ambulances," which allowed first aid to be delivered on the battlefield, contributed to Larrey's reputation as one of history's greatest military surgeons. As Larrey's reputation grew, he was ordered to Toulon in the capacity of chief surgeon of the army of Corsica. There followed a brief campaign in Spain, civilian practice, a short term as professor of surgery at the military school at Val-de-Grâce, and orders to take charge of the flying ambulances with the army of Italy. Larrey accompanied Napoleon I on his expedition into Egypt, Palestine, and Syria, where Larrey became the first to point out the contagious nature of trachoma in his *Memoire Sur L'Ophthalmie Regnante En Egypte* (1802). In 1805 Larrey was made surgeon-in-chief and inspector general of the French army. Then came adventurous campaigns under the direct command of Napoleon I, including those into Germany and Poland and the disastrous retreat from Moscow. Throughout these marches the ingenuity Larrey exhibited and his solicitude for his sick and wounded comrades added immeasurably to his stature. It was said that Napoleon commanded no more love and respect from his troops than Larrey did. In 1810 Napoleon made Larrey a commander of the Legion of Honor and bestowed upon him the title of baron. In 1812 he was appointed surgeon-in-chief of the Grande Armée. The many lessons Larrey learned from his military experiences were preserved for his surgical colleagues in the famous five-volume *Memoires De Chirurgie Militaire, Et Campagnes* (1812-1817). In these works Larrey was one of the first to describe the therapeutic effect of maggots on wounds, and he detailed his performance of one of the first successful amputations at the hip joint (1812). Larrey participated in 25 military campaigns, 60 battles, and more than 400 skirmishes. Larrey was one of the few who stood by Napoleon at the time of his abdication and was waiting for him on his return in

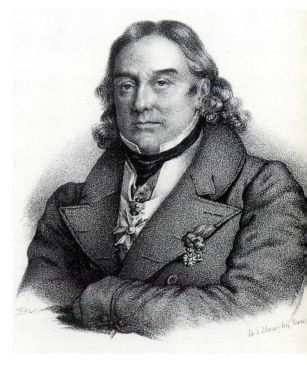

249. Dominique Larrey. *(Historical Collections, College of Physicians of Philadelphia.)*

1815. As a consequence, at the battle of Waterloo after having been shot and left for dead, Larrey was captured by the Prussians, who sentenced him to be executed. Larrey was eventually recognized and brought before Gebhard Blucher (1742-1819), the Prussian field marshal. Blucher's son had previously been captured by French forces, and Larrey had exerted his efforts and saved the young man's life. In return for this gesture, Blucher commuted Larrey's sentence and provided him safe escort to Belgium and freedom. The restoration of the monarchy found Larrey lonely and dispirited, although his reputation for valor and humanity had not dimmed. He continued to write, composing the monumental military treatise *Clinique Chirurgicale, Exercée Particulierement Dans Les Camps Et Les Hôpitaux Militaires Depuis 1792 Jusqu'en 1829* (1829-1836). The *Clinique Chirurgicale* was the most comprehensive of his surgical treatises and the only one of his works that was extensively illustrated. Larrey's name remains linked with an amputation at the shoulder joint, Mediterranean yellow fever, and ligation of the femoral artery immediately below Poupart's ligament.

The second period of prelisterian nineteenth-century French surgery centers around the professional life of Guillaume Dupuytren (1777-1835). Dupuytren's reputation was diminished by his contentious personality and seeming indifference to the welfare of his teachers and friends. He was born in the village of Pierre-Bouffière, the son of a constantly struggling lawyer. His early childhood was not marked by any evidence of scholastic abilities. In 1793, however, his father forced him to enroll in the medical-surgical school of the St. Alexis Hospital in Limoges with the authoritarian injunction that he would become a surgeon. Dupuytren acceded to his father's wishes but decided to pursue his education in Paris. He developed a great aptitude for anatomical dissection and by competitive examination won a position as prosector in the Academy of Medicine. In 1801 Dupuytren became chief of the department of anatomy. At the same time, he obtained the position of second surgeon at the Hôtel Dieu, again by *concours*. By 1808 Dupuytren was head of the surgical department; 4 years later he was appointed to the chair of operative surgery, and in 1815 he became surgeon-in-chief to the Hôtel Dieu. As professor of surgery in the Faculty of Medicine, Dupuytren was acknowledged to be the outstanding teacher of his generation. He was a merciless, obsessive-compulsive personality, an absolute perfectionist in everything he did, including operative surgery. Despite all his achievements and the recognition they brought him, he remained austere, arrogant, cold, and calculating. He was made a baron by Louis XVIII after becoming his personal surgeon. Dupuytren had an enormous practice that made him one of the wealthiest medical men in France. At his death he was a millionaire several times over: he bequeathed a substantial sum of money to establish a chair in pathological anatomy. His most important treatises included a two-volume work on military surgery, *Traité Théorique Et Pratique Des Blessures Par Armes De Guerre* (1834) and his four-volume *Leçons Orales De Clinique Chirurgicale* (1832-1834). Among his outstanding clinical feats were the first successful excision of the lower jaw (1812), some of the earliest ligations of the external iliac artery (1815) and subclavian artery (1819), and the treatment of torticollis by subcutaneous section of the sternocleidomastoid muscle (1822). Dupuytren was the first surgeon to successfully treat an aneurysm by compression with a tourniquet-like instrument (1818). In 1828 he invented an enterotome, or cutting forceps, for use in an operation for artificial anus (1828), and 3 years later he described an operation for the treatment of a nodular proliferation of fibrous tissue of the palmar fascia that led to flexure contractures of the fingers, especially the fourth and fifth. Among his most important clinical observations were a description of a fracture of the lower part of the fibula with dislocation of the ankle (1819), a clear pathological account of congenital dislocation of the hip joint (1826), and a detailed paper on an abscess of the right iliac fossa (1829). Dupuytren also classified burns in his *Leçons Orales De Clinique Chirurgicale* (1832). He is eponymically associated with an amputation of the arm at the shoulder joint, the palmar aponeurosis, a bilocular hydrocele in which the sac fills the scrotum and also extends into the abdominal cavity beneath the peritoneum, a clinical sign in

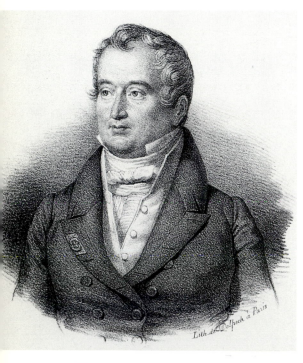

250. Guillaume Dupuytren. *(Historical Collections, College of Physicians of Philadelphia.)*

which there is free up-and-down movement of the head of the femur when traction is applied to it in cases of congenital dislocation, and a crackling sensation on pressure over the bone in certain cases of sarcoma.

Jacques Delpech (1777-1832) was a native of Toulouse and received his medical education at Montpellier (1801). By competitive examination he was appointed professor of surgery at his alma mater (1812), where he became celebrated as a clinical surgeon and teacher. In 1823 Delpech performed the first successful rhinoplasty by the Indian forehead-flap method in France. He was also the first to restore the lower lip by means of a skin graft from the neck. Delpech founded a large orthopedic institute at Montpellier and is considered the father of French orthopedic surgery. In his *Chirurgie Clinique De Montpellier* (1823), Delpech described the beneficial effect of section of the Achilles tendon for clubfoot. Although not the first surgeon to perform such an operation, Delpech was able to conclusively demonstrate the value of tenotomy in the correction of contracture deformities of the extremities. His most important work was the two-volume *De L'Orthomorphie* and accompanying atlas (1828). In this comprehensive treatise on deformities of the bones and joints Delpech established the tuberculous nature of certain cases of spondylitis and described the function of his orthopedic hospital. His name is also associated with a type of abscess that appears suddenly but with only slight inflammatory symptoms in patients with marked debility. Delpech was assassinated by a deranged patient who mistakenly thought Delpech had rendered him sexually impotent.

251. Illustration from Delpech of an orthopedic piano. At his orthopedic institution in Montpellier (1828) Delpech devised several innovative devices for the correction of spinal deformities. Among them was this piano: the patient's back and neck are supported and stretched while she plays. The large bird is a fine artistic touch. *(Jeremy Norman & Co., Inc.)*

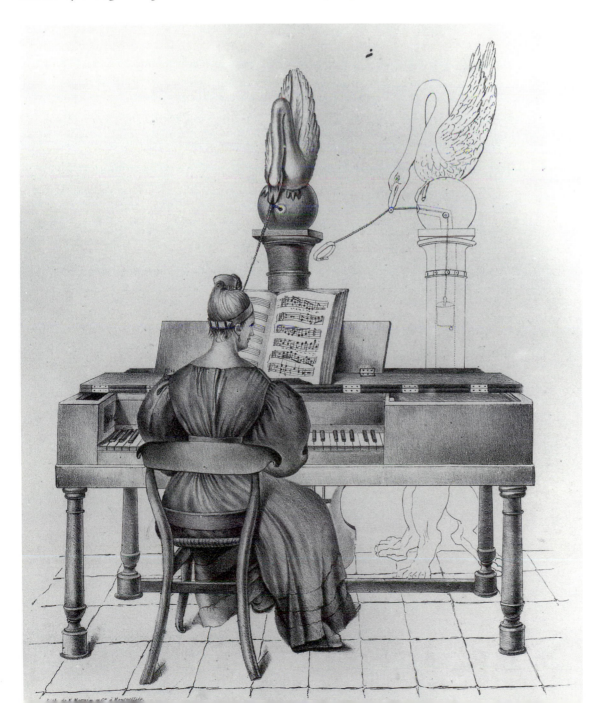

Jean Marjolin (1780-1850) was born in Ray-sur-Saone and received his surgical education in Paris. From 1801 to 1809 he passed through the various surgical grades via *concours*. In 1806 Marjolin was appointed prosector in the Faculty of Medicine of Paris. Ten years later he was named second surgeon of the Hôtel Dieu but soon left the position because of his contentious relationship with Dupuytren. In 1819 Marjolin was elected professor of surgical pathology while serving as surgeon to the king. Later he became surgeon-in-chief of the Hôpital Beaujon. His name remains connected with a malignant, verrucose, ulcerating growth occurring in cicatricial tissue or at the epithelial edge of a chronic benign ulcer.

Philibert Roux (1780-1854) was the successor to Bichat, who had served as his mentor. Roux became surgeon at the Charité in 1810 and professor of surgery in the Faculty of Medicine in 1820; he succeeded Dupuytren at the Hôtel Dieu in 1835. His most important literary work was the two-volume *Quarante Années De Pratique Chirurgicale* (1844-1855). Roux performed a staphylorrhaphy in 1819 on the medical student John Stephenson (1797-1842), who later reported on his experience as part of his graduation thesis (1820). Roux also gained fame for his method of resection of bone (1830) and the suturing of a ruptured perineum in a woman (1832). His name remains linked with a method of division of the inferior maxilla in the median line, which acts to facilitate the operation of ablation of the tongue.

Gilbert Breschet (1784-1845) was born at Clermont-Ferrand and educated at the Faculty of Medicine in Paris (1812). In 1818 he was appointed surgeon to the Central Bureau of that city and in the following year, surgeon-in-chief of the Foundling Hospital. Breschet eventually achieved the position of surgeon-in-ordinary to the Hôtel Dieu. On the retirement of Pierre Beclard (1785-1825) Breschet was appointed professor of anatomy at his alma mater. He became known as an outstanding surgical pathologist and anatomist, and his name remains linked with numerous anatomical structures.

During the 1790s a number of individuals were born who would eventually fill the void left after Dupuytren's death. For the most part, they were the last of the preanesthetic and prelisterian French surgeons. Jules Cloquet (1790-1883) was a native Parisian and received his early education at the Lycée Napoleon. In 1807 he went to study anatomy in Rouen, and 2 years later he was appointed to the Faculty of Medicine in his native city. Like every other young surgeon in postrevolutionary France, Cloquet had to advance within the hierarchical surgical system by a series of competitive examinations. In turn he became assistant surgeon to the Hospital St. Louis and *agregé* to the Faculty of Medicine. In 1831 Cloquet was named professor of surgical pathology at the Hôpital des Cliniques, and 2 years later he assumed the chair of clinical surgery as successor to Dubois. His most important written works were a monograph on hernia (*Recherches Sur Les Causes Et L'Anatomie Des Hernies Abdominales,* 1819) and a five-volume anatomical atlas (1821-1831). The *Anatomie De L'Homme* was the first anatomical atlas illustrated by lithography and contained 300 plates in folio format. Cloquet is eponymically linked with a femoral hernia that perforates the aponeurosis of the pectineus muscle and insinuates itself between this aponeurosis and the muscle.

Claude Lallemand (1790-1853) was a native of Metz and studied in that city's military medical school. In 1811 he moved to Paris and became an assistant to Dupuytren. Eight years later Lallemand was appointed professor of clinical surgery at Montpellier; after the death of Delpech, Lallemand was considered the premier surgeon in southern France. He is best known as the author of the three-volume *Des Pertes Seminales Involontaires* (1836-1842), in which he described small, gelatinoid concretions occasionally found in seminal fluid.

Jacques Lisfranc (1790-1847) studied at Lyon and Paris and received his medical degree in 1813. He served briefly as a military surgeon but eventually settled permanently in Paris. In 1825 Lisfranc became second surgeon at La Pitie and shortly thereafter, chief surgeon. He remains particularly well known for his contributions to orthopedic surgery. In his most important work, *Nouvelle Méth-*

ode Operatoire Pour L'Amputation Partielle Du Pied Dans Son Articulation Tarso-Metatarsienne (1815), Lisfranc described an amputation of the foot at the tarso-metatarsal joint, with the sole being preserved to make a flap. In addition, his name remains linked with the tarsometatarsal joint and a strong ligament between the lower part of the external surface of the first cuneiform bone and the lower two thirds of the internal surface of the base of the second metatarsal bone, and a tubercle of the anterior scalene muscle.

Jean Civiale (1792-1867) was born in Thierzac, the son of poor parents. His early education was entirely neglected, and he did not receive a medical degree until 1820. Civiale was greatly interested in diseases of the genitourinary system, and his first book, *Nouvelles Considerations Sur La Retention D'Urine* (1823), signified his desire to specialize in the field. This work was followed by *Sur La Lithotritie* (1826), which described his invention of a lithotriptor for crushing stones inside the bladder. In 1828 two wards at the Hôpital Necker in Paris were set aside for Civiale's studies, especially those of bladder calculus. Among his important treatises were the two-volume *Traité Pratique Sur Les Maladies Des Organes Genitourinaires* (1837) and *Traité Pratique Et Historique De La Lithotritie* (1847).

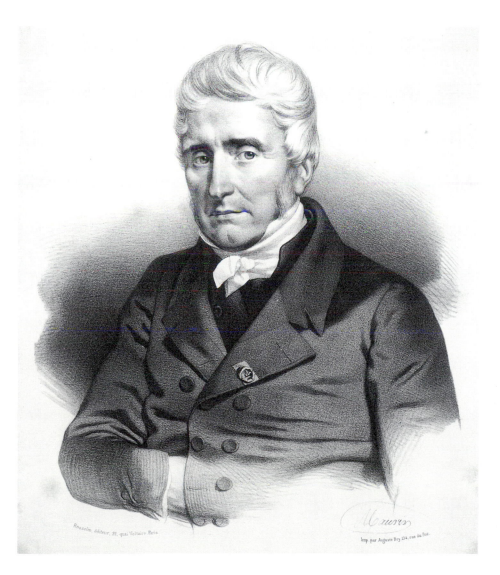

252. Jacques Lisfranc, orthopedic surgeon. Lithograph by Maurer. *(Historical Collections, College of Physicians of Philadelphia.)*

Alfred Velpeau (1795-1867) was born at Breche, the son of a village black-smith. Although he initially learned the trade of his father, at the age of 20 years Velpeau decided to study medicine in Tours with Pierre Bretonneau (1778-1862). In 1820 Velpeau settled in Paris, where he became an assistant to Cloquet and received his degree from the Faculty of Medicine (1823). Eight years later Velpeau became surgeon to the Hôpital St. Antoine and in 1830, to La Pitie. He remained in the latter institution until 1834, when he was appointed to the chair of clinical surgery in the Faculty of Medicine, as successor to Boyer. Velpeau contributed many important works to surgical literature, commencing with his *Traité D'Anatomie Chirurgicale* (1823). In 1831 he wrote a paper in which the first operative treatment of an aneurysm was described. In the following year Velpeau wrote his three-volume *Nouveaux Elements De Médecine Operatoire,* which was considered one of the most comprehensive works on operative surgery in France. His treatise on tumors of the breast (*Traité Des Maladies Du Sein Et De La Région Mammaire,* 1854) was a most important work in its time and provided a good account of hyperplastic cystic disease of the breast. Velpeau's name remains linked with a bandage that serves to immobilize the arm to the chest wall, a femoral hernia in which the intestine is in front of the blood vessels, and the ischiorectal fossa.

253. *A Lesson of Alfred Velpeau.* Lithograph by Louis Eugène Pirodon after the painting by François Feyen-Perrin, circa 1865. Velpeau stands with his hands outspread just before opening the cadaver. He wears an apron over his business suit. The artist has placed himself just behind Velpeau with sketches in his hands. *(Jeremy Norman & Co., Inc.)*

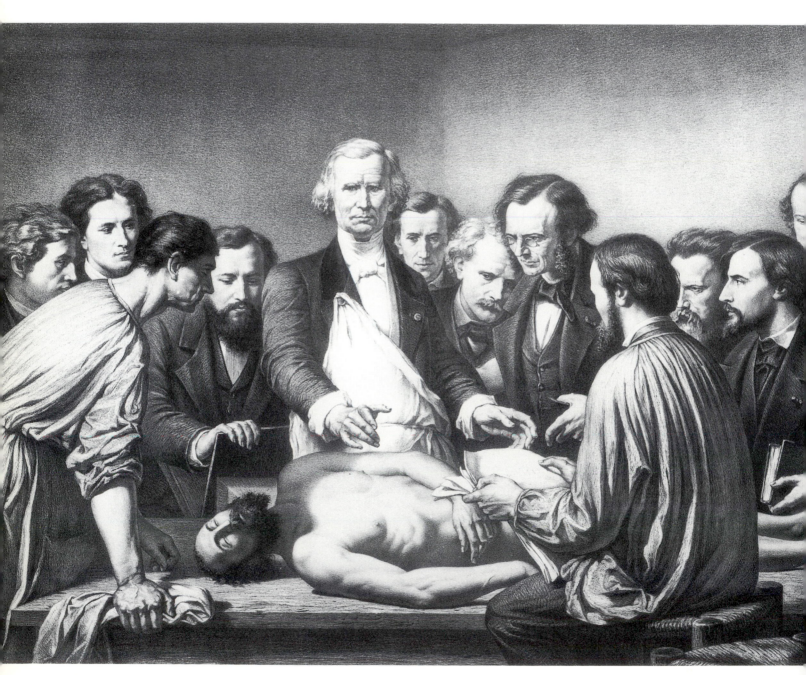

Jean Amussat (1796-1856), the son of a country physician, entered the army medical service in 1814. After gaining experience as a military surgeon, Amussat settled in Paris, where he received his formal medical degree in 1826. Amussat never held an academic title and spent most of his professional life in private practice. He was quite a prolific writer and in 1839 authored a treatise that established lumbar colostomy as the method of choice for obstruction of the colon. His name is associated with the spiral valves of the cystic duct and an abnormal fold of the urethral mucous membrane.

Pierre Gerdy (1797-1856) received his medical degree in Paris in 1823, after having served as a military surgeon. In 1828 Gerdy became second surgeon to La Pitie, where he worked under Lisfranc. Five years later, as a result of the political machinations of Dupuytren to undo Velpeau, Gerdy was unexpectedly named professor of the principles of surgery at the Faculty of Medicine. In 1839 Gerdy, hardly one of the best technical surgeons in France, was appointed surgeon to La Charité. His most important surgical publications were the *Anatomie Des Formes Exterieures Du Corps Humain* (1829) and the two-volume *Traité Des Bandages Et Des Pansements* (1837-1839). Gerdy's name is associated with a thin fibrous band stretching across the roots of the palmar surface of the four fingers; the sagittal fontanel; an aponeurotic band bounding the anterior fold of the axilla; a muscular fasciculus in the interatrial septum of the heart, passing backward from the atrioventricular groove; and a bony tubercle on the lateral side of the upper end of the tibia giving attachment to the iliotibial tract and some fibers of the anterior tibial muscle.

Antoine Jobert De Lamballe (1799-1867) was born in Lamballe and began his medical education with a country physician in his native city. Recognizing the need for further studies, Jobert moved to Paris, where he began the long, arduous passage through various minor positions that a young surgeon in France was compelled to undertake. By 1828 he was appointed a surgeon of the Central Bureau. Three years later Jobert was named surgeon to the Hôtel Dieu, and in 1854 he succeeded Roux as professor of surgery in the Faculty of Medicine. His reputation had been secured when he authored the two-volume *Traité Théorique Et Pratique Des Maladies Chirurgicales Du Canal Intestinal* (1829). His other important works included *Traité De Chirurgie Plastique* (1849) and *Traité Des Fistules Vesico-Uterines* (1852). In later life Jobert began to suffer from mental illness and was institutionalized in an insane asylum, where he died. Jobert is eponymically linked with a fossa formed by the adductor magnus and the sartorius and gracilis muscles, closure of a vesicovaginal fissure by autoplasty, and an interrupted intestinal suture used for invaginating the margins of the intestines in circular enterorrhaphy.

Stanislaus Laugier (1799-1872) was born in Paris, where he studied medicine (1828). He soon became a surgical intern under Dupuytren and eventually, an *agregé*. Laugier became surgeon to the Hôpital Necker in 1832, to Hôpital Beaujon 4 years later, and professor of clinical surgery in the Faculty of Medicine in 1848. Laugier later succeeded Roux as surgeon to the Hôtel Dieu. His name is associated with a hernia passing through an opening in the lacunar ligament and with a clinical sign that in fracture of the lower portion of the radius the styloid processes of the radius and of the ulna are on the same level.

In general it was French surgeons born after 1800 who developed their country's practice of surgery during the period between the introduction of anesthesia and the acceptance of listerian techniques. That proved to be a time of scientific transition, although the process of professionalizing French surgery in its socioeconomic status within medicine had been previously accomplished.

Jules Guerin (1801-1886) was a native of Bossu and became a pupil of Boyer and Roux in Paris (1826). In 1830 Guerin founded the *Gazette Médicale De Paris* and remained its editor for 40 years. Most of Guerin's surgical career was dedicated to orthopedic surgery, since he had established a private orthopedic hospital in Paris. In 1838 he authored a monograph on deformities of the osseous system; in 1840 he described an operation for strabismus.

Auguste Bérard (1802-1846) received his medical education in Paris (1829) and became surgeon to the Central Bureau by *concours* in 1831. He subsequently held surgical posts in several Parisian hospitals, and in 1842 he succeeded Sanson as professor of clinical surgery in the Faculty of Medicine. His most important treatise, on parotid tumors, was *Maladies De La Glande Parotide Et De La Region Parotidienne* (1841). Bérard's name is associated with a type of arteriovenous aneurysm in the tissues outside of the injured vein.

Amedée Bonnet (1802-1858) studied at Paris (1832) and in the following year obtained the position of surgeon at the Hôtel Dieu in Lyon by *concours*. His principal works were *Traité Des Sections Tendineuses Et Musculaires Dans La Strabisme, La Myopie* (1841), the two-volume *Traité Des Maladies Des Articulations* (1845), and *Traité De Therapeutique Des Maladies Articulaires* (1853). Bonnet is eponymically remembered for an operation for enucleation of the eyeball and for pain on adduction of the thigh in sciatica.

Antoine Lembert (1802-1851) studied with Dupuytren and was his assistant when Lembert provided a description of a new type of intestinal suture (1826). His method, which ensured that serous surface is applied to serous surface in suturing intestine, became the foundation of all modern gastric and intestinal surgery.

Jean Baudens (1804-1857) was born in Aire, initially studied medicine in Paris, and matriculated in 1823 at the military medical school in Strassburg. After graduation (1829), Baudens served in Africa from 1830 to 1837, and in 1838 he became professor in the hospital at Lille. Three years later he received the rank of chief of the military school and hospital at Val-de-Grâce. Baudens made numerous important contributions to military surgery, especially in his writings, which included *Clinique Des Plaies D'Armées A Feu* (1836) and the authoritative medical survey of the Crimean War, *La Guerre De Crimee, Les Campements, Les Abris, Les Ambulances, Les Hôpitaux* (1857).

Edouard Chassaignac (1804-1879) studied medicine at Nantes and Paris (1835). He never received a position as professor of surgery; instead, he became surgeon to the Lariboisière (1852). Chassaignac was an ingenious experimenter and a designer of instruments. In his two-volume *Traité Pratique De La Suppuration Et Du Drainage Chirurgicale* (1859) he introduced tubes of india rubber to drain abscesses and provided the subject of surgical drainage with a solid scientific and methodical foundation. Chassaignac's name is associated with a strong steel chain snare used for crushing through the pedicle of a tumor, also known as an *ecraseur,* and with an anatomical space between the pectoralis major muscle and the mammary gland.

Charles Sédillot (1804-1883), a native of Paris, studied with Boyer and Roux. He graduated in 1829 and entered the military service. In 1836 Sédillot was appointed professor of operative surgery at the military school in Val-de-Grâce. Five years later he became professor of surgery in Strassburg by *concours*. Sédillot remains best known for performing the first recorded gastrostomy (1849).

Joseph Malgaigne (1806-1865) was born at Charme-sur-Moselle. His father was a poor country physician. Consequently Malgaigne was forced to earn money to pay his expenses while studying medicine in Paris (1831). After a short term of service as a military surgeon in Poland he resettled in Paris where, after a competitive examination, he was appointed a surgeon of the Central Bureau (1835). At the same time, Malgaigne was granted authority to give public lectures at the Ecole Pratique on surgical anatomy. He soon gained numerous appointments at hospitals throughout Paris, including the Charité. In 1850 Malgaigne won by *concours* the chair of operative surgery in the Faculty of Medicine. His first important book was the *Manual De Médecine Operatoire* (1834), which was translated into Arabic, English, German, and Italian and soon was followed by the two-volume *Traité D'Anatomie Chirurgicale Et De Chirurgie Experimentale* (1838). His greatest work was the two-volume *Traité Des Fractures Et Des Luxations* (1847-1855), which was accompanied by an atlas and included his description of a bilateral vertical fracture of the pelvis. Malgaigne, a skillful, efficient

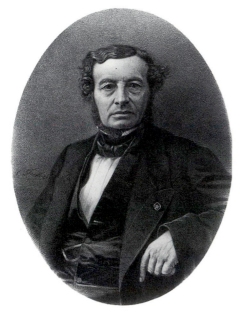

254. Joseph-François Malgaigne. *(Jeremy Norman & Co., Inc.)*

surgical technician, described a two-flap method for repair of cleft lip (1844). He is widely regarded as among the greatest of surgical historians, having edited the best edition then known of Paré's works (1840-1841); the introduction of the three-volume set included the *Histoire De La Chirurgie En Occident Depuis De VIe Jusqu'au XVIe Siècle, Et Histoire De La Vie Et Des Travaux D'Ambroise Paré* (1840), an outstanding history of surgery that included a masterful biography of Paré. Malgaigne is eponymically linked with a subastragalar amputation, a double-inclined plane for treatment of fracture of the femur, an infantile hernia preceding the descent of the testis, metal hooks that seize the upper and lower fragments of a fractured patella and are then approximated by screws, and a luxation of the head of the radius beneath the annular ligament.

255. Maxillofacial surgery. From *Traité Complet De L'anatomie De L'homme Comprenant La Médecine Opératoire* by Bourgery and Jacob. (eight volumes, 1866-1867). *(Jeremy Norman & Co., Inc.)*

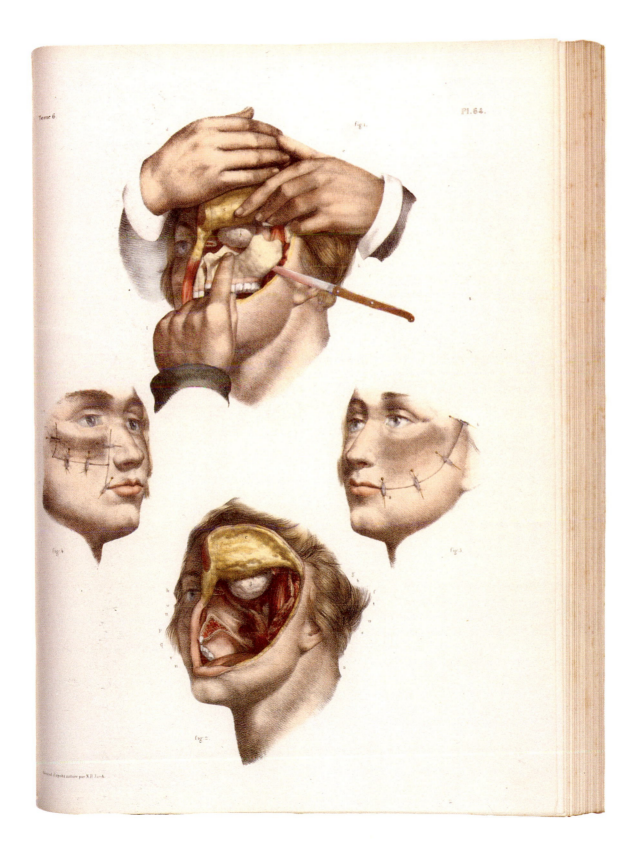

256. A selection of state-of-the-art surgical instruments, including elaborate cranked chain saws for cutting through bone, as depicted in Bourgery and Jacob's *Traité Complet De L'anatomie De L'homme Comprenant La Médecine Opératoire*. (Jeremy Norman & Co., Inc.)

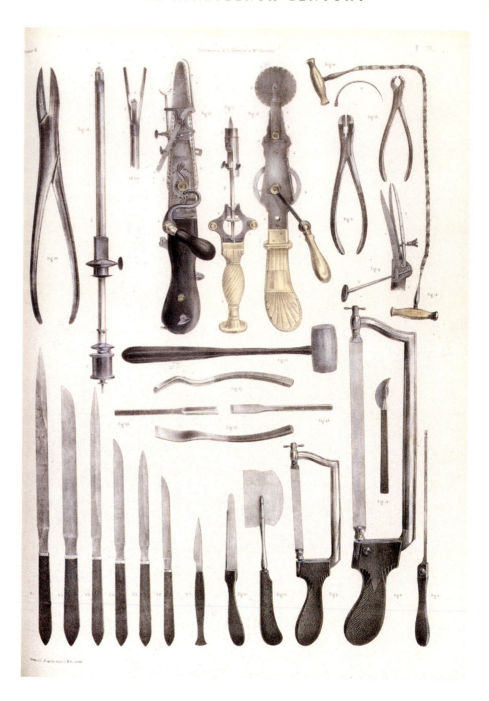

Auguste Nélaton, (1807-1873) the son of a French soldier, was born in Paris. He studied with Dupuytren at the Hôtel Dieu and at the Foundling Hospital (1836). Nélaton was soon made *agregé* and in 1851 became professor of surgery to the Faculty of Medicine. For many years both he and Malgaigne were colleagues at the Hôpital St. Louis, from which he resigned in 1867. Nélaton was among the most popular of Paris surgeons, and his skills as diagnostician, teacher, and surgical technician were considered unsurpassed. His principal published works included the exhaustive five-volume *Eléments De Pathologie Chirurgicale* (1844-1859) and *De L'Influence De La Position Dans Les Maladies Chirurgicales* (1851). In 1852 Nélaton provided a classic description of pelvic hematocele. His name is associated with a flexible catheter of red rubber; a porcelain-tipped probe for bullets; a fracture-dislocation in which the astragalus is wedged between the widely separated tibia and fibula; an anatomical line drawn from the anterior superior spine of the ilium to the tuberosity of the ischium, within which the greater trochanter normally lies but above which the trochanter is palpated in cases of dislocation of the hip or fracture of the neck of the femur; an inconstant band of circular muscular fibers in the wall of the rectum approximately 3 or 4 inches above the anal verge; and a fibrous tumor, or sarcoma, lying between the peritoneum and the muscles of the abdominal wall.

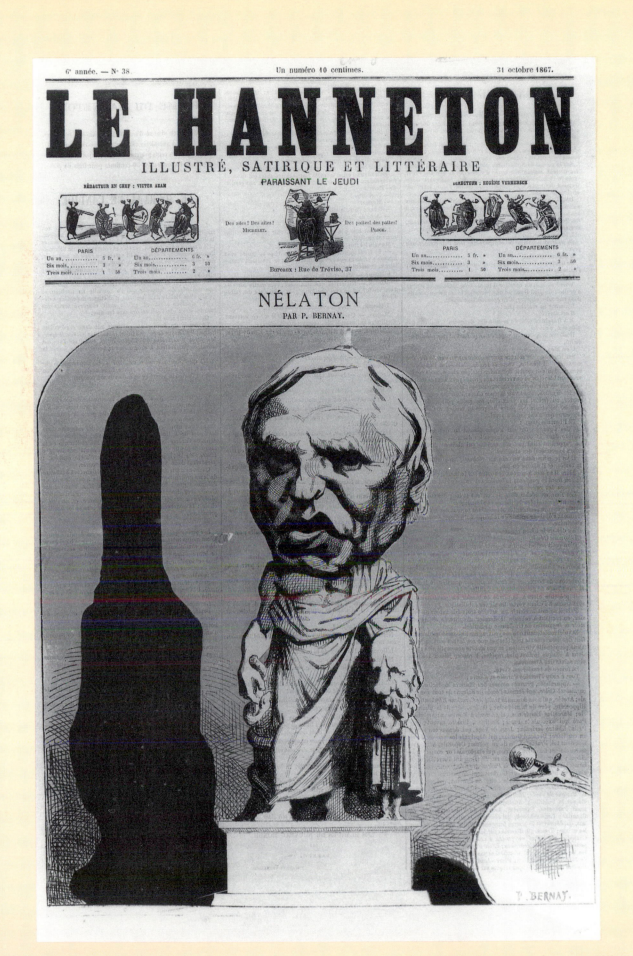

6ᵉ année. — N° 38.   Un numéro 10 centimes.   31 octobre 1867.

LE HANNETON

ILLUSTRÉ, SATIRIQUE ET LITTÉRAIRE

PARAISSANT LE JEUDI

RÉDACTEUR EN CHEF : VICTOR AZAM   DIRECTEUR : EUGÈNE VERMERSCH

Des ailes ! Des ailes !
MICHELET.

Des pattes ! des pattes !
PLOCK.

Bureaux : Rue de Tréviso, 37

PARIS		DÉPARTEMENTS	
Un an..........	5 fr. »	Un an..........	6 fr. »
Six mois..........	3 »	Six mois..........	3 50
Trois mois..........	1 50	Trois mois..........	2 »

PARIS		DÉPARTEMENTS	
Un an..........	5 fr. »	Un an..........	6 fr. »
Six mois..........	3 »	Six mois..........	3 50
Trois mois..........	1 50	Trois mois..........	2 »

NÉLATON
PAR P. BERNAY.

P. BERNAY.

257. Caricature of Auguste Nélaton as the new Asclepios, on the cover of the satirical magazine, *Le Hanneton,* 1867. This marked Nélaton's appointment as surgeon to Napoleon III and his entrance into medical immortality. *(Jeremy Norman & Co., Inc.)*

Charles Denonvilliers (1808-1872) studied medicine in Paris (1837) and within 3 years was appointed surgeon to the Central Bureau. In 1842 he attained the important positions of chief of the School of Practical Anatomy and surgeon at the Hôtel Dieu. A decade and a half later Denonvilliers was named professor of surgery. His interests tended to be more in anatomy than in clinical surgery, although he performed his most important service to French medicine when he was appointed inspector general of public instruction for medicine (1858). Denonvilliers's name remains associated with the rectovesical aponeurosis and the puboprostatic ligament.

Athanase Gosselin (1815-1887) studied medicine in his native city of Paris (1843). He soon became associated with a number of hospitals and in 1858 was named professor of surgery to the Faculty of Medicine. A decade later Gosselin was appointed attending surgeon to La Charité. His name is associated with a V-shaped fracture of the distal end of the tibia.

Alphonse Guerin (1816-1895) practiced in Paris; his major interest was in urologic surgery. His name is associated with a valve in the fossa navicularis of the urethra; a fracture of the facial bones in which there is a horizontal fracture at the base of the maxillae above the apices of the teeth; and a gland within the meatus of the female urethra.

Aristide Verneuil (1823-1895) practiced in Paris, where he introduced the use of forcipressure in the control of hemorrhage (1875). His five-volume *Memoires De Chirurgie* (1877-1888) discussed dry bandaging and iodoform in the treatment of abscesses. Verneuil performed an early gastrostomy in 1876. He is eponymically linked with traumatic spondylopathy, axillary abscess, and a neuroma of the cutaneous nerves.

Paul Broca (1824-1880), the son of an army surgeon, was sent to Paris to obtain all of his education (1849). Immediately after his graduation Broca became prosector at the Ecole Pratique. In 1853 he became assistant professor of surgery to the Faculty of Medicine and 14 years later, professor of surgery and successor to Nélaton. Broca was also on the surgical staff of many hospitals, including St. Antoine's, La Pitie, Des Cliniques, and Hôpital Necker. He remains best known as an anatomist, especially of the brain. During the latter part of his life, when he was devoted to the study of anthropology, he authored the three-volume *Memoires D'Anthropologie* (1871-1877) and the renowned *Memoires Sur Le Cerveau De L'Homme Et Des Primates* (1888). Broca originated modern craniometry and devised numerous craniometric and cranioscopic instruments. In 1861 he claimed that the third left frontal convolution of the brain was the center for articulate speech. Using his techniques of localization, Broca was the first to perform trephination for a cerebral abscess; he is considered an early pioneer in neurologic surgery. He also introduced the term *motor aphasia*.

Louis Ollier (1825-1900) was the son of a physician and studied medicine in Lyon and Montpellier (1856). In 1860 he was called to the chair of clinical surgery in Lyon and appointed senior surgeon to the Hôtel Dieu. There he gained his reputation as a masterful reconstructive and plastic surgeon. In 1858 Ollier described the osteogenetic layer of the periosteum. He also wrote about dyschondroplasia (1890). Ollier's most important paper concerned the transplantation of free skin (1869). He is eponymically associated with a theory of compensatory growth, which holds that after resection of the articular extremity of a bone the articular cartilage of the other bone entering into the structure of the joint takes on an increased growth.

Eugene Koeberle (1828-1915) practiced in Strassburg, where he established an excellent reputation for his work in ovariotomy. In the early 1860s he helped introduce the operation in France. In 1863 Koeberle performed the first successful excision of both the uterus and the ovaries for cancer. His name is associated with a type of hemostatic forceps.

Ulysse Trélat (1828-1890) was a native of Paris, where he studied medicine (1854). He became prosector in 1856 and assistant professor in surgery to the Faculty of Medicine in 1857. In 1860 Trélat was made surgeon to the Central Bureau and served in a number of successive hospitals, including Maternité, St.

Antoine's, St. Louis's, La Pitie, and La Charité. He was named professor of surgical pathology to the Faculty of Medicine in 1872. Trélat's major written works were *Leçons De Clinique Chirurgicale* (1877) and the two-volume *Clinique Chirurgicale* (1891). His name is associated with a bivalve rectal speculum and with a glairy stool streaked with blood in proctitis.

Listerian antisepsis had been generally accepted by most younger French surgeons by 1875. Thus the surgeons born after 1830 would bring France into the modern age of surgery and guide its destiny into the twentieth century. Jules Péan (1830-1898) was one of the most important French gynecologists of his time. He was a native of Chateaudun and studied at Paris (1860). After holding various hospital appointments, Péan organized the Hôpital International. Quite skilled as a surgical technician, he performed the first known pylorectomy for carcinoma, albeit unsuccessfully (1879). In 1886 Péan described a method for removing a tumor of the uterus by nipping or crushing off little bits at a time, known as *morcellement*. He performed a total prosthetic replacement of the shoulder in 1894 and in the following year became the first surgeon to operate on diverticula of the bladder (1895). His name is associated with a clamp intended to obtain hemostasis by forcipressure.

258. *Doctor Péan Operating* by Henri de Toulouse-Lautrec, 1891-1892. Oil on cardboard. In 1891 Lautrec shared an apartment with his friend Dr. Henri Bourges and quickly struck up friendships with many other members of the Parisian medical community. At the same time Lautrec's cousin Gabriel Tapié de Céleyran arrived in Paris, where he completed his medical training with Dr. Jules Emile Péan. Perhaps that is how Lautrec was invited to observe Péan operating. The type of procedure being performed is unknown. *(Sterling and Francine Clark Art Institute, Williamstown, Mass.)*

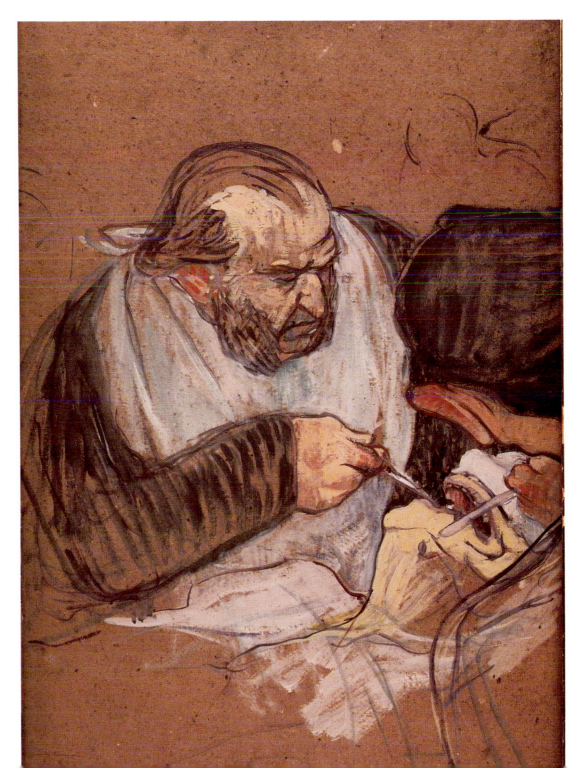

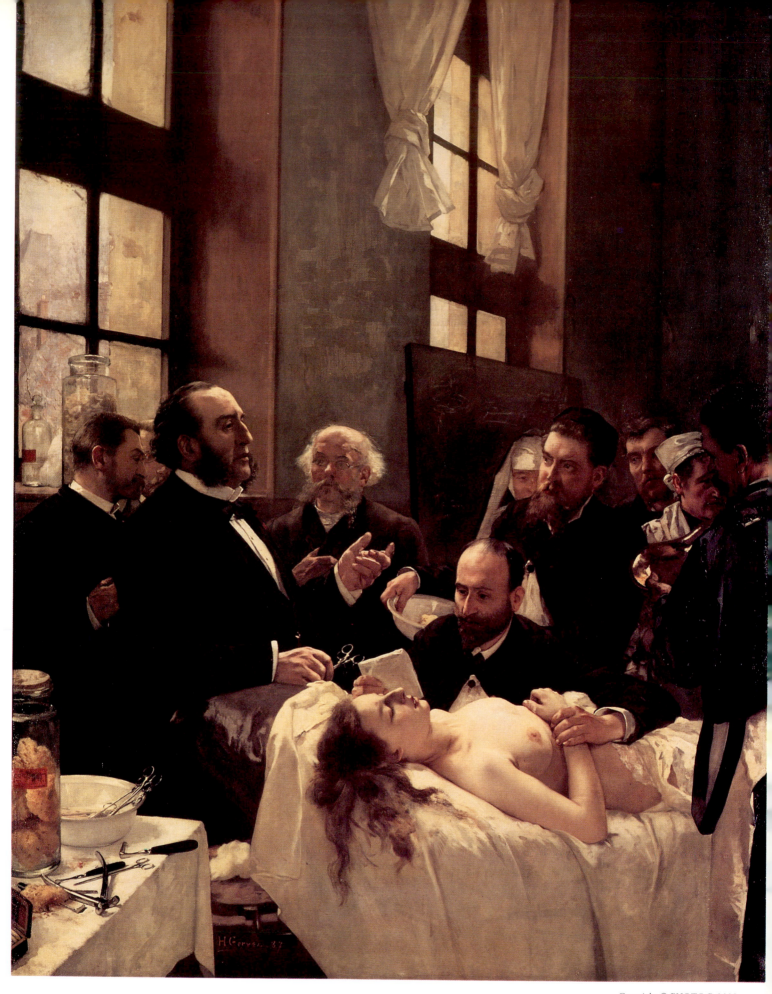

259. *Before the Operation Where Dr. Péan, Chief at l'Hôpital Saint-Louis, Discovered the Clamping of Bloodvessels,* 1887. Painting by Henri Gervex (1852–1929). *(Musée d'Orsay, Paris.)*

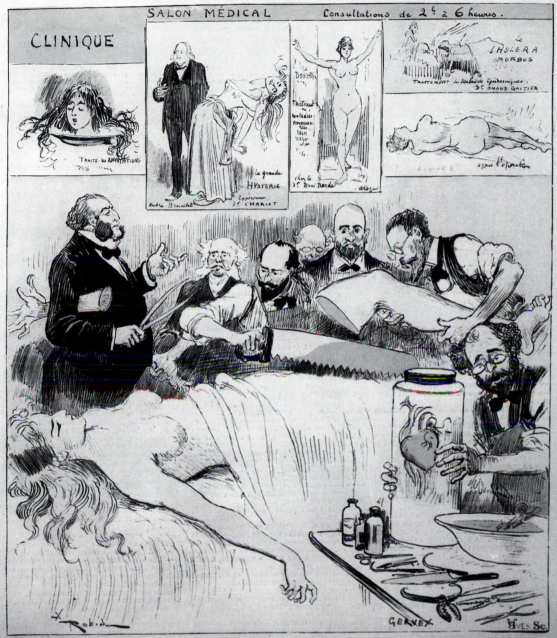

260. Caricatures of Gervex's painting of Péan and other medical discoveries of the time, such as Charcot's work on hysteria by A. Robida, 1887. The caption points out that the armless Venus de Milo would not be jealous of this beauty undergoing amputation after an accident in a carriage. (*The William H. Helfand Collection.*)

Jean Guyon (1831-1920) was educated at Nantes and Paris (1858). He soon became a urological surgeon at the Hôpital Necker and in 1890 was named professor of genitourinary surgery at the University of Paris. His major written works were *Leçons Cliniques Sur Les Maladies Des Voies Urinaires* (1881) and *Leçons Cliniques Sur Les Affections Chirurgicales De La Vessie Et De La Prostate* (1888). Guyon's name is associated with an amputation of the foot above the malleoli, the uterine isthmus, an operative treatment of ingrowing toenail by the excision of a wedge-shaped piece from the side of the great toe, and the ballottement of the kidney in cases of nephroptosis, especially when there is a concurrent renal tumor.

Odilon Lannelongue (1840-1911) of Paris performed the first thyroid transplantation for treatment of cretinism in 1890. His name is associated with venous openings into the right atrium of the heart, a fibrous band passing from the anterior surface of the pericardium to the sternum, and a decompression operation consisting of the removal of segments of bone from the roof of the skull.

Just Lucas-Championière (1843-1913) obtained his medical education in Paris (1870). Just before receiving his degree, he spent time in Lister's service in Glasgow, where he became imbued with the concept of listerian antisepsis. In 1876 Lucas-Championière authored his *Chirurgie Antiseptique,* the first authoritative work on antiseptic surgery, which allowed him to introduce such methods into French surgery. Among his other important works was a classic account of hernia, *Cure Radicale Des Hernies* (1887). Lucas-Championière's name is associated with fibrinous bronchitis.

Samuel Pozzi (1846-1918) studied under Broca in Paris. In 1877 Pozzi received the post of *agregé,* and 6 years later he became surgeon to the Hôpital de Loureine. He was later elected to the chair of gynecology in that city (1901). Pozzi was quite active in organized medicine and served as the secretary general to the French Congress of Surgery from 1885 to 1894. He founded the journal *Revue De Gynecologie Et De Chirurgie Abdominale* and remained its editor for many years. His name is linked with the minor extensor muscle of the fingers. Pozzi, an ardent student of the history of medicine, was fatally shot by a mentally deranged patient in his Paris office.

Antonin Poncet (1849-1913) spent most of his professional life in Lyon. There he described tuberculous rheumatism in 1897. Poncet was a superb technician; his name is associated with an operation for lengthening the Achilles tendon in tip foot, a perineal urethrostomy, and perineal cystotomy in prostatic disease.

Edouard Quenu (1852-1933) received his surgical training in Paris. He was particularly interested in colorectal surgery and wrote the two-volume *Chirurgie Du Rectum* (1895-1899). Quenu's name is linked with the lymphatic plexuses in the anal skin; an excision of the rectum with removal of the neighboring lymph glands for cancer; a clinical sign in a case of aneurysm in which when the main artery of a limb is compressed and a puncture is made at the periphery, it is assumed that if blood flows, the collateral circulation is well maintained; and a resection of the ribs to allow retraction of the thorax in the treatment of empyema.

Marin-Theodore Tuffiér (1857-1929) was born in Belleme and educated in Paris (1885). He later was lecturer in surgery to the Faculty of Medicine and also taught at the Sorbonne. Tuffiér described the first cure of tuberculosis by removal of the lung apex in his *Chirurgie Du Poumon En Particulier Dans Les Cavernes Tuberculeuses Et La Gangrene Pulmonaire* (1897). He remained active in thoracic surgery, having perfected a method of extrapleural pneumolysis (1910), and performed the first successful experimental operation for the relief of chronic valvular disease. In 1914 Tuffiér operated successfully in a case of aortic stenosis. He was also the first to attempt to visualize the urinary tract by the combination of an opaque ureteral styletted catheter and X rays (1899).

Eugene Doyen (1859-1916) of Reims studied in Paris, where he later established his own private surgical clinic. In 1913 he was the first to attempt surgical relief of valvular disease of the heart. Doyen was among the earliest surgeons to make motion pictures of his operative procedures.

Joaquin Albarran (1860-1912) was born in Cuba, studied medicine in Spain, and settled in Paris, where he began research under Louis Ranvier (1835-1922). Albarran eventually became acquainted with Guyon and decided to specialize in urological surgery. He succeeded Guyon as urological surgeon at the Hôpital Necker in 1906. His clinics became world renowned and attracted students from all countries. His important written works included *Les Tumeurs De La Vessie* (1891), in which he described subtrigonal glands in the bladder and introduced a classification of bladder tumors based on embryological origin. Other works were *Exploration Des Fonctions Renales* (1905) and his acknowledged masterpiece, *Médecine Operatoire Des Voies Urinaires* (1909). In 1896 Albarran performed the first planned nephrostomy, and 9 years later he introduced a method for nephropexy. Eponymically he is linked with a clinical polyuria test for renal insufficiency.

Henri Hartmann (1860-1952) received his education in Paris (1887) and eventually became professor of surgery at the Hôtel Dieu, where he served from 1909 to 1930. He is best remembered for the two-stage colectomy he devised for colonic cancer or diverticulitis. Hartmann's experience with that technique was summarized in his *Chirurgie Du Rectum* (1931).

Mathieu Jaboulay (1860-1913) studied at Lyon, where he became surgeon to that city's hospital in 1892. A decade later he was named professor at the city's surgical clinic. In his most important text, *Chirurgie Du Grand Sympathique Et Du Corps Thyroide* (1900), he reported the first sympathectomy for the relief of vascular disease. In 1892 Jaboulay introduced a side-to-side gastroduodenostomy, and 2 years later he performed the first known interilioabdominal amputation. His name is associated with a method of suturing arteries by splitting the cut ends for a short distance and then suturing the intimal flaps together.

Hippolyte Morestin (1869-1919) was a native of Martinique and studied in Paris (1894). In 1902 he introduced a method of mammaplasty. During World War I, Morestin devoted himself to the restoration of shattered faces. As a result, many of the early techniques in plastic and reconstructive surgery are credited to him. His name is linked with the posterior anal nerve.

261. Preoperative and postoperative photographs of reconstructive surgery of the face from Hippolyte Morestin's personal case records (1899-1914). *(Jeremy Norman & Co., Inc.)*

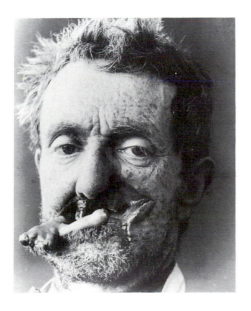
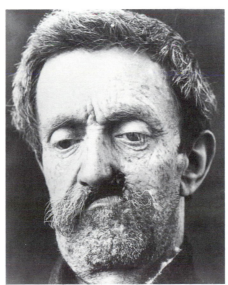
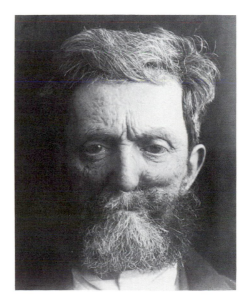

427

ITALY

During the rule of Napoleon I, Italy was invaded by his armies and was made a French dependency with Napoleon as king of Italy. This political subordination was especially evident when Napoleon named his brother Joseph Bonaparte (1768-1844) as king of Naples in 1806. Joachim Murat (1771-1815), married to Napoleon I's sister Caroline (1782-1839), became the next king of Naples (1808-1814) when Joseph was later appointed king of Spain. In 1811 Napoleon I proclaimed his newborn son, Napoleon II, the king of Rome. Pope Pius VII (1742-1823) was kidnapped and held captive in France until Napoleon's downfall in 1814.

In 1815 the Congress of Vienna left large portions of Italy under the rule of Austria and the pope. Concurrently the House of Savoy was restored in the kingdom of Sardinia, and the Bourbons were returned to Sicily. Although wishes for Italian unity and independence were effectively stalemated by Austria, the desire for freedom was growing.

During the 1850s and 1860s the modern country of Italy was forged through the efforts of Giuseppe Garibaldi (1807-1882), Camillo Cavour (1810-1861), and Victor Emmanuel II (1820-1878), first king of the unified Italy. The task of preserving peace and organizing the new state was carried on by Humbert I (1844-1900), son of Victor Emmanuel II. Although greatly admired, Humbert I was assassinated, and his son Victor Emmanuel III (1869-1947) succeeded him.

Italian leadership in the medical sciences, which had endured for nearly a millennium, had clearly waned by the beginning of the nineteenth century. Few individuals excelled in surgery and anatomy: Antonio Scarpa (1752-1832) was one of them. He was born in northern Italy, just south of the Tyrol. An uncle who was a priest took charge of his early education. Accordingly, by the age of 15 years, Scarpa was an excellent Latinist and had passed the entrance examinations to the famed University of Padua. There he began the study of medicine and came under the tutelage of Morgagni. Morgagni died in 1771, but during his final years Scarpa became his personal secretary and confidant. Scarpa received his degree in 1770 and within 2 years, after receiving Morgagni's recommendation, was appointed professor of anatomy and clinical surgery at the University of Modena. Some of Scarpa's most important anatomical research was completed during the 10 years he spent in Modena. In 1772 he authored *De Structura Fenestrae Rotundae Auris, Et De Tympano Secundario Anatomicae Observationes,* in which he elucidated the membranous labyrinth of the inner ear. From 1779 to 1782 Scarpa embarked on a tour of all the major medical centers in Europe. While in Austria, he met Brambilla, who was surgeon to the Austrian monarch, Joseph II. From this friendship came an invitation to assume the chair of anatomy at the University of Pavia (1783). In 1787 the chair of clinical surgery was also given to Scarpa. He remained there for the rest of his professional career, and the university became preeminent in Europe. His most important clinical work was completed in Pavia, and his proclivity for writing became legendary. In *Anatomicae Disquisitiones De Auditu Et Olfactu* (1789) Scarpa recorded important research concerning the auditory and olfactory apparatuses of fishes, birds, reptiles, and humans. In 1794, his greatest work, the *Tabulae Neurologicae,* was published; it included the first proper delineation of the nerves of the heart. Five years later, Scarpa authored a treatise on the ear, *De Penitiori Ossium Structura Commentarius.* By the beginning of the nineteenth century Scarpa had become quite wealthy and lived in a grand manner. He was said to have been a favorite of Napoleon I, who appointed him an imperial surgeon and conferred the Cross of the Legion of Honor and the Order of the Iron Crown upon him. Scarpa won universal admiration as a lecturer and an orator, and although he retired from active teaching in 1813, he continued writing for many years. His *Saggio Di Osservazioni E D'Esperienze Sulle Principali Malattie Degli Occhi* (1801) was a beautifully illustrated work on ophthalmology and the first book on the subject to be published in the Italian language. In 1803 he provided the first accurate

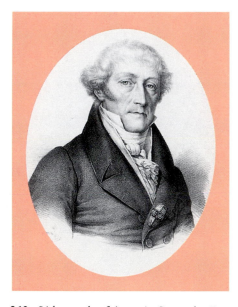

262. Lithograph of Antonio Scarpa by Frey after Maurer, 1835. *(Historical Collections, College of Physicians of Philadelphia.)*

description of the pathological anatomy of congenital clubfoot (1803). In *Sull' Aneurisma* (1804), Scarpa distinguished true from false aneurysms and introduced the concept of arteriosclerosis. He authored an important monograph on herniorrhaphy, *Sull' Ernie, Memorie Anatomico-Chirurgiche* (1809), and a treatise on the arteries, *Memoria Sulla Legature Delle Principali Arterie Degli Arti* (1817). In *Sull' Ernia Del Perineo* (1821) Scarpa detailed perineal hernia and provided a classic description of sliding hernia. In 1825 the first volume of his *Opusculi De Chirurgia* was published; it was intended to be a series of works on various surgical topics. Scarpa remained a bachelor throughout his life, although he was said to have fathered several illegitimate sons. Scarpa remained a power at Pavia after his retirement and exercised his authority in a ruthless, tyrannical manner. As permanent director of the Faculty of Medicine, he was able to control every facet of medical education and remained vindictive toward several individuals. Bitterness and hatred surrounded Scarpa, and when he died at 80 years of age, his reputation was attacked and his achievements were derogated.

Giovanni Monteggia (1762-1815) was professor of anatomy and surgery in Milan (1795). He was associated with Scarpa in the preparation of the five-volume *Istituzioni Di Chirurgia* (1802-1803). Monteggia's name is linked with a fracture of the ulna with simultaneous dislocation of the head of the radius.

Eduardo Bassini (1844-1924) was born in Pavia, where he received his medical degree in 1866. He initially participated in the unification movement of Italy and during one battle sustained a bayonet wound of the groin. A fecal fistula resulted and was successfully treated by Luigi Porta (1800-1875). After Bassini's recovery he served as second assistant to Porta. At the suggestion of his mentor, Bassini went to Vienna, where he worked in Billroth's clinic; he also visited renowned medical centers in Berlin and London. In 1874 Bassini was invited to return to Pavia to serve as first assistant to Porta. Porta died during the following year, but his chair was not given to Bassini. Bassini was deeply disappointed, and

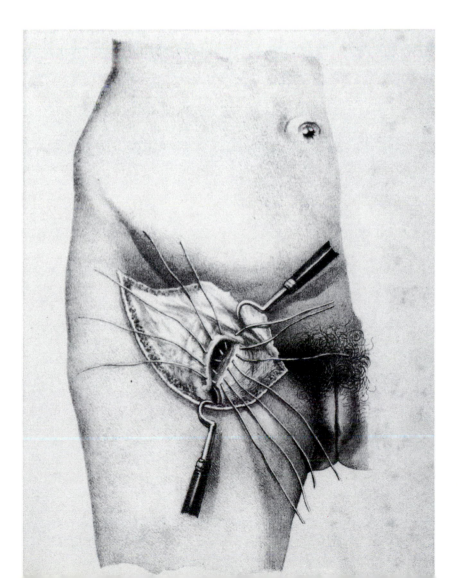

263. After Bassini's success in repairing inguinal hernias he applied his revolutionary operating techniques to crural or femoral hernia in *Nuovo Methodo Operativo Per La Cura Radicale Dell'ernia Crurale* (1893). *(Jeremy Norman & Co., Inc.)*

429

he resigned from the university and returned to London for 6 months. He was soon appointed lecturer in surgery at Parma and in 1877 became head of the department of surgery at Spezia. Bassini was an early advocate of listerian techniques and was instrumental in introducing these concepts into Italian surgery. In 1882 he was appointed to the chair of surgical pathology at the University of Padua, where he spent the next 40 years. During the early 1880s Bassini proposed a method of nephropexy. In 1887 he first presented his operation for the radical cure of inguinal hernia, and 4 years later he detailed a surgical operation for femoral hernia in *Nuovo Metodo Operativo Per La Cura Radicale Dell' Ernia Crurale*.

Antonio Ceci (1852-1920) is credited with the development of scientific surgery in Pisa, where he was professor at the surgical clinic. He had also previously served as professor of surgical pathology in Genoa (1883). He is remembered for being the first surgeon to perform an amputation in which the musculature above the stump was used to form a motor unit for artificial limbs (1906).

Leonardo Gigli (1863-1908) was professor of gynecology in Florence. In 1894 he proposed a surgical saw that was first used for pubiotomy. Indications for the use of the so-called Gigli saw were eventually broadened to include craniotomy (1898). In 1902 Gigli substituted pubiotomy for symphysiotomy.

RUSSIA

In the 1820s the death of Alexander I (1777-1825) led to a revolt of discontented nobles and guardsmen, which marked the first appearance in Russia of a revolutionary force: later revolutionaries would trace their origins to these so-called Decembrists. Nicholas I (1796-1855) succeeded his brother, Alexander I. The 30-year rule of Nicholas I was one of extreme repression during which attempts were made to eliminate progressive thinking. In many ways this conservative leadership reflected the status of Russian medicine, which was not nearly as advanced as medicine in other European countries.

Alexander II (1818-1881), son of Nicholas I, began his reign as a reformer. In 1861 Alexander proclaimed freedom for the serfs and set out to modernize and improve Russian medicine. His relatively enlightened changes, however, were not adequate to meet the increasing demands of certain groups, and he was assassinated by a terrorist bomb in the center of St. Petersburg. After his death an era of reaction continued through the reigns of the last two Romanovs, Alexander III (1845-1894) and Nicholas II (1868-1918).

Little in the way of surgical education and training existed in Russia before the middle of the nineteenth century. In general the priests served as dispensers of medical care for the masses. If the wealthy needed specialized attention, an individual was usually brought from another country for the service of the court.

The modern era of Russian surgery began with Nikolai Pirogoff (1810-1881). Through the efforts of a family friend he was admitted to the Medical Faculty at Moscow in 1824. Eight years later Pirogoff received his degree, after which he studied in Berlin and Gottingen for 2 years. In 1836 he was appointed to the chair of surgery at Dorpat. Four years later Pirogoff was elected professor of surgery in the Medico-Chirurgical Academy in St. Petersburg, where he remained until 1856, when he permanently retired from teaching and hospital work. The bulk of Pirogoff's most important research was completed in St. Petersburg. In 1847 Pirogoff became the first surgeon known to practice rectal etherization; his monograph *Recherches Pratiques Et Physiologiques Sur L'Etherisation* showed that he was one of the earliest surgeons in Europe to adopt ether anesthesia. Pirogoff's three-volume *Klinische Chirurgie* (1851-1854) was among the most important surgical works published in the mid-nineteenth century. Interestingly, this German edition predates the publication of the Russian volume. The eight-part *Anatome Topographica Sectionibus Per Corpus Humanum Congelatum Triplici Directione Ductis Illustrata* (1852-1859) represented the first important use of frozen sections in anatomical illustration. His clinical skills were considerable, and in 1854 Pirogoff authored a paper that outlined a method of complete osteoplastic amputation of the foot. Later in his professional career Pirogoff became most interested in improving medical sanitation. His attempts to improve the conditions at his military hospital in St. Petersburg created so much ill feeling that the medical director of the hospital branded Pirogoff insane and forced him to resign his professorship. During the Crimean War Pirogoff organized medical aid and helped develop basic principles of field surgery. He was also instrumental in introducing the help of women during the war effort, which ultimately led to the formation of the Russian Red Cross. After the war Pirogoff began to condemn the restrictions on education for the poor and for non-Russian citizens and supported education for women. His name is associated with an anatomical triangle formed by the intermediate tendon of the digastric muscle, the posterior border of the mylohyoid muscle, and the hypoglossal nerve.

Russian surgeons born after 1830 were the ones who guided their country into the postlisterian age. Robert Wreden (1837-1893) was an otologist in St. Petersburg. He was attending surgeon to the czars and was the first to call special attention to otomycosis (1867). He is eponymically remembered for a clinical sign that in a stillborn child a gelatinous material completely fills the external auditory meatus. Vladimir Vladimirov (1837-1903) is best remembered for his osteoplastic resection of the ankle after which the patient walks on tiptoe.

Carl Reyher (1846-1890) was a native of Riga and received his medical education at Dorpat (1870). He soon enlisted in the Prussian army to serve as a surgeon during the Franco-Prussian War. In 1872 Reyher joined the clinic of Bergmann at his alma mater. There he remained until 1877, when, over the protests of his mentor, he entered the Russian army medical service. During the Russo-Turkish conflict Reyher began his work with debridement of war injuries. Through his efforts a controlled study of the value of debridement in contaminated gunshot wounds was undertaken (1881). In 1883 Reyher became chief of surgery at the Semenov Hospital in St. Petersburg. Like many innovators, he met unlimited opposition, especially regarding the introduction of listerian techniques. This opposition, compounded by instability in his marriage, drove him to commit suicide while on a hunting expedition.

Peter Dyakonov (1855-1908) was professor of surgery at the University of Orel and a founder of the annual congresses of Russian surgeons that began in 1888. Dyakonov was also editor of the first Russian surgical journal, *Kirurgiya* (1897-1908).

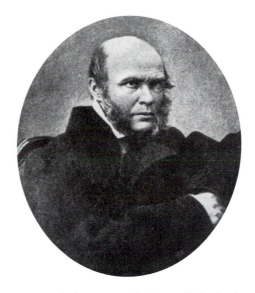

264. Nikolai Ivanovitch Pirogoff, the leading Russian surgeon of his era, made many innovations in surgical technique. *(Jeremy Norman & Co., Inc.)*

SCANDINAVIA

At the beginning of the nineteenth century the Academia Chirurgica in Denmark had been functioning for almost 20 years as a major source of education for Danish surgeons, including Henry Callisen (1740-1824). He was a native of Holstein and a pupil of Krueger. After passing his preliminary graduation examination (1767), Callisen studied in London with William Hunter and in Paris. Returning to Copenhagen, he became chief naval surgeon and in 1773, professor of surgery at his alma mater. Callisen's most important writings included *Institutiones Chirurgicae Hodiernae* (1777) and *Systema Chirurgicae Hodiernae* (1778).

Adolf Callisen (1787-1866), a nephew of Henry Callisen, graduated from the university in Kiel in 1809. He was professor of surgery at the surgical academy in Copenhagen (1817). A quarter of a century later he was appointed professor at the University of Copenhagen. Callisen's best-known work was the 33-volume *Medicinisches Schriftsteller-Lexicon Der Jetzt Lebenden Arzte* (1830-1845), the era's greatest medical bibliography, which provided a complete review of the medical and surgical literature from about 1780 to 1830. It is considered one of the greatest written achievements of a single surgeon.

Niels Rovsing (1862-1927) was the most renowned Danish surgeon at the beginning of the twentieth century. He was appointed professor of operative surgery at Copenhagen in 1899. Five years later he was named senior surgeon of Frederiks Hospital. Rovsing was one of the founders of the Danish Surgical Society. His name is linked to a clinical sign in which pain in the right lower quadrant of the abdomen is induced in cases of acute appendicitis by exerting pressure over the descending colon.

In Sweden the most important surgeon in the early part of the nineteenth century was Peter Bjerkin (1755-1818). He had studied with John Hunter and served in the Finnish army as a military surgeon. Bjerkin was appointed chief of surgery in Stockholm in 1809. He wrote little of major consequence. Carl Santesson (1819-1886), a native of Gothenburg, was a graduate of Uppsala University (1846). He was the leading Swedish surgeon during the second half of the nineteenth century, serving as professor of surgery in Stockholm. In 1878 Adolf Lindstedt (1847-1915) and Johan Waldenstrom (1839-1879) detailed the first recorded operation for sigmoid volvulus. Waldenstrom's name is associated with a test for porphyrin in the urine and with a clinical syndrome in which macroglobulins are present in the circulating blood.

NETHERLANDS

In 1795 the Austrian Netherlands was annexed into the French Republic. The medical schools in Belgium were shut down, much as those in France had been. Consequently each large town attempted to regulate its medical practitioners by local examinations. The schools they established, decidedly inferior, were devoted strictly to providing instruction in surgery and obstetrics to relatively uneducated individuals. In 1815 the Netherlands was reorganized, the universities of Ghent and Liege were established, and the old university in Louvain was reopened. Instruction was given in Latin, although German influence was heavy. The result was educational failure, and most Belgian medical students preferred to study in Paris. Political unrest in the early 1830s caused the universities to close. In 1835 they were reestablished but with a greater French influence than previously.

Christian Tilanus (1796-1883) graduated from the university in Utrecht in 1819. He then studied in Paris with Dupuytren and Lisfranc. In 1828 Tilanus was appointed professor of surgery and obstetrics in Amsterdam, where he was the first to give clinical bedside teaching in surgery.

UNITED STATES

The practice of surgery in the United States during the nineteenth century consisted of several distinct periods, each characterized by conditions sufficiently different to constitute separate surgical eras. The initial decades (1800 to 1825) were in most respects an extension of medicine as it had developed in the 13 colonies. Few physicians or surgeons in early nineteenth-century America had become qualified to practice through a systematic course of education, since academic facilities in the United States were limited and an extensive medical education generally required attendance at a European medical school. Few American students had the financial means necessary for such an expensive undertaking. To meet existing conditions, most future practitioners were compelled to become apprentices to practicing physicians in America and to "read medicine and surgery" while working in the physicians' offices.

Pioneer conditions resulted in a general backwardness of American medicine. Standards for physicians were nonexistent, and almost no means were available for disseminating medical knowledge. There were no universities of British or Continental pattern, and few hospitals. Virtually any American who dared to call himself a surgeon had to travel to London or Edinburgh to receive specialized training.

During the earliest period of nineteenth-century American medicine, surgery remained merely a "technical mode" of medical treatment: there was little to suggest that it had become a branch of "scientific medicine." Unlike in Europe, where Hunter and Bichat were practicing, there were no individuals in the United States who could be considered "scientific surgeons." However, several developments during the early nineteenth century indicated progress toward the professionalizing of American surgery.

Increasing numbers of young Americans were beginning to matriculate at leading European medical centers, especially those in Great Britain. Americans who managed to study abroad came to form a considerable proportion of the leading surgeons in sparsely settled America. Among these individuals were Wright Post (1766-1822), Valentine Mott (1785-1865), and J. Kearny Rodgers (1793-1851) of New York City. Post studied with John Sheldon (1752-1808) in London; Mott and Rodgers worked with Astley Cooper and John Abernethy. The Philadelphia surgeons Philip Syng Physick (1768-1837), his nephew John Syng Dorsey (1783-1818), and William Gibson (1768-1868) took lengthy periods of training in London and Edinburgh. Physick's training was of particular importance, since he was with John Hunter for 4 years and became Hunter's most prominent American pupil. Both Ephraim McDowell (1771-1830) and Benjamin Winslow Dudley (1785-1870) returned, after studying in Edinburgh, to practice medicine and surgery in the wilds of Kentucky. The renowned John Collins Warren (1778-1856) of Boston received his medical degree from Edinburgh in 1802.

Because of the medical education and training that the young Americans received in Great Britain, the first surgical era in nineteenth-century America was strongly influenced by the hunterian principles of surgery. Among the most prominent of these concepts was the application of anatomical and pathological studies to achieve a better understanding of surgical treatment. Despite the growing cadre of well-trained physicians, actual surgical procedures, in both the United States and Europe, remained largely limited to operations on the vascular and osseous systems.

The American surgeons devised an almost unlimited variety of vascular ligations and bone and joint operations. Among the vascular highlights were Dorsey's ligation of the external iliac artery (1811); Post's ligation of the common carotid artery (1814) and the subclavian artery (1817); Mott's tying off of the innominate artery (1818), the common iliac (1827), and the internal iliac artery (1837); and Gibson's account of the first known attempt to ligate the common iliac artery (1812). Among the most well-known osseous operations were Mott's removal of the right half of the mandible (1822), his first reported amputation at the hip joint in America (1827), and his resection of the left clavicle (1828).

265. John Syng Dorsey's original manuscript, with drawing, of his operation for aneurysm of the external iliac artery. Dorsey was the first surgeon in America to ligate the external iliac artery successfully. *(Historical Collections, College of Physicians of Philadelphia.)*

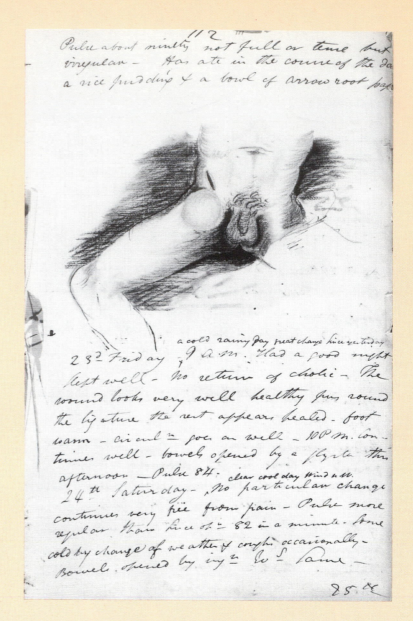

266. *Below,* Various incisions and methods used to ligate blood vessels, as drawn on stone by W.K. Hewitt for the famous American lithographer Nathaniel Currier (1813-1888), of Currier & Ives. Originally Figure 29 in Augustus Doane's (1808-1852) *Surgery Illustrated,* New York, 1836. Illustrations on medical subjects are rare in Currier's prolific output of lithographs. *(From the author's collection.)*

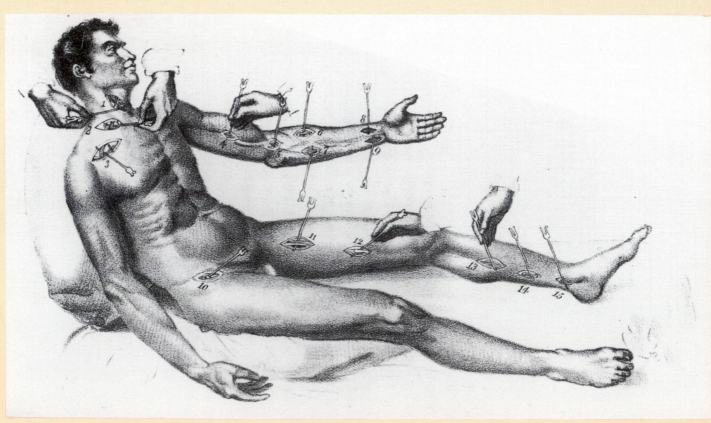

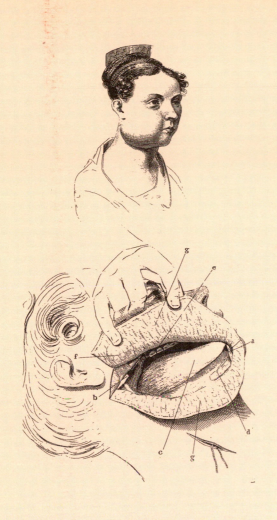

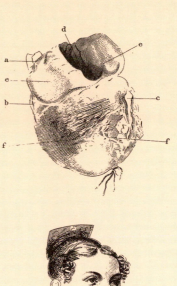

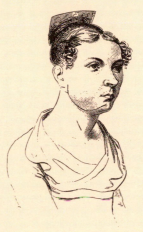

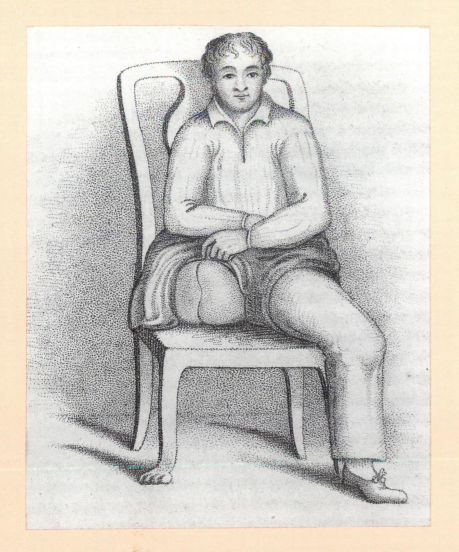

267. *Above,* Top left, Valentine Mott disarticulated the right side of the mandible of this patient suffering from osteosarcoma in 1822. Mott was the first surgeon to disarticulate half of the lower jaw during resection. In his early operations for head and neck tumors, Mott deemed it necessary to ligate the carotid artery a few days before the resection. Subsequent experience proved this step unnecessary and complicating. Top right, The tumor and, below this, the patient after the operation. *(From* New York Medical and Physical Journal, *vol 1, pp 385-393, 1822.)*

268. Appearance of the stump after healing in the first successful amputation at the hip joint undertaken in America by Valentine Mott, 1827. *(From* Philadelphia Journal of the Medical and Physical Sciences, *vol 14, pp 521-523, 1827.)*

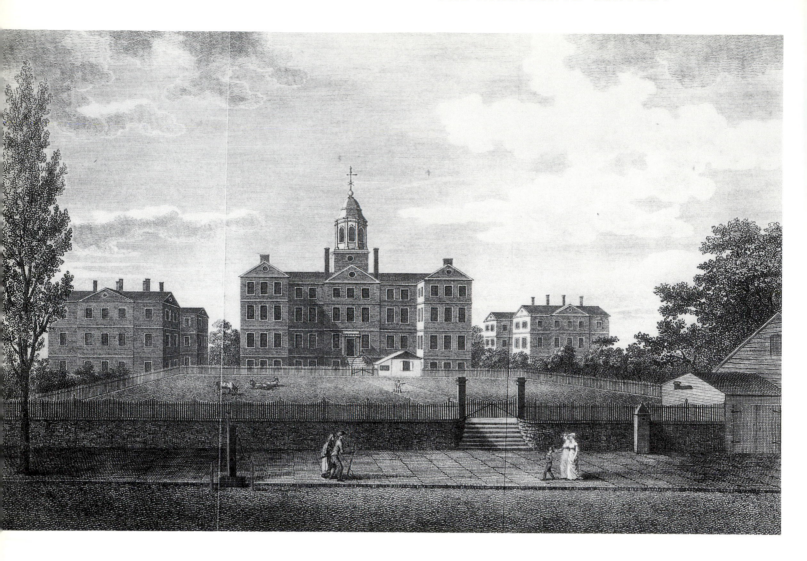

269. View of the New York Hospital as it looked in the early nineteenth century. *(Historical Collections, College of Physicians of Philadelphia.)*

The years from the mid-1820s to 1846, when ether anesthesia was introduced, can also be considered a distinct period in the history of American surgery. During that time, because of the vast proliferation of medical schools throughout the country, nearly every important physician and surgeon in the United States initially studied at an American medical school. From the few scattered eighteenth-century institutions in Boston, New York, and Philadelphia to myriad schools that were opened during the nineteenth century, medical education became widely available (see the box on p. 437).

As British influence in the world of surgery faded, especially after the Napoleonic Wars and the War of 1812, an increasing number of young Americans ventured to Paris and entered the lecture rooms of Larrey and Dupuytren. In contrast to earlier American students, individuals in this second generation of students were already physicians, having obtained their basic education in the fledgling American medical schools.

The overwhelming allure of France is described in F. Campbell Stewart's (1815-1899) *The Hospitals and Surgeons of Paris* (1843). Stewart had received his medical degree from the University of Pennsylvania in 1837; he then went to Europe, where he studied until 1843 in Paris. He returned to commence a practice in New York City but soon noticed a growing demand for information about opportunities for medical study in Paris. To provide a practical guide for those Americans wishing to study in France, he wrote his book. Stewart provided details on all the general and specialty hospitals in Paris and the school of medicine. Like any modern travel book, Stewart's furnished miscellaneous information on hotels, lodging houses, boarding houses, restaurants, and cafés in the city. He even detailed what the anticipated expenses should be for a student wishing to remain in Paris for 1 year. The monograph concluded with bio-

AMERICAN MEDICAL SCHOOLS OPENED IN THE EARLY NINETEENTH CENTURY

∾

UNIVERSITY OF MARYLAND (1807)
COLLEGE OF PHYSICIANS AND SURGEONS IN NEW YORK (1810)
YALE UNIVERSITY (1813)
FAIRFIELD IN NEW YORK (1812)
TRANSYLVANIA UNIVERSITY IN KENTUCKY (1817)
MEDICAL COLLEGE OF OHIO IN CINCINNATI (1819)
MEDICAL DEPARTMENT OF BOWDOIN COLLEGE IN MAINE (1820)
MEDICAL COLLEGE OF SOUTH CAROLINA (1824)
JEFFERSON MEDICAL COLLEGE IN PHILADELPHIA (1826)
RUSH MEDICAL COLLEGE IN CHICAGO (1827)
GENEVA IN NEW YORK (1835)
BERKSHIRE MEDICAL INSTITUTION IN WESTERN MASSACHUSETTS (1837)
ALBANY IN NEW YORK (1838)
BELLEVUE HOSPITAL MEDICAL COLLEGE IN NEW YORK CITY (1841)
BUFFALO IN NEW YORK (1846)

graphical information and descriptions of Stewart's own encounters with 20 Parisian physicians and surgeons. Among other provocative comments, he wrote:

> Cloquet . . . is one of the very few foreign surgeons, who think highly enough of American authorities to quote them, which he frequently does—speaking, on such occasions, with the greatest respect and kindness of the distinguished scientific men of our country . . .
>
> Lisfranc . . . notwithstanding his many good qualities . . . is unpopular with a number of his fellow practitioners in Paris; he has made enemies of many by being too plain spoken, and overbearing in his manner towards them; his enmity to Velpeau leads him occasionally to indulge in abuse of so gross a character as rather to reflect upon himself, than injure the person against whom it is directed . . .
>
> Velpeau . . . is much liked by his friends, and heartily detested by his enemies, of whom he has many, owing in a great measure to his origin and wonderful talents, which render others jealous and envious of his success and reputation. His manner towards his public patients, is sometimes inexcusable and harsh in the extreme, whilst his treatment of the young men placed under him in the hospital, is occasionally such, as to give rise to a strong feeling of indignation on the part of the spectator. I state this circumstance so unworthy of Velpeau, hoping that when it comes to be seen by him, it may have the good effect of causing him to be more considerate of the sensitive feelings of his young assistants, and more mindful of what is due to all, who, less fortunate than himself, are placed in a dependent position . . .

Two other surgical travel books, albeit lacking in practical information, were also written by American surgeons during the 1840s: William Gibson's *Rambles in Europe in 1839, with Sketches of Prominent Surgeons* (1841) and Valentine Mott's *Travels in Europe and the East* (1842). These lengthy texts provided information about surgical conditions throughout the Continent. Their chatty reminiscences of many important surgeons were particularly insightful.

Despite the rapid increase in the number of new medical schools in the United States, there was a deterioration in the existing quality of medical care during the 1830s and 1840s. Much of the authority to license physicians had been previously given to the various state medical societies. As new states were added to the Union, some of them enacted laws either granting to the new medical colleges the authority to license their own graduates or authorizing medical societies to examine and license those who sought the privilege to practice medicine. These new laws proved totally ineffective in improving the quality of American medicine. For instance, in Philadelphia it was reputed that two of every three physicians and surgeons were neither members of the local medical society nor graduates of a bonafide medical school.

From 1847 through 1860, when the Civil War began, a third era in nineteenth-century American surgery occurred, a period dominated by the increasing use of surgical anesthesia and tempered by the continued inability to control infection. The surgeon's technical regard of operations changed markedly. Whereas the trademark of the bold surgeon had always been operative speed (for example, completing an amputation in less than 60 seconds), the advent of anesthesia enabled the operator to remove his focus from speed alone and to be more precise in his methods. Numbers of surgical operations were increasing, and some surgeons were beginning to pursue scientific investigation.

The foremost example of the new type of American surgeon was Samuel Gross (1805-1884). He was adamant in his use of animal models to understand surgical diseases and therapies. Gross authored the first exhaustive, systematic study of pathological anatomy in English, the two-volume *Elements of Pathological Anatomy* (1839). He was the first to precede each description of the morbid anatomy of an organ with an account of its healthy color, weight, size, and consistency founded on original research. In 1843 Gross wrote *An Experimental and Critical Inquiry into the Nature and Treatment of Wounds of the Intestines.* This rare monograph reported a series of animal experiments conducted to determine the best way to treat traumatic intestinal wounds.

Despite the growing sophistication of American surgery, formalized attempts to organize surgeons were few. Unlike their European brethren, American physicians continued to provide care without undue interference by any examining bodies or other public or private societies. Most of the states had begun to withdraw the licensing privileges from medical societies, and any attempts at governmental examining boards lacked the professional and public support necessary to make them effective. During the 1840s and 1850s the American practice of medicine and surgery was essentially open to all who cared to call themselves doctors. Efforts to deal with this problem resulted in the creation of the American Medical Association (1847). Its initial recommendations regarding educational standards, however, were regarded as an ill-conceived and deceptive attempt to destroy most of the existing proprietary medical colleges.

Of unquestioned importance in the development of an American profession of surgery was the tragic experience of the Civil War (1861-1865). This armed struggle produced a huge number of casualties, and the concomitant need for surgical care constituted a unique fourth era in the development of surgery in the United States during the nineteenth century. The contributions to surgical treatment that developed during the Civil War have never been fully appreciated, probably because antiseptic techniques remained unknown and more deaths and suffering resulted from infectious processes than from battlefield injury. Yet, the specific accomplishments that did occur in surgical practice should not be overlooked.

The Civil War was the first major armed struggle in which the rifle was the real killer. More than 90% of the wounds suffered in the conflict were inflicted by bullets. The increasingly sophisticated weapons of war radically altered the manner in which surgical care was rendered. To deal with the enormous number of wounded (in the Union Army alone, 100,000 soldiers were killed in battle, 225,000 died of disease, and 25,000 succumbed to accidents, suicides, and so forth), a system of managing mass casualties was developed that included battlefield aid stations, field hospitals, and general hospitals.

The aid station served each regiment and was staffed by a regimental surgeon. Typical treatment was confined to the control of bleeding, the bandaging of wounds, and the administration of opiates and whiskey for pain and shock. By 1864 an efficient horse-drawn ambulance corps had been developed to evacuate the wounded from the aid station to the field hospital, which was located within 2 miles of the battle site.

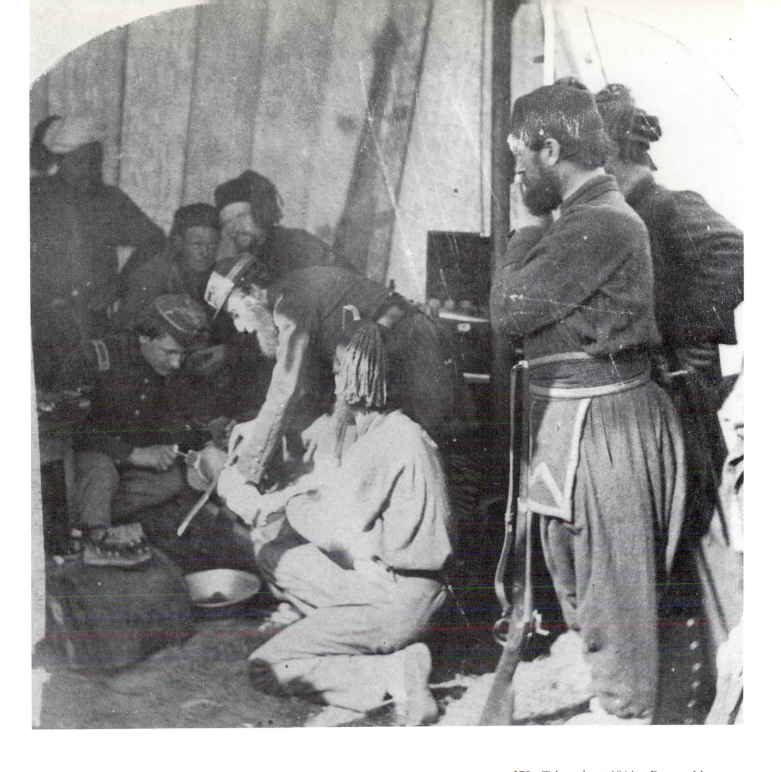

270. Taken about 1864 at Fortress Monroe, this informal photograph shows two unknown Union surgeons about to amputate a leg. One surgeon holds the amputation knife; the other steadies the leg with a forked retractor. A catch basin is placed to collect blood. The medicine chest is in the background. There is no visible evidence of any attempt at anesthesia. The unusual uniforms in the foreground, which included tasseled fez hats, are those of soldiers from Union Zouave units. This is one of only a handful of photographs taken of actual operations during the American Civil War. The wet collodion glass-plate negatives were exposed for so long that all photographs of this type had to be posed. *(Courtesy of the Edward G. Miner Library, Rochester, N.Y.)*

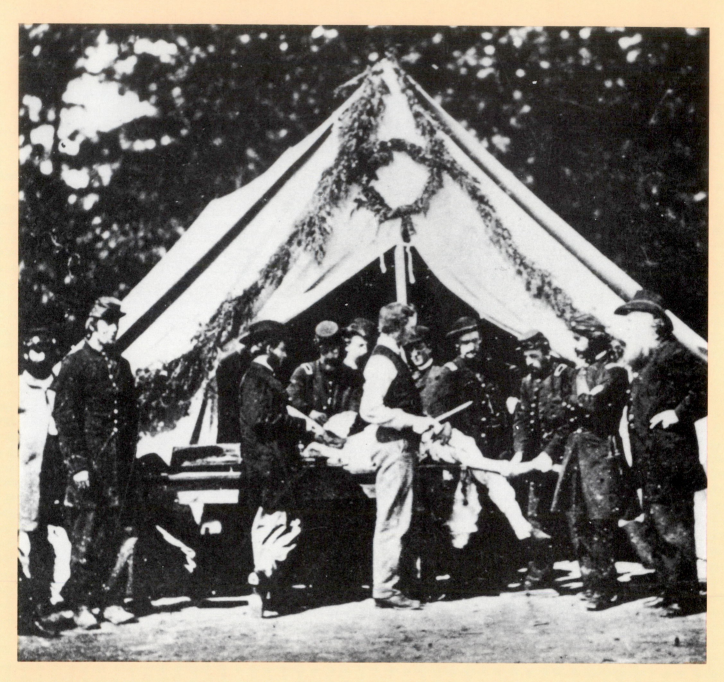

271. Leg amputation at a field hospital in Gettysburg, Pennsylvania, on July 3, 1863. The patient was probably Major General Daniel E. Sickels, commander of the Third Army Corps, who was struck by a cannonball at Gettysburg. It is thought that Sickels wanted his amputation recorded for posterity. The surgeon was James T. Calhoon of Rahway, New Jersey. The photographer is unknown. After the amputation Major General Sickels remained in his command until the end of the Civil War. He preserved his amputated leg, and after the war he presented it in a small coffin to the Army Medical Museum, Washington, D.C., where it remains on display. *(Courtesy of the Edward G. Miner Library, Rochester, N.Y.)*

440

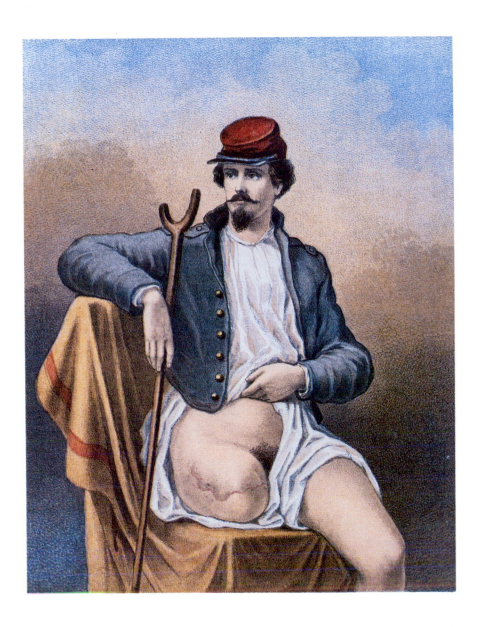

272. An artistic rendering of one of the countless amputees in the Union Army who lost limbs chiefly as a result of gunshot wounds. In the Civil War both sides absorbed enormous losses caused by wounds and disease. Between 1861 and 1865, 300,000 men died for the Union and 200,000 for the Confederacy. Among the Union forces there were 400,000 cases of wounds and injuries. Without the ability to fight infection, amputation was the treatment of choice for any serious wounds of the extremities. Chromolithograph by F. Morag after a drawing by Faber. From the United States War Department, *Report on Amputations at the Hip Joint*, 1867. *(From the author's collection.)*

The field hospital was most often a barn, church, or private home that had been commandeered by the medical corps. Once a battle began, the wounded initially arrived at the field hospital in manageable numbers. During the continuing carnage, however, the flow of wounded increased so dramatically that these temporary hospitals were instantly transformed into scenes of great human suffering. Surgeons were on their feet for 12 hours at a time, working by natural light or flickering lamplight, performing amputation after amputation. It was always easy to recognize a busy field hospital, since enormous piles of severed limbs were tossed into a heap in the plain sight of everyone.

As the wounded arrived at the field hospital, they were lifted from the ambulance and placed on an operating table for complete evaluation. In many cases the operating table was little more than wooden planks laid across two barrels. The injured underwent a complete evaluation, which included the probing of wounds with dirty instruments and dirty fingers, followed by the removal of detritus and an attempt at debridement. If a soldier had sustained a head or an abdominal wound, his chances of survival were less than 10%. These unfortunate victims were laid out in neat rows, given as much opium and morphine as possible, and made comfortable until their death, often a slow and hideously painful process.

For individuals with wounds that were not deemed mortal, definitive treatment was carried out immediately, since empirical observations, in both the United States and Europe, were beginning to demonstrate that delayed operation led to higher rates of morbidity and mortality. Amputations and other types

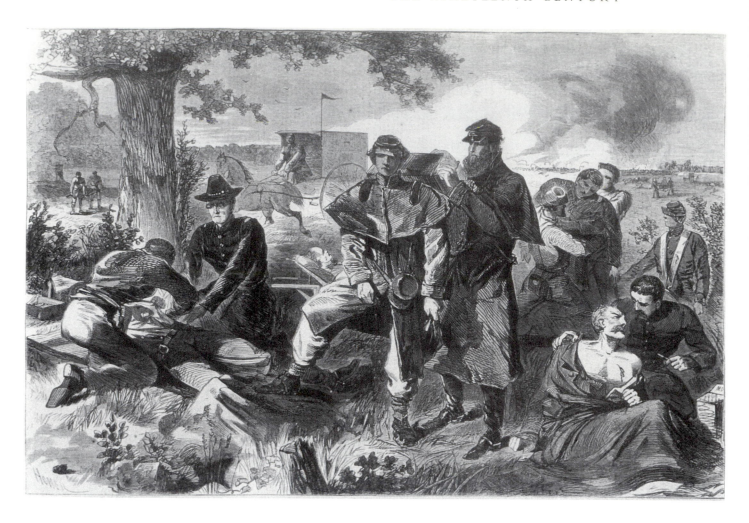

273. A Union surgeon at work *(lower right)* at the rear of the battle. The celebrated artist, Winslow Homer, captured action far more realistically than any Civil War photographer could, since the bulky, wet collodion glass-plate negatives used at the time required lengthy exposures and posed photographs. Cameras were cumbersome, and immediately after exposure the plates had to be developed in the confines of a darkroom, which in the field was outfitted in the wagon in which the photographer traveled. Wood engraving published in *Harper's Weekly,* July 12, 1862. *(National Library of Medicine, Bethesda, Md.)*

of heroic surgical operations were usually accomplished within the first day after injury. These decisions to operate as soon as possible undoubtedly played an important role in improving results under circumstances in which antisepsis and asepsis were unknown and could not be practiced.

General hospitals were situated in the large urban areas and provided a final health care facility for the injured or seriously ill. In many instances the wounded and postoperative patients were taken from the field hospitals and loaded onto the floors of railroad freight cars, which were covered with layers of straw. These trains were marked, in enormous red letters, *U.S. HOSPITAL TRAIN,* and the locomotive boiler and tender were painted red. After the dreadful horrors of the field hospital and the painful, lurching journey aboard a hospital train or steamboat, the general hospital proved to be an improvement for the wounded.

The general hospitals were designed in a pavilion style; interconnected buildings had excellent ventilation. This plan ensured the maximum amount of light and air, and separate areas were created for laundries, kitchens, dispensaries, operating rooms, and nurses' quarters. Each separate building was its own ward, with high vaulted ceilings and large air vents, and usually accommodated about 60 patients. Cross-contamination was minimized by maintaining adequate space between beds. The success of these large, airy institutions was evident: federal hospitals cared for more than a million men during the war, and less than 10% of them died.

At the beginning of the Civil War, whether the use of anesthesia was appropriate in a battlefield setting was controversial. Some physicians believed that the "excitement" of the severely wounded soldier would be adequate to carry him through the most serious operation. Shock after injury was thought to be aggravated by anesthesia, and the patient's pain was considered an appropriate stimulus to prevent or modify his shock. Despite these discussions, anesthesia was extensively applied throughout the war effort by both the North and the South.

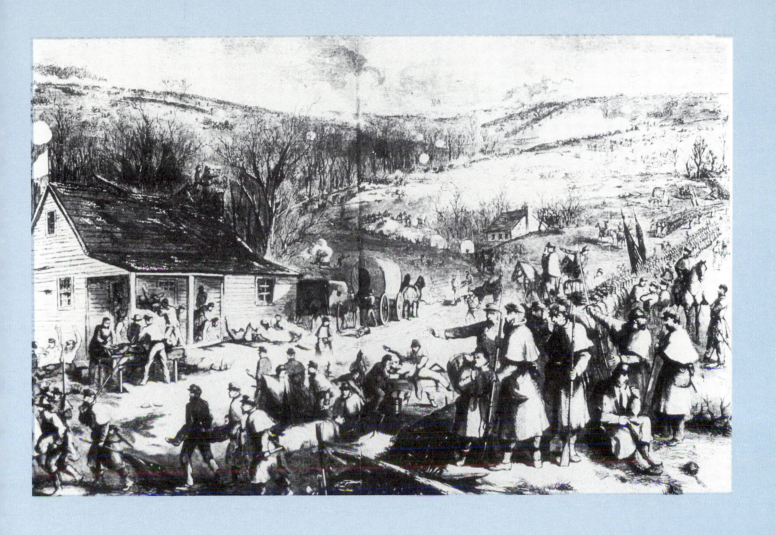

274. Operations by the roadside during a battle. A dramatic scene of Civil War military surgery and treatment of the wounded, as recorded by the noted artist Thomas Nast (1840-1902). Operations are occurring on both sides of the street in the midst of great confusion. In the background a fierce battle is being waged just a short distance away. Wood engraving from *Harper's Weekly*, 1862. *(National Library of Medicine, Bethesda, Md.)*

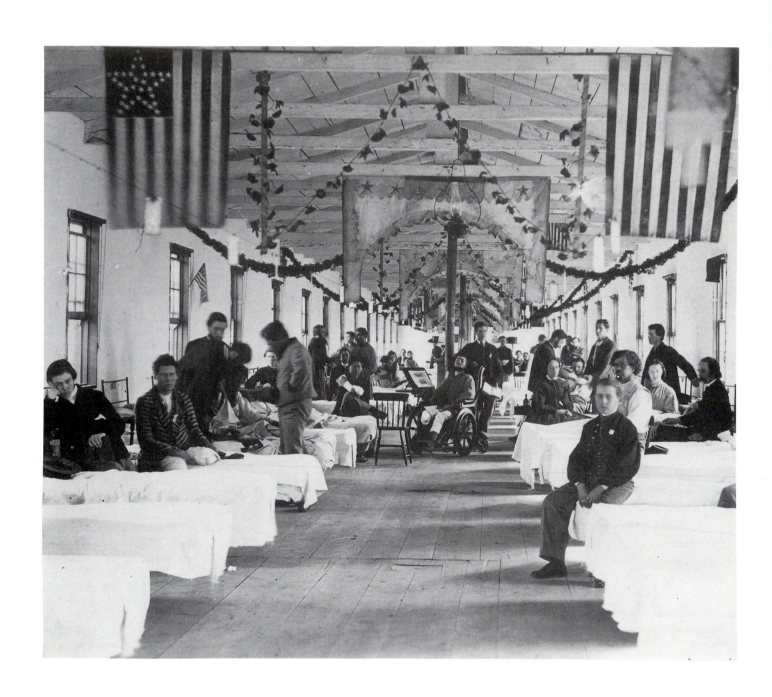

275. Wounded veterans of the Civil War in the Armory Square Hospital. Photograph by Mathew Brady (1823-1896). *(Metropolitan Museum of Art, Harris Brisbane Dick Fund, 1933 [33.65.307].)*

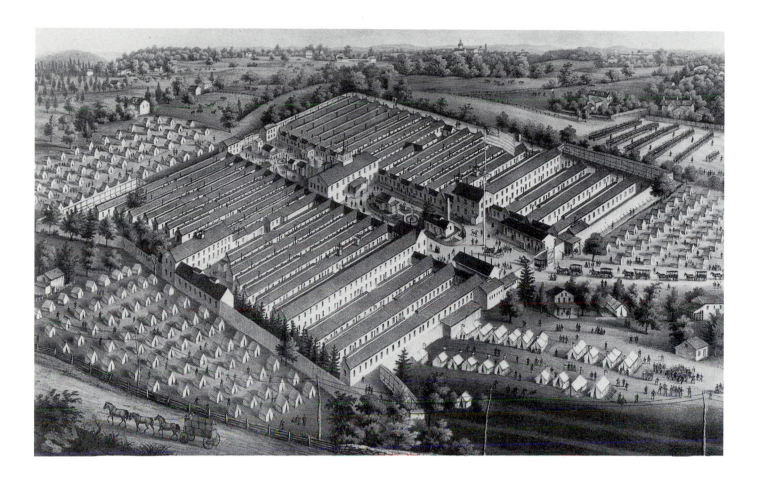

Chloroform was the agent of choice in the field hospitals because of its rapid onset of action and because it was not flammable. Ether was used as an anesthetic more commonly in the general hospitals, but only in 14% of the cases. Records from the Union army indicate that nearly 80,000 surgical operations were completed in which general anesthesia was used.

The major complications of wounds during the Civil War were hemorrhage and infection. As ligatures pulled away in infected amputation sites, severe bleeding inevitably occurred. Secondary hemorrhage 3 or 4 days after injury was quite frequent and carried a death rate of more than 60%. When stables were used as hospitals, tetanus was a major problem. Erysipelas occurred in epidemics in some hospitals and carried a mortality rate of almost 90%. Hospital gangrene was particularly feared and appeared to be a synergistic infection of aerobes and anaerobes.

One of the important indirect effects of the Civil War was the great number of physicians who were introduced to basic principles of surgery. At the beginning of the conflict the competence of the medical corps, particularly those termed "surgeons," was questionable. Most of the medical volunteers had no operative training and were capable only of general medical practice. Because they were inept, they frequently botched the simplest of surgical operations and caused wounded soldiers more harm than good. Yet, because so many war injuries had to be treated during the course of a 1- or 2-day battle (for example, at Antietam 5510 were killed and 25,815 wounded; at Chickamauga 4033 were killed and 22,674 wounded; and at Gettysburg 6334 were killed and 28,209 wounded), the surgical experience of thousands of physicians was broadened. These "surgeons" were introduced to new ideas and standards of care and became familiar with anesthetic agents. After this on-site surgical education and training, American surgical practice evolved rapidly.

276. Lithograph showing bird's-eye view, by Charles Magnus of Satterlee U.S.A. General Hospital, West Philadelphia, 1864. The caption to the print states, "This is perhaps the largest and most complete Army Hospital in the world. It covers 16 acres of ground. There are 34 wards, containing 4500 beds. The length of the buildings is 900 feet. There are altogether 7 acres of floors. It was opened for the reception of our brave sick and wounded soldiers, June 9, 1862. Admitted up to May 27, 1864, 12,773. Deaths, 260. Since the great battles of the Wilderness and Spottsylvania there have been several hundred tents put up outside of the enclosure, as the accommodations are not sufficient for the large number of patients daily arriving from the field." (Jeremy Norman & Co., Inc.)

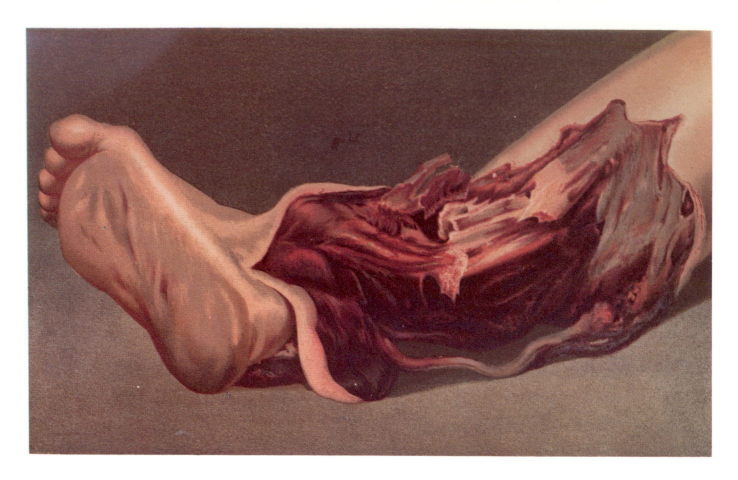

277. Laceration of the right leg by solid shot. A dramatic painting of exactly the sort of wound that without antiseptic techniques would be cured in the Civil War by only one means: amputation. Chromolithograph by T. Sinclair and Son after the painting by Edward Stauch of the Army Medical Museum, for the *Medical and Surgical History of the War of the Rebellion,* part III, vol II, p 478 (1883). *(From the author's collection.)*

SURGICAL MANUALS PUBLISHED DURING THE CIVIL WAR

∾

Confederate Army

JOHN JULIAN CHISOLM (1830-1903)
A Manual of Military Surgery (1861)

EDWARD WARREN (1828-1893)
An Epitome of Practical Surgery for Field and Hospital (1863)

SAMUEL PRESTON MOORE (1813-1889)
A Manual of Military Surgery Prepared for the Use of the Confederate States Army (1863)

Union Army

SAMUEL GROSS (1805-1884)
A Manual of Military Surgery; or Hints on the Emergencies of Field, Camp and Hospital Practice (1861)

FRANK HAMILTON (1813-1886)
A Practical Treatise on Military Surgery (1861)

CHARLES TRIPLER (1806-1866)
AND GEORGE BLACKMAN (1819-1871)
Handbook for the Military Surgeon (1861)

STEPHEN SMITH (1823-1922)
Hand-Book of Surgical Operations (1862)

JOHN HOOKER PACKARD (1832-1907)
A Manual of Minor Surgery (1863)

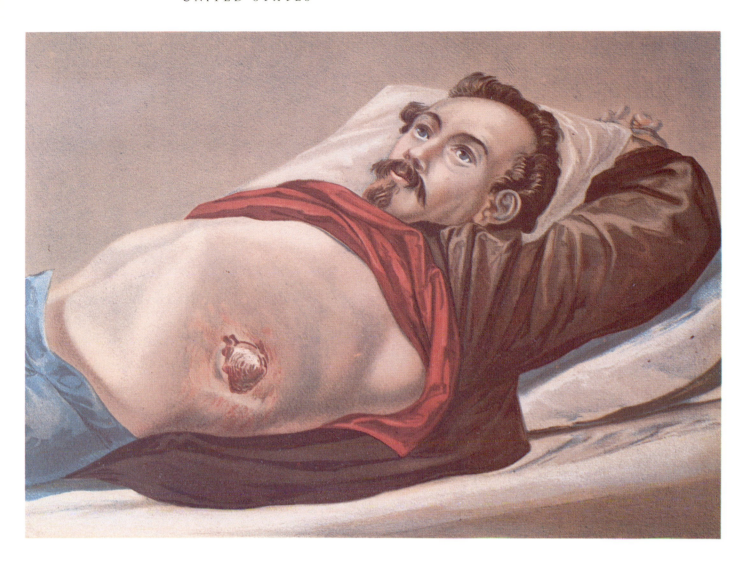

The Civil War proved to be the greatest single influence in the development of American surgery after the founding of the nation. Literally thousands upon thousands of the most difficult surgical cases imaginable were handled in a short time; as many cases would not have occurred in many years of peace. The experiences of the medical and surgical personnel were carefully noted, and for the first time the accumulation of adequate records and detailed reports provided a complete military medical history. The six-volume *Medical and Surgical History of the War of the Rebellion* (1870-1888) was published, and in Europe these volumes were soon considered the first major academic accomplishment of American medicine and the country's first comprehensive medical book.

American medical literature proliferated during the Civil War. Many surgical manuals that supplied "how-to-do-it" directions for the novice physician-surgeon were published (see the box on p. 446).

A fifth era of American surgery in the nineteenth century occurred from 1865 through the late 1870s. Rapid advances were being made in medical sciences, and new state licensing laws were being passed. Such laws were deemed necessary not only to protect the public but also to force medical colleges to modernize their curricula and upgrade standards. Boards of medical examiners were created in Texas (1873), Kentucky and New York (1874), New Hampshire (1875), and Vermont and California (1876). The medical degree had become widely accepted as a license to practice, and it was commonly thought that the hundreds of proprietary medical schools, because of their pecuniary interest in graduating as many students as possible, had failed to withhold the degree from those who were not qualified to practice. Consequently American medicine of the 1870s was dominated by various medical sects, including homeopathic, eclectic, and other sectarian schools. In many instances bogus di-

278. Shot wound of the thorax and abdomen, with hernia of the lung. Chromolithograph by T. Sinclair & Son after the painting by Edward Stauch of the Army Medical Museum, for the *Medical and Surgical History of the War of the Rebellion,* part I, vol II, p 515 (1875). "The patient, Captain Robert S—, survived the wound well enough to walk half a mile after receiving the round musket ball. Five days after receiving the gunshot wound he voided the musket ball at stool. . . ." *(From the author's collection.)*

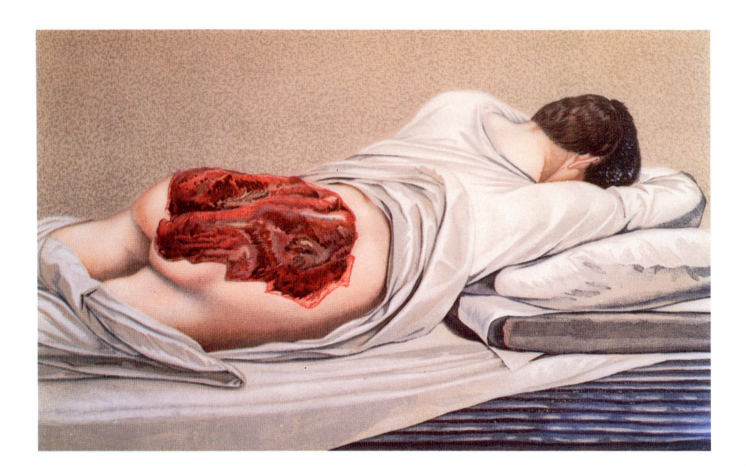

279. Laceration of the buttocks by a shell fragment. The American Civil War was the first war in which huge quantities of medical and surgical records were preserved and vast quantities of statistics tabulated and published. Publication of the medical records of the war continued for more than a decade after the war ended. Chromolithograph by T. Sinclair and Son after the painting by Edward Stauch of the Army Medical Museum, for the *Medical and Surgical History of the War of the Rebellion,* part II, vol II, p 430 (1877). *(From the author's collection.)*

ploma mills were established that licensed thousands of unscrupulous individuals as physician-surgeons.

During the 1870s, for the first time, a substantial number of surgical textbooks and monographs by American surgeons were published (see the box on p. 450).

That American surgery had reached a new level of sophistication was evident both in the growth of surgical literature and in the number of well-respected practitioners. However, there still remained no clear delineation between physician and surgeon. By the mid-1870s the defining of an American surgeon had become a particularly difficult task. At the time of the country's centennial (1876) Samuel Gross wrote a report on the status of American surgeons. An astute observer of the American surgical scene, he noted that:

> . . . although this paper is designed to record the achievements of American surgeons, there are, strange to say, as a separate and distinct class, no such persons among us. It is safe to affirm that there is not a medical man on this continent who devotes himself exclusively to the practice of surgery.

Clearly there was a difference between the European concept of a surgeon and the American counterpart. The European medical community had an established history of groups of physicians who performed little but surgical operations, whereas such specialization would not be attained in America until after the 1880s. Therefore it is likely that most "surgeons" practicing in the United States from 1865 through the 1870s practiced more nonsurgical medicine and derived greater income from their medical therapies than their surgical operations.

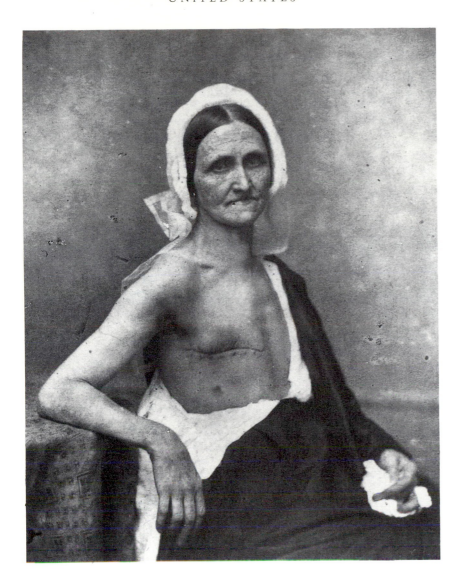

280. Postoperative photograph of a mastectomy, as published in one of the most bizarre early American treatises on surgery, *Earth as a Topical Application in Surgery . . . (1872)* by Addinell Hewsen (1828-1889). The author describes successful application of "earth" directly on wounds in 93 cases treated at the Pennyslvania Hospital during 1869. Was there, unknown to Hewsen, some kind of mold with antibiotic properties in the earth he was using? Such a concept was too advanced for the medicine of Hewsen's time. This photograph also represents one of the earliest uses of photomechanical reproduction of photographs, in this case, Woodburytypes, in an American medical book. *(From the author's collection.)*

Only toward the end of the nineteenth century was surgery in the United States increasingly performed by those who considered themselves specialists in surgery. Whereas most general practitioners continued to perform minor surgical operations (such as those for simple fractures, minor skin trauma, and hernia), the more difficult procedures such as abdominal operations were being completed by these new specialists in surgery. This distinction between surgeon and physician was most evident in the large urban areas of the United States.

In rural America the turn toward specialists in surgery would not occur until well into the twentieth century. A major part of this delay can be attributed to the large number of rural physicians who received surgical training during the Civil War and to their desire to remain physician-surgeons as a means of augmenting their income. In addition, physicians in rural America were in short supply and these general practitioner–surgeons were obligated to provide the only surgical expertise available for many miles.

Some of the most important breakthroughs in American surgery were performed by the rural general practitioner–surgeon. For example, the first successful extirpation of the entire thyroid gland in America was completed by E. L. Marshall, a general practitioner–surgeon from Keithsburg, Illinois (1867). John Bobbs (1809-1870) practiced in rural Indiana, where he performed the world's first cholecystotomy for removal of gallstones (1867). B. B. Allen, a little-known rural physician, reported the first known operation on the pancreas, both in America and worldwide (1876).

By the conclusion of the 1870s surgery was being practiced with about equal success on both sides of the Atlantic Ocean. The major difference between the two continents was that in most instances any evidence of advanced scientific

TEXTBOOKS AND MONOGRAPHS
WRITTEN BY AMERICAN SURGEONS
DURING THE 1870s

❧

General Textbooks

JOHN PACKARD (1832-1907)
A Handbook of Operative Surgery (1870)

JOHN ASHHURST (1839-1900)
The Principles and Practice of Surgery (1871)

FRANK HAMILTON (1813-1886)
The Principles and Practice of Surgery (1872)

JAMES GILCHRIST (1842-1906)
The Homeopathic Treatment of Surgical Diseases (1873)

DAVID HAYES AGNEW (1818-1892)
Principles and Practice of Surgery
(in three volumes) (1878-1883)

JAMES EWING MEARS (1838-1919)
Practical Surgery (1878)

LEWIS STIMSON (1844-1917)
A Manual of Operative Surgery (1878)

ANDREW HOWE (1825-1892)
The Art and Science of Surgery (1879)

STEPHEN SMITH (1823-1922)
Manual of the Principles and Practice
of Operative Surgery (1879)

Specialty Monographs

HENRY ANGELL (1829-1911)
A Treatise on Diseases of the Eye (1870)

BENJAMIN JEFFRIES (1833-1915)
The Eye in Health and Disease (1871)

JACOB DASILVA SOLIS-COHEN (1838-1927)
Diseases of the Throat (1872)

LAURENCE TURNBULL (1821-1900)
A Clinical Manual of the Diseases of the Ear (1872)

DANIEL ST. JOHN ROOSA (1838-1908)
A Practical Treatise on the Diseases of the Ear (1873)

GURDON BUCK (1807-1877)
Contributions to Reparative Surgery (1876)

CHARLES BURNETT (1842-1902)
The Ear (1877)

LEWIS SAYRE (1820-1900)
Lectures on Orthopedic Surgery and Diseases of the Joints (1876)

EDMUND PEASLEE (1814-1878)
Ovarian Tumors (1872)

THOMAS ADDIS EMMET (1828-1919)
The Principles and Practice of Gynaecology (1879)

WILLIAM GOODELL (1829-1894)
Lessons in Gynecology (1879)

JOHN GOULEY (1832-1920)
Diseases of the Urinary Organs (1873)

WILLIAM VAN BUREN (1819-1873)
A Practical Treatise on the Surgical Diseases of the Genito-Urinary Organs
(1874) and *Lectures upon Diseases of the Rectum* (1870)

research was still concentrated in the older, established European university and hospital centers, not in the United States. In 1874 John Erichsen, the well-known London surgeon, made an extended trip to several major cities in America. Erichsen was much impressed by what he saw and described a very high level of excellence in surgery in the United States. He considered both the British and the American surgeon practical rather than scientific. He also cogently commented on the relative social status of the medical profession in America:

. . . it appears to me that medicine occupies a far higher social status than it does in Britain. The reason for this seems tolerably obvious. In the absence of an exalted hierarchy in an established church and of great dignitaries of the law, these professions do not offer sufficient inducement for men of the highest intellectual caliber to enter them. Medicine, therefore, stands prominent as probably the best-educated, certainly the most scientific, and, consequently, in a country where education is so widely diffused and so much regarded, the most respected of the professions. And in the absence of all titled classes, it can socially more than hold its own in competition with the trading and financial elements which are such prominent constituents of the society of most of the American cities. Perhaps, also, the high position that medicine occupies is owing, in some respect, to the greater uniformity of practice that prevails amongst medical men in America than with us. For, just as in the law there is no division into barristers and solicitors, so in medicine there is none into physicians, surgeons, and general practitioners. Special aptitude, inclination, or opportunity will necessarily lead men to a greater eminence in particular departments of the profession. But the subdivision into classes and specialties, which is so prevalent here, is unknown in the United States.

The penultimate evolutionary stage of American surgery in the nineteenth century, including the existence of well-supported and adequately supplied hospitals and research institutions, occurred during the decade of the 1880s, the sixth era in surgical development. These 10 years brought about a final acceptance of the germ theory in America and with it the introduction of crude antiseptic and aseptic techniques into many of the country's operating rooms.

For various reasons Lister found widespread enthusiastic support for his beliefs among the surgeons of the European continent. In his own country, however, and in the United States, surgeons had turned to listerian techniques slowly and, at times, with reluctance. Almost a quarter of a century passed before the surgical profession in the United States was willing to unequivocally accept Lister's 1867 discovery and the necessity for cleanliness in surgery.

Before the 1880s few American surgeons had a sufficient appreciation of cleanliness to recognize the implications of the germ theory in general or Lister's beliefs in particular. More important, there was less infection in America's spacious general hospitals than in the exceptionally crowded charity hospitals of Europe. Consequently the clinical need for listerian principles was not as great in the United States as in Europe. The antisepsis controversy was discussed throughout the American surgical literature; Samuel Gross served as its greatest detractor. In 1876 he wrote that:

. . . little, if any faith, is placed by any enlightened or experienced surgeon on this side of the Atlantic in the so-called carbolic acid treatment of Professor Lister, apart from the care which is taken in applying the dressing, or, what is the same thing, in clearing away clots and excluding air from the wound.

During the late 1880s a number of European scientists had extended Koch's work of relating specific microorganisms to specific diseases. Certain micrococci were then shown to be the cause of most surgical infections. The bacteriologist's laboratory demonstrations were confirmed in clinical practice, and as a result, during the 1880s and 1890s Germany entered a golden age of surgery. Once it was recognized that operations could be performed without threat of an infection, there appeared to be no limit to what could be attempted. This change in surgeons' attitudes appeared in Europe about 10 years earlier than it did in America; the only reason it occurred at all in America was because young American students brought back German attitudes and techniques.

During the late 1880s several surgical texts appeared that brought about the final acceptance of Lister's techniques in the United States. The most important of these American publications was Arpad Gerster's (1848-1923) *The Rules of Aseptic and Antiseptic Surgery* (1888). It was the first American surgical text based on listerian principles and was so popular that two more editions were published within 3 years. The book's importance rested not only with its contents but also with the efforts that were expended in its production. It was printed on heavy calendered paper and contained many halftone illustrations, which were then rare in scientific books. In addition, Gerster, who had mastered the technique of photography, had made his own plates at a time when photography by an amateur was unusual. Using the slow film of that day and with the assistance of his residents at the German Hospital in New York City, Gerster took a camera into the operating room and for the first time took pictures of actual operations and surgical dressings in which listerian techniques had been used.

In 1889 Nicholas Senn (1844-1908) wrote *Surgical Bacteriology,* which was the first American surgical work on the subject. Senn had recently returned from a trip to Europe, where he had studied bacteriology in its relation to surgery. Senn's book provides evidence that bacteriology was strictly a European discipline. American surgeons had little knowledge of the subject, and Senn's text brought them the latest advances. In that same year Henry Marcy (1837-1924) wrote *A Treatise on Hernia, the Radical Cure by the Use of the Buried Antiseptic Animal Suture.* Marcy had been Lister's first American pupil (1870) and on his return to the United States was the first to introduce Lister's antiseptic methods in surgery. Marcy devoted many years to a continuous study of microorganisms in wounds, which culminated in his use of antiseptic ligatures in the radical cure of hernia.

Two other events during the 1880s were also crucial in the professionalizing of American surgery. In 1880 Samuel Gross founded the American Surgical Association, and 3 years later the initial volume of the *Annals of Surgery* was edited by Lewis Pilcher (1845-1934). With a growing confidence in American surgery, Gross felt the need for a surgical society that would enable those with similar interests to encourage both the expansion of boundaries and the growing use of surgery as an increasingly effective means of therapy. His object was to:

> . . . foster surgical art, science, education and literature, to cultivate good feeling in the profession, and to unite the prominent surgeons of the country in one harmonious body.

The American Surgical Association held its first scientific session in 1881 at the Hotel Brighton in Coney Island, New York. The need for such an organization was apparent in that American surgeons had already begun to organize themselves into various surgical specialty societies, including the American Ophthalmological Society (1864), American Otological Society (1868), American Gynecological Society (1876), American Association of Genito-Urinary Surgeons (1886), and American Orthopedic Association (1887). The importance of the unification of American surgeons into a single entity was becoming paramount if surgery was to exist as a viable profession within the practice of medicine.

For the surgeon the *Annals of Surgery* represented the most influential and important of all American medical journals of the nineteenth century. It was the first American periodical devoted solely to the practice of surgery, and its pages recorded the advancement of American surgery more accurately than did any other written source. By having their own society and journal, American surgeons finally achieved some measure of the social and political organization that European surgeons had had for almost a century.

By the beginning of the 1890s it was evident that both American and European surgery had been affected more profoundly than any other area of nineteenth-century medical practice by achievements in the medical sciences. The discovery of useful anesthetics and the development of a method to prevent wound infection revolutionized surgical practice. From a crude and dangerous art, surgery rapidly became an influential, prestigious medical specialty in the nineteenth century. During the final era in the development of surgery in the nineteenth century, American surgery finally achieved its status as a distinct medical specialty.

The last developmental era began in May 1889, when William Halsted initiated his work in the newly opened Johns Hopkins Hospital in Baltimore. Halsted, like many other young American physicians after the Civil War, had traveled to the major German cities for his postgraduate education. By the 1870s France had been displaced as the European center of medical expertise, and American physicians were returning home imbued with a sense of German educational tradition.

The advent of The Johns Hopkins Hospital and its School of Medicine (1893) marked a new era of American medicine, in which American surgery would be guided into the twentieth century by individuals who ensured its rightful place in the history of world surgery. John Shaw Billings (1838-1913), who founded the surgeon general's library and the index catalogue of the library (1880), which is the forerunner of the *Index Medicus*, and served for 17 years as director of the New York Public Library, summarized the situation of American surgery in 1893:

281. *The Agnew Clinic. Portrait of David Hayes Agnew*, 1889, by Thomas Eakins (1844-1916). Painted 14 years after Eakins's celebrated painting, *The Gross Clinic*, this monumental work (74½ by 130½ inches) offers several striking contrasts to the earlier masterpiece. Reflecting the acceptance of antiseptic techniques, which were not widely accepted in America at the time of Eakins's painting of Samuel D. Gross, Agnew and his assistants are in operating gowns, not business suits. They are using sterilized instruments but no gloves or masks. The operation is a mastectomy for breast cancer. In contrast to *The Gross Clinic*, in which the only woman shown was a suffering relative of the patient, an operating room nurse is prominently portrayed as a member of the operative team. *(Courtesy of the University of Pennsylvania School of Medicine, Phiadelphia.)*

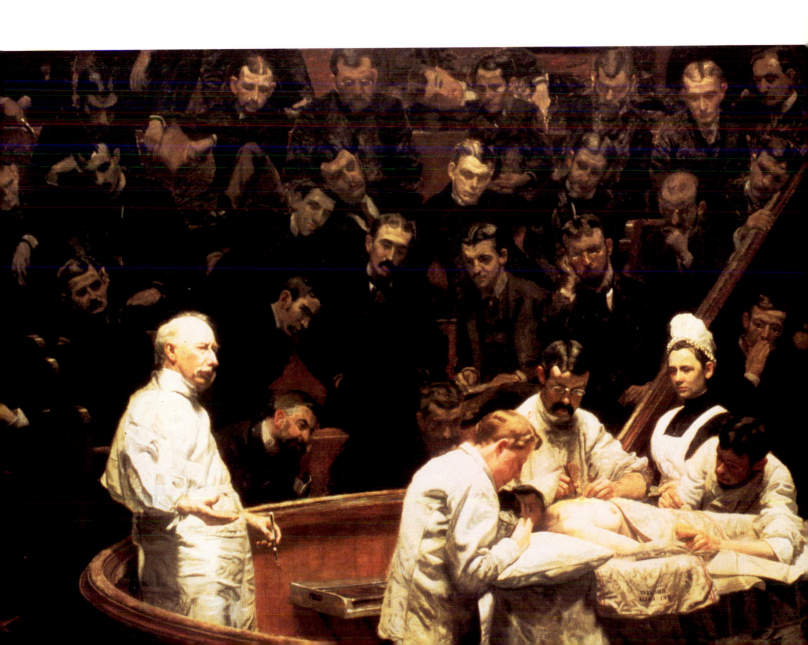

282. The Johns Hopkins Hospital and School of Medicine, designed by John Shaw Billings, soon after their founding in 1893. The remarkable association of talented, innovative professors of medicine and surgery at this new institution brought about extraordinary achievements in American medicine and surgery almost immediately after it opened. Founders of the medical school of particular note were William Osler, Professor of Medicine, William H. Welch, Professor of Pathology, Howard A. Kelly, Professor of Obstetrics and Gynecology, and William S. Halsted, Professor of Surgery. *(The Alan Mason Chesney Medical Archives of The Johns Hopkins Medical Institutions Baltimore, Md.)*

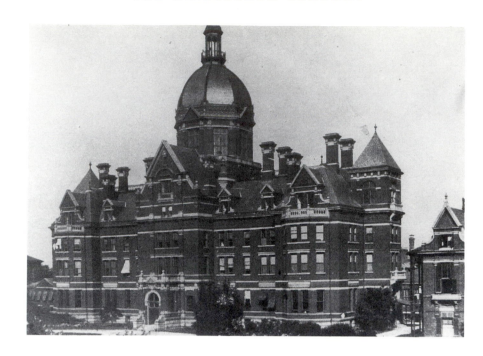

The most important improvements in practical medicine made in the United States have been chiefly in surgery, in its various branches. We have led the way in the ligation of some of the larger arteries, in the removal of abdominal tumors, in the treatment of diseases and injuries peculiar to women, in the treatment of spinal affections and of deformities of various kinds. Above all, we were the first to show the uses of anesthetics—the most important advance in medicine made during the century. In our late war we taught Europe how to build, organize and manage military hospitals, and we formed the best museum in existence illustrating modern military medicine and surgery. Our contributions to medical literature have been many and valuable, and our government possesses the largest and best working medical library in the world.

Although other surgeons had more international reputations, it was Halsted who set the tone for the final period of American surgical history in the nineteenth century. His work reveals the beginning of a new American surgery based as much on physiology as on anatomy. Halsted moved surgery from the heroics of the operating "theater" to the relative sterility of the operating "room" and the privacy of the research laboratory. American surgery was becoming a true science, and the recognition of surgery's true therapeutic powers would follow.

William Halsted (1852-1922) was born in New York City into a well-to-do merchant family whose members had originally emigrated from England in the 1640s. He graduated from Yale University in 1874 and soon matriculated at the College of Physicians and Surgeons in his native city. Halsted was an excellent student and ranked among the top ten members of his medical school's graduating class in 1877. According to the rules of the college, each student was assigned as a preceptee to a faculty member. Halsted's preceptor was Henry Sands (1830-1888), who was professor of anatomy and a highly regarded surgeon. In addition, Halsted became student assistant to John Dalton (1825-1889), a pioneer experimental physiologist. These two men would have a important influence on Halsted's later role as an experimental surgeon.

Halsted served an 18-month internship at Bellevue Hospital and a short stint as house surgeon to the New York Hospital. Financial means were available, so Halsted departed for Europe to further his education. In a letter he wrote to William Welch (1850-1934), professor of pathology at Johns Hopkins and his lifelong confidant, Halsted provided some idea of the depth and variety of his contacts and experiences during his European stay:

In the Fall of 1878 I sailed for Europe . . . anatomy was my chief work . . . took a train arriving in Vienna . . . attended the clinics of Billroth . . . My work with the embryologist Schenck was chiefly valuable because it led to friendly relations with Wolfler, Billroth's first assistant. We dined together not infrequently, and he gave me unrestricted entrée to the surgical wards . . . What impressed me chiefly was the magnitude of the operations, the skill of Billroth and his assistants, particularly Mikulicz, and the great number of artery forceps used . . . leaving Vienna in the Spring of 1879 I went to Würzburg and attended the clinics of von Bergmann regularly . . . returned to Vienna in the Autumn . . . soon after Easter I deserted Vienna for Leipzig . . . I enjoyed the clinics of Thiersch although his operations were generally minor ones . . . traveled to Halle where with Volkmann I spent several profitable weeks . . . Volkmann invited me to his house several times . . . from Halle I went to Berlin, Hamburg (Schede), and I think, Kiel (Esmarch) . . . returned, via Paris and London, to New York early in September 1880 . . .

The 2 years spent in Europe made a profound impression on Halsted. He could not help but notice the stark contrast between the American and German standards of surgical training. Although a few so-called teaching hospitals existed in the United States, their approach to surgical education consisted mainly of limited operating-room work, with almost no integration of the fundamental sciences with clinical diagnoses and treatment. Inevitably, therefore, most American surgeons were self-taught. The self-made surgeon was not overly eager to hand down the valuable, hard-earned skills to younger men who wished to learn but were certain to become competitors.

It is difficult to assign the role to one particular German surgeon of having provided the major influence on Halsted and his educational philosophies. More likely, the entire scholastic milieu of Germany in the mid-nineteenth century had the most enduring influence on Halsted's later surgical and educational beliefs. The young, impressionable American surgeon, in making his first tour of the German-speaking countries, could not have failed to notice the overwhelming success of the German educational system in training surgeons of the highest order. These impressions would later be translated into a new order of American surgery based on Halsted's principles.

Halsted returned to New York in September 1880. He immediately was appointed demonstrator of anatomy at his alma mater and accepted an offer by Sands to become his associate in surgical practice at the Roosevelt Hospital. There Halsted established the outpatient department and began his work with cocaine and local anesthesia.

The early 1880s were wondrous years for the young surgeon. Unlike his later years, when his addiction to cocaine had changed his personality into that of a socially distant and overwhelmingly reserved individual, these early years in New York were filled with an active social life. Between 1882 and 1886 Halsted published or presented more than 20 scientific papers on a wide variety of topics. In late 1884 or 1885 Halsted and several of his Roosevelt colleagues quite innocently became habituated to the use of cocaine. As the effects of addiction became worse, Halsted was threatened with professional extinction. In periods of agitation engendered by the drug he turned to morphine and alcohol. His attendance at meetings dropped off, and by April 1885 he could no longer deliver a series of lectures in competition for the chair of surgery at his alma mater. Halsted's health steadily declined; in February 1886 he took an extended sailing trip to the Windward Islands in the hope of restoring his former self. The effort was to no avail, and in May, with the encouragement of his friends and family, he voluntarily committed himself to the Butler Hospital in Providence, Rhode Island, a leading mental hospital that included alcoholics and drug addicts on its patient lists.

Halsted was discharged in November 1886 after 7 months of inconclusive treatment. It is likely that during this time he was weaned from cocaine but became dependent on morphine. Halsted realized that his career in New York was over and accepted an invitation by his old friend Welch to come to Baltimore and work in his new laboratory at The Johns Hopkins University. It is interest-

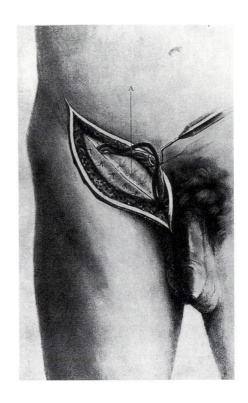

283. William S. Halsted's repair of inguinal hernia remains among the most misunderstood of the operations he devised. The drawing shows the aponeurosis of the external oblique muscle after it had been reapproximated with interrupted sutures. The spermatic cord was then transposed above this layer, forming the Halsted I repair. (From The Johns Hopkins Hospital Bulletin, vol 4, pp 17-24, 1893.)

ing, in view of Halsted's later prominence and surgical accolades, that when Halsted first went to Baltimore it was neither to accept a professorship nor to assume chairmanship of a department but to accept the offer of a friend who wanted to help him in dire times. Welch was fully aware of Halsted's tragic problems but also sensed his potential. All was not well, however, and in April 1887 Halsted reentered the Butler Hospital after stopping at the Harvard Medical School to present his work on the circular suture of the intestines, which stressed the importance of the submucosal layer. This time, Halsted remained at the Butler Hospital for 9 months, until the last day of 1887. His problems had been "treated"; he was listed as recovering from the opium habit.

Halsted returned to Baltimore in January 1888 and began working once again in Welch's laboratory. He began to see patients and perform surgery at various hospitals around the city. It was his hope to become a staff member of the about-to-open Johns Hopkins Hospital. Finding a professor of surgery for the institution was difficult, and finally, in February 1889, after apparent improvement in his health, Halsted was appointed surgeon-in-chief to the outpatient dispensary and acting surgeon to the hospital. Later that year he was made associate professor, but he was not named professor of surgery until 1892. Regardless of historical conjecture and innuendo, it is a fact that Halsted continued to use morphine throughout his life. Other than the definite change from the former *joi de vivre* of his personality, there was no apparent physical or mental deterioration, despite his 40-year drug addiction. From 1889 until his death in 1922 Halsted directed a department that produced an impressive array of surgical talent, which in turn brought his own philosophy to chairs of surgery throughout the United States.

Halsted never wrote a textbook of surgery, a monograph, or a treatise. All his written contributions were made to the periodical literature. By 1889 Halsted had devised a modern operation for the treatment of inguinal hernia. During the 1890s he authored a series of papers describing a method of radical mastectomy as treatment for breast cancer. In 1892 Halsted completed the first successful ligation of the left subclavian artery. A decade and a half later, in 1909, he introduced a metal band in place of a ligature for the occlusion of arteries. In that same year Halsted performed some of the earliest work on the autotransplantation and isotransplantation of parathyroid glands. He is eponymically associated with many things, including a stitch placed through the subcuticular fascia for exact skin approximation.

The resident system of training surgeons, which Halsted inaugurated at The Johns Hopkins Hospital, was not merely the first program of its kind in America; it was unique in its primary purpose. Above all other concerns Halsted desired to establish a school of surgery that would eventually disseminate throughout the surgical world the principles and attributes he considered sound and proper. His aim was to train surgical teachers, not merely competent operating surgeons. During the 33 years he spent as director of his system of surgical training, Halsted appointed 17 resident surgeons. Of these men, seven became professors of surgery, including Harvey Cushing (1869-1939) at Harvard; Stephen Watts (1877-1953) at Virginia; George Heuer (1882-1950) at Cincinnati and Cornell; Mont Reid (1889-1943) at Cincinnati; John Churchman (1877-1937) at Yale; Robert Miller (1886-1960) at Pittsburgh; and Emile Holman (1890-1977) at Stanford. Roy McClure (1882-1951) was named surgeon-in-chief at the Henry Ford Hospital in Detroit; James Mitchell (1871-1961) became professor of clinical surgery at George Washington University; Joseph Bloodgood (1867-1935) and Walter Dandy (1886-1946) remained on staff at Johns Hopkins.

Fifty-five men served as assistant resident surgeons under Halsted, and as a group they exerted a profound influence on American surgery, especially in the surgical specialties. Prominent among these men were Hugh Young (1870-1945), professor of urologic surgery; William Baer (1872-1931), professor of orthopedic surgery; and Samuel Crowe (1883-1955), professor of otolaryngologic surgery, all of whom remained at Johns Hopkins.

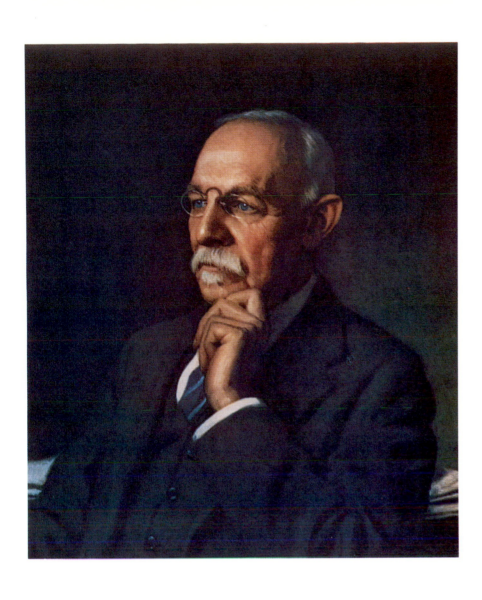

284. William Stewart Halsted in an oil painting copy of John H. Stocksdale's photograph from winter 1922. Halsted brought laboratory science into American surgery. A brilliant innovator and an awe-inspiring teacher, he more than any other American surgeon created the foundation on which the American school of surgery rests. *(From the author's collection.)*

285. The first published photograph of William Halsted's wound for radical mastectomy. The open portion of the incision is completely filled with a blood clot. *(From The Johns Hopkins Hospital Reports, vol 2, pp 225-314, 1890-1891.)*

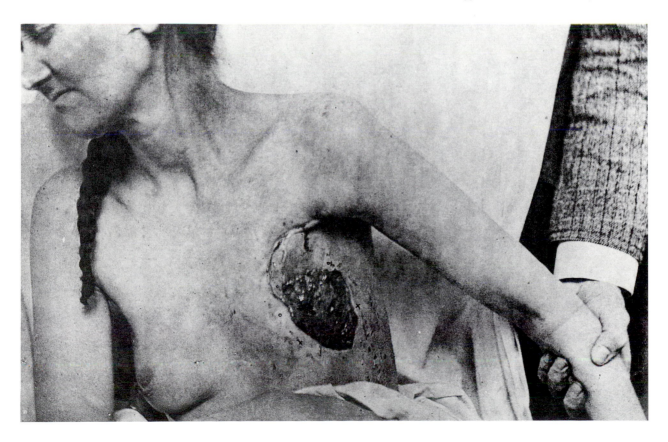

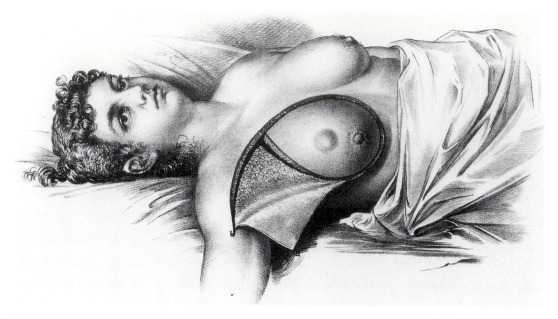

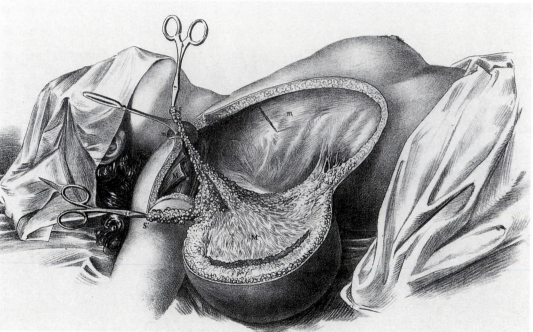

286. These engravings represent the earliest presentations of Halsted's radical mastectomy in pictorial form (1894). They reproduce drawings by the renowned anatomical illustrator Max Brödel (1870-1941) and are among the first illustrations he prepared in his new department of anatomical illustration at The Johns Hopkins Hospital. *(From* The Johns Hopkins Hospital Reports, *vol 4, pp 297-350, 1894-1895.)*

By the end of the nineteenth century, American surgery had sufficiently matured to acquire a professionalism of its own. Great surgical centers were being constructed in every section of the United States, and the practice of surgery was proliferating and progressing. What American surgeons lacked was a cohesiveness brought about by some type of educational organization similar to the Royal Colleges in Great Britain or the Academy of Surgery in France. Although such societies as the American Medical Association (1847), the American Surgical Association (1880), and the various surgical specialty groups had been established, they held no overt regulatory powers. They were primarily educational alliances with no control over licensure. Lack of an organized system of surgical education, training, and licensure would plague American surgery well into the twentieth century.

Like their European counterparts, American surgeons were great individual achievers. It is impossible to fully understand the evolution of surgery in the United States without knowing something of the surgeons' personal lives. Nathan Smith (1762-1829) was a native of Rehoboth, Massachusetts, who studied at Harvard Medical School, graduating in 1790. Quite early in his career he became interested in medical education and, communicating with the trustees of Dartmouth College, convinced them of the advisability of establishing a medical

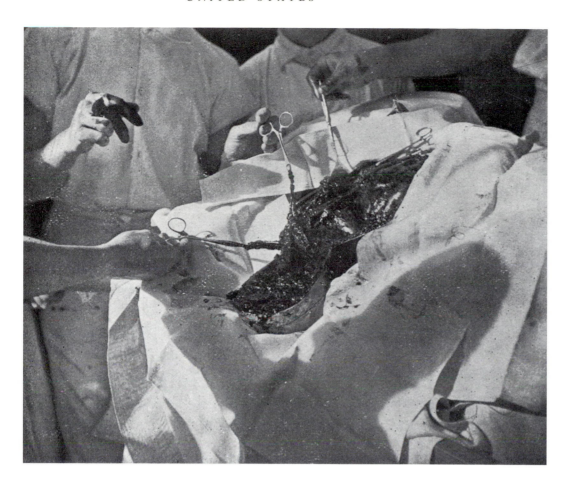

287. The earliest photograph of a Halsted radical mastectomy, taken just before the final severance of the breast, pectoral muscles, and axillary contents. The photograph was the first in a medical journal depicting the use of rubber gloves in surgery. Although Halsted may not have conceived the idea of rubber gloves in surgery, he was the first to actively promote their use and he may be credited for stimulating their initial wide acceptance. (From The Johns Hopkins Hospital Reports, *vol 4, pp 297-350, 1894-1895.*)

school on their campus. With his plans essentially approved, Smith traveled to Edinburgh and London to receive further postgraduate training and better qualify himself for the task that lay ahead. He returned in the fall of 1797 and shortly thereafter commenced a course of medical lectures at Dartmouth. Smith, serving as the entire faculty, repeated his lecture series for many years. In 1813 he was invited to help organize a medical school at Yale University and become professor of physic, surgery, and obstetrics. Smith also founded the medical department of Bowdoin College in Maine in 1820. He wrote little and left no great treatises. His written contributions were mostly to the periodical literature and included the second reported ovariotomy in America (1822), the first amputation of a knee joint in that country (1825), and an early account of osteomyelitis (1827). Smith also recognized the contagious nature of typhoid in his classic *A Practical Essay on Typhous Fever* (1842).

Wright Post (1766-1822) apprenticed under Richard Bayley (1745-1801), a physician in New York City. From 1784 to 1786 Post studied in London; a few years after his return he was appointed professor of surgery at Columbia College (1792). In 1811 he transferred to the chair of anatomy in the newly organized College of Physicians and Surgeons. He wrote nothing beyond a few accounts of his cases, which included America's first ligation of the common carotid artery for aneurysmal disease (1814); a description of the second ligation of the external iliac artery (1814); and the first successful ligation of the subclavian artery to be reported in the United States (1817).

John Davidge (1768-1829) studied medicine with James (1739-1819) and William (1751-?) Murray, brothers who practiced in Annapolis. He then attended lectures in Philadelphia, Edinburgh, and Glasgow, where he received his medical degree in 1793. After practicing briefly in England, Davidge moved to Baltimore. He was instrumental in establishing the University of Maryland School of Medicine, where he occupied the chair of anatomy and surgery from 1807 to 1829. In 1823 he reported the first case in America of an extirpation of the parotid gland.

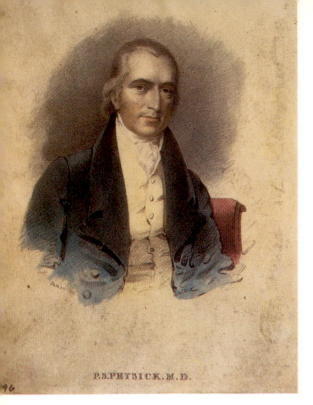

288. Philip Syng Physick as depicted in this hand-colored lithograph by Inman, Philadelphia, 1821. Physick was a brilliant surgical innovator; however, he did not consider himself a competent writer, so virtually all of his contributions to surgery were written by his nephew, John Syng Dorsey. *(Historical Collections, College of Physicians of Philadelphia.)*

Philip Syng Physick (1768-1837) was born in Philadelphia and received his college education at the University of Pennsylvania. He apprenticed in the office of Adam Kuhn (1741-1817) for 3 years. In 1789 Physick went to London, where he became a pupil of John Hunter and lived with his family. Three years later, after attending a year-long course of instruction in Edinburgh, Physick received his medical degree (1792). Shortly after returning to his native city, Physick was appointed surgeon to the Pennsylvania Hospital (1794), and a decade later he was named to the newly established chair of surgery at the University of Pennsylvania. In 1819 he transferred to the chair of anatomy, where he remained for 12 years, until his retirement. Physick never considered himself a competent writer, although he remained a creative, respected surgeon. Among his many contributions, he was first in the United States to introduce the use of a seton in the treatment of an ununited fracture (1804) and in the treatment of a fracture of the mandible (1822). He published the first American report of treatment in which mechanical countertraction was used for the reduction of a dislocated femur (1805) and the first report of an arteriovenous fistula to be surgically repaired in America (1805). He was responsible for the introduction and popularization of the gastric tube as a means of removing unwanted substances from the stomach (1813), the development of dissolving buckskin and kid ligatures (1816), the establishment of a colocutaneous fistula to treat strangulated hernia (1826), and the development of an instrument that was the progenitor of all tonsil guillotines (1828). Physick is eponymically remembered for a proctitis with mucous discharge and burning pain that primarily involves the sacculations or pouches between the rectal valves and for an iridectomy with the formation of a circular opening.

David Hosack (1769-1835) received his medical degree from the University of Pennsylvania in 1791 and then spent 2 postgraduate years in Edinburgh and London. From 1796 to 1811 Hosack served as professor of botany and materia medica at the College of Physicians and Surgeons in New York City, and during the last 4 of those years he also lectured on surgery. In 1811 he transferred to the chair of theory and practice of physic and clinical medicine, where he remained until 1826, when he helped found the Rutgers Medical College in New York City. Hosack received an honorary degree in 1815 from Union College in Schenectady, New York, the nation's first nondenominational college. Although Hosack originated no new surgical procedures, he was considered an outstanding clinical surgeon. In 1798 he introduced to American surgeons the method of treating hydrocele by injection. A decade and a half later he authored an article describing the importance of leaving wounds open to the air to heal and provided the first case report in an American periodical of a mastectomy.

Ephraim McDowell (1771-1830) was a native of Virginia who apprenticed with a local physician. In 1793 McDowell traveled to Edinburgh, where he attended the lectures of John Bell. Returning to the United States in 1795, McDowell commenced practice in Danville, Kentucky, where he not only was a general practitioner but also acquired a reputation for his surgical skills. One interesting case of his was the extraction of a bladder stone from James Polk (1795-1849), who later became the President of the United States. In December 1809 McDowell introduced ovariotomy to the world as a successful operation for treatment of ovarian tumors. He disliked writing, which explains why this first ovariotomy was not reported until 1817. Like many of the most influential contributions to surgery, his paper received scant notice and roused little interest among contemporary surgeons.

Horatio Jameson (1778-1855) graduated from the University of Maryland in 1811. He remained in Baltimore, where he became an influential member of the community and a respected surgeon. In 1827 Jameson founded the Washington Medical College and served as professor of surgery. He is best remembered for the first known report of a resection of the superior maxillary bone (1821); the first known attempt in America, albeit unsuccessful, to remove a cancerous uterus via the vagina (1824); and an important paper on various methods used to control hemorrhage (1827).

John Collins Warren (1778-1856) was the eldest son of John Warren. After a short apprenticeship with his father, Warren studied further in London and Paris and received his formal medical degree from Edinburgh in 1802. In that year he returned to Boston because of his father's illness and assumed his private practice. From 1806 to 1815 Warren served as adjunct professor in anatomy and surgery at Harvard. He was promoted to full professor in 1815 and remained in that position until 1847, when he retired. Warren was a founder of the Massachusetts General Hospital (1821), the *Boston Medical and Surgical Journal* (1812), and the American Medical Association (1847). He performed the first surgical operation in which ether anesthesia was administered (1846). Among Warren's most important treatises were America's first text on surgical oncology, *Surgical Observations on Tumours* (1837); two monographs on ether anesthesia, *Etherization with Surgical Remarks* (1848) and *Effects of Chloroform and of Strong Chloric Ether, as Narcotic Agents* (1849); and a lengthy work, *Dislocation of the Hip Joint* (1824). His most important paper concerned cleft palate repair (1828).

Reuben Mussey (1780-1866) graduated from Dartmouth College in 1803, apprenticed with Nathan Smith, and received his medical degree from the University of Pennsylvania in 1809. In his peripatetic career he was professor of anatomy and surgery and of medical theory and practice at Dartmouth (1814-1838), professor of surgery at the Medical College of Ohio (1838-1852), and professor of surgery at the Miami Medical College in Cincinnati (1852-1857). In 1850 Mussey served as president of the American Medical Association. His only contributions to surgical literature were case reports published in various journals. The most prominent included the ligation of both common carotid arteries within a few days of each other as treatment for an ulcerated vascular tumor of the scalp (1829) and the earliest reported scapulectomy in America (1838).

John Syng Dorsey (1783-1818) was the nephew of Philip Syng Physick, with whom he apprenticed. While working in his uncle's office, Dorsey also attended medical lectures at the University of Pennsylvania, where he received his medical degree (1802). In 1803 he traveled to London and Paris to receive postgraduate training. After returning to the United States, Dorsey commenced private practice in Philadelphia, and in 1807 he was named adjunct professor of surgery at his alma mater. Shortly thereafter, he was appointed surgeon to the Pennsylvania Hospital. Physick, who occupied the chair of surgery, never became a competent writer. He therefore asked Dorsey to organize his lectures into the form of a surgical handbook, and in response to this request Dorsey authored the two-volume *Elements of Surgery,* the first systematic treatise on surgery to be written by an American surgeon, in 1813. In that same year Dorsey was appointed to the university's chair of materia medica, and in 1818 he succeeded Caspar Wistar (1761-1818) in the chair of anatomy. In 1812 Dorsey reported the first successful ligation of the external iliac artery in America. Dorsey's success was short lived: within a few days of delivering his first anatomical lecture he died of typhus.

John Ball Brown (1784-1862) apprenticed under various general practitioners in New England. In 1812 he moved to Boston, where he soon married the daughter of John Collins Warren. At the urging of his father-in-law, Brown began to specialize in orthopedic operations. In 1838 he open the Orthopedique Infirmary, eventually renamed the Boston Orthopedic Institution, the first such specialty hospital in America. Brown wrote little of consequence.

Benjamin Dudley (1785-1870) was a native of Virginia and matriculated at the University of Pennsylvania, where he received his medical degree in 1806. He spent the next few years in Europe at various clinical centers and returned to Lexington, Kentucky, in 1814. He acquired a reputation locally as an outstanding general practitioner and surgeon. By 1817 Dudley was able to establish the medical department of Transylvania University, where he remained as professor of anatomy and surgery for his entire professional career. Dudley was renowned for his expertise in lithotomy and summarized his clinical cases in a short monograph, *Observations on the Nature and Treatment of Calculous Diseases* (1836). He also authored an important paper on head injuries (1828).

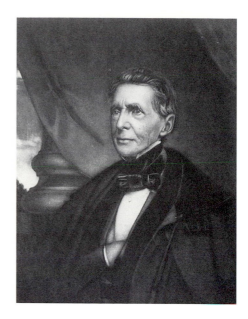

289. John Collins Warren, one of the greatest of the Warren dynasty of physicians and surgeons in Boston. John Collins Warren may be best remembered today for performing the first surgical operation in which anesthesia was used (1846). *(Historical Collections, College of Physicians of Philadelphia.)*

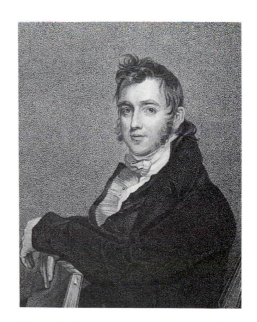

290. John Syng Dorsey, nephew of Philip Syng Physick, who apprenticed at an early age to his uncle. Because Physick, a prolific surgical innovator, did not consider himself a competent writer, it was left to Dorsey to compose many of Physick's original contributions. *(Historical Collections, College of Physicians of Philadelphia.)*

461

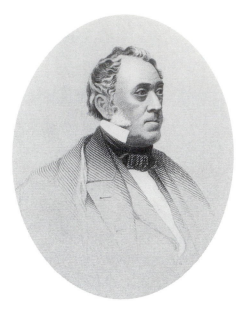

291. Valentine Mott, a student of Astley Cooper, was a major surgical innovator in America before the Civil War. *(Historical Collections, College of Physicians of Philadelphia.)*

Valentine Mott (1785-1865) was among the most prominent of early American surgeons. He had initially apprenticed with a cousin, Valentine Seaman (1770-1817), a well-known New York City practitioner. Seaman authored the unrecognized but important *Pharmacoepia Chirurgica In Usum Nosocomii Novi Eboracencis* (1811), an account of the clinical practices of the surgical department of New York Hospital. After Mott obtained his medical degree from Columbia College (1806), he decided to remain for another year under Seaman's tutelage. That year's experience persuaded Mott to become a surgeon and to seek further education in London and Edinburgh. Mott became a student under Astley Cooper and was so well regarded that Cooper made him "dresser of wounds" for all his patients. In 1808 Mott worked with Thomson and Bell in Edinburgh. Having received a great deal of technical experience, Mott returned to New York City in 1809. Almost at once he began to teach a course of private instruction in surgery, which attracted a large student following. In 1811 Mott was elected professor of surgery at his alma mater. In the following year the medical department of Columbia College was united with the College of Physicians and Surgeons of the University of New York. This new College of Physicians and Surgeons represented the major medical institution in New York City, and Wright Post nominated Mott to the first chair of surgery. For political reasons Mott resigned from his position in 1826 and helped found the Rutgers Medical College in New York City. He occupied the chair of operative surgery until he resigned in 1834 because of poor health. In early 1835 Mott left for an extended stay in Europe that lasted 7 years. During his travels Mott was received by the most famous of European surgeons; he described his experience in *Travels to Europe and the East* (1842). Before returning home in 1841, Mott was informed that he had been elected to the new chair of surgery at the recently established University Medical College, which was associated with New York University. The presence of Mott on the faculty guaranteed that the school would be an immediate success, and during the next 10 years Mott enjoyed one of the busiest surgical practices in the United States. In 1850 ill health again forced him to retire, and he set out once more for Europe. After a year-long sojourn, Mott felt better and reaccepted his old position at the University Medical College. Although his health was fine, he decided to retire in 1853 and assumed an emeritus position. Mott's later years were spent in humanitarian pursuits. In 1862, at the request of the United States Sanitary Commission, a civilian body that aided Civil War soldiers, he prepared two papers on the use of anesthetics and the treatment of hemorrhage from gunshot wounds. Mott made numerous contributions to the advancement of clinical surgery. Although he never authored a surgical textbook, he did edit the American version of Velpeau's three-volume New Elements of *Operative Surgery* (1847). Mott wrote many journal articles, including the first reported attempt to ligate the innominate artery (1818), an early case of common carotid ligation and mandibular resection (1822), the first successful ligation of the common iliac artery in the United States (1827), the first reported amputation at the hip joint in America (1827), the earliest resection of the clavicle in the United States for an osteosarcoma (1828), the first reported use of Brasdor's technique for treatment of aneurysmal disease (1829), a case of external iliac ligation (1831), the first attempt in America to ligate the subclavian artery within the scalenus muscle (1833), the second successful reported ligation of the internal iliac artery in the United States (1837), and an operation to remove a fibrous growth from the nostril by division of the nasal and maxillary bones (1843).

John Mettauer (1787-1875) received his medical degree from the University of Pennsylvania in 1809. He soon returned to his home state of Virginia, where he remained for most of his professional life. For 1 year, from 1835 to 1836, Mettauer was professor of surgery at Washington Medical College in Baltimore. He opened his own medical institute in 1837, and a few years later it became part of Randolph-Macon College. Mettauer was an outstanding clinical surgeon who reported the first successful repair of a lacerated perineum and rectovaginal septum in America (1833). This achievement assumed particular importance because he espoused the use of metallic sutures during such an operation. Mettauer followed his initial paper with numerous other reports during the 1840s and 1850s.

292. The surgical kit of John Mettauer, who is remembered for his use of metallic sutures in the first successful repair in America of a lacerated perineum and rectovaginal septum in 1833. Metallic sutures from Mettauer's surgical set are visible in the lower left corner of the photograph. The ivory handles on Mettauer's instruments, although beautiful to look at, could not be sterilized. They confirm that his surgical set dates from the period before antisepsis, which did not become widely accepted in America until the 1880s. *(Mütter Museum, College of Physicians of Philadelphia.)*

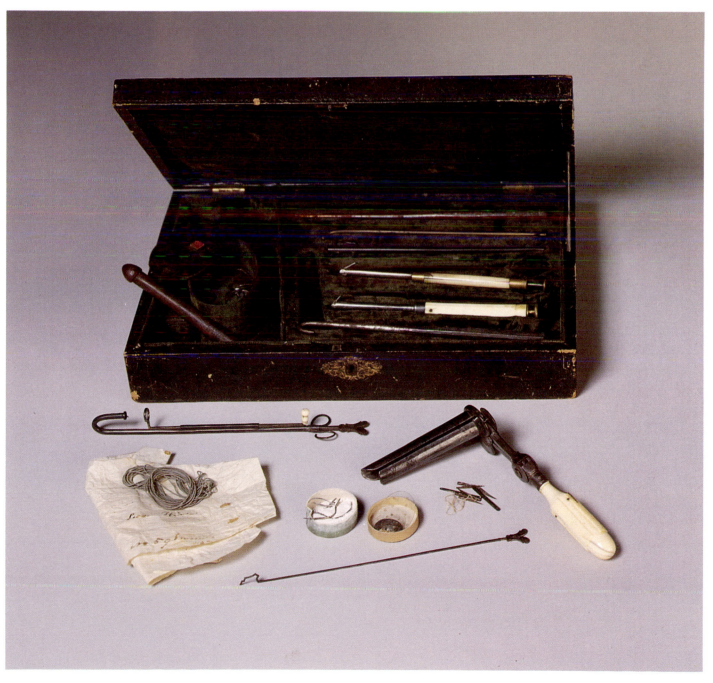

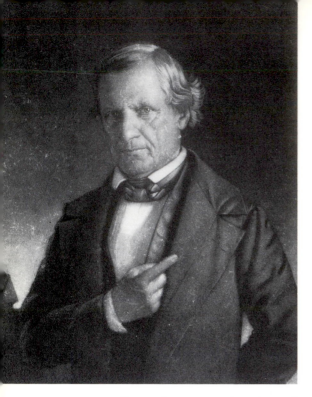

293. William Gibson. *(From the author's collection.)*

William Gibson (1788-1868) studied in Edinburgh, where he received his medical degree in 1809. After returning to the United States, he was appointed to the chair of surgery at the University of Maryland. After Physick's retirement Gibson was appointed his successor at the University of Pennsylvania and remained there until his own retirement in 1855. In 1824 Gibson authored the two-volume *Institutes and Practice of Surgery,* the second systematic American textbook of surgery. Among his surgical accomplishments were the first known performance of a ligation of the common iliac artery (1820) and the first recorded instance of the same woman having two successful cesarean sections (in 1835 and 1838). Gibson also wrote a popular travel book, *Rambles in Europe in 1839, with Sketches of Prominent Surgeons* (1841).

Jonathan Knight (1789-1864) attended medical lectures at the University of Pennsylvania but never received a formal medical degree. At the founding of the Yale Medical School, Knight was named professor of anatomy and physiology (1813-1838), and subsequently transferred to the chair of surgery (1838-1864). Among his honors was the presidency of the American Medical Association (1853). Knight wrote sparingly; his most important paper presented the first reported cure of aneurysm by means of digital compression worldwide (1848).

Alexander Stevens (1789-1869) attended Yale College and received his medical degree from the University of Pennsylvania in 1811. In 1814 he was appointed professor of surgery at the New York Medical Institute, and 4 years later he became one of the visiting surgeons to the New York Hospital. In 1826 he succeeded Mott as professor of surgery at the College of Physicians and Surgeons of New York City. Stevens also served as the second president of the American Medical Association (1848). Although he was not a prolific medical author, he did write the first American treatise on urologic surgery, *Lectures on Lithotomy* (1838), and the first major paper on trauma in the United States surgical literature (1837).

George Hayward (1791-1863) received his medical education at the University of Pennsylvania, graduating in 1812. He spent time abroad, working with Astley Cooper, but returned to Boston and founded a private medical school with John Collins Warren. Hayward is most remembered for being the first American surgeon to perform a major surgical operation with ether anesthesia, an amputation of the thigh, on November 7, 1846. His most important publication was *Surgical Reports and Miscellaneous Papers* (1855). His most memorable contribution to the periodical literature was a report of a successful operative cure of vesicovaginal fistula (1839).

George Bushe (1793-1836) was born in Ireland and received his medical and surgical training in Europe. He was brought to America in 1828 by the faculty of Rutgers Medical College, to serve as professor of anatomy. He was widely regarded as a surgeon and gave daily office lectures on surgery for almost 3 years. Bushe's most impressive text was *A Treatise on the Malformations, Injuries, and Diseases of the Rectum and Anus* (1837), the first book to deal solely with colon and rectal surgery in the United States. Bushe died of tuberculosis immediately after completing the text, before it was published.

George Frick (1793-1870) graduated from the University of Pennsylvania in 1815 and spent several years in Vienna studying under George Beer (1763-1821). Frick later returned to Baltimore, where he became ophthalmic surgeon at Baltimore General Dispensary. He authored the first American ophthalmologic text, *A Treatise on the Diseases of the Eye* (1823). In 1840 Frick abandoned the practice of medicine and spent the rest of his life in Europe.

J. Kearny Rodgers (1793-1851) studied medicine with Post and graduated from the College of Surgeons and Physicians in New York City in 1816. He spent time in Europe and on his return to America was appointed surgeon to the New York Hospital. His most important paper presented the earliest successful wiring of an ununited fracture of the humerus to be found in the American periodical literature (1827).

John Rhea Barton (1794-1871) was an 1818 graduate of the University of Pennsylvania. Shortly thereafter, he became surgeon to the Pennsylvania Hospital. He is best known as the originator of the osteotomy for joint ankylosis (1826). Barton's name is associated with a figure-of-eight bandage that provides support below and anterior to the lower jaw; an obstetrics forceps with one fixed, curved blade and a lunged anterior blade for application to a high transverse position of the head; and a fracture of the lower articular extremity of the radius.

Alden March (1795-1869) attended medical lectures on anatomy and surgery in Boston during 1818 and received his medical degree from Brown University in 1820. In 1834 he established a proprietary medical school in Albany, New York. Five years later March was the principal organizer of the Albany Medical College, which later became affiliated with Union College; he served as professor of surgery until his death. March was president of the American Medical Association in 1864. He wrote no great texts but did author a number of reports in the periodical literature, including those of a splint for hip disease (1853) and the invention of a forceps used in repair of cleft lip (1855).

Alban Goldsmith (1795-1876), an interesting personality in American surgical history, had his name changed from Smith by an act of the New York State legislature in 1839. Goldsmith never received a formal medical degree. Instead, he apprenticed with both Ephraim McDowell and a Philadelphia surgeon, Joseph Parrish (1779-1840). Because of Goldsmith's early association with McDowell, it is believed that Goldsmith was present at the first ovariotomy in 1809. In 1833 Goldsmith was appointed professor of surgery at the Medical College of Ohio. Four years later, because of his irascible personality, his contract was not renewed. Shortly thereafter, the regents of the College of Physicians and Surgeons in New York City offered him the chair of surgery. Goldsmith's academic career in New York was short lived. He resigned after only 2 years and remained in private practice for the rest of his life. Goldsmith's most important text was *Diseases of the Genitourinary Organs* (1857).

George McClellan (1796-1847) studied with John Syng Dorsey and received his medical degree from the University of Pennsylvania in 1819. McClellan remained in Philadelphia and helped found the Jefferson Medical College, where he served as professor of surgery from 1826 to 1838. After McClellan's death his son John (1823-1874) posthumously published McClellan's lectures, notes, and other material in the *Principles and Practice of Surgery* (1848), which contained an excellent description of shock.

Nathan Ryno Smith (1797-1877) studied medicine under the direction of his father, Nathan Smith, and in 1823 received his medical degree from Yale. Smith began practicing in Burlington, Vermont, and with his father's assistance founded the medical school at the University of Vermont (1825). He served as its first professor of anatomy and surgery but soon was called to the chair of anatomy at Jefferson Medical College. In 1827 Smith became professor of surgery at the University of Maryland. Except for a short interval spent at Transylvania University, Smith remained in Baltimore for 40 years. Smith authored *Surgical Anatomy of the Arteries* (1830) and *Treatment of Fractures of the Lower Extremity by the Use of the Anterior Suspensory Apparatus* (1867). Among his most important case reports were the first thyroidectomy in America (1835), and his invention of the anterior or suspensory splint for the treatment of lower-extremity fracture (1860).

John Atlee (1799-1885) was a native of Lancaster, Pennsylvania, and graduated from the University of Pennsylvania in 1820. His entire professional life was spent in private practice in his native city, where he was on the faculty of anatomy and physiology at Franklin and Marshall College. In 1843 Atlee's widely noted report of a successful case revived the operation of ovariotomy in America. In the following year he performed the first known bilateral oophorectomy.

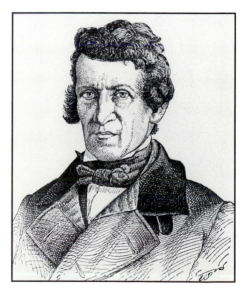

294. George McClellan. *(From the author's collection.)*

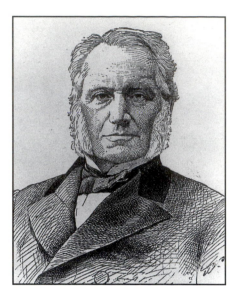

295. Willard Parker. *(From the author's collection.)*

Homer Bostwick (?-1862), a little-known New York surgeon, may have been the first urological specialist in the United States. He practiced in New York City, where he authored *A Treatise on the Nature and Treatment of Seminal Diseases, Impotency, and Other Kindred Affections* (1847) and *A Complete Practical Work on the Nature and Treatment of Venereal Diseases, and Other Affections of the Genito-Urinary Organs of the Male and Female* (1848).

Dixi Crosby (1800-1873) received his medical degree from Dartmouth in 1824. He was professor of surgery at his alma mater from 1838 to 1870. In 1839 Crosby resected the entire arm and scapula and three fourths of the clavicle for a reported osteoma. This monumental operation, performed in preanesthestic America, was not reported in the literature until 1875 by Crosby's son Alpheus (1832-1877). Dixi Crosby remains best known in the United States as the defendant in the first malpractice suit brought against a consulting surgeon. Crosby lost the initial suit, although the decision was reversed on appeal in 1854.

Willard Parker (1800-1884) was a private pupil of John Collins Warren and graduated from Harvard (1830). After serving for 1 year as house surgeon to the Massachusetts General Hospital, Parker was appointed professor of anatomy at the Bershire Medical College in Pittsfield, Massachusetts. In 1836 he transferred to the chair of surgery at the Medical College of Ohio, and 3 years later he accepted the professorship of surgery at the College of Physicians and Surgeons in New York City. He remained there until his retirement; he also joined the staffs of Bellevue Hospital (1845) and New York Hospital (1856). Parker never wrote a true textbook of surgery, although after his death his son compiled manuscript notes and had them published as *Cancer: A Study of Three Hundred and Ninety-Seven Cases of Cancer of the Female Breast* (1885). Parker remains well known for a number of surgical triumphs. In 1851 he initiated cystotomy as a treatment of irritable bladder. Parker reported the ligature of the left subclavian, the common carotid, and the vertebral arteries (1864) and advocated the opening of appendicular abscesses at an early stage (1867). He is eponymically remembered for an oblique incision nearly parallel with the inguinal ligament over the area of dullness in an appendiceal abscess.

Horace Green (1802-1866) is considered the father of American laryngology and the first specialist in the United States to devote his practice exclusively to diseases of the throat. He received his medical degree from Castleton Medical College in Vermont in 1824. After pursuing a general practice in Vermont, Green traveled to Europe and acquired an interest in laryngology. From 1840 to 1843 he was connected with his alma mater as professor of medicine. In 1850 he was among the founders of the New York Medical College. Green was the recepient of an honorary degree from Union College. Green became a controversial and colorful figure in American surgery when he announced in 1840 that he was able to pass a sponge-tipped probang into the larynx and thus directly apply medication to the laryngeal mucosa. For the next 20 years he was involved in stormy, often acrimonious debate concerning this research. He authored the first laryngology text in America, *A Treatise on Diseases of the Air Passages* (1846). Green also wrote *Observations on the Pathology of Croup* (1849), *On the Surgical Treatment of Polypi of the Larynx, and Oedema of the Glottis* (1852), and *A Practical Treatise on Pulmonary Tuberculosis* (1864).

Joseph Pancoast (1805-1882) was a native of New Jersey and an 1828 graduate of the University of Pennsylvania. He began teaching practical anatomy and surgery in Philadelphia in 1831 and 7 years later was elected professor of surgery at Jefferson Medical College. However, in 1841 he was reassigned to the chair of general, descriptive, and surgical anatomy, where he remained until his retirement in 1874. Pancoast authored the outstanding *A Treatise on Operative Surgery* (1844), which became one of the most popular surgical atlases in America in the mid-nineteenth century. He is distinguished for his repair of an exstrophy of the bladder (1859) and for his procedure of sectioning the second and third branches of the fifth pair of cranial nerves as they emerge from the base of the brain (1872). Pancoast's name is linked with a suture that provides for the union of two edges in plastic repair by means of a tongue-and-groove arrangement.

Alfred Post (1805-1885), the nephew of Wright Post, graduated in medicine from the College of Physicians and Surgeons in New York City (1827). He continued his studies in Berlin, Edinburgh, and Paris. Post returned to New York in 1829 to begin the practice of surgery. He was one of the founders of the medical department of the University of the City of New York and held its chair of surgery from 1851 to 1875. Post's only treatise was *Observations on the Cure of Strabismus* (1841). He was the first in America to successfully perform and report on plastic operations to correct lid deformities (1842).

Louis Dugas (1806-1884) was one of the leading surgeons of the South. An 1827 graduate of the University of Maryland, he soon traveled to Europe, where he continued his medical training for another 4 years. After returning to the United States, he settled in Augusta, where in 1832 he was one of the founders of the Medical College of Georgia. From 1855 to 1883 Dugas served there as professor of principles and practice of surgery. His most noteworthy contribution to surgery was an 1856 report in which he described a clinical test to determine shoulder dislocation: if the elbow cannot be made to touch the chest while the hand rests on the opposite shoulder, the injury is a dislocation, not a fracture of the humerus.

Paul Eve (1806-1878), a native of Augusta, Georgia, received his medical education at the University of Pennsylvania in 1828. He studied in Europe for 3 years and on his return was appointed professor of surgery at the newly founded Medical College of Georgia. In 1850 Eve transferred to the chair of surgery at the University of Louisville but left after one session to accept the professorship of surgery at the University of Nashville. In 1857 he was president of the American Medical Association. During the Civil War, Eve was chief surgeon to the Confederate army. His most interesting text was the entertaining *A Collection of Remarkable Cases in Surgery* (1857).

Gurdon Buck (1807-1877), a native of New York City, graduated from that city's College of Physicians and Surgeons in 1830. He served as a house surgeon at the New York Hospital for 1 year and then left for 2 years to study in Berlin, Paris, and Vienna. On his return to the United States Buck was appointed attending surgeon to the New York Hospital, where he remained until his death. Buck was considered an outstanding clinical surgeon and authored the important *Contributions to Reparative Surgery* (1876), the first American text on plastic and reconstructive surgery. In addition, Buck wrote numerous case reports, including those in which ligatures were simultaneously applied to the common and internal carotid arteries (1855) and to the femoral, profunda, external, and common iliac arteries (1858). Among his spectacular surgical feats was the restoration of an ankylosed right-angled knee joint to a straight position (1845) and the first known operation in America for a cancer of the larynx to be treated by an external incision (1853). In 1862 Buck described the traction device he used in extremity fractures. He is eponymically remembered for the fascial sheath of the penis (1848).

Henry Gassett Davis (1807-1896) was among a small group of American surgeons who brought orthopedic surgery from a tenuous obscurity to its position as a special branch of the surgical sciences. He was a graduate of Yale School of Medicine (1839) and later practiced in New York City. His greatest contribution to orthopedic surgery was the application of the principle of "continuous elastic extension." He wrote numerous articles on his system of traction, but his only textbook was *Conservative Surgery, As Exhibited in Remedying Some of the Mechanical Causes That Operate Injuriously Both in Health and Disease* (1867).

John Watson (1807-1863), a native of Ireland, was brought to America as a young child. He received his medical degree from the College of Physicians and Surgeons in New York City (1832). In the following year Watson was appointed to the staff of the New York Dispensary, where he served as attending surgeon from 1839 to 1862. In 1838 he also joined the staff of the New York Hospital, where he introduced regular clinical instruction in surgery. Watson remains best known for the first report of an esophagotomy in the American periodical literature (1844). He never wrote a lengthy text but did author an obscure historical monograph, *The Medical Profession in Ancient Times* (1856).

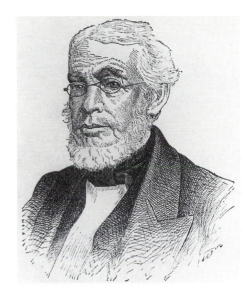

296. Paul Eve. *(From the author's collection.)*

467

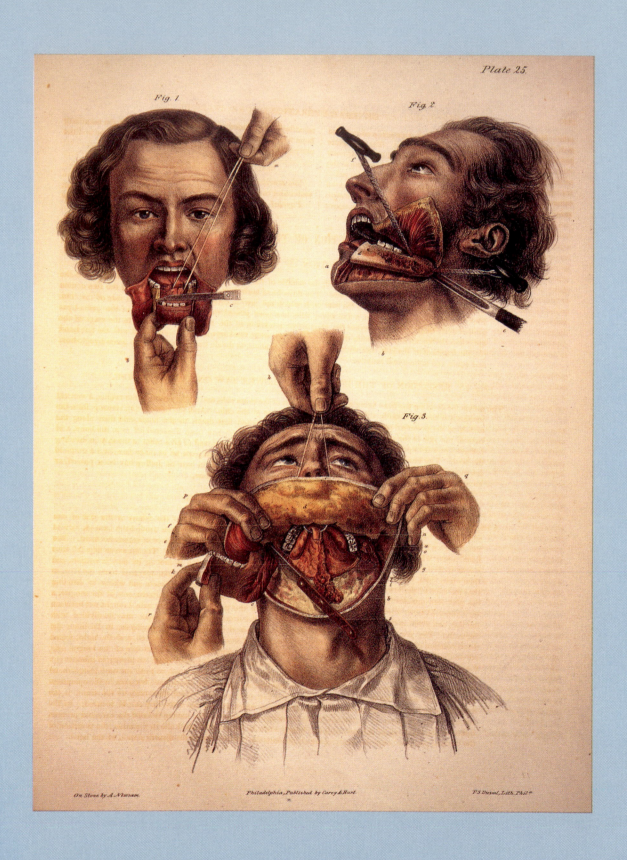

297. Maxillofacial surgery drawn on stone by A. Newsam for Joseph Pancoast's *Treatise on Operative Surgery* (1844). Following in a long tradition of surgical illustrations, the idealized patient is depicted as placid and wide awake while undergoing an operation that must have been completely unbearable before surgical anesthesia, which was not discovered until 1846. *(Historical Collections, College of Physicians of Philadelphia.)*

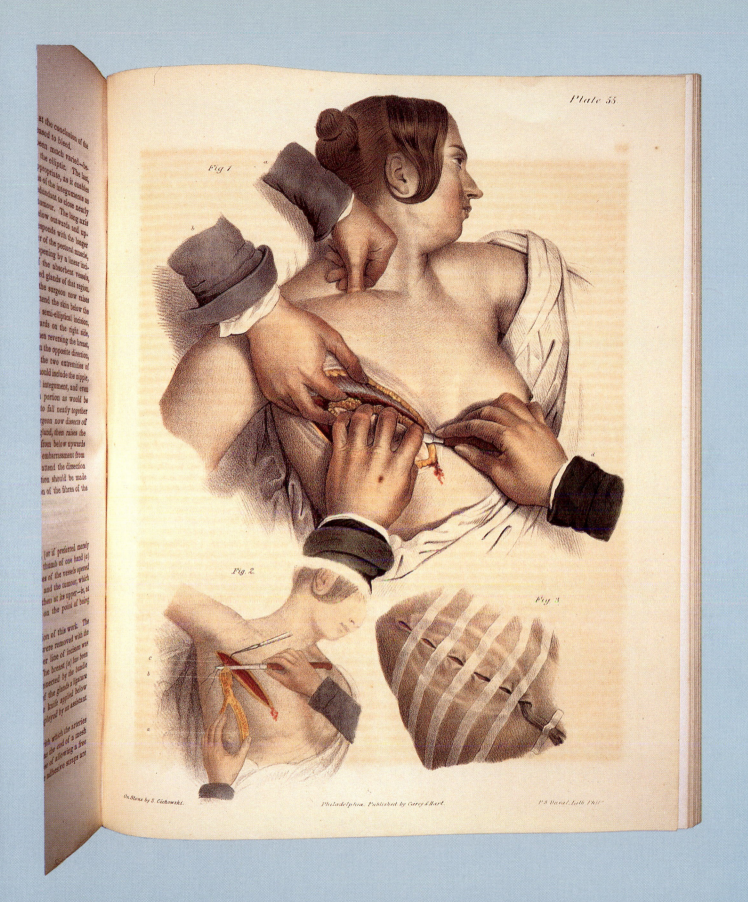

298. Mastectomy drawn on stone by S. Cichowski for Joseph Pancoast's *Treatise on Operative Surgery* (1844). With 80 full-page lithographs, Pancoast's work was the first American surgical treatise to be extensively illustrated. Most copies were issued with black and white plates. Hand-colored copies such as those reproduced here are particularly rare. (*Historical Collections, College of Physicians of Philadelphia.*)

A

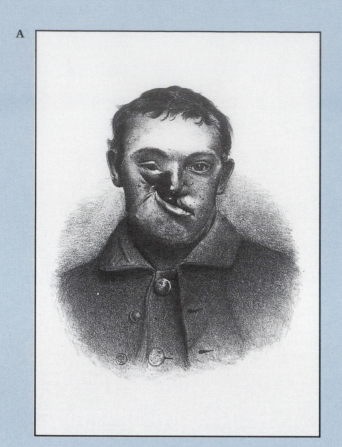

B

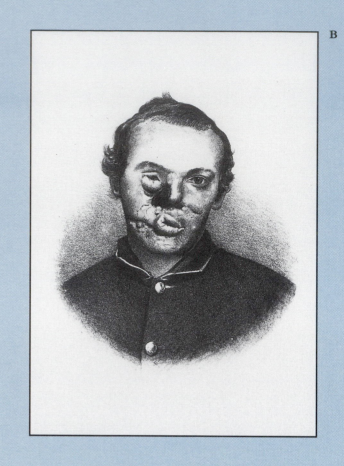

C

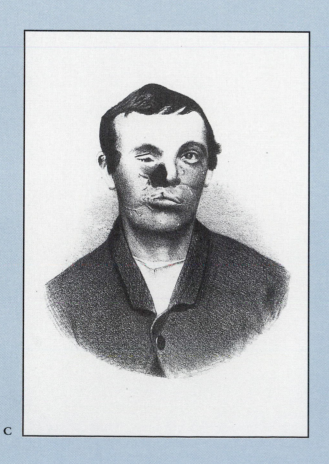

D

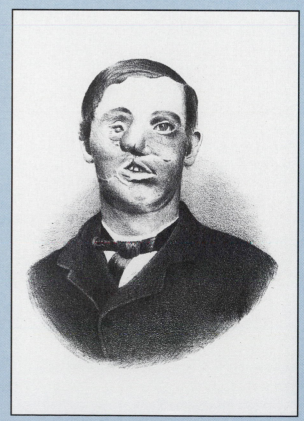

Washington Atlee (1808-1878), brother of John Atlee, graduated from Jefferson Medical College (1829). The early part of his professional career was spent in Lancaster, Pennsylvania. After 1844 he practiced in Philadelphia, where he was on the medical chemistry faculty of the Medical College of Philadelphia. He and his brother reestablished the operation for ovariotomy in the United States. Atlee was a founder of the American Gynecological Society. In 1873 he summarized his life's operative work in *General and Differential Diagnosis of Ovarian Tumors, with Specific References to the Operation of Ovariotomy, and Occasional Pathological and Therapeutical Considerations.* Atlee, a prolific contributor to the surgical literature, wrote an 1851 article that detailed all known operations of ovariotomy from 1701 to 1851, a study of the surgical removal of uterine fibroids (1853), and the description of an operation for vesicovaginal fistula (1860).

William Bodenhamer (1808-1905) graduated from the Worthington Medical College of Ohio University (1839). America's first specialist in anal and rectal diseases, he is in many respects a nineteenth-century American version of the European itinerant surgeon who traveled from city to city performing rectal surgery. Bodenhamer made it known to the public that he divided his time between Louisville and New Orleans so that he could bring his medical advice to as many people as possible. A prolific writer, he authored six treatises: *Practical Observation on Some of the Diseases of the Rectum, Anus, and Contiguous Textures* (1847), *A Practical Treatise on the Etiology, Pathology, and Treatment of the Congenital Malformations of the Rectum and Anus* (1860), *Practical Observations on the Etiology, Pathology, Diagnosis, and Treatment of Anal Fissure* (1868), *The Physical Exploration of the Rectum* (1870), *An Essay on Rectal Medication* (1878), and *A Theoretical and Practical Treatise on the Hemorrhoidal Disease* (1884).

William Detmold (1808-1900) was born in Germany, where he received most of his medical education and training. He emigrated to the United States in 1837 and soon established his reputation as one of New York City's earliest orthopedic surgeons. Detmold authored the first paper in the United States on the treatment of clubfoot by the division of the Achilles tendon (1838). In 1850 he reported the earliest known instance of opening the lateral ventricles of the brain for treatment of a cerebral abscess.

George Norris (1808-1875) was a graduate of the University of Pennsylvania (1830). After 2 years' service in the Pennsylvania Hospital he went to Paris and studied with Dupuytren, Roux, and Velpeau. After returning to the United States, Norris became surgeon to the Pennsylvania Hospital. In 1848 he succeeded John Rhea Barton as professor of clinical surgery at his alma mater. Norris's sole full-length clinical text was *Contributions to Practical Surgery* (1873). His only other book of note, *The Early History of Medicine in Philadelphia* (1886), was published posthumously. Norris remains most remembered for the numerous statistical compilations of data about surgical operations that he published in the 1830s and 1840s.

Warren Stone (1808-1872) was an 1831 graduate of the Berkshire Medical Institute in Massachusetts and had also studied with Amos Twitchell (1781-1850). Twitchell, a family practitioner in Vermont and a well-respected surgeon, had performed the first ligation of the common carotid artery for traumatic injury in America (1807). Stone had difficulty establishing a practice in New England and resettled in New Orleans. There he became associated with the medical department of the University of Louisiana. In 1836 Stone was appointed lecturer on surgery and within a few years, professor of surgery. He wrote little but did report the first use of metallic sutures in the ligation of an artery (1859).

John Bobbs (1809-1870) received his medical degree from Jefferson Medical College (1836). After settling in Indianapolis he helped establish Indiana Central Medical College (1849), serving as its dean and professor of surgery. Two decades later Bobbs became the founder of the Medical College of Indiana. Bobbs wrote sparingly and was typical of that era's surgeon in being both a general practitioner and, occasionally, a surgical operator. In 1868 he reported the world's first known account of a cholecystotomy for the removal of gallstones.

299. *Facing page,* Gurdon Buck's reconstruction of Carleton Burgan's deformed face, requiring five separate surgical procedures performed over 6 months, was one of the greatest operative triumphs of nineteenth-century American surgery. These four illustrations show, **A,** Burgan before the first operation; **B,** Burgan after the initial procedure during which the mouth was reconstructed; **C,** the improvement of the right angle of the mouth after the second operation; and, **D,** a front view of the final result of all the operations. A rapidly spreading ulcer had developed on the right side of the patient's face while he was serving in the Civil War. The massive tissue loss probably resulted from treatment with mercurials for presumed venereal disease. *(From* Transactions of the Medical Society of the State of New York *pp 173-186, 1864.)*

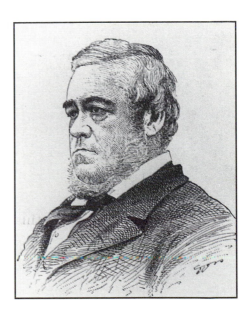

300. Warren Stone. *(From the author's collection.)*

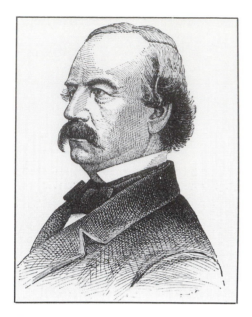

301. Daniel Brainard. *(From the author's collection.)*

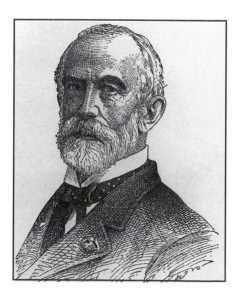

302. Frank Hastings Hamilton. *(From the author's collection.)*

James Knight (1810-1887) graduated from Washington Medical College in Baltimore in 1832. Having come under the influence of Mott, he soon began to devote himself to the study of orthopedic surgery. Knight is remembered for establishing the Hospital for the Ruptured and Crippled in New York. He wrote little; his only major text was *Orthopaedia, or a Practical Treatise on the Aberrations of the Human Form* (1874).

Thomas Mütter (1811-1859) graduated from the University of Pennsylvania (1831) and then studied medicine in Paris. He eventually became professor of surgery at Jefferson Medical College (1841) and remained there for 15 years, until ill health forced his retirement. His only significant treatise was the loosely written *A Lecture on Loxarthrus or Clubfoot* (1839). In addition, as professor of surgery he had published a *Syllabus of the Course of Lectures on the Principles and Practice of Surgery* (1843). Mütter remains most remembered for his extensive experience in many areas of plastic and reconstructive surgery.

Jonathan Mason Warren (1811-1867) was the son of John Collins Warren. After studying with his father and graduating from Harvard (1832), Warren received further education in both London and Paris. He returned to the United States in 1835 and immediately began to assist his father at the Massachusetts General Hospital. A decade later he was elected a visiting surgeon to that institution. Warren's only major text was *Surgical Observations, with Cases and Operations* (1867). He is particularly remembered for his extensive experience with rhinoplastic operations (1837) and cleft palate repair (1843).

Daniel Brainard (1812-1866) graduated from Jefferson Medical College (1834). He spent the next few years in practice in Chicago, but he eventually decided to travel to Paris in the hope of furthering his medical knowledge. On his return to America in 1841, Brainard again settled in Chicago, where he founded Rush Medical College and became its first professor of surgery. A versatile surgeon, Brainard reported on intravenous treatment of cancer (1852), did experimental work regarding snake bites (1854), and authored a short essay on the treatment of ununited fractures (1854).

John Homer Dix (1813-1884), a native of Boston, graduated from Jefferson Medical College in 1836. He soon returned to his native city and began to practice medicine, giving special attention to diseases of the eye. He became one of America's earliest ophthalmologists and a founder of the American Ophthalmological Society. His works included *Treatise on Strabismus, or Squinting and the New Mode of Treatment* (1841) and *Treatise upon the Nature and Treatment of Morbid Sensibility of the Retina, or Weakness of Sight* (1849).

Benjamin Lord Hill (1813-1871) was professor of surgery and later professor of anatomy at the Eclectic Medical Institute in Cincinnati. Eclecticism was a botanical movement that first flourished in the 1840s and was strongest in the Midwest. Hill's important *Lectures on the American Eclectic System of Surgery* (1850) was the first textbook of surgery to come out of this movement and the first nonallopathic surgical work to be published in America. By the early 1850s, like many other Eclectic physicians, Hill had turned his attention to homeopathic medicine. He became professor of obstetrics and diseases of women and, later, professor of surgery at Western Homeopathic College in Cleveland, where he authored *The Homeopathic Practice of Surgery, Together with Operative Surgery* (1855).

Frank Hastings Hamilton (1813-1886) received a classical undergraduate education at Union College in Schenectady, New York, and graduated with a degree in medicine from the medical department of the University of Pennsylvania in 1833. Hamilton served in a number of chairs of surgery, including the medical institute in Geneva, New York (1840), Buffalo Medical College (1846), Long Island College Hospital (1860), and Bellevue Hospital Medical College (1868). Hamilton was one of mid–nineteenth century America's most versatile surgeons and produced an influential body of written work. His major texts included *Monograph On Strabismus* (1845), *A Practical Treatise on Fractures and Dislocations* (1860), *A Practical Treatise on Military Surgery* (1861), *A Treatise on Military Surgery and Hygiene* (1865), *The Principles and Practice of Surgery* (1872), and *Fracture of the Patella*

(1880). He also edited the massive two-volume *Surgical Memoirs of the War of the Rebellion: Collected and Published by the United States Sanitary Commission* (1870-1871). Among Hamilton's most important journal articles were the earliest description of a crossleg pedicle flap as a treatment for chronic ulcer (1854) and a description of deformities after fractures (1855). His name is linked with a tropnic affection of the subcutaneous connective tissue marked by a circumscribed swelling that may become indurated and red but never suppurates and with a clinical test whereby in axillary dislocation of the shoulder a rod touches both the acromion process and the outer condyle of the humerus.

J. Marion Sims (1813-1883) was born in South Carolina and received his medical degree from Jefferson Medical College (1835). Through his efforts modern gynecological surgery began to unfold, and his international standing made him one of America's most prominent clinicians. He initially went into practice in Alabama, where he had much difficulty because of poor health and what he felt to be his inadequate medical knowledge. As years passed, Sims was able to attract a growing patient base by the success of his surgical operations, which was most evident in his influential article reporting the cure of a series of vesicovaginal fistulas (1852). Beginning in 1845, after repeated fruitless attempts at that procedure, Sims ultimately succeeded with the aid of silver sutures, improved exposure provided by the knee-chest position, and a vaginal speculum of his own design. For various reasons Sims became disillusioned with practicing in the South and resettled in New York City (1853). Within 2 years he had convinced several benefactors to assist him in establishing the Woman's Hospital in the State of New York. In that facility, where he was joined by such men as Edmund Peaslee (1814-1878), Thomas Addis Emmet (1828-1919), and Theodore Gaillard Thomas (1831-1903), many advances were made in gynecological surgery, such as those presented in Sims's treatise, *Silver Sutures in Surgery* (1858), and in his paper on a method of cervical amputation (1861). After the outbreak of the Civil War Sims, disgusted with the growing political strife, left the United States. His reception in Europe, especially in London and Paris, was overwhelming. He was America's first surgeon with a truly international reputation. So great was Sims's reputation that he was called to all parts of Europe to operate and to enter consultation for treatment of various maladies. Sims continued his writing while in Europe, authoring an important paper on vaginismus (1862) and his most impressive text, *Clinical Notes on Uterine Surgery* (1866). At the close of the Civil War Sims returned to New York City, where his reputation was becoming tarnished by his lengthy travels and by management difficulties at the Woman's Hospital. After the outbreak of the Franco-Prussian war, Sims again sailed for Europe and organized the Anglo-American Ambulance Corps, serving as surgeon-in-chief. From then until his death Sims lived alternately in Europe and in the United States, busily engaged in his clinical practice wherever he found himself. Sims served as president of the American Medical Association in 1876 and of the American Gynecological Society in 1880. While in Paris, he performed and reported the last of his important surgical operations, an unsuccessful cholecystotomy (1878). Sims's name is linked with a position used to facilitate vaginal examination, in which a woman lies on her side with her lower arm behind her back, and the thighs flexed, the upper one more than the lower; and with a double "duckbill" vaginal speculum.

James Wood (1813-1882) initially apprenticed with David Rogers (1799-1877), a little-known surgeon from New York City who performed an early excision of the superior maxillary bone (1824), and authored *Surgical Essays and Cases in Surgery* (1849). Wood received his medical degree from Castleton Medical College in Vermont (1834). He soon established a private practice in New York City and in 1847 was appointed to the Medical Board of Bellevue Hospital. Fourteen years later he was instrumental in establishing the Bellevue Hospital Medical College. Wood was the first professor of operative surgery and surgical pathology at the new school. He wrote little, but among his most important articles were those on phosphorus poisoning (1856) and carotid ligation (1859).

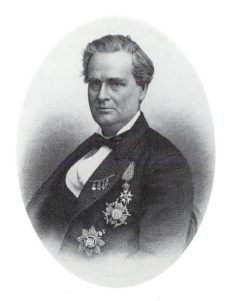

303. J. Marion Sims, perhaps the first great American gynecologist, wearing the decorations he had received from European royalty. A southerner working in New York, where he founded the Women's Hospital, Sims chose not to take sides during the American Civil War and practiced in London and Paris throughout the conflict. Thus he became the first American surgeon to develop a truly international reputation. *(Historical Collections, College of Physicians of Philadelphia.)*

Louis Bauer (1814-1898) was born in Prussia and settled in the United States in 1853. In the following year he founded the Orthopedic Institution of Brooklyn, the first orthopedic hospital in the New York City area. Eventually Bauer helped establish the German Dispensary, which later became the Long Island College Hospital and Medical School. His most important publications were *Lectures on Orthopedic Surgery* (1864) and *Lectures on Causes, Pathology, and Treatment of Joint Diseases* (1868).

Edmund Peaslee (1814-1878) is one of the forgotten heroes of American surgery. A graduate of Yale Medical School (1840), he pursued further studies in Europe and in 1843 was appointed lecturer and, later, professor of anatomy and surgery at Bowdoin College Medical School in Maine. In 1858 Peaslee moved to New York City, where he remained until his death. He became associated with Sims at the Woman's Hospital and also held the chair of gynecology at the Bellevue Hospital Medical College. Peaslee had one of the largest practices in the United States and was particularly interested in ovarian pathology. He wrote the influential *Ovarian Tumors: Their Pathology, Diagnosis, and Treatment, Especially by Ovariotomy* (1872).

Henry Smith (1815-1890) graduated from the University of Pennsylvania in 1837, after which he studied in London and Paris. Smith was the son-in-law of William Horner and eventually succeeded William Gibson as professor of surgery at his alma mater (1855). Among Smith's many texts were *Minor Surgery* (1843), *Anatomical Atlas* (1844), *A System of Operative Surgery: Based upon the Practice of Surgeons in the United States* (1852), *Syllabus of the Lectures on the Principles and Practice of Surgery* (1855), *A Treatise on the Practice of Surgery* (1856), and the two-volume *The Principles and Practice of Surgery, Embracing Minor and Operation Surgery* (1863). The latter work is especially important to surgical historians, since it contains a detailed history of surgery in the United States and a bibliography of American works on surgery from 1783 to 1860.

Henry Bigelow (1818-1890), a native of Boston, obtained his medical degree from Harvard (1841) and spent 3 years in Europe, mostly in Paris. In 1845 he was appointed instructor of surgery at the Tremont Street Medical School in his native city. In the following year he was elected surgeon to the Massachusetts General Hospital. In 1849 the two Harvard chairs of surgery and clinical surgery that had been previously held by Warren and Hayward were united, and Bigelow was named professor of surgery. Bigelow was a major contributor to the advancement of American medicine, especially in orthopedic surgery. In 1845 he wrote the first comprehensive monograph on orthopedic surgery in the United States, *Manual of Orthopedic Surgery* (1845). Seven years later Bigelow became the first American surgeon to excise the head of the femur. In his classic treatise, *The Mechanism of Dislocation and Fracture of the Hip with the Reduction of the Dislocation by the Flexion Method* (1869), he described in detail the structure and function of the accessory Y, or iliofemoral, ligament of the acetabulum, which clarified the pathology of dislocation of the hip. In an 1875 paper he identified the calcar femorale, which is a bony spur springing from the underside of the neck of the femur above and anterior to the lesser trochanter, which adds strength to this portion of the bone. Bigelow provided the world with its first detailed understanding of ether anesthesia in his important papers on insensibility during surgical operations produced by ether inhalation (1846). He followed these with another group of articles discussing the discovery of ether and chloroform and their physiological effects (1848). Of Bigelow's many contributions to American surgery, his improvement of the lithotrite used for crushing bladder stones and development of a large-caliber evacuation tube to effectively remove bladder debris during the operation were considered major advances (1878).

David Prince (1816-1889) received his medical education at the Medical College of Ohio (1838), where his mentor was Reuben Mussey. From 1840 to 1843 Prince practiced in Illinois, but he eventually left to accept the chair of anatomy and surgery at the newly created medical department of Illinois College. After 5 years he accepted the professorship of surgery at the St. Louis Medical College in Missouri. Prince resigned this professorship in 1852 and settled in

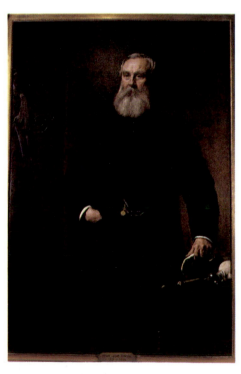

304. Henry Jacob Bigelow. *(Boston Medical Library.)*

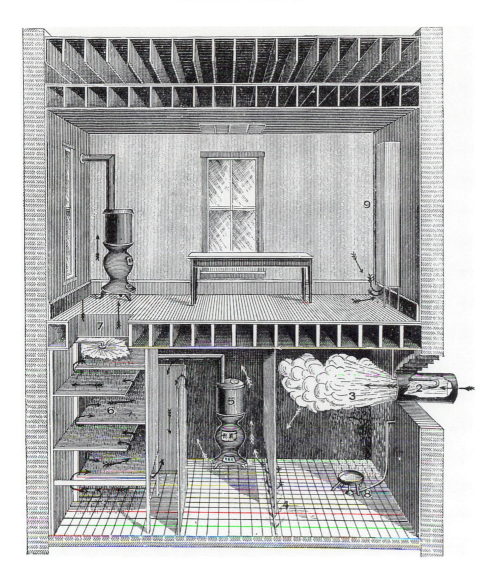

305. After Lister's introduction of antisepsis, the presence of bacteria in the air was thought to be a major source of infections in the operating room. Rather than limit himself to the use of carbolic acid mist in the operating room, as prescribed by Lister, David Prince developed in 1885 an elaborate system for purifying operating-room air. In Prince's system, which was installed in his private hospital in Jacksonville, Illinois, the air was taken into the operating room through a steam jet, which brought the air into a hot-air room, through a spray of water, through a series of soaked muslin sheets, and finally into the stove-heated operating room. (From Transactions of the American Surgical Association, *vol 3, pp 390-395, 1885.*)

Jacksonville, Illinois, where he spent the remainder of his life in the practice of general medicine and surgery. Prince's most important works were *Orthopedics: A Systematic Treatise upon the Prevention and Correction of Deformities* (1866) and *Plastics and Orthopedics* (1871).

William Byford (1817-1890) was a founder of the American Gynecological Society. Known primarily as a gynecologist, he received his medical education from the Medical College of Ohio (1845). From 1859 to 1879 Byford was on the faculty of the Chicago Medical College, where he served as professor of obstetrics and diseases of women. From 1870 to 1890 he also served on the gynecology faculty of Rush Medical College. His two most important texts were *A Treatise on the Chronic Inflammation and Displacement of the Unimpregnated Uterus* (1864) and *The Practice of Medicine and Surgery, Applied to the Diseases and Accidents Incident to Women* (1865).

John Carnochan (1817-1887), a student of Valentine Mott, graduated from the College of Physicians and Surgeons in New York City (1836). He spent most of his professional career in New York, where he was surgeon-in-chief to the State Emigrant Hospital on Ward's Island, then the largest hospital in the United States. He also served as professor of surgery at the New York Medical College. Carnochan was a daring operator who excised the entire mandible (1852) and in 1858 reported the first excision of the superior maxillary nerve for the treatment of facial neuralgia. His book-length works were *A Treatise on the Etiology, Pathology and Treatment of Congenital Dislocations of the Head of the Femur* (1850) and *Contributions to Operative Surgery, and Surgical Pathology* (1877).

David Hayes Agnew (1818-1892) was a graduate of the University of Pennsylvania (1838). After establishing a general medical and surgical practice, he became head of the Philadelphia School of Anatomy (1852). In 1863 Agnew left that position to become demonstrator of anatomy at his alma mater. Eight years later he was named professor of surgery. Agnew was a highly skilled anatomist and an unusually dexterous surgeon who acquired immense practical experience in all forms of surgical diseases. His life's work was embodied in his massive three-volume *Principles and Practice of Surgery* (1878-1883), which was translated into Japanese in 1888. His other important text was *Lacerations of the Female Perineum; and Vesico-Vaginal Fistula; Their History and Treatment* (1873). Agnew also authored the lengthy *History and Reminiscences of the Philadelphia Almshouse and Philadelphia Hospital* (1890).

Charles Pope (1818-1870) was a graduate of the University of Pennsylvania (1839). He served as professor of surgery at the St. Louis Medical College and as president of the American Medical Association (1853). He wrote little of consequence.

George Blackman (1819-1871) graduated with a degree in medicine from the College of Physicians and Surgeons in New York City (1840). He spent many years studying in London and Paris and on his return to America was appointed professor of surgery at the Medical College of Ohio. He made voluminous contributions to the periodical literature, but his only monograph, jointly authored with Charles Tripler (1806-1866), was *Handbook for the Military Surgeon* (1861).

Buckminster Brown (1819-1891) was the son of John Brown and the grandson of John Collins Warren. He followed in his father's footsteps by assisting him in the practice of orthopedic surgery at the Boston Orthopedic Institution. Buckminster Brown left a considerable sum of money to found the first professorship of orthopedic surgery at Harvard Medical School. He wrote little of consequence, although his short pamphlet, *Cases of Orthopedic Surgery* (1868), represents the first American orthopedic text to be illustrated with actual photographs.

William Van Buren (1819-1883) was a graduate of the University of Pennsylvania (1840). While studying in Paris, he made the acquaintance of Valentine Mott, who was then on an extended sojourn in Europe. In 1845, after having served as an assistant surgeon in the United States Army, Van Buren joined Mott in New York City as his prosector. With his surgical skills well honed at the side of Mott, who had since become his father-in-law, Van Buren was named to the chair of anatomy at the University of New York. In 1866, he was elected professor of surgery for the newly established department of diseases of the genitourinary system at the Bellevue Hospital Medical College. Van Buren was an extremely versatile surgeon who wrote *Contributions to Practical Surgery* (1865), *Lectures upon Diseases of the Rectum* (1870), *A Practical Treatise on the Surgical Diseases of the Genito-Urinary Organs* (1874), and *Lectures on the Principles of Surgery* (1884). Van Buren is eponymically linked with fibrous cavernitis of the penis.

Lewis Sayre (1820-1900) graduated from the College of Physicians and Surgeons of New York City in 1842. In the same year, he was appointed prosector to the chair of surgery at his alma mater, a position he held until 1852. In 1853 Sayre was appointed one of the visiting surgeons to Bellevue Hospital, and in 1861 he was one of the founders of the Bellevue Hospital Medical College. At his suggestion a professorship of orthopedic surgery was established, which was subsequently assigned to him. He held this position until 1897, when ill health forced him to resign. Sayre is particularly remembered for reporting the first successful resection of a hip for ankylosis in the United States (1855). Undoubtedly his greatest original contribution to orthopedic surgery was the use of plaster-of-paris as a support for the spinal column in scoliosis and tuberculosis of the spine (1877). Sayre's name is linked with a plaster-of-paris jacket applied while the patient is suspended by the head and axillae and with a tripod derrick suspension apparatus with rope and pulley for head traction during the application of a plaster-of-paris jacket. Among Sayre's surgical textbooks were *A Practical Manual of the Treatment of Club Foot* (1869), *Lectures on Orthopedic Surgery and Diseases of the Joints* (1876), and *Spinal Disease and Spinal Curvature, Their Treatment by Suspension and the Use of the Plaster-of-Paris Bandage* (1877). The latter monograph, a landmark in American medical photography, is the first surgical textbook known to contain actual mounted photographs.

306. Among the first albumin photographic prints used to illustrate an American surgical textbook, these portraits of a 10-year-old girl with Pott's disease of the cervical and upper dorsal vertebrae appear in Lewis Sayre's *Spinal Disease and Spinal Curvature, Their Treatment by Suspension and the Use of the Plaster of Paris Bandage* (1877). When first examined by Sayre in Guy's Hospital, London, the girl could neither sit nor stand except by bearing her weight upon her hands. After placement of a plaster-of-paris bandage she was able to ambulate alone. *(From the author's collection.)*

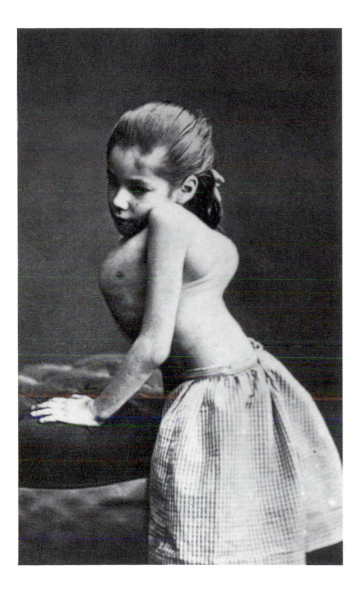

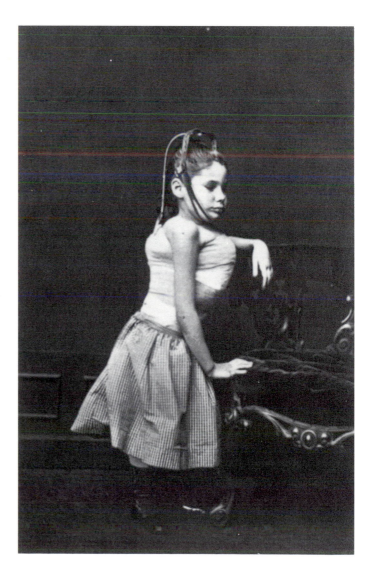

477

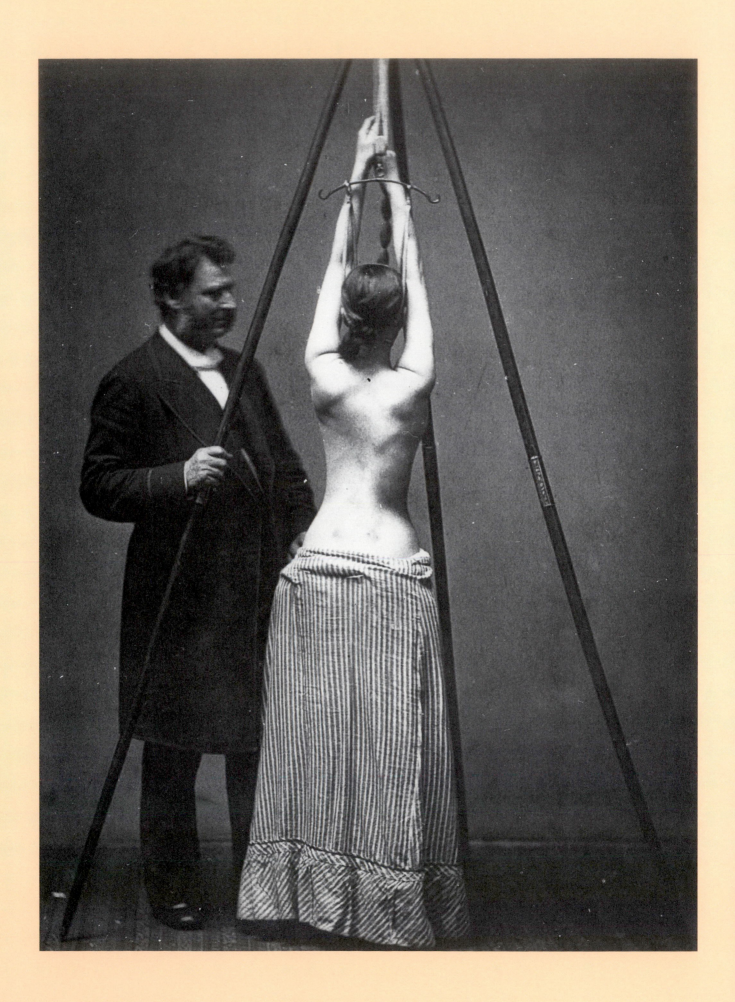

Laurence Turnbull (1821-1900) was a native of Scotland who graduated from Jefferson Medical College (1845). In 1857 Turnbull was elected one of the physicians for the ear and eye at the Western Clinical Infirmary in Philadelphia. He spent most of 1859 in Europe to obtain further training in otology and ophthalmology. In 1878 Turnbull was appointed aural surgeon at the Jefferson Hospital. His two texts on anesthesia, *The Advantages and Accidents of Artificial Anesthesia* (1878) and *The New Local Anaesthetic; Hydrochlorate of Cocaine,* were the first book-length works written by an American surgeon to discuss anesthesia and its applications in depth. He also authored *A Clinical Manual of the Diseases of the Ear* (1872) and *Imperfect Hearing and the Hygiene of the Ear* (1881).

Henry Williams (1821-1895) is one of America's best-known early ophthalmologists. He was a graduate of Harvard (1849) and became interested in ophthalmological surgery while studying in Europe. Williams established a private practice in Boston (1850), and eventually he was appointed first professor of ophthalmology at his alma mater. He was a founder of the American Ophthalmological Society (1864) and served as its president from 1868 to 1875. His chief texts were *A Practical Guide to the Study of the Diseases of the Eye* (1862), *Recent Advances in Ophthalmic Science* (1866), *Our Eyes and How to Take Care of Them* (1871), and *The Diagnosis and Treatment of the Diseases of the Eye* (1882).

Daniel Ayres (1822-1892) was a graduate of the medical department of the University of the City of New York (1845). He settled in Brooklyn, where he spent his entire professional life. Ayres was a founder of the Long Island College Hospital and served as professor of clinical surgery and surgical pathology. He authored no textbooks but did report the first successful repair in the United States of an exstrophy of the bladder in women (1859).

Edward Franklin (1822-1885) is one of the least known but most prolific of nineteenth-century American surgeons. Although trained by Valentine Mott, he became an adherent of homeopathic medicine and was appointed professor of surgery at Hahnemann Medical College in Chicago in 1862. Three years later he was nominated professor of surgery at the Homeopathic Medical College of Missouri. There he authored his two-volume *The Science and Art of Surgery, Embracing Minor and Operative Surgery* (1867-1873). The volumes were huge and contained an interesting general descriptive history of surgery, with a specific section on surgery in the United States. Franklin soon transferred to the surgical chair at the Homeopathic College of the University of Michigan, where he wrote *The Homoeopathic Treatment of Spinal Curvatures According to the New Principle* (1878), *A Complete Minor Surgery* (1882), *The Practitioner's and Student's Manual of the Science of Surgery* (1882), and *A Manual of Venereal Diseases* (1883).

Moses Gunn (1822-1887) received his medical degree from the Geneva Medical College in 1846. He immediately moved to Ann Arbor, Michigan, where he established a private practice and began to lecture on anatomy. Within 10 years he held the chair of anatomy and surgery at the University of Michigan. In 1867 Gunn accepted the chair of surgery at Rush Medical College. He wrote little of major consequence.

Stephen Smith (1823-1922), a native of upstate New York, received his medical education at the College of Physicians and Surgeons in New York City (1850). He served on the resident staff of Bellevue Hospital, and by 1855 he was elected one of the attending surgeons at that institution. In 1861 Smith was one of the founders of the Bellevue Hospital Medical College, and he served as professor of surgery from 1861 to 1865. He eventually transferred to the chair of anatomy, where he remained until 1874, when he became professor of clinical surgery in the medical department of New York University. Interestingly, Smith did not gain his place in American medical history because of his career as a surgeon. Instead, Smith is remembered as a pioneer public health officer and sanitary reformer. He was New York City's commissioner of health from 1868 to 1875 and through this position helped found the American Public Health Association. Smith's major written works were the *Hand-Book of Surgical Operations* (1862) and the *Manual of the Principles and Practice of Operative Surgery* (1879). In addition to his clinical contributions, Smith is also known for his remarkable

307. *Facing page,* Portrait of the orthopedic surgeon Lewis Sayre with a young woman patient, who is in his self-suspension device for treatment of lateral curvature of the spine. During the nineteenth century it was not unusual for physicians or surgeons to pose with their patients in illustrations that accompanied serious medical monographs. From Sayre's *Spinal Disease and Spinal Curvature. . . .* (1877). *(From the author's collection.)*

essay on the evolution of American surgery, which appeared in 1906 as the first chapter in the eight-volume *American Practice of Surgery* written by Joseph Bryant (1845-1914) and Albert Buck (1842-1922).

Edmund Andrews (1824-1904) was a graduate of the University of Michigan in 1852. In 1853 he founded the *Peninsular Journal of Medical and Collateral Sciences*. Most of his professional career was spent at Chicago Medical College and at Northwestern University, where he was professor of clinical surgery. He pioneered and reported on the use of an oxygen–nitrous oxide mixture as an anesthetic agent (1868).

John Hodgen (1826-1882) received his medical degree from Missouri Medical College in 1848. He began his career at his alma mater as a demonstrator of anatomy. During the Civil War Hodgen joined the faculty of the St. Louis Medical College, where he served as dean and professor of surgical anatomy. Among his most memorable accomplishments was the invention of a wire suspension device that offered a supportive role for traction in fractures of the middle or lower end of the femur.

Nathan Bozeman (1825-1905) was a colorful nineteenth-century American surgeon. He received his medical degree from the University of Louisville (1848). He was soon professionally associated with Sims in Alabama, and the relationship led to one of the most bitter rivalries in American medicine. Sims would later claim that Bozeman stole his concepts for repair of vesicovaginal fistula; Bozeman would later trumpet his "button-suture" as having nothing to do with Sims's work (1853). After the Civil War Bozeman moved to New York City, where he practiced for the remainder of his life. From 1878 to 1889 Bozeman was on the surgical staff of the Woman's Hospital of the State of New York. During those years he specialized in ureteral, kidney, and bladder surgery. Among the most difficult surgical conditions to treat was chronic pyelitis caused by vesical and fecal fistulas. Bozeman used all his talents in the treatment of this complication by means of catheterization of the ureter through a vesicovaginal opening (1887 and 1888). Because of those efforts his name is linked with a slightly curved double-current uterine catheter with several openings at the tip; the operation of hysterocystocleisis for uterovaginal fistula, in which the cervix is attached to the bladder, opening into its cavity; the knee-elbow position; and a bivalve vaginal speculum in which the long blades remain parallel when separated so that the vagina is evenly dilated.

Andrew Howe (1825-1892) was considered the foremost surgeon of eclectic medicine in nineteenth-century America. He received his medical education from Worcester Medical Institute in Massachusetts (1855). In 1861 Howe was named to the chair of surgery at the Eclectic Medical Institute in Cincinnati. He was quite a prolific writer, and the only nineteenth century American surgeon to have written books about four different specialties: *A Practical and Systematic Treatise on Fractures and Dislocations* (1870), *Manual of Eye Surgery* (1874), *The Art and Science of Surgery* (1879), and *Operative Gynecology* (1890).

Fessenden Nott Otis (1825-1900) obtained his undergraduate education at Union College in Schenectady, New York (1849). He received his medical degree from New York Medical College in 1852. Otis was in private practice in New York City from 1862 to 1871. From 1871 to 1890 he served as professor of genitourinary and venereal diseases at his alma mater. Among his treatises were *Stricture of the Male Urethra, Its Radical Cure* (1878), *Practical Clinical Lessons on Syphilis and the Genitourinary Diseases* (1883), and *The Male Urethra, Its Diseases and Reflexes* (1888). Otis is best remembered for his paper describing attempts to use local anesthesia in urological surgery (1884).

Robert Kinloch (1826-1891) was a native of Charleston, South Carolina, and graduated with a degree in medicine from the University of Pennsylvania (1848). He pursued further education in Edinburgh, London, and Paris. After the Civil War Kinloch became professor of surgery at the Medical College of South Carolina. He was among the most prominent surgeons in the South, although he wrote no major texts. His claim to distinction concerned numerous surgical feats, including being the first to treat fractures of the jaw by wiring the fragments together (1859).

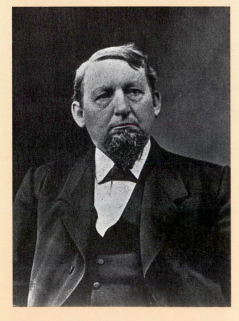

308. Andrew Howe. *(From the author's collection.)*

Claudius Mastin (1826-1898) spent most of his professional life in Mobile, Alabama, after his graduation from the University of Pennsylvania (1849). He founded the American Association of Genito-Urinary Surgeons and served as president of the American Surgical Association (1890). He wrote only for the periodical literature; his most important paper described the use of metallic sutures to ligate aneurysmal arteries (1866). Mastin was the nephew of Henry Levert, who performed America's first published series of experiments on the use of metallic sutures in surgery as part of his graduation thesis for the University of Pennsylvania (1829).

Emil Noeggerath (1827-1895) received his medical education in Bonn, Germany (1852). Five years later he emigrated to the United States, where he eventually began a practice in gynecology in New York City. Noeggerath was appointed professor of obstetrics and diseases of women at the New York Medical College. In 1886, because of poor health, he returned permanently to Germany. Noeggerath's most important treatise was *Die Latente Gonorrhoe Im Weiblichen Geschlecht* (1872), in which he was the first to point out the late effects of gonorrhea in women, particularly its role in the production of sterility. In 1858 he authored a paper that reintroduced epicystotomy, or suprapubic cystotomy, to the American surgeon.

Charles Fayette Taylor (1827-1899) was one of America's preeminent orthopedic surgeons. He received his medical degree from the University of Vermont (1856), after which he studied in London. There Taylor was introduced to the concept of kinesipathy, or the "Swedish movement" system of Per Henrik Ling (1776-1839). On returning to the United States, Taylor introduced this system to American surgeons, especially at his New York Orthopedic Dispensary and Hospital. His texts were *Theory and Practice of the Movement-Cure* (1861), *Infantile Paralysis, and Its Attendant Deformities* (1864), and *On the Mechanical Treatment of Disease of the Hip-Joint* (1873).

Robert Battey (1828-1895) was a native of Augusta, Georgia, and received his medical education at Jefferson Medical College in 1857. He commenced practice in that year in Rome, Georgia, where he would remain continuously, except between 1859 and 1860, when he studied in Paris, and from 1872 to 1875, when he was professor of obstetrics at the Atlanta Medical College. Among Battey's many honors was the presidency of the American Gynecological Society (1888). His name remains linked with a surgical operation in which normal ovaries are removed to induce an artificial menopause for the cure of uterine fibroids and other ill-defined conditions. It was his conviction that to excise the ovaries, whether diseased or not, would do away with disturbances of menstruation accompanied by various nervous manifestations (such as severe headaches, pelvic pain, and hysteroepileptic attacks). Battey thus contributed to the development of pelvic and abdominal surgery and helped establish both the functional relationship between the ovaries and menstruation and the beginnings of surgical endocrinology. Although Battey never authored a major surgical text, he contributed numerous articles to the surgical literature, particularly regarding his operation (1872).

Thomas Addis Emmet (1828-1919) was one of the great pioneers of modern American gynecology. He was born at the University of Virginia, where his father, John Emmet (1797-1842), was professor of chemistry and materia medica. Emmet received his medical degree from Jefferson Medical College in 1850. He moved to New York, where he became a resident physician at the Emigrant Refuge Hospital on Ward's Island. In 1855 Emmet first met Sims, who invited his soon-to-be protégé to join the staff at the Woman's Hospital. He remained Sims's assistant for 5 years. Sims then departed for Europe, and the 33-year-old Emmet was named surgeon-in-chief. He stayed in that position through 1872, when his one-man autocratic rule was challenged by the hospital's board of governors. Although removed as chief, Emmet retained his connection with the institution as a visiting surgeon through 1902. He was a founder of the American Gynecological Society and later served as its president (1882). Emmet, an extremely prolific writer, authored important papers on the treatment of

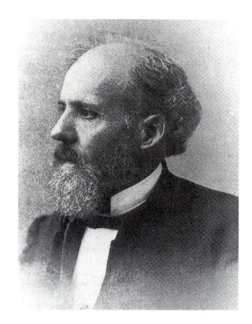

309. Robert Battey. *(From the author's collection.)*

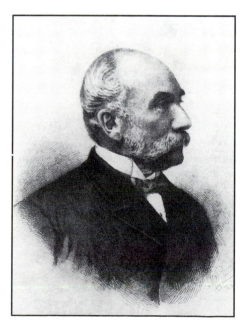

310. Thomas Addis Emmet. *(From the author's collection.)*

481

dysmenorrhoea and sterility (1865), cervical surgery (1869), chronic cystitis (1872), and repair of perineal lacerations via perineorrhaphy (1884). His treatises included *Vesico-Vaginal Fistula from Parturition and Other Causes* (1868) and *The Principles and Practice of Gynaecology* (1879).

Edward Warren (1828-1893) was one of the most flamboyant nineteenth-century American surgeons. An 1851 graduate of Jefferson Medical College, he served as professor of surgery at two small proprietary medical schools in Baltimore. In 1873 he left the United States for the Middle East, where he became chief surgeon of the general staff of the Khedive of Egypt. From 1875 to 1893 Warren practiced medicine and surgery in Paris. His most important written work was *An Epitome of Practical Surgery for Field and Hospital* (1863), which he authored while in the service of the Confederate army.

Levi Cooper Lane (1833-1902) received his undergraduate education at Union College in Schenectady, New York. In 1851, he obtained his medical degree from Jefferson Medical College. His uncle was the renowned San Francisco surgeon Elias Cooper (1822-1862), who founded the first medical college on the Pacific Coast. Lane joined his uncle at the Cooper Medical College in San Francisco and served as professor of surgery. His most important text was *The Surgery of the Head and Neck* (1896), the first American work on the topic.

Emmeline Cleveland (1829-1878) is one of the few women in nineteenth-century America to achieve prominence as a surgeon. She was an 1855 graduate of the Woman's Medical College of Pennsylvania, where she later was professor of obstetrics and diseases of women (1862-1878). In 1875 Cleveland performed an ovariotomy and became the first woman known to complete that operation.

Cornelius Rea Agnew (1830-1888) graduated from the College of Physicians and Surgeons in New York City (1852). He was eventually appointed surgeon at the New York Eye Infirmary and served as clinical professor of diseases of the eye and ear at his alma mater. His most important paper described an operation for divergent strabismus (1866). Agnew's name is linked with an incision used to release pus in the lacrimal sac in acute phlegmonous dacryocystitis.

Julian John Chisolm (1830-1903) was a key figure in the surgical hierarchy of the Confederate army. He studied at the Medical College of South Carolina (1850) and in Europe. Most of his early career was devoted to general surgery; before the Civil War Chisolm served as professor of surgery at his alma mater. During the conflict he authored *A Manual of Military Surgery, for the Use of Surgeons in the Confederate Army* (1861). At the conclusion of hostilities, Chisolm resumed practice in Charleston, South Carolina. However, in 1869, worsening financial difficulties forced him to move to Baltimore, where he was appointed professor of operative surgery and diseases of the eye and ear at the University of Maryland.

Henry Sands (1830-1888) received his medical degree from the College of Physicians and Surgeons in New York City (1854). After further studies in Paris Sands became professor of anatomy and then of surgery at his alma mater. He was also on the staff of the Bellevue, New York, and Roosevelt Hospitals. Sands was a "prime mover" in America for more aggressive surgical treatment of appendicitis. His 1880 paper detailed plans for opening appendiceal abscesses earlier than had been previously advocated. His other important contribution to the periodical literature concerned a laryngectomy for papillomas (1865).

David Cheever (1831-1915) was a graduate of Harvard Medical School (1854) who also obtained additional medical training in Europe. He was made visiting surgeon of the Boston City Hospital in 1864 and concurrently joined the faculty of his alma mater. In 1875 Cheever was elected professor of clinical surgery, and 7 years later he succeeded Henry Bigelow as professor of surgery. Cheever remained a dominant figure at Harvard after his retirement from active teaching (1893). Cheever was president of the American Surgical Association in 1889. His only textbook was *Lectures on Surgery* (1894).

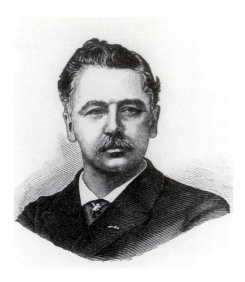

311. Edward Warren. *(From the author's collection.)*

Theodore Gaillard Thomas (1831-1903) was one of nineteenth-century America's most prominent gynecological surgeons. He received his medical degree from the Medical College of South Carolina in 1852 and spent the next 3 years in Dublin and Paris. When he returned to the United States, Thomas commenced practice in New York City. He was named professor of obstetrics and the diseases of women (1863-1879) and professor of gynecology (1879-1890) at the College of Physicians and Surgeons. Thomas became attending surgeon to the Woman's Hospital in 1872, where he completed most of his clinical work. In 1868 he authored *A Practical Treatise on the Diseases of Women,* which was considered the most authoritative text of its day. Thomas is also remembered for his journal articles concerning the first reported vaginal ovariotomy (1870) and an extraperitoneal cesarean section (1871). He also wrote an interesting chapter on the history of American obstetrics and gynecology for Edward Clarke's (1820-1877) *A Century of American Medicine, 1776-1876* (1876).

John Gouley (1832-1920) was one of America's earliest and most renowned genitourinary specialists. He received his medical degree from the College of Physicians and Surgeons in New York City (1853). Most of his professional life was spent in New York City, where early in his career he was an assistant to Van Buren. In 1866 Gouley was named professor of clinical surgery and genitourinary diseases at the University of the City of New York. From 1876 to his retirement he was professor of diseases of the genitourinary system. His most prominent texts were *Diseases of the Urinary Organs* (1873), *Diseases of the Urinary Apparatus; Phlegmasic Affections* (1892), and *Surgery of Genito-Urinary Organs* (1907). Gouley is eponymically linked with a solid, curved catheter used to pass through a urethral stricture.

Henry Noyes (1832-1900) was professor of ophthalmology and otology at Bellevue Hospital Medical College and surgeon at the New York Eye and Ear Infirmary. He studied at the College of Physicians and Surgeons (1855) and entered private practice in 1859. Noyes wielded great influence in American ophthalmology, being one of the founders of the American Ophthalmological Society (1864) and serving as president from 1878 to 1884. He was among the earliest in America to understand the relationship between retinitis and glycosuria (1869) and reported on the use of cocaine as a local anesthetic in eye operations (1884). Noyes's texts included *Diagnosis of Those Diseases of the Eye Which Can Be Seen without the Ophthalmoscope* (1876), *A Treatise on Diseases of the Eye* (1881), and *A Textbook on Diseases of the Eye* (1890).

John Packard (1832-1907) was an 1853 graduate of the University of Pennsylvania. He never held an academic position but was on the surgical staff of the Episcopal Hospital and other Philadelphia institutions. He was the father of the well-known surgical historian Francis Randolph Packard (1870-1950). Among Packard's writings were *A Manual of Minor Surgery* (1863), *Lectures on Inflammation* (1865), and *A Handbook of Operative Surgery* (1870).

William Tod Helmuth (1833-1902) was the most prominent homeopathic surgeon of his era. Because homeopathic medicine vanished from the American scene after allopathic medicine came to the forefront, he remains little known. At the age of 22 years, after studying with his uncle (William S. Helmuth [1801-1880], professor of the theory and practice of medicine in the Homoeopathic Medical College of Pennsylvania), Helmuth was made professor of anatomy at the Homoeopathic Medical College in Philadelphia. At that early stage of his career he authored his first text, *Surgery and Its Adaptation into Homeopathic Practice* (1855). In 1858 Helmuth moved to St. Louis, where he founded the Homeopathic Medical College of Missouri, served as professor of surgery, and completed *A Treatise on Diphtheria* (1862). In 1870 Helmuth accepted an offer to assume the chair of surgery at the New York Homoeopathic Medical College and Flower Hospital. Three years later he authored *A System of Surgery* (1873). Helmuth was a vigorous defender of antiseptic and aseptic surgical procedures; as early as 1875 he was performing operations using antiseptic technique.

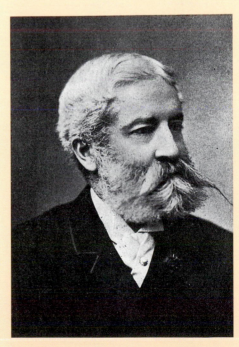

312. William Tod Helmuth. *(From the author's collection.)*

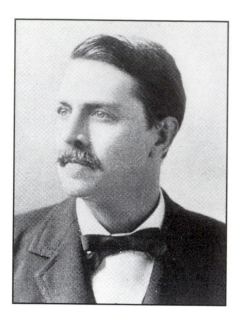

313. Hunter Holmes McGuire. *(From the author's collection.)*

Hunter Holmes McGuire (1835-1900) achieved most of his fame quite early in life, as medical director of the Army of the Shenandoah under the command of Stonewall Jackson (1824-1863). At the end of hostilities, McGuire was nominated to the chair of surgery at the Medical College of Virginia. Among his many honors were the presidencies of the American Surgical Association (1886) and the American Medical Association (1893). He wrote no major texts but did report the first known attempt in America to ligate the abdominal aorta for aneurysmal disease (1868).

Thomas Morton (1835-1903) graduated from the University of Pennsylvania (1856) and became professor of clinical and operative surgery at the Philadelphia Polyclinic. He was also on staff at the Pennsylvania Hospital and authored *Surgery in the Pennsylvania Hospital* (1880). This lengthy text remains unique in American surgical history because it provided an in-depth look at colonial and early to mid–nineteenth century surgical practices. Morton is also remembered for a number of important clinical contributions, including a description of neuralgia of an interdigital nerve of the foot (1876) and one of the earliest correct preoperative diagnoses of appendicitis (1887).

Oscar Allis (1836-1931) received his medical degree from Jefferson Medical College (1866). He soon became one of the original staff surgeons at the Presbyterian Hospital in Philadelphia. Allis is eponymically remembered for a clinical sign in fracture of the neck of the femur in which the trochanter rides up and relaxes the fascia lata so that a finger can be sunk deeply between the great trochanter and the iliac crest. Allis's interest in hip disease was further evidenced when he won the Samuel Gross prize from the Philadelphia Academy of Surgery for *An Inquiry into the Difficulties Encountered in the Reduction of Dislocations of the Hip* (1896). Allis is most remembered for his description of a surgical clamp that remains part of the modern surgeon's armamentarium.

Louis Elsberg (1836-1885), one of the preeminent figures in American laryngology, graduated from Jefferson Medical College (1857) and later founded and served as the first president of the American Laryngological Association. For 17 years Elsberg was professor of laryngology at the University Medical College in New York City. He was also editor of the short-lived *American Archives of Laryngology* (1880-1884). His best known treatises were *Laryngoscopal Surgery* (1866) and *The Throat and Its Functions* (1880).

John Homans (1836-1903) was a pioneer ovariotomist who graduated from Harvard Medical School in 1862. After serving in the Civil War, he returned to Boston and began to practice at a number of hospitals. Homans's only academic appointment was as clinical instructor in the diagnosis and treatment of ovarian tumors at his alma mater. He did little writing; his most important work was a monograph, *Three Hundred and Eighty-Four Laparotomies for Various Diseases* (1887). His son was John Homans (1877-1954), who described a clinical sign of slight pain at the back of the knee or calf when the ankle is forcibly dorsiflexed, indicating an incipient or established thrombosis in the veins of the leg.

Beriah Watson (1836-1892) received his medical degree from New York University in 1861. After the Civil War he settled in Jersey City, where he was instrumental in the formation of St. Francis and Christ Hospitals. Although Watson is little known, he was one of the earliest advocates of Lister's techniques in the United States. His massive *Treatise on Amputations of the Extremities and Their Complications* (1882), was dedicated to Lister and actually predated Arpad Gerster's textbook on antiseptic surgery. Watson performed some of the most unique and important surgical experimentation of nineteenth-century American surgeons, and he published a paper on cardiac sensitivity to chloroform anesthesia (1887) and a monograph, *An Experimental Study of Lesions Arising from Severe Concussions* (1890).

Samuel Weissell Gross (1837-1889), the son of Samuel Gross, was an important Philadelphia surgeon in his own right. Gross graduated from Jefferson Medical College in 1857. He served on the surgical faculty of his alma mater and is well known for writing the first comprehensive report on bone sarcoma (1879). His two major texts were *A Practical Treatise on Tumors of the Mammary Glands* (1880) and *A Practical Treatise on Impotence, Sterility, and Allied Disorders of the Male Sexual Organs* (1881). After his early death, Gross's widow married William Osler (1849-1919).

William Williams Keen (1837-1932), a brilliant, innovative surgeon, gained worldwide recognition for a number of formidable surgical operations. He received his medical education at Jefferson Medical College (1862) and accomplished postgraduate studies in Berlin and Paris. During the Civil War Keen was an assistant surgeon in the United States Army and worked with Silas Weir Mitchell (1829-1914) at a special hospital for neurological casualties in Philadelphia. A classic monograph, *Gunshot Wounds and Other Injuries of Nerves* (1864), was derived from their collaborative efforts. This work provided the first detailed study of traumatic neuroses and introduced the concept of causalgia. From 1866 to 1875 Keen taught pathological anatomy at his alma mater. He eventually was appointed professor of surgery at Women's Medical College (1884), and 5 years later he succeeded Samuel Weissel Gross as professor of surgery at Jefferson. In 1892 Keen and James White (1850-1916) jointly edited the impressive *American Text-Book of Surgery,* an important work because of its strong advocacy of listerian principles and because it was the first surgical text written by multiple contributors in which only American surgeons were involved. Keen, an exceptionally prolific writer, also authored *The Surgical Complications and Sequels of Typhoid Fever* (1898) and the eight-volume *Surgery, Its Principles and Practice* (1906-1921). The latter work became the "clinical bible" of American surgeons in the first few decades of the twentieth century. Keen's contributions to the periodical literature were also legendary and included the description of a clinical sign of increased width at the malleoli in Pott's fracture of the fibula (1872). Keen remains particularly renowned as one of the major contributors to early neurological surgery. He performed a successful resection of a brain tumor (1888) and the first tapping of the lateral cerebral ventricles (1888). He used a linear craniotomy incision (1891), and he removed the trigeminal ganglion for the treatment of tic douloureux (1894). Among his many other operative accomplishments, Keen will long be eponymically linked with a procedure for the treatment of torticollis in which sections of the posterior branches of the spinal nerves to the affected muscles and the spinal accessory nerve itself are removed. Keen assisted Joseph Bryant in the performance of a "secret" operation on President Grover Cleveland (1837-1908) for sarcoma of the left upper jaw in 1893. Keen is also recognized as a historian, having written the well-known *Sketch of the Early History of Practical Anatomy* (1874). Among his many honors were the presidencies of the American Surgical Association (1899) and the American Medical Association (1900). In 1900 he was in the first group of American surgeons to be elected to honorary fellowship in the Royal College of Surgeons of England. Although he retired from active practice in 1907, Keen remained intellectually vigorous. In 1917 he wrote a monograph, *The Treatment of War Wounds,* which detailed the development and progress of surgery during World War I. In addition, he was an effective spokesman for various causes, advocating, for example, the theory of evolution and the importance of animal experimentation in the progress of biomedical research. During his later years Keen authored *Animal Experimentation and Medical Progress* (1914), *Medical Research and Human Welfare* (1917), *I Believe in God and Evolution* (1922), and *Everlasting Life: A Creed and a Speculation* (1924). A kind, compassionate person with deep spiritual beliefs, Keen wrote a 511-page history of the Baptist church entitled *The Bicentennial Celebration of the Founding of the First Baptist Church of the City of Philadelphia* (1899).

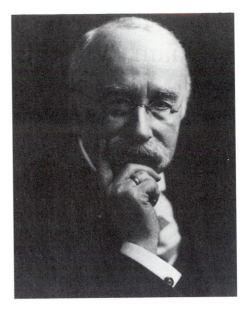

314. William William Keen. *(From the author's collection.)*

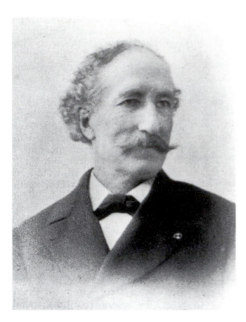

315. Henry Marcy. *(From the author's collection.)*

Henry Marcy (1837-1924) graduated from Harvard Medical School (1864) and in Europe soon became Lister's first American pupil. Upon his return to America, Marcy was the first to introduce antiseptic methods in surgery. He practiced in Massachusetts, where he established a private hospital in Cambridge for the treatment of surgical diseases of women. In 1892 Marcy served as president of the American Medical Association. He wrote two major texts, *A Treatise on Hernia, the Radical Cure by the Use of the Buried Antiseptic Animal Suture* (1889) and the monumental *Anatomy and Surgical Treatment of Hernia* (1892). He also wrote numerous journal articles, including several on the use of carbolized catgut ligatures (1878).

Alexander Johnston Skene (1837-1900) was born in Scotland and emigrated to America in 1857. Six years later he received his medical degree from the Long Island College Hospital Medical School. All of his professional career was spent in Brooklyn. From 1868 to 1893 Skene served on the faculty of his alma mater. He was a founder of the American Gynecological Society and served as its president in 1887. Skene was also professor of gynecology at the New York Post-Graduate Medical School. His name is forever linked with his description of the paraurethral glands in women (1880). Among his major texts were *Diseases of the Bladder and Urethra in Women* (1878), *Treatise on the Diseases of Women* (1888), *Medical Gynecology* (1895), and *Electrohaemostasis in Operative Surgery* (1899).

James Ewing Mears (1838-1919) was a graduate of Jefferson Medical College (1865) and later served as professor of anatomy and surgery in the Pennsylvania College of Dental Surgery. Mears was a charter member of the American Surgical Association and served as its president in 1894. He was the first surgeon to suggest trigeminal ganglionectomy as treatment for trigeminal neuralgia (1884). His only textbook was *Practical Surgery* (1878).

Jacob DaSilva Solis-Cohen (1838-1927) helped establish laryngology as a surgical specialty in the United States. He received his medical education at the University of Pennsylvania, graduating in 1860. All of his professional life was spent in Philadelphia, where he served as lecturer on laryngoscopy and diseases of the throat and chest at Jefferson Medical College. From 1880 to 1882 Solis-Cohen was president of the American Laryngological Society. In 1867 he reported the removal of a cancerous polyp from the inferior surface of the right vocal cord with the aid of a laryngoscope. Among his book-length works were *Inhalation: Its Therapeutics and Practice* (1867), *Diseases of the Throat* (1872), *Croup, in Its Relation to Tracheotomy* (1874), and *The Throat and the Voice* (1879).

Robert Weir (1838-1927) was a prominent New York City surgeon who received his medical degree from the College of Physicians and Surgeons in 1859. He was on the staff of numerous city hospitals and served as professor of surgery at his alma mater. All his written contributions were to the periodical literature, including articles on his technique for sterilization of the hands by scrubbing for 5 minutes with green soap, creating friction with calx chlorinata for 5 minutes, and rinsing with carbonate of soda and running water (1878); a method of appendicostomy (1887); and a logical, step-by-step rhinoplasty (1892).

John Ashhurst (1839-1900) completed his medical studies at the University of Pennsylvania in 1860. In 1863 he was appointed a surgeon to the Episcopal Hospital, where he began to write voluminously. Ashhurst became professor of surgery at his alma mater in 1888 and held the John Rhea Barton chair until his death. Among Ashhurst's textbooks and monographs were *Injuries of the Spine* (1867), *The Principles and Practice of Surgery* (1871), and the six-volume *International Encyclopedia of Surgery* (1881-1886). The latter played an important role in the evolution of American surgery because it introduced the concept of a multiauthor surgical textbook. Previously all surgical texts had been based on the cumulative experience of one individual. As a result of his efforts in this project, Ashhurst became recognized as one of the nineteenth century's greatest authorities on surgical bibliography.

Christian Fenger (1840-1902) was born in Denmark and received all of his education and training in Denmark. In the late 1870s he emigrated to Chicago, where he became a pathologist at the Cook County Hospital. He taught surgery at both the Northwestern University and the Rush Medical College. Fenger was a versatile surgeon who reported many types of cases. His most important paper detailed an operation for stenosis of the ureter at the ureteropelvic junction (1894). Many of Chicago's later renowned surgeons received much of their clinical knowledge from Fenger.

Albert Buck (1842-1922), the son of Gurdon Buck, graduated from the College of Physicians and Surgeons in New York City (1867). After studying the physiology of the ear in Europe, Buck became aural surgeon at the New York Eye and Ear Infirmary and instructor in otology at his alma mater. He later was named clinical professor of the diseases of the ear at the College of Physicians and Surgeons. Buck was a prominent figure in American otorhinolaryngological surgery and served as president of the American Otological Society (1879-1880). His most prominent clinical texts were *Diagnosis and Treatment of Ear Diseases* (1880), *A Manual of Diseases of the Ear* (1889), and *First Principles of Otology* (1899). Among his other medical works were the two-volume *A Treatise on Hygiene and Public Health* (1879) and the eight-volume *American Practice of Surgery* (1906-1911), which he jointly edited with Joseph Bryant. Buck is also remembered as a masterful medical historian who authored *The Growth of Medicine from the Earliest Times to About 1800* (1917) and *The Dawn of Modern Medicine* (1920).

Charles Burnett (1842-1902) received his medical degree from the University of Pennsylvania (1867). He was always interested in the study of hearing and commenced practice in Philadelphia in 1872, devoting his work to diseases of the ear and eye. Burnett was eventually named aurist to the Pennsylvania Institution for the Deaf and Dumb and to the Presbyterian Hospital. He served as president of the American Otological Society in 1884 and 1885 and for many years edited the department of progress of otology in the *American Journal of the Medical Sciences*. Among Burnett's textbooks were *The Ear; Its Anatomy, Physiology, and Diseases* (1877), *Hearing and How to Keep It* (1879), *Diseases and Injuries of the Ear* (1889), and the two-volume *System of Diseases of the Ear, Nose, and Throat* (1893).

Berthold Hadra (1842-1908) was born in Germany and received his medical education at the University of Berlin (1866). He soon emigrated to Texas (1872), where he practiced in various cities. Hadra eventually settled in Galveston, where he held the chair of surgery at the Texas Medical College and Hospital. His only treatise was the detailed *Lesions of the Vagina and Pelvic Floor* (1888). Hadra remains best remembered as the first surgeon to plan and successfully complete spinal immobilization through the wiring of the vertebrae in cervical fracture (1891).

Edward Keyes (1843-1924), one of the pioneers of American urological surgery, received his medical education at the University of the City of New York (1866). He studied for a year in Paris and returned to New York City to serve as an assistant to William Van Buren. Keyes later was named professor of genitourinary surgery at the Bellevue Hospital Medical College. Among his many accomplishments was the founding of the American Association of Genito-Urinary Surgeons; he served as its first president (1887). In collaboration with Van Buren, Keyes authored *A Practical Treatise on the Surgical Diseases of the Genito-Urinary Organs, Including Syphilis* (1874), a work that exerted enormous influence on the urological practice of the ensuing generation of American surgeons. Keyes also wrote *The Venereal Diseases, Including Strictures of the Male Urethra* (1880) and *Diseases of the Genito-Urinary Organs* (1910).

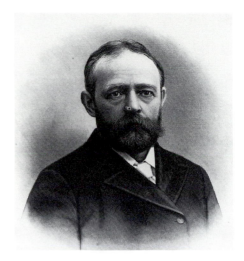

316. Christian Fenger. *(From the author's collection.)*

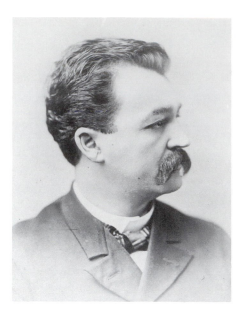

317. Nicholas Senn, pioneer intestinal surgeon, was as prolific a writer of travelogues as of surgical textbooks. *(Historical Collections, College of Physicians of Philadelphia.)*

Francke Bosworth (1843-1925) is credited with having developed the science of laryngology and rhinology in the United States as a well-defined surgical specialty. He received his medical degree from the Bellevue Hospital Medical College in 1868. In 1871 Bosworth was appointed to the surgical faculty of his alma mater and became professor in 1881. When Bellevue merged with New York University Medical College in 1898, Bosworth became its first professor of laryngology. His most important paper concerned the physiology and pathology of the sinuses and nasal obstruction (1891). Among his textbooks were *Handbook upon Diseases of the Throat* (1879), *A Manual of Diseases of the Throat and Nose* (1881), the influential two-volume *A Treatise on Diseases of the Nose and Throat* (1889-1892), and *A Textbook of Diseases of the Nose and Throat* (1896).

Nicholas Senn (1844-1908) was born in Switzerland and brought to the United States in 1852. He was an 1868 graduate of the Chicago Medical College and initially practiced in Wisconsin. By 1878 Senn was unhappy with his medical training and went to Germany for further studies. He returned to Chicago (1880) and was named to the professorship of surgery at his alma mater. In 1888 Senn was appointed professor of surgery and surgical pathology at Rush Medical College, 3 years later occupying the chair of surgery formerly held by Charles Parkes (1842-1891). Around this same time Senn was also elected professor of surgery and military surgery at the University of Chicago. Senn was a pioneer in intestinal surgery and did much animal experimentation in this field. He was among the most prolific of nineteenth-century surgeon-authors, and his texts included: *Experimental Surgery* (1889), *Intestinal Surgery* (1889), *Surgical Bacteriology* (1889), *Principles of Surgery* (1890), *Tuberculosis of Bones and Joints* (1892), *The Pathology and Surgical Treatment of Tumors* (1895), *Tuberculosis of the Genito-Urinary Organs, Males and Females* (1897), *Practical Surgery for the General Practitioner* (1902), and *A Nurses's Guide for the Operating Room* (1902). Among Senn's most important papers were those on surgery of the pancreas (1886) and the use of rectal insufflation to test for colonic perforation (1888), as well as one that presented a historical review of intestinal sutures and anastomosis (1893). In 1897 Senn was president of the American Medical Association, and in the following year he served in Cuba during the Spanish-American War as chief surgeon. He did much to improve military surgery, such as his founding of the Association of Military Surgeons of the United States (1891). Senn wrote about his military experiences in two texts, *War Correspondence* (1899) and *Medico-Surgical Aspects of the Spanish American War* (1900). In his later years Senn became an indefatigable world traveler who documented his journeys in a series of books entitled *Around the World Via Siberia* (1902), *Surgical Notes from Four Continents and the West Indies* (1903), *Around the World Via India, a Medical Tour* (1905), *Tahiti, the Island Paradise* (1906), and *In the Heart of the Arctics* (1907).

Lewis Stimson (1844-1917) graduated from Bellevue Hospital Medical College in 1874. He occupied numerous academic positions in New York City medical schools but was most closely affiliated with New York Hospital. When Cornell University Medical College was organized in 1898, Stimson became its first professor of surgery. Stimson's son, Henry L. Stimson (1867-1950), was secretary of war under President William Howard Taft (1857-1930) and secretary of state under President Herbert Hoover (1874-1964). Lewis Stimson's book-length works included *A Manual of Operative Surgery* (1878), *A Treatise on Fractures* (1883), *A Treatise on Dislocations* (1888), and *A Practical Treatise on Fractures and Dislocations* (1899).

Joseph Bryant (1845-1914) rose to prominence not only as a surgeon but also as sanitary inspector and health commissioner of New York City and commissioner of the New York State Board of Health. He graduated from Bellevue Hospital Medical College (1868) and later became professor of anatomy and clinical surgery at his alma mater. Bryant is best remembered for having performed a "secret" operation on President Grover Cleveland for sarcoma of the left upper jaw in 1893. His assistant in this operation was William W. Keen, who wrote about the famous case in *The Surgical Operations on President Cleveland in 1893* (1917). Bryant's textbooks included the two-volume *Manual of Operative*

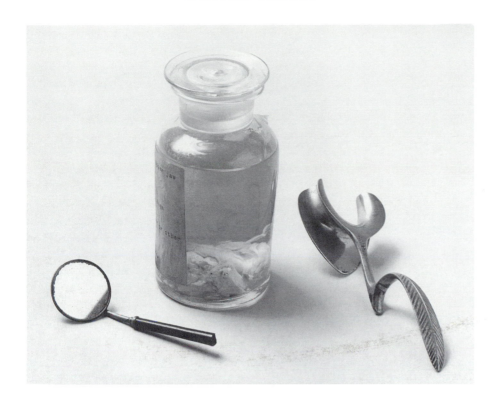

Surgery (1884) and the massive eight-volume *American Practice of Surgery* (1906-1911). He was also the first American surgeon to report on a surgical approach to the posterior mediastinum (1895).

Matthew Mann (1845-1921) was a pioneer American gynecologist who served as professor of obstetrics and gynecology at the University of Buffalo (1882-1910). Because of the esteem in which he was held in Buffalo medical circles, he acted as chief surgeon in charge of President William McKinley (1843-1901) after the assassination attempt on McKinley. Mann was president of the American Gynecological Society in 1895. His two-volume text, *A System of Gynecology by American Authors* (1887-1888), crystallized and successfully promulgated many operative techniques new to American physicians.

Charles McBurney (1845-1913) was born in Massachusetts and graduated from the College of Physicians and Surgeons in New York City (1870). He then went abroad for further study in Berlin, London, Paris, and Vienna. When McBurney returned to the United States (1873), he became demonstrator of anatomy at his alma mater. He progressed through the academic ranks to serve as professor of surgery from 1889 to 1894 and, from 1894 to 1907, as professor of clinical surgery. Most of his clinical work was completed at Roosevelt Hospital, including his famous studies on appendicitis. McBurney's classic report on early operative interference in cases of appendicitis was presented before the New York Surgical Society in 1889. In it he described the area of greatest abdominal pain in this disease process as determined by the pressure of one finger and located an inch and a half to two inches from the anterior spinous process of the ilium on a straight line drawn from that landmark to the umbilicus. Five years later, McBurney set forth in another paper the incision that he used in cases of appendicitis, which parallels the course of the external oblique muscle, one or two inches from the anterior superior spine of the ilium.

Lewis Pilcher (1845-1934) was an 1866 graduate of the University of Michigan Medical School. Beginning in 1872 Pilcher entered private practice in Brooklyn, where he was on the staff of various local hospitals. From 1885 to 1895 he served as professor of clinical surgery in the New York Post-Graduate Medical School. Pilcher was the first editor of the *Annals of Surgery* (1885-1934), which made him one of the most influential surgeons in the United States. His most important clinical text was *The Treatment of Wounds; Its Principles and Practice* (1883). Pilcher was also a well-known surgical bibliophile; in 1918 he authored a lengthy annotated bibliography of his own rare-books collection.

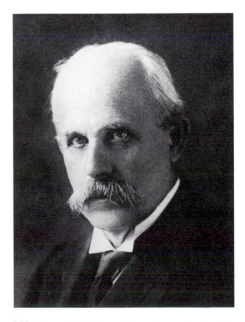

319. Lewis Pilcher. *(From the author's collection.)*

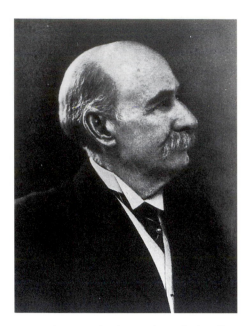

320. John Wyeth. *(From the author's collection.)*

John Wyeth (1845-1922) is little remembered, but his contributions relative to the founding of the New York Polyclinic Hospital and Medical School (1882) were extremely important in the evolution of the education and training process of American surgeons. Wyeth was born in Alabama and graduated from the medical department of the University of Louisville (1869). After spending a few years in private practice, he traveled to New York in the hope of securing further medical training. Much to his consternation, Wyeth discovered that there were few formal courses for graduate students in medicine. After 2 years of study in Europe Wyeth returned to New York City (1878) and began to promote his plans for a postgraduate school of medicine. The concept received wide support, and the Polyclinic Hospital and School was opened. Its founding marked the introduction of systematic postgraduate medical instruction in America and was an important factor in the movement to revolutionize the teaching and practice of medicine and surgery. Its success was overwhelming, and by 1914 the Polyclinic had provided postgraduate instruction for more than 25,000 physicians. Wyeth devoted most of his professional life to the Polyclinic, serving first as surgeon-in-chief and later as president. He made a number of original contributions to clinical surgery, including a bloodless amputation of the hip in which hemorrhage was controlled by a strong elastic tube held in place by long needles transfixing the tissues above the joint (1892). Wyeth wrote extensively and authored four texts, *Essays in Surgical Anatomy and Surgery* (1879), *Handbook of Medical and Surgical References* (1873), *Textbook on Surgery: General, Operative and Mechanical* (1887), and *Surgery* (1908). He was active in numerous medical organizations and served as president of the American Medical Association in 1901. Despite all he accomplished, Wyeth was never able to attain membership in the American Surgical Association because of his lack of a true academic title.

Benjamin Baer (1846-1920) did not graduate from the medical department of the University of Pennsylvania until he was 30 years old. He soon became an assistant to William Goodell (1829-1894), professor of clinical gynecology at his alma mater, and served as an instructor in gynecology from 1878 to 1885. Baer became a professor of gynecology at the Philadelphia Polyclinic in 1885 and remained there for the rest of his professional life. His most important contribution to gynecologic surgery concerned his simplified approach to abdominal hysterectomy (1892).

Newton Shaffer (1846-1928) received his medical degree from the New York University Medical College in 1867. He took his initial training at the New York Orthopaedic Dispensary under Charles Taylor. In 1872 St. Luke's Hospital established an orthopedic surgical service, the first large general hospital in the United States to do so, and Shaffer was named chief surgeon. Four years later he succeeded Taylor at the Dispensary. In 1900 Shaffer became the first professor of orthopedic surgery at Cornell University Medical College. Among his texts were *Pott's Disease, Its Pathology and Mechanical Treatment* (1879), *The Hysterical Element in Orthopaedic Surgery* (1880), and *Brief Essays On Orthopedic Surgery, Including a Consideration of Its Relation to General Surgery* (1898). Shaffer was one of the principal organizers and second president of the American Orthopedic Association (1887).

DeForest Willard (1846-1910) was one of America's pioneer orthopedic surgeons. A graduate of the University of Pennsylvania (1867), he was appointed lecturer in orthopedic surgery at his alma mater in 1887. Willard served as clinical professor of orthopedic surgery (1889-1903) and, later, as full professor. He was president of the American Surgical Association (1901) and the American Orthopedic Association (1890). Willard's most important text was *The Surgery of Childhood, Including Orthopedic Surgery* (1910). He also authored *Artificial Anaesthesia and Anaesthetics* (1891).

Virgil Gibney (1847-1927) received his medical degree from Bellevue Hospital Medical College in 1871. After graduation he obtained a position at the Hospital for the Ruptured and Crippled under James Knight. Gibney literally lived in the hospital for 13 years. During that time he authored *The Hip and Its*

Diseases (1884). He became surgeon-in-chief of that institution after Knight's death and remained active through 1924. In 1894 Gibney was also appointed the first professor of orthopedic surgery at Columbia University's College of Physicians and Surgeons. In a paper written in 1875 Gibney described for the first time hereditary multiple exostoses. His name is linked with a fixation bandage used in the treatment of sprains of the ankle.

Fernand Henrotin (1847-1906) was born in Brussels and brought to America at the age of 10 years. He graduated from Rush Medical College (1868) and soon joined his father in practice. Eventually he became professor of gynecology at the Chicago Polyclinic. He remains best known for his papers on vaginal hysterectomy (1892) and drainage of parauterine and periuterine abscesses through the vagina (1895).

Joseph Mathews (1847-1928) was an 1877 graduate of the University of Louisville School of Medicine. He became interested in the specialty of proctology after studying in London. Mathews returned to Louisville in 1880 and was appointed professor of surgery at the Kentucky School of Medicine. Three years later a department of proctology was organized, and Mathews was appointed surgeon-in-chief. He helped organize the American Proctological Society (1899) and served as president of the American Medical Association (1899). Mathews is considered America's first formal proctologist and is credited with taking proctology out of the hands of itinerant quacks and charlatans and placing it on a firm scientific basis. His most important clinical text was *A Treatise on Diseases of the Rectum, Anus, and Sigmoid Flexure* (1892).

Edward Bradford (1848-1926) was born in Boston and graduated from Harvard Medical School in 1872. He spent 2 years in Europe, where he studied with Hugh Owen Thomas. After returning to the United States, Bradford worked for several years with Buckminster Brown; in 1880 Bradford was appointed clinical instructor in surgery at his alma mater. Twenty-three years later he was named the first John Ball and Buckminster Brown professor of orthopedic surgery. Among his many contributions to organized medicine was his service as a founder and president (1889) of the American Orthopedic Association. His most important text, jointly written with Robert Lovett (1859-1924), was *A Treatise on Orthopedic Surgery* (1890), considered the standard American orthopedic textbook of its day. Bradford's name is linked with an oblong rectangular frame made of pipe over which are stretched transversely two strips of canvas, the device thus permitting the trunk and lower extremities to move as a unit; this device was used for patients with deformities of the spine.

George Fowler (1848-1906) was an 1871 graduate of Bellevue Hospital Medical College. He practiced in Brooklyn and New York City and became professor of surgery in the New York Polyclinic Hospital and surgeon-in-chief of the Brooklyn Hospital. Fowler was a founder and first president of the Brooklyn Red Cross (1884) and introduced first-aid instruction to the New York National Guard. He authored a *Syllabus of a Course of Lectures on First Aids to the Injured* (1887). Fowler is best remembered for completing the first known thoracoplasty (1893) and for describing an inclined patient position obtained by raising the head of the bed by as much as two to two and a half feet to ensure better dependent drainage after an abdominal operation (1900). Among his textbooks were the first American work to deal exclusively with appendicitis, *A Treatise on Appendicitis* (1894), the two-volume *A Treatise on Surgery* (1906), and *The Operating Room and the Patient* (1906).

Arpad Gerster (1848-1923) was born in Hungary and graduated in 1872 from the University of Vienna. He immediately left for the United States and settled in Brooklyn. In 1878 Gerster was made surgeon to the German Hospital, and in the following year he joined the staff of the Mount Sinai Hospital. Gerster accepted the professorship of clinical surgery at the College of Physicians and Surgeons of Columbia University in 1910. From 1882 to 1895 he also held the chair of surgery at the New York Polyclinic Medical School. In 1896 he was president of the American Surgical Association. Gerster was an outstanding pioneer of listerian surgery and one of the first American surgeons to actively use antisepsis for all his opera-

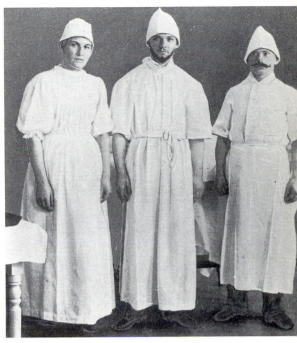

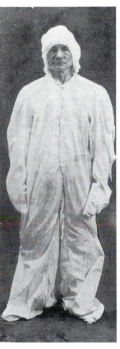

321. Aseptic operating-room attire, vintage 1895, designed by Carl Beck (1856-1911). Costumes for a female nurse, a male surgeon, a male nurse, and a patient are shown. From Beck's *Manual of the Modern Theory and Technique of Surgical Asepsis* (1895). *(From the author's collection.)*

tions. His *Rules Of Aseptic and Antiseptic Surgery* (1888) was the first American surgical text based on listerian principles. The book caused a furor, since at that time suppuration was still basically considered a natural sequence of every surgical procedure. Gerster also authored a little-known paper that occupies an influential place in the history of oncological surgery in the United States (1885). He described how surgical incision of tumors promotes metastases in the earliest discussion of the concept of surgically induced metastases to be found in American surgical literature (1885).

William Bull (1849-1909) was one of New York City's leading surgeons. He received his medical education at the College of Physicians and Surgeons (1872). After completing an internship at Bellevue Hospital and traveling throughout Europe, Bull was placed in charge of the New York Dispensary. Afterward he worked at numerous institutions throughout the city, including Chambers Street Hospital, where he reported a case of gunshot wound of the intestine that had a profound effect on the evolution of American surgery. In 1884 Bull intentionally opened the peritoneal cavity of a patient with a gunshot wound of the abdomen and repaired seven perforations in the small intestine and one in the sigmoid colon, and the patient survived. This widely reported surgical triumph electrified American surgeons and provided the major impetus for further emergency laparotomies for intestinal injuries. Bull was appointed professor of the practice of surgery and clinical surgery at his alma mater in 1888.

Frederic Dennis (1850-1934) was a native of Newark, New Jersey, and a graduate of Bellevue Hospital Medical College (1874). He practiced in New York City and was elected professor of the principles and practice of surgery at his alma mater. Dennis served as president of the American Surgical Association in 1895. His most important text was the four-volume *System of Surgery* (1895-1896), the first multivolume American general surgical textbook in which the various authors received credit for each individual chapter. The most prominent section was that by John Shaw Billings (1838-1913) on the history and literature of surgery.

James White (1850-1916) was an 1871 graduate of the medical department of the University of Pennsylvania. Within a few years he became assistant to David Hayes Agnew and was appointed professor of genitourinary diseases at his alma mater (1886). White was elected to the chair of clinical surgery in 1889, and from 1900 to 1910 he occupied the John Rhea Barton chair of surgery. He will be long remembered in the annals of urological surgery for his concept of orchiectomy as a means of bringing about atrophy of the prostate (1893). White's texts included *An American Text-Book of Surgery* (1892), written with William W. Keen, and *Genito-Urinary Surgery and Venereal Diseases* (1897).

Robert Abbe (1851-1928) was an attending surgeon to St. Luke's Hospital, consulting surgeon to the Hospital for the Ruptured and Crippled, and professor of surgery in the Post-Graduate School and Hospital in New York City. He was an extremely versatile surgeon who performed a widely acclaimed posterior root section (rhizotomy) for brachial neuralgia (1889), introduced the use of catgut rings for supporting the ends of intestine during an anastomosis (1892), and described a lip-switch flap operation for treatment of bilateral cleft lip (1898). Abbe wrote no major textbooks.

Marie Mergler (1859-1901) was born in Bavaria but was brought to the United States in 1863. She attended the Woman's Medical College in Chicago and graduated as valedictorian in 1879. In 1881 she became a surgical assistant to William Byford at the Woman's Hospital. In the following year Mergler was appointed professor of materia medica at her alma mater and served until 1890, when she succeeded her mentor in the chair of gynecology. Considered among the most highly esteemed women in nineteenth-century American surgery, Mergler served as editor of the *Medical Woman's Journal*. Her *Guide to the Study of Gynecology* (1893) was one of only two books written by American women surgeons in the nineteenth century. The other was written by Gertrude Annie Walker (1863-?), an ophthalmologist in Philadelphia.

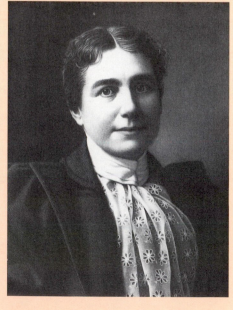

322. Marie Mergler. *(From the author's collection.)*

Roswell Park (1852-1914) graduated from the Northwestern University Medical School in 1876. He became instrumental in promulgating listerian techniques to American surgeons and served as professor of surgery at the University of Buffalo from 1884 to 1914. Park was also a founder of the Gratwick Laboratory, which later became the New York State Institute for the Study of Malignant Diseases. Among his textbooks were *The Mütter Lectures on Surgical Pathology* (1892), the two-volume *A Treatise on Surgery by American Authors* (1896), and *The Principles and Practice of Modern Surgery* (1907). Park was highly regarded as a medical historian, having written *An Epitome of the History of Medicine* (1897).

John Roberts (1852-1924) was an 1874 graduate of Jefferson Medical College. In 1882 he proposed and assisted in the establishment of the Philadelphia Polyclinic and College for Graduates in Medicine. He later was appointed professor of surgery at the Women's Medical College of Pennsylvania. Active in many surgical organizations, Roberts served as president of the American Surgical Association (1921). Of Roberts's clinical achievements, those concerning cardiac surgery are his least known but most important. In 1880 he authored the important monograph, *Paracentesis of the Pericardium, a Consideration of the Surgical Treatment of Pericardial Effusions.* His major conclusion, which contributed to the advancement of cardiac surgery in the United States, was that paracentesis of the pericardium is indicated in every case of pericardial effusion that does not respond readily to medical care. Among his textbooks were *The Compend of Anatomy* (1881), *The Field and Limitation of the Operative Surgery of the Human Brain* (1885), *A Manual of Modern Surgery* (1890), *A Clinical, Pathological, and Experimental Study of Fracture of the Lower End of the Radius* (1897), *Notes on the Modern Treatment of Fractures* (1899), *Surgery of Deformities of the Face* (1912), and *Treatise on Fractures* (1916).

George Edebohls (1853-1908) was born in New York City, where he attended the College of Physicians and Surgeons and graduated in 1875. After postgraduate studies in Europe he returned to his native city and was appointed visiting gynecologist to St. Francis Hospital. Edebohls was later named professor of the diseases of women at the New York Post-Graduate Medical School and Hospital. He is eponymically remembered for a position for vaginal operations in which the woman lies on her back at the edge of the table, with her hips and knees partly flexed and the feet held up and apart by supports attached to the table. It was Edebohl's version of nephrocapsectomy that brought him the most fame. This consisted of exposing the diseased kidneys and stripping off their fibrous coverings to treat various forms of glomerulonephritis. Although the operation received much negative comment, Edebohls persisted in its use. His most renowned papers were on "floating" kidney and his operation of nephropexy (1893 and 1899). Edebohls also introduced the operation of renal decortication for the treatment of chronic nephritis (1901). His most important text was *The Surgical Treatment of Bright's Disease* (1904).

Joseph Price (1853-1911) received his undergraduate education at Union College in Schenectady, New York. He then attended the University of Pennsylvania (1877) and a year later was named head of the obstetrical department in the Philadelphia Dispensary. Price was a founder of the American Association of Obstetricians and Gynecologists and its president in 1896. He is best remembered for his reports on abdominal drainage after surgical operations (1890).

Francis Watson (1853-1942) was one of the premier urological surgeons in Boston. Early in his career he was surgeon to outpatients at Boston City Hospital and instructor in minor surgery and the surgery of the urinary organs at Harvard Medical School. Watson remained associated with these two institutions for his entire professional life. He is best known for his paper describing the first median perineal prostatectomy in 1889. His major written works were *The Operative Treatment of the Hypertrophied Prostate* (1888) and the two-volume *Disease and Surgery of the Genito-Urinary System* (1908).

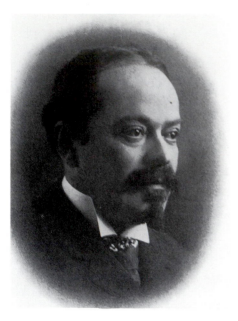

323. Augustus Bernays. *(From the author's collection.)*

Augustus Bernays (1854-1907) was born in Germany and received his medical degree from the University of Heidelberg (1876). He soon emigrated to the United States and settled in St. Louis, where he was appointed professor of anatomy at the St. Louis College of Physicians and Surgeons. He was prolific in his contributions to the periodical literature, but his only major text was *Golden Rules of Surgery* (1906), the first work to be published by the then newly formed C. V. Mosby Medical Book Company.

John Deaver (1855-1931) was an 1878 graduate of the University of Pennsylvania. He later was appointed professor of the practice of surgery at his alma mater and eventually filled the John Rhea Barton chair of surgery (1911). In 1886 he became a surgeon to the German Hospital of Philadelphia and chief of the department 10 years later. At this institution he made many contributions to American surgery. Among his surgical texts were *A Treatise on Appendicitis* (1896), the three-volume *Surgical Anatomy* (1899-1903), *Surgical Anatomy of the Head and Neck* (1904), *Enlargement of the Prostate* (1905), the two-volume *Surgery of the Upper Abdomen* (1913), and *The Breast, Its Anomalies, Its Diseases, and Their Treatment* (1917). Deaver is eponymically remembered for a technique used for appendectomy in which a vertical incision is made in the right lower abdominal quadrant with medial retraction of the rectus muscle and for a retractor used in abdominal operations.

George Goodfellow (1855-1910) was one of the most colorful nineteenth-century American surgeons. He graduated from the medical department of Wooster University in Cleveland (1876). Goodfellow first practiced in Tombstone, Arizona Territory, until 1892, when he took a position as surgeon with the Southern Pacific Railroad. His surgical fame was attributable to his aggressive, innovative approach to gunshot wounds of the abdomen. Aided by the general lawlessness of the western territories, Goodfellow had plenty of patients who needed his expertise in this area. Later in his career, he fought in the Spanish-American War and eventually settled in San Francisco, where he reported on one of America's earliest perineal prostatectomies (1904).

William Jarvis (1855-1895) graduated from the medical department of the University of Maryland in 1875. He practiced in New York City, where he worked as an assistant to Francke Bosworth on the nose-and-throat service in the outpatient department of Bellevue Hospital. From 1881 to 1893 Jarvis was on the laryngology faculty of the University of the City of New York. He was an innovative laryngologist who developed a wire snare that could be tightened by a screw in the handle and was used to cut off polyps and other sessile growths in the nose and other accessible cavities (1881). His device, which was nothing more than a cold wire ecraseur and quite simple in design, created a new era in intranasal surgery. Jarvis also presented a plan for illumination of the upper air passages by the application of electric light bulbs at the focus of the head mirror and at the shank of a laryngoscope handle (1885).

William Belfield (1856-1929) graduated from Rush Medical College in 1878, where he served as associate professor of surgery (1899-1908), and professor of genitourinary surgery (1909-1923). In 1902 Belfield was president of the American Association of Genito-Urinary Surgeons. He is eponymically remembered for the operation of vasostomy. His most important treatise was *Diseases of the Urinary and Male Sexual Organs* (1884). In 1886 Belfield performed the first suprapubic prostatectomy in the United States.

Frank Hartley (1856-1913) was a native of Washington, District of Columbia, and received his medical degree from the College of Physicians and Surgeons in New York City (1880). He interned for 2 years at Bellevue, afterward doing postgraduate work in Berlin, Heidelberg, and Vienna. On his return to New York City Hartley was named demonstrator of anatomy at his alma mater. He later became clinical professor of surgery. Hartley is best known for his operation of intracranial neurectomy for facial neuralgia (1892).

Edward Jackson (1856-1942) was one of America's most prominent ophthalmologists. He graduated from Union College in Schenectady, New York, and received his medical degree from the University of Pennsylvania (1878). Jackson settled in Philadelphia, where he became professor of diseases of the eye at Philadelphia Polyclinic and College for Graduates in Medicine. There he authored the *Essentials of Refraction and the Diseases of the Eye* (1890). In 1898 Jackson relocated to Denver and from 1905 to 1921 served as professor of ophthalmology at the University of Colorado. He held many important positions in American medical organizations, including the chairmanship of the American Board of Ophthalmology for the first 5 years of its existence (1914-1919). In addition, Jackson was editor of the *American Journal of Ophthalmology* from 1918 to 1928. Among his other texts were *Skiascopy and Its Practical Applications to the Study of Refraction* (1895) and *A Manual of the Diagnosis and Treatment of the Diseases of the Eye* (1900).

Casey Wood (1856-1942) is remembered not only as an ophthalmologist but also as an influential ornithologist and bibliophile. He received his medical degree in Montreal (1877) and was trained at the New York Eye and Ear Infirmary. He spent 2 years at the Royal London Ophthalmic Hospital as a clinical assistant. On returning to America in 1890, Wood settled in Chicago, where he eventually became professor of clinical ophthalmology at Northwestern University. Among the positions he held in ophthalmology were the presidency of the American Academy of Ophthalmology and Otolaryngology, and editor of the *Annals of Ophthalmology* (1896-1898) and the *Ophthalmic Record* (1897-1918). In 1918 Wood was appointed to the editorial board of the *Annals of Medical History*. His clinical texts included *Lessons in the Diagnosis and Treatment of Eye Diseases* (1891), *The Eye, Ear, Nose and Throat Yearbook* (1902), *The Common Diseases of the Eye* (1904), *A System of Ophthalmic Therapeutics* (1909), the two-volume *System of Ophthalmic Operations* (1911), and the 18-volume *American Encyclopedia and Dictionary of Ophthalmology* (1913-1921). He also wrote *The Fundus Oculi of Birds, Especially as Viewed by the Ophthalmoscope* (1917).

Franklin Martin (1857-1935) played a key role in several aspects of American surgery; most notably he was the driving force behind the founding of the American College of Surgeons. Born in Wisconsin, Martin received his medical degree from Chicago Medical College in 1880. He practiced obstetrics and gynecology in that city for his entire professional life. After organizing the Clinical Congress of Surgeons of North America in 1910, Martin merged the organization 3 years later into the American College of Surgeons. During World War I he served on the Council of National Defense and was a member of the General Medical Board, which oversaw the military mobilization of physicians, surgeons, and dentists. He founded and edited the monthly journal *Surgery, Gynecology and Obstetrics,* and was on the editorial board of the *American Journal of Obstetrics and Gynecology*. Martin served as professor of gynecology at the Post-Graduate Medical School and as attending surgeon at the Woman's Hospital. His clinical texts included *Electricity in Diseases of Women and Obstetrics* (1892), *Lectures on the Treatment of Fibroid Tumors of the Uterus* (1897), and *A Treatise on Gynecology*. An inveterate world traveler, he also authored *South America from a Surgeon's Point of View* (1922) and *Australia and New Zealand, a Monograph* (1924).

John Benjamin Murphy (1857-1916), an enigmatic, colorful personality, was one of the most prominent nineteenth-century American surgeons. He received his medical education from Rush Medical College (1879). After serving 18 months as an intern at Cook County Hospital, he went into private practice until 1882, when he went to Europe. He obtained 2 years of postgraduate studies in Berlin, Heidelberg, Munich, and Vienna. On his return to the United States he reestablished his office for the practice of surgery in Chicago. Murphy's brilliant, indomitable spirit allowed him to pioneer many fields. His career as a surgical teacher began with his appointment as lecturer in surgery at his alma mater (1884). In 1892 Murphy was made professor of clinical surgery at the College of Physicians and Surgeons. He remained there for a decade, and he was elected professor of surgery at Northwestern University Medical School (1901). Murphy stayed at Northwestern through 1905, when he moved back to Rush as professor of surgery. In 1908 Murphy made his last career transfer and returned to Northwestern. He was also chief of the surgical staff at Mercy Hos-

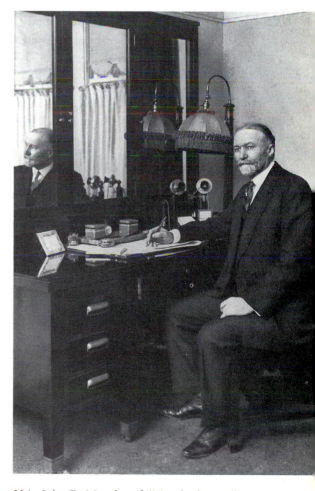

324. John B. Murphy of "Murphy button" fame in 1914, with twin telephones on his desk. It was highly unusual to have two telephone lines at that time. *(From the author's collection.)*

325. The Murphy button with and without its spring-cup attachment. The device revolutionized surgery by demonstrating the feasibility of joining portions of the intestine without sutures and by demonstrating that it was within the scope of any competent surgeon's practice to do so. In its time the Murphy button was considered the greatest mechanical aid in surgery. As improved suturing techniques were introduced, it fell into disuse. (From The Medical Record vol 42, pp 665-676, 1892.)

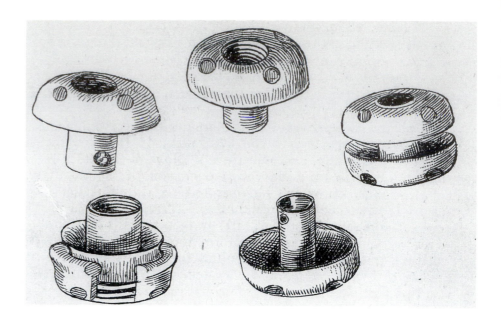

pital in Chicago, where he accomplished most of his achievements. Murphy served as president of the American Medical Association in 1911. In 1892 he startled the surgical world by introducing a mechanical device, or "button" that allowed the approximation of hollow viscera without sutures. Four years later he published a report on research and clinical work in sutures of arteries and veins, including a description of one of the earliest repairs of a lacerated femoral artery. Although Murphy never wrote a general textbook of surgery, he did edit the first *Year Book Of General Surgery* (1901), and he served as editor-in-chief of the journal *Surgery, Gynecology and Obstetrics*. Murphy was considered an outstanding teacher of surgery, especially in the operating room, where his clinical presentations were exceedingly popular. The demand for publication of his weekly conferences led to the organization of *The Surgical Clinics Of John B. Murphy* from 1912 to 1916. These volumes were the direct forerunner of the *Surgical Clinics of North America*.

Royal Whitman (1857-1946) received his medical degree from Harvard in 1882. From the middle to late 1880s he practiced in Boston, where he was surgeon to the orthopedic department of the Boston Dispensary. In 1889 he moved to the Hospital for the Ruptured and Crippled in New York City, where he remained for the rest of his life. Whitman, president of the American Orthopedic Association in 1895, was quite well known, and his work bridged the gap between the nineteenth century and the twentieth century in American orthopedic surgery. His most prominent text, *A Treatise on Orthopaedic Surgery* (1901), served as the standard orthopedic textbook in the United States for many years.

George DeSchweinitz (1858-1938) was one of America's leading ophthalmologists. He received his medical education at the University of Pennsylvania (1881) and eventually was appointed professor of ophthalmology at his alma mater (1902). Among his many honors were presidencies of the American Ophthalmological Society (1916) and the American Medical Association (1922). His *Diseases of the Eye* (1892), one of the most popular ophthalmological textbooks in the United States, went through 10 editions. DeSchweinitz's other works were *The Toxic Amblyopias* (1896), *An American Text-Book of Diseases of the Eye, Ear, Nose and Throat* (1899), and *Pulsating Exophthalmos* (1908).

Howard Kelly (1858-1943) is a major figure in the development of gynecological and abdominal surgery in the United States. He received his medical degree from the University of Pennsylvania in 1882. Within 7 years Kelly had advanced to the position of professor of obstetrics at his alma mater. In 1889 he moved to Baltimore, where he began his lengthy association with The Johns Hopkins Hospital and School of Medicine in his capacity as professor of gynecology. Kelly served as president of the Southern Surgical and Gynecological Association (1906) and the American Gynecological Society (1912). Among his many contributions to the surgical literature were papers on hysterorrhaphy (1887), the introduction of aeroscopic examination of the bladder in women and catheterization of the ureters (1893), a method of ureteroureteral anastomosis that included the use of the catheter as a temporary ureteral splint (1894), the removal of pelvic inflammatory masses by the abdomen after bisection of the uterus (1900), the use of wax on a bladder catheter tip so that it registers any pressure resulting from sharp stones, thus providing an important means of diagnosing calculi (1901), and the design of various rectal and vesical speculums (1903). Kelly, a prolific author, wrote the two-volume *Operative Gynecology* (1898), *The Vermiform Appendix and Its Diseases* (1905), the two-volume *Gynecology and Abdominal Surgery* (1907), *Medical Gynecology* (1908), *Myomata of the Uterus* (1909), *Diseases of the Kidney, Ureters, and Bladder* (1914), and *Electrosurgery* (1932). Also an influential medical historian, he authored the two-volume *Cyclopedia of American Medical Biography* (1912), *Some American Medical Botanists* (1914), and *A Dictionary of American Medical Biography* (1928). He is eponymically linked with a tubular speculum with an obturator for rectal and sigmoid examination and with an operation in which retroversion of the uterus is corrected by affixing it to the anterior abdominal wall.

Alexander Duane (1858-1926) graduated as valedictorian of his class from Union College in Schenectady, New York (1878). After receiving his medical degree from the College of Physicians and Surgeons in New York City, he practiced general medicine until 1887. Duane became associated with Hermann Knapp (1832-1911), and his interest soon turned toward ophthalmology. He became prominent in American ophthalmology and served as president of the American Ophthalmological Society (1923). In 1919 he received an honorary doctorate from Union College and became a trustee of that institution. Duane authored *A New Classification of the Motor Anomalies of the Eye* (1897).

Albert Ochsner (1858-1925) was an 1886 graduate of Rush Medical College, and occupied the chair of clinical surgery at the University of Illinois College of Medicine (1900-1925). He accomplished much in the world of American surgical politics, including the presidencies of the Clinical Congress of Surgeons of North America (1910-1912), the American College of Surgeons (1923), and the American Surgical Association (1924). His most important journal article concerned peritonitis as a complication of appendicitis (1901). In that paper he proposed a treatment of appendicitis with which his name remains linked: when operation is not advisable, treatment should consist of intestinal rest obtained by abstention from the use of cathartics and oral intake while gastric lavage and rectal irrigation are being instituted. Among Ochsner's textbooks were *Clinical Surgery* (1902), *A Handbook of Appendicitis* (1902), *The Surgery and Pathology of the Thyroid and Parathyroid Glands* (1910), and the four-volume *Surgical Diagnosis and Treatment by American Authors* (1920). He also wrote *The Organization, Construction and Management of Hospitals* (1907).

William Rodman (1858-1916) received his medical education at Jefferson Medical College (1879). From 1885 to 1893 he served as demonstrator of surgery in the medical department of the University of Louisville. In 1893 Rodman was named to the chair of surgery at the Kentucky School of Medicine. Five years later he moved to Philadelphia, where he assumed the professorship of surgery in the Medico-Chirurgical College of Philadelphia. Among his many accomplishments were the founding of the National Board of Medical Examiners (1915) and his service as president of the Association of American Medical Colleges (1902) and the American Medical Association (1915). His major written work was *Diseases of the Breast with Special Reference to Cancer* (1908). Rodman's name is linked with a surgical technique for radical mastectomy.

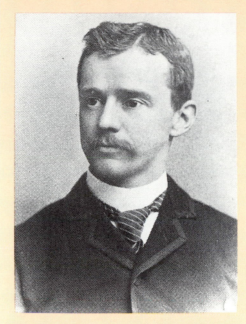

326. Howard Kelly. *(From the author's collection.)*

327. James Cornish shown after an operation for a stab wound of the heart, which was performed by Daniel Williams in 1897. A founder of the Provident Hospital in Chicago, the first hospital in the United States operated by Afro-Americans, Williams was a charter member of the American College of Surgeons and a founder of the National Medical Association. *(From* The Medical Record *vol 51, pp 437-439, 1897.)*

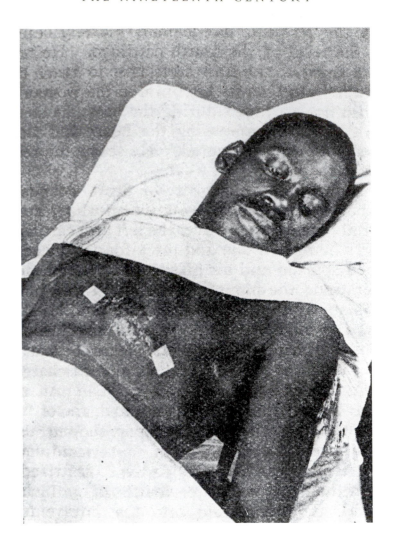

Daniel Williams (1858-1931) was a graduate of Chicago Medical College (1883) and became a founder of the Provident Hospital in Chicago, the first hospital in the United States opened by African Americans. From 1893 to 1898 Williams was surgeon-in-chief at the Freedmen's Hospital in Washington, District of Columbia. He was a charter member of the American College of Surgeons and, later, a founder of the National Medical Association. Williams received considerable notoriety when he reported the successful suturing of the pericardium for a stab wound of the heart (1897). His paper had substantial impact on the future course of American cardiac surgery by opening up new vistas in thoracic surgery.

Edwin Cragin (1859-1918) took his medical education at the College of Physicians and Surgeons in New York City (1886). He served an internship in Roosevelt Hospital and in 1889 was appointed assistant gynecologist to that institution. Cragin was also on the staff of the New York Cancer Hospital. He was named professor of obstetrics and attending obstetrician to the Sloane Maternity Hospital in 1899 and later added the professorship of gynecology. Cragin was frequently criticized for writing so few scientific reports. However, he did write *Essentials of Gynaecology* (1890) and *The Practice of Obstetrics* (1913).

Robert Lovett (1859-1924) graduated from Harvard Medical School in 1885. He soon became an assistant to Edwin Bradford, and after advancing through the academic ranks he was named Bradford's successor (1915) as professor of orthopedic surgery at Harvard. Among Lovett's works were *A Treatise on Orthopedic Surgery* (1890), written with Bradford, *The Etiology, Pathology, and Treatment of Diseases of the Hip Joint* (1891), *Lateral Curvature of the Spine and Round Shoulders* (1907), and the monumental *Orthopaedic Surgery* (1923), jointly authored with Robert Jones.

Edward Martin (1859-1938) was a native of Philadelphia; he graduated from the University of Pennsylvania (1883). He became an office assistant to David Hayes Agnew and James White and after practicing medicine, decided to specialize in urological diseases and general surgery. Martin was named professor of clinical surgery at his alma mater (1903) and John Rhea Barton professor of surgery from 1910 to 1918. A founding member of the American College of Surgeons, he is remembered for performing a cordotomy for the relief of intractable pain (1912). Among his many texts were *Questions and Answers of the Essentials of Surgery* (1888), *Essentials of Minor Surgery and Bandaging* (1890), *The Surgical Treatment of Wounds and Obstruction of the Intestines* (1891), *Impotence and Sexual Weakness in the Male and Female* (1895), and *Genito-Urinary Surgery and Venereal Diseases* (1897), cowritten with White.

John Baldy (1860-1934) was professor of gynecology at the Philadelphia Polyclinic. He is best remembered for having performed one of the earliest, albeit unsuccessful, gastrectomies in the United States (1898) and for modifying John Webster's (1863-1950) method of treating retrodisplacement of the uterus (1903). Baldy edited one of the most successful gynecological texts in the United States, *An American Textbook of Gynecology, Medical and Surgical* (1894).

Rudolph Matas (1860-1957) received his medical education at the University of Louisiana (1876). He had such a long, distinguished career that his many accomplishments are astounding. Among his honors were presidencies of the American Surgical Association (1909), the South Surgical Association (1911), the American Association for Thoracic Surgery (1920), and the American College of Surgeons (1924). Most of his professional life was spent on the surgical faculty of Tulane University, where he held the chair of surgery. Although Matas never authored a textbook of surgery, he did make numerous contributions to the periodical literature. In 1888 he reported the first known aneurysmorrhaphy worldwide. A decade later Matas performed the first successful preplanned attempt at intraspinal cocainization.

Clayton Parkhill (1860-1902) was a graduate of Jefferson Medical College (1883). After initial postgraduate training, he returned to his native city of Denver, where he eventually assumed the position of professor of surgery at the University of Colorado. Parkhill remains best known to American surgeons for his introduction of external fixation in fractures (1898).

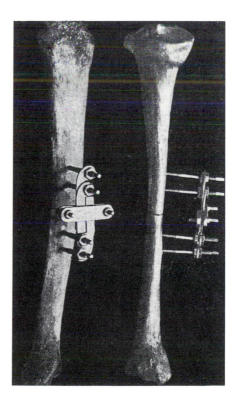

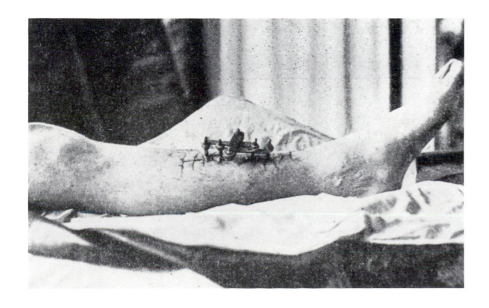

328. The first bone clamp for the external fixation of fractures, as introduced in 1898 by its inventor, Clayton Parkhill. The top photograph shows the clamp joining a fractured tibia. The clinical photograph, *left,* shows the clamp's appearance at the time of first dressing, 6 weeks after it had been applied. (*From* The Annals of Surgery *vol 27, pp 553-570, 1898.*)

William Mayo (1861-1939) is one of the most famous figures in American surgery. He was born in Rochester, Minnesota, and attended the University of Michigan School of Medicine (1883). Mayo immediately went to New York City to receive postgraduate education. Although his formal training was modest, Mayo, beginning in 1889, took annual study leaves, both in the United States and abroad. His entire professional life was spent in practice with his father, William Worrall Mayo (1819-1911), and his brother Charles (1865-1939). The three men made the Mayo Clinic one of the world's foremost centers for surgical care, training, and research. William Mayo's professional career included close associations with numerous medical organizations, including the presidencies of the American Medical Association (1906), the Society of Clinical Surgery (1911), the American Surgical Association (1913), and the American College of Surgeons (1925). His name is linked with a number of operations, including an excision of the pylorus and exclusion of the duodenum with posterior gastrojejunostomy (1900), the cure of umbilical hernia (1901), and the excision of the rectum with removal of the neighboring lymph glands for cancer (1910). Mayo is eponymically associated with the prepyloric vein. He never wrote a textbook of surgery but contributed more than 600 papers to the periodical literature.

329. William and Charles Mayo, founders of the Mayo Clinic, Rochester, Minnesota. *(By permission of the Mayo Foundation.)*

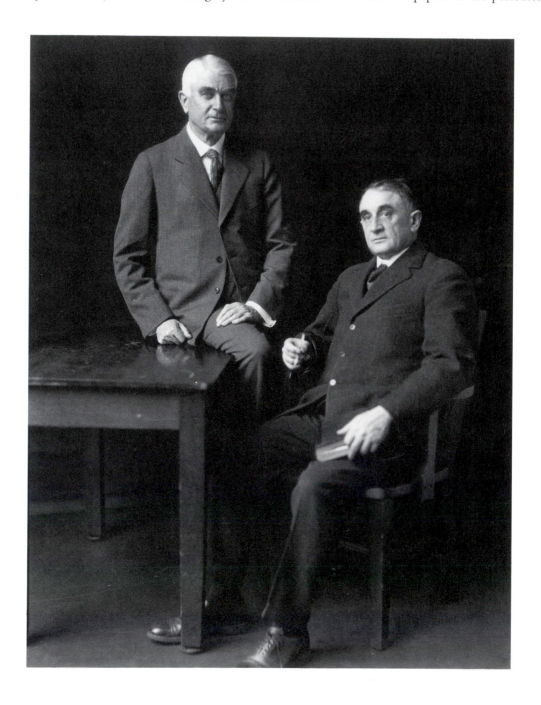

William Coley (1862-1936) was a graduate of Harvard Medical School (1888). Most of his professional life was spent in New York City, where he was on the surgical faculty of Cornell University Medical College and the Hospital for the Ruptured and Crippled. Coley's most important accomplishment was the development of a toxin consisting of the killed cultures of *Streptococcus erysipelatis* combined with the toxins of *Bacillus prodigiosus,* which he used for the treatment of certain types of malignant tumors, especially sarcoma (1891). In many respects his research represented the beginning of adjuvant immunotherapy for cancer. Coley's name is remembered for the stitch placed lateral to the internal ring to provide further support in an inguinal hernia repair.

Charles Penrose (1862-1925) received his medical education at the University of Pennsylvania (1884), where he eventually became professor of gynecology (1893-1899). Penrose retired from active surgical practice at the age of 37 years because of cardiac disease. His name is remembered in surgery for his description of a rubber tissue, or "cigarette drain" (1890). By enclosing a length of absorbent guaze in a thin rubber sheath, Penrose was able to provide for capillary drainage in abdominal operations. His written texts included *Syllabus of the Lectures on Gynecology* (1896) and *A Textbook of Diseases of Women* (1897).

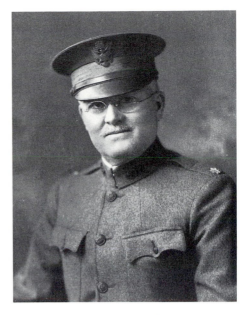

330. George Crile. *(From the author's collection.)*

George Crile (1864-1943) typified the late nineteenth-century American surgeon, who provided the leadership and intellectual guidance to ensure America's position in twentieth-century surgery. Crile was born in Ohio and received his medical degree from the University of Wooster in Cleveland (1887). After serving as an intern for a year at the University Hospital, Crile began his practice of medicine in that city. However, his practice was interrupted by three extended trips abroad for postgraduate surgical study: in 1893 he went to Vienna, in 1895 he studied in London, and in 1897 Crile traveled to Paris. In London he worked on problems of surgical shock, performing numerous experiments to observe the effects of hemorrhage, anesthesia, and physical stresses on surgical outcomes. His career was characterized by ambition, industry, and an intense curiosity regarding the role of physiology and emotional factors in successful surgery. Crile became associated with his alma mater as professor of physiology (1890-1893) and professor of the principles and practice of surgery (1893-1900). He was later appointed professor of clinical surgery at the same university, which was renamed Western Reserve. Crile's other institutional affiliations included the Lakeside Hospital, and he was founder and chief surgeon of the Cleveland Clinic. A prodigious writer, he authored 24 books, among them *An Experimental Research into Surgical Shock* (1899), *Experimental Research into the Surgery of the Respiratory System* (1899), *An Experimental and Clinical Research into Certain Problems Relating to Surgical Operations* (1901), *Blood-Pressure in Surgery* (1903), *Hemorrhage and Transfusion* (1909), *Anemia and Resuscitation* (1914), *Anoci-Association (1914), The Kinetic Drive, Its Phenomena and Control* (1916), *Surgical Shock and the Shockless Operation through Anoci-Association* (1920), *The Physical Interpretation of Shock, Exhaustion, and Restoration* (1921), *The Thyroid Gland* (1922), *Notes on Military Surgery* (1924), *Problems in Surgery* (1927), and *The Surgical Treatment of Hypertension* (1938). His most important journal article concerned the kinetic theory of shock and its prevention through anociassociation (shockless surgery) (1913). Crile's honors were numerous, among them the presidencies of the American College of Surgeons (1916) and the American Surgical Association (1924).

Charles Mayo (1865-1939) was the brother of William (1861-1939) and one of the Mayo family members who established the Mayo Clinic. He received his medical education at the Chicago Medical College (1888). After a period of postgraduate study at the New York Polyclinic and New York Post-Graduate Medical School, Mayo went into practice with his brother. Although not as prolific or surgically innovative as his brother, Mayo was well regarded and served as president of the American Medical Association (1916) and the American College of Surgeons (1924). His name is associated with the operative treatment of tic douloureux, in which the affected nerve branch is exsected and the foramen of exit in the skull is plugged by a silver screw to prevent reunion, and with a bunionectomy, the principal feature of which is the resection of the first metatarsal head.

Ernest Codman (1869-1940) was a leading crusader for the reform of hospital standards. He was born in Boston and attended Harvard Medical School (1895). After completing a house officership at the Massachusetts General Hospital, he joined the surgical staff there and became a member of the Harvard faculty. He lost his staff privileges there in 1914 in a dispute over evaluating the competence of surgeons, which resulted from his zealous efforts to improve and promote standardization of hospital treatment nationally. Thus, to test his management concepts, Codman was forced to develop his own private hospital. His ideas were enumerated in two privately printed pamphlets, *A Study in Hospital Efficiency* (1915 and 1920). In the early 1920s Codman established the first bone tumor registry in the United States, which set the precedent for a national exchange of information on bone tumor cases. This effort culminated in his authoring *Bone Sarcoma, an Interpretation of the Nomenclature* (1925). Codman was also the first American expert on diseases and injuries of the shoulder, described subdeltoid bursitis, and authored *The Shoulder: Rupture of the Supraspinatus Tendon and Other Lesions in or about the Subacromial Bursa* (1934). Codman's name is linked with a clinical sign of hunching of the shoulder that occurs when the deltoid muscle contracts in the absence of rotator cuff function and with a chondroblastoma.

331. Harvey Cushing writing his postoperative notes, as photographed by Walter Willard Boyd (1928). *(Arthur E. Lyons Collection.)*

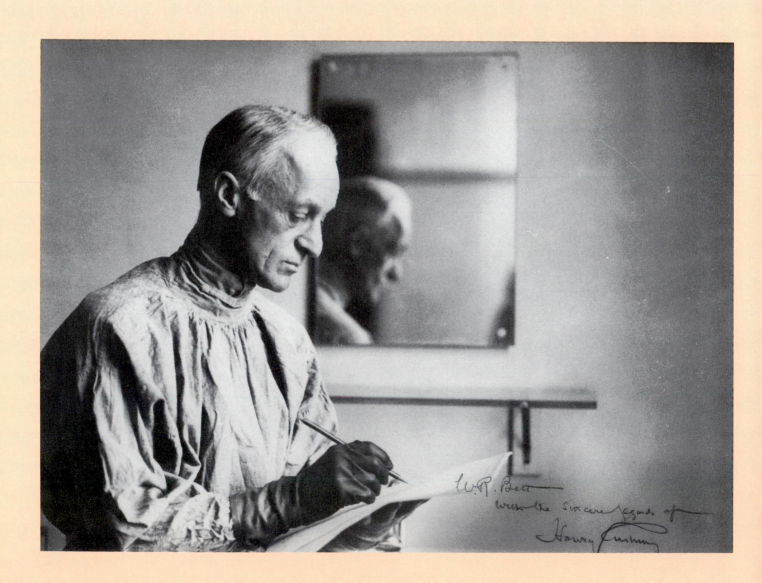

It is a fitting tribute to Harvey Cushing (1869-1939) that he is the final surgeon to be listed in this review of nineteenth-century American surgery. Through his industriousness, foresight, and obsessive attention to detail, he led surgery into the modern era. Cushing's efforts provided a foundation for the supremacy of American surgery in the twentieth century. He graduated from Harvard Medical School in 1895. Shortly thereafter, Cushing began his surgical residency under William Halsted. In 1900 Cushing completed his training and left for a year-long sojourn in Europe, where he worked with Theodor Kocher and Victor Horsley. On returning to the United States, Cushing rejoined the surgical staff of the Johns Hopkins Hospital, where he began his neurosurgical studies. In 1912 he was appointed professor of surgery at Harvard and surgeon-in-chief of the newly built Peter Bent Brigham Hospital. There he remained until 1933, when he was forced to resign. Cushing was a pioneer neurosurgeon who developed many of the basic techniques and procedures used in surgery of the brain and spinal cord. All his clinical texts dealt with neurosurgery, including *The Pituary Body and Its Disorders* (1912), *Tumors of the Nervus Acusticus* (1917), *A Classification of the Tumors of the Glioma Group* (1926), *Studies in Intracranial Physiology and Surgery* (1926), *Tumors Arising from the Blood-Vessels of the Brain* (1928), *Papers Relating to the Pituitary Body, Hypothalamus and Parasympathetic Nervous System* (1932), *Intracranial Tumors* (1932), and *Meningiomas* (1938). Among his most important papers were those on an operative method of extirpating the trigeminal ganglion (1900), infiltration anesthesia (1902), operative intervention in intracranial hemorrhage of the newborn (1905), the use of iatrogenically induced cerebral hernia as a decompressive measure for inaccessible brain tumors (1905), sexual infantilism (1906), the functions of the pituitary body (1910), experimental hypophysectomy (1910), the introduction of electrocoagulation in neurosurgery (1928), and basophil adenomas of the pituitary body (1932). He also devised, with Ernest Codman, an "ether chart" for the operating room, on which pulse, respiration, blood pressure, and other vital signs could be recorded (1895). Cushing had a profound impact on the training of young surgeons by establishing the Hunterian Laboratory of Experimental Medicine at Johns Hopkins (1905) and a widely respected residency program at Harvard. In addition to his clinical work, Cushing found time to write the two-volume *Life of Sir William Osler* (1925), for which he was awarded the Pulitzer prize in 1926. Cushing was a renowned medical and surgical historian and bibliophile. His extensive collection was bequeathed to Yale University and summarized in *The Harvey Cushing Collection of Books and Manuscripts* (1943).

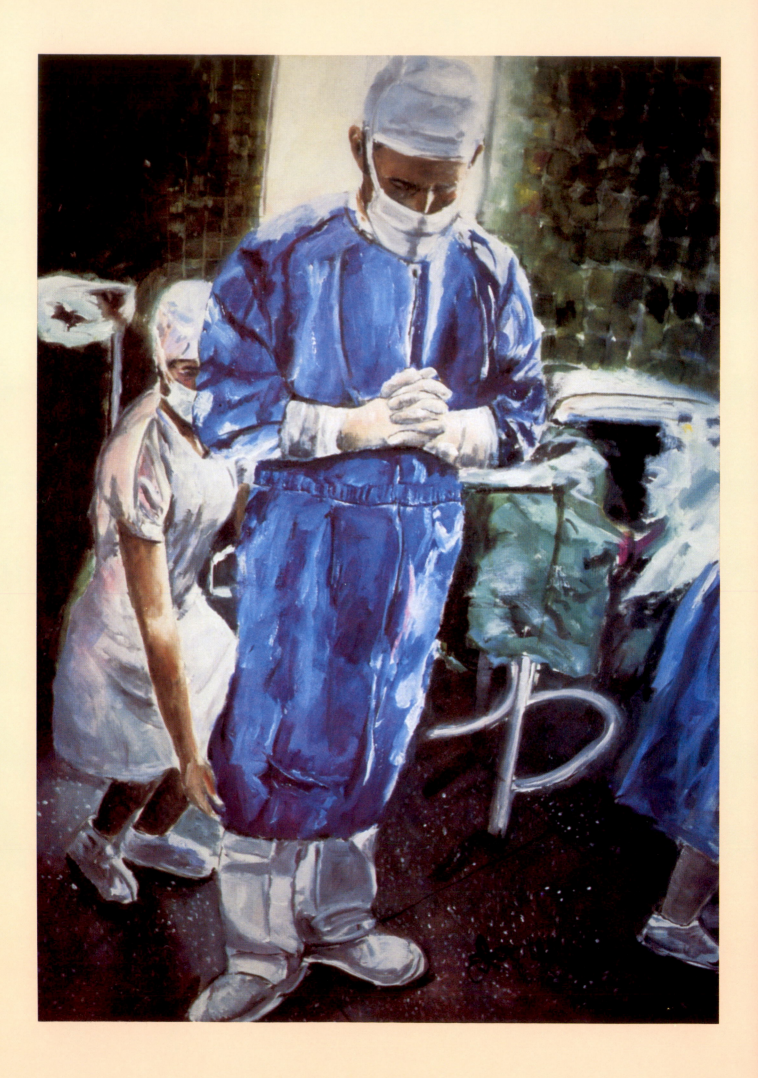

CHAPTER 12

THE TWENTIETH CENTURY

Although it may be easier for us to relate to the "modern" surgery of this century than to the more primitive practices of prior periods, since the closer we come to the present the closer surgical practices resemble those of our own time, writing the history of modern surgery is in some respects more difficult than writing the history of the development of surgery before the twentieth century. One reason for this is the ever-increasing pace of scientific development. The craft of surgery is in constant flux, and the more rapid the change, the more difficult it is to obtain a satisfactory historical perspective. Only the passage of time permits a truly valid historical analysis. Therefore, the history of the recent evolution of surgery cannot be written in stone. However, distinct themes have become apparent in the surgery of the past 94 years.

Three phases of surgical development are noted during the twentieth century—from 1900 to 1918, from 1919 to 1945, and from 1946 to the present. Within each period significant events have transpired that have affected the history of surgery. The first 20 years represent a direct continuation of the tremendous revolution that had occurred within the surgical sciences during the last quarter of the nineteenth century. Many advances in surgery have been made during armed conflict. Not unexpectedly, therefore, World War I provided a signpost for surgery during the remainder of the twentieth century.

The exigencies of the First World War brought about the final maturation and equitable standing of surgery and surgeons within the medical community. Before 1914, surgeons still felt a need to justify their own practice, as noted in comments made by Theodor Kocher to the Swiss Society of Surgery (1913):

> It is still very popular today to deprecate the surgeon as a mere specialist . . . however, the surgeons have by now become the true physicians for they have, on the basis of studying the physiology of the internal organs, conquered the therapy of these, and, in fact, they are often more knowledgeable about the inside of the body, thanks to their interventions in brain, lungs, hearts, stomach, and kidneys, than the official internist physicians.

A certain sense of social discomfort on the part of surgeons led to continued mockery by "scientific" physicians, who often disqualified surgeons as nonthinkers and surgery as an inferior craft. By 1900, surgeons had basically explored all the cavities of the body. Nonetheless, operative surgery had not yet been accepted by physicians who were not oriented to surgery or, most important, by patients and society. Even in the 1990s, the immediate consequences of surgical operations, such as discomfort and associated complications, often are of more concern to patients than the positive knowledge that surgery can eliminate potentially devastating disease processes.

By the early twentieth century it was becoming evident that research models, theoretical concepts, and valid clinical applications would be necessary to demonstrate the scientific basis of surgery to the public and that, to devise new op-

332. *Facing page, Contemplation Before Surgery,* 1987, by Joseph R. Wilder. One of numerous paintings in The Surgeon at Work series. Formerly director of surgery at the Hospital for Joint Diseases and Medical Center, New York, and professor emeritus of surgery at Mount Sinai School of Medicine, New York, Wilder has distinguished himself as an athlete, a surgeon, and a painter. *(Courtesy Joseph R. Wilder.)*

333. *Facing page*, Aviator Charles Lindbergh (1902-1974) posing with the surgeon Alexis Carrel and the perfusion pump that they developed together, on the cover of *Time* (June 1938). In 1931, the year before his son's sensational kidnapping, Lindbergh began working with Carrel at the Rockefeller Institute on a perfusion pump that would allow the cultivation of whole organs in vitro. Lindbergh's pump maintained a sterile, pulsating circulation of fluid through excised organs and enabled Carrel to keep alive and functioning such organs as the thyroid gland and kidney. The perfusion pump is a forerunner of today's heart pump. *(Copyright 1983 Time Inc. Reprinted by permission.)*

erative methods, experimental surgery was necessary. Most important, a scientific basis for therapeutic surgical recommendations consisting of empirical data collected and analyzed according to internationally accepted rules and set apart from individual authoritative appreciations would have to be developed. Surgeons needed to allay society's fear of the surgical unknown and present surgery as an accepted part of the established medical armamentarium. The most consequential achievement for twentieth-century surgeons was the eventual social acceptability of surgery.

Although success and acceptability in the biomedical sciences are difficult to determine, one measure of both in the twentieth century has been the annual Nobel prize in medicine and physiology. Since the inception of the award in 1901, nine surgeons have been named laureates (see the box below).

At the beginning of the twentieth century internationalization was one of the underlying themes in the practice of surgery. William Halsted and Hermann Küttner (1870-1932), director of the surgical clinic in Breslau, had instituted the first known official exchange of surgical residents in 1914. This experiment in surgical education, which involved George Heuer (1882-1950) of Baltimore and Felix Landois (1879-1950) of Breslau, was meant to underscore the true international spirit that had engulfed surgery. Halsted firmly believed that young surgeons achieved greater clinical maturity by observing the practice of surgery in other countries as well as in their own.

As part of the internationalization process, the many differences evident in each country's surgical past became less obvious as the twentieth century progressed. As industrialized nations have grown in economic strength, less diversity has been evident in surgical practice within each country. Therefore the details of each country's separate surgical evolution are not crucial to an understanding of surgery in the twentieth century and are not reviewed here.

SURGEONS WHO HAVE RECEIVED THE NOBEL PRIZE IN MEDICINE AND PHYSIOLOGY

THEODOR KOCHER (1841-1917) of Switzerland
Thyroid surgery (1909)

ALLVAR GULLSTRAND (1862-1930) of Sweden
Ocular dioptrics (1911)

ALEXIS CARREL (1873-1944) of France and the United States
Vascular surgery (1912)

ROBERT BÁRÁNY (1876-1936) of Austria
Vestibular disease (1914)

FREDERICK BANTING (1891-1941) of Canada
Insulin (1922)

WALTER HESS (1881-1973) of Switzerland
Midbrain physiology (1949)

WERNER FORSSMANN (1904-1979) of Germany
Cardiac catheterization (1956)

CHARLES HUGGINS (born 1901) of the United States
Oncology (1966)

JOSEPH MURRAY (born 1919) of the United States
Transplantation (1990)

FIFTEEN CENTS • June 13, 1938

TIME

The Weekly Newsmagazine

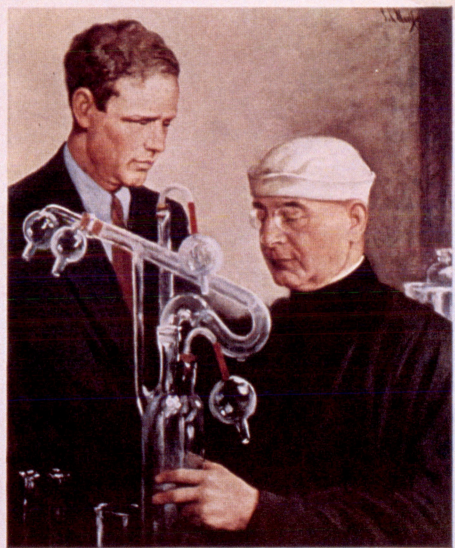

Painted for TIME *by S. J. Woolf*

Volume XXXI

LINDBERGH, CARREL & PUMP

They are looking for the fountain of age.

(See MEDICINE)

Number 24

Among the difficulties in studying twentieth-century surgery is the abundance of famous names and important written contributions. It becomes a difficult and an invidious task to attempt any selection of representative personalities along with their significant journal or book-length writings, particularly after World War I, when the evolution of surgery became more affected than ever before by socioeconomic events and technological advances rather than by unique individual clinical achievements. The vast social transformation of surgery and medicine has controlled the fate of the individual practitioner in the twentieth century to a much greater extent than the clinicians as a collective force were able to control it by their attempts to direct their own profession.

For American surgeons the years just before World War I were a time of active coalescence into various social and educational organizations. The most important of these societies was the American College of Surgeons, founded by Franklin Martin in 1914. Patterned after the Royal Colleges of Surgeons of England, Ireland, and Scotland, the American College of Surgeons established professional, ethical, and moral standards for every authorized graduate in medicine who practiced surgery, and conferred the designation *Fellow of the American College of Surgeons (F.A.C.S.)* on its members.

On an international level surgeons were confronted with the lack of any organizational body. The International College of Surgeons was founded in 1935 in Geneva. At its inception it was intended to serve as a liaison for the existing colleges and surgical societies in the various countries of the world. However, its goals of elevating the art and science of surgery, creating greater understanding among the surgeons of the world, and affording a means of international postgraduate study never came to fruition, in part because the American College of Surgeons opposed the establishment of the American chapter of the International College of Surgeons.

334. John Deaver operating in 1914 with a predominantly female surgical team at Women's Medical College, Philadelphia. At that time few women were admitted to coeducational medical schools in the United States. Fewer still were admitted to surgical residencies. *(Historical Collections, College of Physicians of Philadelphia.)*

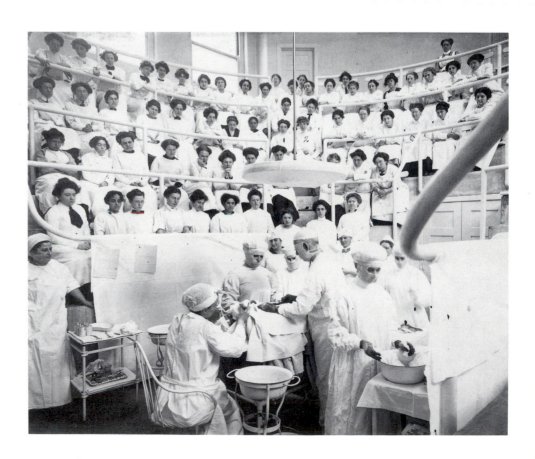

The American College of Surgeons was viewed as an elitist organization when it was founded and for several decades afterward. Because surgeons who were immigrants, females, or members of particular religious and racial minorities were granted fellowships sparingly, many prominent American surgeons were never permitted the "privilege" of membership. Among those individuals was Max Thorek (1880-1960), a well-known Chicago surgeon and author of an important textbook, *Plastic Surgery of the Breast and Abdominal Wall* (1942). He felt that the injustice of exclusion must be rectified, and to do so he organized an American chapter of the International College of Surgeons. Members, most of whom had been refused fellowship in the American College of Surgeons, quickly began to designate themselves fellows of the International College of Surgeons and to use the initials *F.I.C.S.* so that the perceived discrimination of the American College could be partially alleviated.

After World War II the American College of Surgeons became a more democratic organization. As time passed and individuals died, the internecine surgical "war" between the American and International Colleges of Surgeons was forgotten. Nonetheless, at present there is still no international body that represents all surgeons and coordinates their educational, social, economic, and cultural affairs.

Because of the enormous growth of the surgical sciences, no one surgeon could understand and incorporate into surgical practice all the intricacies of new achievements in the surgical sciences during the twentieth century. The well-trained surgeon who limited his or her work to general surgery or to one of the other specialties, particularly in the United States, was rarely differentiated from the majority of doctors who were inadequately trained in surgery and were practicing general medicine and surgery. The leaders of various American surgical societies saw a need for examining boards that had the authority to test future surgical specialists and certify them after necessary requirements were fulfilled so that surgeons would be more unified and their standards of care better delineated.

Although accreditation by an American surgical specialty board has no legal basis, it can be an asset. More and more hospitals are restricting privileges in specialty fields to those who have obtained the certificates of the specialty boards, and many governmental, voluntary, and other agencies are required to send referrals only to surgeons with specialty certificates.

Austria-Hungary and Germany continued as the dominating forces in world surgery until World War I began. However, the results of the conflict proved disastrous to the central powers (Austria-Hungary, Bulgaria, Germany, and the Ottoman Empire) and especially to German-speaking surgeons. Europe took on a new look after the signing of the Peace of Paris. Three independent countries, Austria, Czechoslovakia, and Hungary, emerged from the defeated Austro-Hungary. Allied diplomats created a new Poland out of old Austrian, German, and Russian territories. Yugoslovia was formed, and the area of Romania was doubled. The Ottoman Empire lost most of its land in the Middle East, and its territorial claims in Africa were dismissed. Estonia, Finland, Latvia, and Lithuania declared their independence from Russia.

The demise of Germany's status as the world leader in surgery occurred after the war. Economic ruin and deprivation were evident throughout the land. Erwin Payr (1871-1946), professor of surgery and director of the university clinic in Leipzig, wrote in a letter to Halsted in 1919:

> . . . there are only sad things to report. The saddest is that in each nation a few hot-blooded politicians and radical nationalists exert more influence on the masses than 99% of the rational thinking intellectuals. When in the years to come the truth is told about the origin of the war, you will see that our only fault was stupidity which lured us into a well prepared trap. This stupidity destroyed a nation which was capable to excel intellectually in any area for 50 years or more . . . Our science is heavily threatened by poverty. Perhaps people will start writing poetry and philosophize again, at least they don't cost anything. Undoubtedly, technology, the natural sciences and medicine are finished . . .

As with most armed conflicts, because of the massive destruction, especially the battlefield injuries, tremendous strides were made in virtually every area of surgery. Undoubtedly the greatest surgical achievement was in the treatment of wound infection. Trench warfare in soil contaminated by decades of cultivation and animal manure made every wounded soldier a potential carrier of any number of pathogenic bacilli. On the battlefront sepsis was inevitable. Any attempt at aseptic technique was impossible, but the treatment of infected wounds by antisepsis was becoming a pragmatic reality.

Surgeons experimented with numerous antiseptic solutions and various types of surgical dressings. A principle of wound treatment applied by means of debridement and irrigation eventually evolved. Henry Dakin (1880-1952), an English chemist, and Alexis Carrel, the Nobel prize–winning French-American surgeon, were the principal protagonists in the development of this extensive system of wound management.

Under Dakin's direction the tedious process of testing solutions for the needed properties of maximal bacterial antisepsis and minimal wound irritation was begun. After several months of preliminary trials, Dakin settled on a solution of sodium hypochlorite buffered with sodium bicarbonate (1915). Carrel concurrently set forth his system of wound management, which included mechanical cleansing, surgical debridement of injured and necrotic tissue, and adequate chemical sterilization by means of copious irrigation with Dakin's new antiseptic solution. Carrel also thought that a bacteriological smear of the wound should be taken daily and that secondary closure should not be performed until the cultures demonstrated complete absence of bacterial growth (1915).

335. *The Large Operation,* drypoint (1914) by Max Beckmann (1884-1950). When World War I began in 1914, Beckmann, a solitary figure within the movement known as German Expressionism, volunteered as a medical corpsman rather than bear arms. In this starkly realistic print he captured some of the grim urgency of war surgery. At the right rear corner, a face bearing a striking resemblance to the artist appears over the surgeon's shoulder. *(Philadelphia Museum of Art: Smith Kline Beecham Corporation Fund.)*

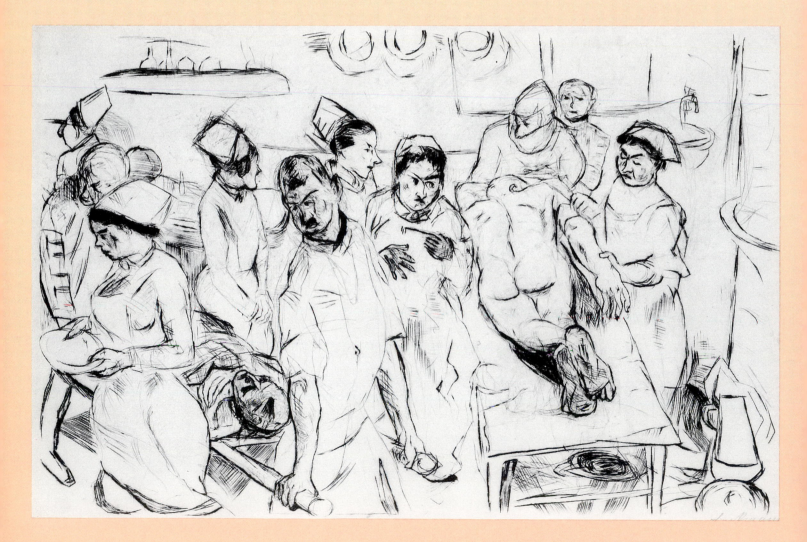

The work of Carrel and Dakin was supported by two English surgeons, Henry Gray (1870-1938) and James Morison (1853-1939), who helped revive debridement of wounds but felt that attempted primary closure of a wound should be performed as soon as possible after adequate épluchage. Morison remains well known to surgeons for his eponymic link with the hepatorenal space and its need for drainage after hepatic or biliary surgery.

Many of the surgical triumphs of World War I are admirably described in Keen's *The Treatment of War Wounds* (1917) and Carrel's *The Treatment of Infected Wounds* (1917). The best account of the day-to-day existence of a wartime surgeon is given in Cushing's *From a Surgeon's Journal, 1915-1918* (1936). In addition to the successes with wound infection, surgical advances were made in the use of X rays in the diagnosis of battlefield injuries, and remarkable operative ingenuity was evident in reconstructive facial surgery and the treatment of fractures resulting from gunshot wounds.

Despite the war's aftermath of worldwide economic depression, the 1920s and 1930s signaled the ascent of American surgery to its current position of international leadership. The rise of scientific surgery in the United States was sparked by the tremendous reforms that engulfed American medical schools in the years before World War I. During that period the poor quality of clinical training, not only for medical students but also for those receiving postgraduate training, became obvious. Among the major contributions to the betterment of medical education was the 1910 report written by Abraham Flexner (1866-1959), *Medical Education in the United States and Canada*.

The Flexner report had great impact not only because of its findings of incompetency in almost all American medical schools, but also because of the uncompromising language Flexner used to describe the deficiencies. Flexner was also able to recognize that once-formidable medical sects such as eclecticism and homeopathy, from whose members many nontraditional surgeons received their educations, were losing popularity and being absorbed by the allopathic profession. All these defects, Flexner wrote, were particularly evident in the way surgery was taught to medical students:

> In general, the less a school has to offer in the way of clinical facilities, the more heavily is surgery overweighted. Its pedagogical value is relatively slight; for operations are performed in large amphitheaters in which the surgeon and his assistants surround the patient, to whom they give their whole mind, in practical disregard of the students, who loll in their seats without an inkling of what is happening below. Most of the students see only the patient's feet and the surgeon's head. Only in rare cases . . . do designated individuals take turns and become part of the operation . . . Inadequacy in general is thus aggravated by increasing predominance of surgical over medical clinics. Clinical teaching thus tends more and more to concentrate in the amphitheater. The laboratory side sinks further and further into the background; the bedside work becomes more and more contracted. The whole thing is demonstrative—and at steadily increasing remoteness.

As a result of the growing agitation for reforms in medical education, which was instigated primarily by the Flexner report and the American Medical Association, more than 75 medical schools, most of them proprietary, were closed between 1906 and 1920. New medical school curricula were established and included such basic changes as the requirement of a bachelor of science degree for admission and the institution of a 4-year program. The stage was thus set for the blossoming of scientific surgery in the United States, which was highlighted by medical school reforms, Halsted's redefinition of surgical residency programs, and the growth of surgical specialties.

From a historical standpoint it is incorrect to assume that organized "surgical specialists" existed before the last decades of the nineteenth century. Until then most surgeons performed all types of surgical operations. It was the rare individual who was thought of as a gynecological surgeon, orthopedic surgeon, or a urological surgeon. More importantly, the professionalization process for surgical specialties (specialty societies, journals) was not yet in place and therefore unable to embrace a more parochial type of surgical practitioner. Consequently, to write of the existence of "orthopedic surgeons" or "urological surgeons" before the mid-nineteenth century is to provide a spurious account of the hierarchy of surgery and its socioeconomical organization.

It was only during the first two decades of the twentieth century that the broadening aspects of operative surgery forcefully demonstrated a glaring need for the surgical specialist. It had become impossible for any single surgeon to master all the manual skills combined with other knowledge required to perform every known surgical operation. For this reason, the evolution of the well-defined surgical specialty, with numerous individuals restricting their surgical practice to one highly structured field, would become one of the most significant and dominating events in twentieth century surgery.

The entire concept of well-defined surgical specialties, with numerous surgeons restricting their practice to organized, structured specialties, is a product of the twentieth century. Therefore, a surgical historian who writes of the existence of orthopedic surgeons or urological surgeons during the early nineteenth century or before is providing a spurious account of how surgery was socioeconomically organized and practiced.

From 1919 to 1945 the maturation process for surgical specialties gathered tremendous momentum. This clarion call became a vital stage in the evolution of world surgery and constituted the most significant aspect of surgical history during that period. Ironically the United States, which had been much slower than European countries to recognize surgeons as a distinct group of clinicians separate from internists and general practitioners, would spearhead the move toward surgical specialization with great alacrity. The course of surgical fragmentation into specialties and subspecialties continues at unimpeded speed today, particularly in the United States. Unless a clear, demonstrable intercommunication is established between specialties, the survival of surgery as a unified discipline will remain uncertain.

GENERAL SURGERY

General surgery was the substrate on which the surgical sciences flourished. Consequently specialization and the development of subspecialties have made the greatest inroads in the broad territories once presided over by so-called general surgeons. The term "general surgeon" is actually a byproduct of this movement toward surgical specialization. Before specialization a surgeon performed basically all types of operations. Thus the average nineteenth-century surgeon could perform a urological procedure as well as an orthopedic operation. General surgery therefore is a contracting field that currently concerns itself with the abdominal and alimentary tracts, the breast, certain types of organ transplantation, critical care, the endocrine glands, the head and neck, hernias, skin and soft tissue, surgical oncology, trauma, and vascular surgery.

Since specialties and subspecialties no longer depend completely on the "general surgeon" for the instruction and orientation in the principles of surgery of their own young protégés, the field of general surgery undergoes continual redefinition. Like its many offshoots, it is considered a true surgical specialty, although the misnomer of "general" is applied to it. General surgeons do not practice "general" surgery; instead they have been left with whatever the other surgical specialties have not been able to or do not choose to treat. Paradoxically, general surgery continues to have the dominant role in medical faculties and the design of the medical school curricula for the surgical sciences.

Within the constantly changing concept of a general surgeon, definitions vary from country to country. For instance, in Germany and Japan general surgeons continue to maintain collateral interests in other specialties such as urology or orthopedic surgery. Therefore they retain vestiges of the old concept of a "general" surgeon, in contrast to the present day practice of general surgeons in the United States.

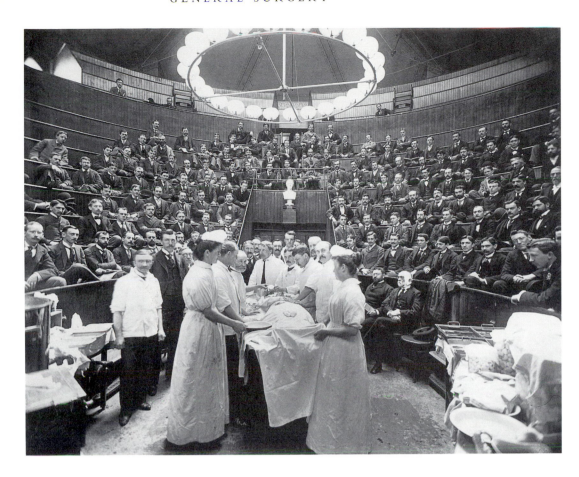

In the United States the public perception of what general surgeons did has always been confused. Until the early 1970s many family physicians also performed simple "general" surgical operations such as appendectomy, cholecystectomy, and herniorrhaphy. As American clinical practice has evolved, however, general internal medicine and family practice have become recognized medical specialties with their own examining boards. In redefining these medical or primary care specialties, family practitioners and internists neither learn nor perform any types of surgical operations. Instead, essentially all surgery in the United States is now conducted by individuals trained in either general surgery or one of the other surgical specialties.

Many of the major extant surgical societies were initially organized during the last 30 years of the nineteenth century and the first 30 years of the twentieth. Although originally intended to encompass all surgeons, these older societies have now assumed the role of serving the general surgeon. Among the most prestigious are the German Society for Surgeons (1872), the American Surgical Association (1880), the Italian Society of Surgery (1883), and the French Surgical Association (1884). Within the United States additional societies have proliferated. The earliest of these included the Southern Surgical Association (1886), the Western Surgical Association (1890), the New England Surgical Society (1916), and the Pacific Coast Surgical Association (1926).

In 1937 general surgery in the United States was accorded official recognition as a surgical specialty when the American Board of Surgery was incorporated as an examining body for all individuals interested in performing general surgical operations. The American Board of Surgery also recently began to offer examinations leading to certificates of special or added qualifications in the subspecialties of pediatric surgery (1975), general vascular surgery (1982), surgical critical care (1986), and surgery of the hand (1989). Before 1980, 25,442 general certificates had been awarded by the American Board of Surgery. During the decade of the 1980s an additional 9492 general certificates and 1682 special or added certificates were given.

336. W.W. Keen operating in the surgical amphitheater at Jefferson Medical College in Philadelphia, 1904. Born in 1837, Keen lived until 1932, witnessing and contributing to the progress of surgery in America from a trade to a profession. In 1932 he was one of the last surviving surgeons to have served in the Civil War. Keen, third from the left, is the slight, bearded figure in the operating team. (*Historical Collections, College of Physicians of Philadelphia.*)

Throughout the twentieth century numerous advances were made in general surgery, especially in surgery of the alimentary tract and the abdomen and its contents. The Belgium surgeon Antoine Depage (1862-1925) reported a method of gastrostomy in which he used a mucous membrane–lined tube formed from the anterior wall of the stomach in 1901. In the following year Robert Weir described an appendicostomy in the surgical treatment of colitis. John Finney (1863-1942) assisted Halsted in the management of the residency program at Johns Hopkins Hospital and authored a paper on a new method of gastroduodenostomy, or widened pyloroplasty (1903). In 1905 Carl Beck (1856-1911) of New York City formed a gastrostomy tube from the greater curvature of the stomach. Donald Balfour (1882-1963) of the Mayo Clinic provided the best account of his important operation for resection of the sigmoid colon in 1910. Eugen Polya (1876-1944), surgeon-in-chief of St. Stephen's Hospital in Budapest, was later murdered by the Nazis. In 1911 he had reported a modification of Billroth's second operation for gastric cancer in which he devised an innovative method of dealing with the duodenal stump. Wilhelm Ramstedt (1867-1963), a German surgeon, described a pyloromyotomy (1912) at the same time that Pierre Fredet (1870-1946) was reporting a similar operation. Franz Torek (1861-1938), an American surgeon, performed the first successful operation for the removal of a carcinoma of the thoracic portion of the esophagus in 1913. In that same year Henry Janeway (1873-1921) of New York City developed a technique for gastrostomy in which he wrapped the anterior wall of the stomach around a catheter and sutured it in place, establishing a permanent fistula. Hans Finsterer (1877-1955), professor of surgery in Vienna, improved Franz von Hofmeister's (1867-1926) description in Germany of a partial gastrectomy with closure of a portion of the lesser curvature and retrocolic anastomosis of the remainder of the stomach to the jejunum (1918). Evarts Graham (1883-1957) was chairman of the department of surgery at Washington University in St. Louis and Warren Cole (1898-1991) one of his residents when they introduced cholecystography (1924). In 1929 Julius Spivack (1889-1956) of Chicago described his tubovalvular gastrostomy. Owen Wangensteen (1898-1981), professor of surgery at the University of Minnesota, first reported on an apparatus for the relief of acute intestinal obstruction in 1932. He followed that work with his classic monograph, *The Therapeutic Problem in Bowel Obstruction* (1937). Allen Oldfather Whipple (1881-1963) was serving as professor of surgery at Columbia University in New York City when he introduced pancreaticoduodenectomy for cancer of the pancreas (1935). Alexander Brunschwig (1901-1969), also of New York City, further modified the operation 2 years later. Lester Dragstedt (1893-1976), professor of surgery at the University of Chicago, reported on the physiology of peptic ulcer disease and the use of vagotomy for operative therapy (1943).

The treatment of breast cancer was radically altered when George Beatson (1848-1933), professor of surgery in Glasgow, proposed oophorectomy and the administration of thyroid extract as a possible cure (1901). Joseph Bloodgood (1867-1935) of Baltimore wrote a paper about his theory of the causation of chronic mastitis in 1906 and followed it with a description of blue dome cysts (1921). William Handley (1872-1962) was surgeon to the Middlesex Hospital in London when he wrote *Cancer of the Breast and Its Treatment* (1906). In that work he advanced the theory that in breast cancer metastasis is due to extension along lymphatic vessels and not to dissemination via the bloodstream. The modern operation of total bilateral mammectomy with transplantation of the nipple and areola for both cancer and gynecomastia was developed by Louis Dartigues (1869-1940), a French surgeon (1928). In 1931 George Cheatle (1865-1951), professor of surgery in London, and Max Cutler (1899-1984), a surgeon from New York, published their important treatise, *Tumours of the Breast*. In that same year Cutler detailed his systemic use of ovarian hormone in the treatment of chronic mastitis. Geoffrey Keynes (1887-1982) of St. Bartholomew's Hospital in London articulated the basis for the opposition to radical mastectomy and his favoring of radium treatment in breast cancer (1932). In 1933 Frank Adair (1887-1982) of New York City gave the first description of plasma cell mastitis.

Alfred Blalock (1899-1964), professor of surgery at The Johns Hopkins Hospital, conducted important research on surgical shock. His papers on experimental shock (1927 and 1930) and his text, *Principles of Surgical Care, Shock and Other Problems* (1940), showed that surgical shock was due not to the elaboration of toxins or to reflex neurological mechanisms but to a decrease in circulating blood volume. In *Treatment of War Wounds and Fractures, with Special Reference to the Closed Method as Used in the War in Spain* (1939), Joseph Trueta (1897-1977), a Spanish surgeon, outlined a method of wound treatment that included the application of closed plaster after packing the excised wound with sterile gauze on which petroleum jelly had been applied.

Among the many triumphs of twentieth-century general surgery have been operative successes in the treatment of endocrine disorders. In 1920 Eugen Steinach (1861-1944), a Viennese surgeon, reported his rejuvenation operation, which consisted of ligation of the vas deferens, for the treatment of impotence and aging. Three years later Serge Voronoff (1866-1951), a Parisian surgeon, authored *Greffes Testiculaires,* which presented his experiments in rejuvenation by means of testicular transplantation. Thomas Dunhill (1876-1957) of London was a pioneer in thyroid surgery, especially in his operation for exophthalmic goiter (1919). Cecil Joll (1885-1945), also professor of surgery in London, described the treatment of thyrotoxicosis by means of a subtotal thyroidectomy in *Disease of the Thyroid Gland, with Special Reference to Thyrotoxicosis* (1932). During the 1930s Frank Lahey (1880-1953) of Boston wrote in numerous papers about the

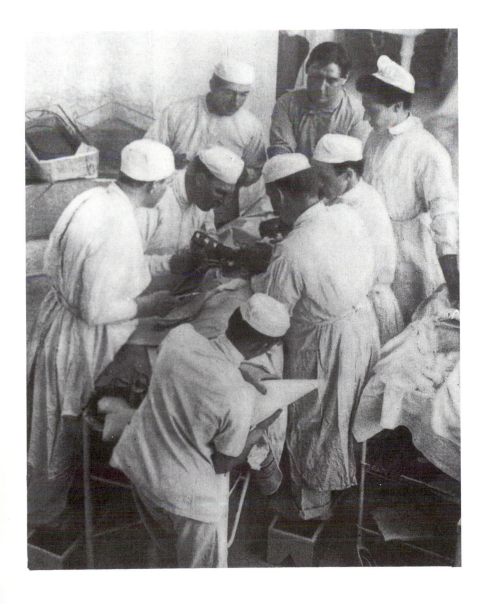

337. William Halsted's first operation in the new surgical amphitheatre at Johns Hopkins Hospital in 1904. Some of Halsted's former residents and staff members returned for the honor of assisting at the first operation in the new building. Among those present were Harvey Cushing (partially visible, second from the right in the foreground), Hugh Young, and J.C. Bloodgood. *(The Alan Mason Chesney Medical Archives of The Johns Hopkins Medical Institutions, Baltimore, Md.)*

importance of identifying the recurrent laryngeal nerve during the course of thyroid surgery. Felix Mandl (1882–1957) of Vienna was the first to successfully treat generalized osteitis fibrosa by extirpation of a parathyroid tumor (1925). In 1906 Hermann Schloffer (1868–1937) of Vienna successfully operated on a pituitary tumor via the nasal route.

Although *Homo sapiens* has long had difficulties with hernias, advances during the last century have greatly simplified the operation. Alexander Ferguson (1853–1912) of Chicago described his methods of herniorrhaphy in *The Technic of Modern Operations for Hernia* (1907). Paul Laroque (1876–1934), a surgeon from Richmond, Virginia, combined a superior transperitoneal gridiron incision with a repair based on the method of Bassini (1919). Bloodgood described his method of transplantation of the rectus muscle in certain cases of inguinal hernia in 1919. In the following year Cheatle became the first surgeon to describe a preperitoneal approach to groin hernias. William Gallie (1882–1959) used sutures fashioned from the fascia lata in herniorrhaphy (1923). The Irish surgeon Arnold Henry (1886–1962) devised an operation for femoral hernia in 1936. Earl Shouldice (1891–1965) of Toronto, Canada, first began to experiment with a repair based on overlapping layers brought together by a continuous wire suture during the 1930s. Norman Tanner (1906–1982) of England used his "slide" operation with a relaxing incision (1942); Chester McVay (1911–1987) popularized a repair based on the pectineal ligament (1948).

The treatment of vascular diseases has become a mainstay of the twentieth-century general surgeon's practice. In 1906 Jose Goyanes (1876–1964) of Madrid used vein grafts to restore arterial flow. Seven years later Bertram Bern-

338. *A Liver Transplant* (1990) by Sir Roy Calne. Professor of surgery at Cambridge University and renowned for his work in immunosuppression, Calne has been drawing and painting for much of his life. *(Private collection. Courtesy of Sheeran Lock Fine Art Consultants.)*

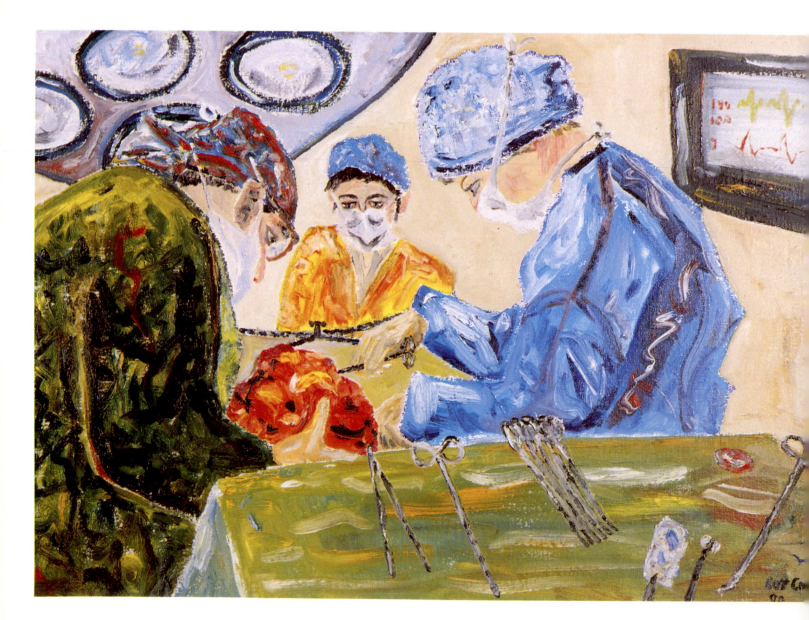

heim (1880-1957), a surgeon from Baltimore, authored America's first textbook on the subject, *Surgery of the Vascular System*. In 1912 Charles Gurthrie authored his renowned monograph, *Blood-Vessel Surgery and Its Applications*, which described the pioneer work he and Carrel did in tissue and organ transplantation. George Vaughan (1859-1948), professor of surgery at Georgetown University, completed a successful ligation of the abdominal aorta for aneurysmal disease in 1921. Barney Brooks (1884-1952), professor of surgery at Vanderbilt University in Nashville, Tennessee, initially introduced clinical angiography and femoral arteriography (1924). Five years later Reynaldo dos Santos (1880-1970), a Portuguese urologist, reported the first translumbar aortogram. In 1929 William Babcock (1872-1963), chief of surgery at Temple University in Philadelphia, proposed his operative decompression of aortic aneurysm by carotid-jugular anastomosis. Friedrich Trendelenburg (1844-1924) first attempted pulmonary embolectomy in 1908, and the procedure was eventually performed successfully by Martin Kirschner (1879-1942), a surgeon in Greifswald, Germany, in 1924. A successful arterial embolectomy was carried out by Ernest Mosny of France in 1911 and by Einar Key (1872-1954) of Vienna in the following year. The first successful embolectomy in Great Britain was reported by Geoffrey Jefferson (1886-1961) in 1925. Max Peet (1885-1949) of Ann Arbor, Michigan, presented his splanchnic resection for hypertension in 1935. René Leriche (1879-1955), one of the outstanding vascular surgeons of the twentieth century, proposed in 1937 an arteriectomy in arterial thrombosis and, later, a periarterial sympathectomy to improve arterial flow. Leriche enunciated a syndrome of aortoiliac occlusive disease in 1940.

COLORECTAL SURGERY

In few countries of the world is colorectal surgery recognized as a surgical specialty distinct from general surgery. In the United States, however, the vagaries of surgical politics conjured the American Board of Colon and Rectal Surgery in 1949. Admittedly the roots of this specialty can be traced back to the itinerant rectal surgeons of medieval Europe. In America the itinerant role was readily assumed by such men as Alexander Brinkerhoff (?-1887) of Ohio. A nuisance and a quack who roamed the Midwest plying his trade of curing piles, Brinkerhoff even privately published a lengthy monograph, *Diseases of the Rectum and New Method of Rectal Treatment* (1881).

Proctology was firmly established in the United States through the efforts of Joseph Mathews; Charles Kelsey (1850-1917), who wrote *Diseases of the Rectum and Anus* (1882), *The Pathology, Diagnosis, and Treatment of Diseases of the Rectum and Anus* (1884), *The Diagnosis and Treatment of Haemorrhoids* (1887), *Surgery of the Rectum and Pelvis* (1897), and *The Office Treatment of Hemorrhoids, Fistula, Etc. without Operation* (1898); and Samuel Gant (1869-1944), who authored *Diagnosis and Treatment of Diseases of the Rectum, Anus, and Contiguous Textures* (1896) and *Constipation and Intestinal Obstruction* (1909).

At the beginning of the twentieth century the specialty was limited to diseases of the anus and rectum. In 1940, surgeons interested in anal and rectal surgery were certified through the American Board of Surgery by a committee of practicing proctologists. Nine years later the American Board of Proctology was granted approval to serve as its own examining body, and in 1961 its name was officially changed to the American Board of Colon and Rectal Surgery.

Today in the United States a recognized specialist in colorectal surgery is a fully trained general surgeon who completes at least 1 additional year of training in colorectal surgery. To become certified, the individual must also have previously passed the certifying examination of the American Board of Surgery. Before 1980, 695 certificates had been awarded by the American Board of Colon and Rectal Surgery, and during the 1980s, 348 more were given.

GYNECOLOGICAL SURGERY

At the beginning of the twentieth century, whether gynecology should remain as a surgical specialty independent of both obstetrics and general surgery was much debated. Many well-intentioned surgeons, particularly Howard Kelly of The Johns Hopkins Hospital wished to keep gynecological surgery separate from obstetrics. At his urging John Whitridge Williams (1866-1931) assumed a separate professorship of obstetrics at that institution. Thomas Cullen (1868-1953) succeeded Kelly and remained vociferous in his resistance to the union of obstetrics and gynecology.

More numerous than the resisters were the proponents of a unified specialty. Thaddeus Reamy (1829-1909) founded the first hospital for women west of the Allegheny Mountains. Franz von Winckel (1837-1911), professor of obstetrics and gynecology in Munich, was particularly outspoken on the subject. In Germany the teachers of obstetrics usually taught gynecology as well. In America, England, and France, however, gynecology was largely practiced by surgeons, who were quite stubborn in their refusal to yield the specialty to obstetricians.

A long struggle preceded the recognition of obstetrics as a specialty, most notably in Great Britain. Obstetrics had always been more closely aligned with medicine than with surgery. English physicians believed that midwives were adequately prepared to deal with parturients and, until well into the twentieth century, that a physician's presence was not necessarily required when a woman gave birth. A royal charter was finally granted to obstetrics in 1942, and the Royal College of Obstetricians and Gynaecologists was later formed. The Royal College of Surgeons, which took the position that obstetricians and gynecologists should have experience in general surgery, was in part responsible for the long delay and opposition.

In late nineteenth-century America there was a growing sense that societies for specialists would be needed to further the professionalization process of practicing physicians. The earliest such organization devoted to obstetrics and gynecology was the American Medical Association's Section on Obstetrics and Gynecology (1860). Many local societies also emerged, including the New York Obstetrical Society (1863), the Obstetrical Society of Philadelphia (1868), the Cincinnati Obstetrical Society (1876), the Chicago Gynecological Society (1878), the Obstetrical Society of Boston (1881), and the Brooklyn Gynecological Society (1890).

The first nationwide organization for gynecologists was the American Gynecological Society (1876), and the founding of the American Association of Obstetricians and Gynecologists (1888) soon followed. In both instances the membership of these two groups was deliberately limited by the founding members. Consequently the rapidly growing corps of obstetrical and gynecological specialists in the United States remained without a politically powerful society to act in its behalf. The problem was not resolved until 1944, when the National Federation of Obstetric-Gynecologic Societies was formed. To become a more egalitarian institution, the federation members decided in 1951 that the organization should be reconstituted into a national body based on individual membership and known as the American Academy of Obstetrics and Gynecology. Five years later the academy changed its name to the American College of Obstetricians and Gynecologists. Although gynecological surgery is no longer recognized as an independent surgical specialty, when combined with obstetrics it becomes the only specialty in America that enjoys both surgical and primary care status.

In America in the mid-twentieth century a few diehards persisted in their efforts to maintain the separate identity of gynecology. As late as 1952, only 78% of American medical schools had combined departments of obstetrics and gynecology. The biggest boost to a joining of these two fields occurred in 1930, when the American Board of Obstetrics and Gynecology was incorporated. As the only officially recognized examining body, it began to award general certificates in obstetrics and gynecology and, later, certificates of special qualifications in gynecological oncology (1974), maternal and fetal medicine (1974), reproductive endocrinology (1974), and critical care (1986). Before 1980, 18,663 general certificates had been awarded; and during the 1980s an additional 10,154 were given. Of the special certificates, 1007 were received during the 1980s.

Many magnificent clinical advances have been made in gynecological surgery during the twentieth century. In 1901 John Webster (1863-1950) of Canada reported his method of treating retrodisplacement of the uterus. James Baldwin (1850-1936) of the United States proposed the formation of an artificial vagina by means of intestinal transplantation in 1904. A relatively infrequent but benign neoplasm of the ovary was described by Fritz Brenner (1877-1963) of Germany, who later practiced in Johannesburg, South Africa. Archibald Donald (1860-1937) of Manchester, England, described an operation for prolapse of the uterus in 1908. In that same year Friedrich Schauta (1849-1919) of Vienna proposed a radical vaginal hysterectomy for carcinoma of the cervix. An outstanding figure in British gynecology and a founder of the Royal College of Obstetricians and Gynaecologists was William Bell (1871-1936). His textbook, *The Principles of Gynaecology* (1910), remained one of the most important treatises on the subject during the first half of the century. The first individual to perform salpingography, in 1914, was William Cary (1883-1969) of the United States. At the same time Isador Rubin (1883-1958) of New York City was conducting his own experimentation on uterotubal insufflation. He expanded on his research 6 years later (1920), when tubal insufflation was used for the diagnosis and treatment of sterility caused by occlusion of the fallopian tubes. William Fothergill (1865-1926) succeeded Donald in Manchester as professor of clinical obstetrics and gynecology. Fothergill modified Donald's operation for uterine prolapse by using anterior colporrhaphy in combination with the amputation of the cervix (1915). Thomas Cullen wrote *Embryology, Anatomy, and Diseases of the Umbilicus Together with Diseases of the Urachus* in 1916. This magnificent volume, with extraordinary illustrations, contained the first reference to a clinical sign of periumbilical darkening of the skin caused by the presence of blood, usually associated with ruptured ectopic gestation. John Sampson (1873-1946) of Albany, New York, first accurately described ovarian endometriosis and its pathognomonic hallmark, the chocolate cyst (1921). Walter Schiller (1887-1960) was born in Vienna, where he worked until the rise of Nazism, which caused him to flee to the United States in 1936. Three years before, he had reported a test to determine carcinoma of the cervix. Irving Stein (1887-1976) and Michael Leventhal (1901-1971) described a syndrome of amenorrhea associated with bilateral polycystic ovaries in 1935. Joe Meigs (1892-1963) reported on the association of fibromyoma of the ovary with hydroperitoneum and hydrothorax (1937). In 1941 George Papanicolaou (1883-1962) observed while working in New York City that he could recognize cancer cells in a microscopic examination of smears of vaginal specimens.

Achievements in the development of the cesarean section included Fritz Frank's (1856-1923) suprasymphyseal transperitoneal technique (1907). Wilhelm Latzko (1863-1945) reported his extraperitoneal lower-segment cesarean section in 1909. He would later be forced to leave his professorship in Vienna because of Nazi oppression and take up residence in New York City. In the third edition of *Operative Gynakologie* (1912) Albert Doderlein (1860-1941) and Bernard Kronig (1863-1917) described a transperitoneal lower-segment cesarean section. Joseph DeLee (1869-1942) proposed his low cervical operation, or laparotrachelotomy, in 1919. Louis Portes (1891-1950), a Parisian obstetrician, reported on the classic cesarean section followed by temporary exteriorization of the uterus (1924). The history of gynecological surgery has been recorded by William McKay (1866-1948) in *The History of Ancient Gynaecology* (1901); Heinrich Fasbender (1843-1914) in *Geschichte Der Geburtshulfe* (1906); James Ricci (1890-1955) in *The Genealogy of Gynaecology* (1943), *One Hundred Years of Gynaecology, 1800-1900* (1945), and *The Development of Gynaecological Surgery and Instruments* (1949); and Richard Leonardo (1895-1959) in *History of Gynecology* (1944).

NEUROLOGICAL SURGERY

At the beginning of the twentieth surgery, neurological surgery was performed primarily by a few general surgeons who had acquired a special interest in the nervous system. These surgeons, including Charles Ballance (1865-1936), Ernst von Bergmann (1836-1907), Harvey Cushing (1869-1939), Charles Frazier (1870-1936), Victor Horsley (1857-1916), William Keen (1837-1932), Fedor Krause (1857-1937), and William Macewen (1848-1924), educated the general practitioner to consult with them about patients with brain tumors. In most cases, however, the general surgeon who performed operations on patients with central nervous system disorders was usually directed by a neurologist.

Cushing provided most of the guidance of the growing specialty during the first 40 years of the twentieth century. He realized the need to develop related sciences such as neuroophthalmology, neuropathology, and neuroradiology. Cushing developed an extensive training program in neurological surgery for surgeons who had already acquired basic training in general surgery.

As the number of neurological surgeons increased, they began to meet to discuss their mutual interests. In 1920 Cushing formed the Society of Neurological Surgeons in Boston. By the 1950s neurological surgery societies were scattered throughout the world.

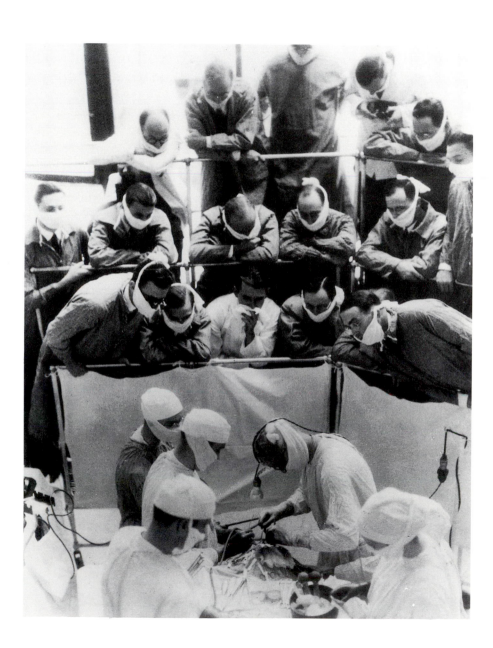

339. Harvey Cushing performing an operation; the Harvey Cushing Society is observing. 1932. Photograph by Richard Upjohn Light. *(Boston Medical Library.)*

As the specialty became more popular, the need for a journal became evident. In 1936 the *Zentralblatt Für Neurochirurgie* was founded, and 8 years later the *Journal of Neurosurgery* appeared in the United States. The American Board of Neurological Surgery was formally established in 1940 to act as an examining body. From 1940 through 1979, 2532 general certificates were awarded. During the 1980s an additional 1078 certificates were given.

Twentieth-century clinical advances in neurological surgery have included the report of William Spiller (1863-1936) of Philadelphia, and Charles Frazier on intracranial trigeminal neurotomy (1901). In 1907 Ballance authored *Some Points on the Surgery of the Brain and its Membranes*. In that treatise he recognized and described subdural hematoma and described a successful operation for it. In the following year Horsley and Robert Clarke (1850-1926) devised an apparatus that opened the way for stereotactic surgery of the brain. Otfrid Foerster (1873-1941) of Germany introduced his operation of rhizotomy for spastic paralysis in 1908, and in that same year Cushing authored his first significant treatise on neurosurgery as part of Keen's eight-volume *Surgery: Its Principles and Practice*. As a result of the publication of Keen's detailed monograph, neurological surgery soon became recognized as a well-defined surgical specialty. From 1908 to 1911 Krause authored his two-volume *Chirurgie Des Gehirns Und Ruckenmarks Nach Eigenen Erfahrungen*. In 1909, Hermann Küttner (1870-1932) reported an operation for tabes dorsalis and Horsley demonstrated that removal of the precentral area in humans abolished athetosis. William Spiller (1863-1940) and Edward Martin (1859-1938) of Philadelphia authored their classic paper on cordotomy for the relief of intractable pain in 1912. William Luckett (1872-1929), a New York City surgeon, observed air in the cerebral ventricles in 1913, which provided Walter Dandy (1886-1946) of The Johns Hopkins Hospital with his idea for ventriculography (1919). In 1913 Hermann Oppenheim (1858-1919) and Fedor Krause (1856-1937) successfully removed a pineal tumor. Three years later René Leriche (1879-1955) performed a periarterial sympathectomy. Harris Mosher (1867-1954) of the United States initiated the modern method of trephinating and draining inflammatory processes of the brain when he devised a wire gauze drain (1916). Dandy first extirpated the choroid plexus of the lateral ventricles in communicating hydrocephalus, thus relieving the swelling, in 1918. Around the same time, Max Peet (1885-1949) of the University of Michigan performed a trigeminal nerve resection with conservation of the motor root for treatment of trigeminal neuralgia. Leonardo Bianchi (1848-1919) of Italy demonstrated that bilateral destruction of the frontal lobes caused personality changes (1920). The technique of sympathetic ramisection was carried out by Norman Royle (?-1944) of Australia in 1924. In that same year Wilfred Trotter (1872-1939) of England performed the first planned operation for intracranial aneurysm, which was diagnosed before surgery. In 1925 Gaston Cotte (1879-1951) of Lyon, France, completed a presacral neurectomy. During the late 1920s Dandy began performing intracranial sections of various cranial nerves, including the trigeminal and glossopharyngeal nerves. Lyudvig Puusepp (1875-1942), a well-known German neurosurgeon, reported his method for removing cerebral tumors (1926). The first successfull operation for traumatic aneurysm of the internal carotid artery was carried out by James Birley (1884-1934) of England in 1928. Herbert Olivecrona (1891-1980) successfully removed an intracranial aneurysm in 1932. Four years later Antonio Egas Moniz (1874-1955) and Walter Freeman (1895-1972) described prefrontal lobotomy as a means of treatment for various mental illnesses. In 1938 Achile Dogliotti (1897-1966) reported the first surgical section of the pain-temperature pathway at the brain stem for the treatment of diffuse, unrelenting pain. Charles Elsberg (1871-1948), an American pioneer in neurosurgery, authored *Surgical Diseases of the Spinal Cord, Membranes, and Nerve Roots* in 1941. Ernest Sachs (1879-1958) wrote a short monograph, *The History and Development of Neurological Surgery,* in 1952.

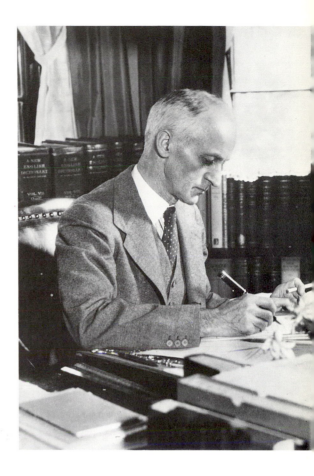

340. Harvey Cushing writing at his desk, circa 1930, his frequently consulted *Oxford English Dictionary* at his elbow. Cushing was the only surgeon to win the Pulitzer prize for his biography of William Osler (1925). *(Boston Medical Library.)*

OPHTHALMOLOGICAL SURGERY

Although ophthalmology enjoys the longest and most distinguished history of all surgical specialties, a definite organizational separation of ophthalmology from the rest of surgery did not occurr until in the mid-nineteenth century.

As ophthalmological data increased and rapidly changing views were advanced, the need for ophthalmological periodicals became evident. The first of lasting significance was the *Archiv Für Ophthalmologie* (1854), founded by von Graefe. In 1884 the *American Journal of Ophthalmology* was initiated under the editorial leadership of Adolf Alt (1851-1920).

The next major organizational movement in ophthalmology after the publication of journals was the creation of specialty societies. In 1864 the American Ophthalmological Society was instigated by Henry Noyes (1832-1900) of New York and Hasket Derby (1835-1914) of Boston and initiations of the Ophthalmological Society of the United Kingdom (1880) and the Societé Française d'Ophthalmologie (1888) soon followed.

Strengthening of ophthalmological organizations in the United States to promote improved research, teaching, and practice standards was a product of the twentieth century. One of the most important organizations was the American Academy of Ophthalmology and Otolaryngology, which was begun in 1903. Around the turn of the century the questions of adequate training and examinations for ophthalmic specialists were being raised by growing numbers of leaders in American ophthalmology. These discussions culminated in 1914 with the formation of a joint committee of the American Academy of Ophthalmology and Otolaryngology, the American Ophthalmological Society, and the Section on Ophthalmology of the American Medical Association to consider ophthalmic education. The committee's report led to the establishment of the American Board for Ophthalmic Examination in 1916. The name was officially changed to the American Board of Ophthalmology in 1933, and the organization became the first established American specialty board. From its beginning through 1979 the Board awarded 12,323 general certificates in ophthalmology. During the 1980s an additional 4711 certificates were given.

341. William Halsted and Theodor Kocher in Inselspital in Bern, Switzerland, performing an operation on a patient with an abdominal aortic aneurysm (1911). Halsted, fourth from the left, is partially visible. Kocher is facing Halsted. Three of Halsted's residents who accompanied him to Europe, Follis, Sowers, and Fisher, form a triangle; the center of the triangle is filled in by the nurse at Kocher's back. *(The Alan Mason Chesney Medical Archives of the Johns Hopkins Medical Institutions, Baltimore, Md.)*

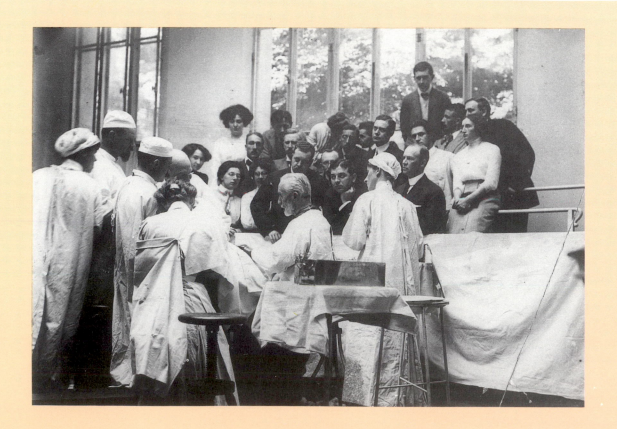

As in other surgical specialties, numerous clinical advances have been made in twentieth-century ophthalmological surgery. From 1899 to 1918 the second edition of Alfred Graefe's (1830-1899) and Edwin Saemisch's (1833-1909) monumental 15-volume collective work, *Handbuch Der Gesamten Augenheilkunde,* was published. In 1900 Allvar Gullstrand (1862-1930), professor of ophthalmology at Uppsala, Sweden, authored a treatise on the general theory of monochromatic aberrations. Henry Smith (1862-1948), a British officer in the Indian Medical Service, had remarkable success with his method of extraction of cataract within the capsule (1901). Among the most important textbooks on ophthalmology at the turn of the century was the four-volume *The Pathology of the Eye* (1904-1908), written by John Parsons (1868-1957) of London. Leopold Heine (1870-1940) introduced cyclodialysis in the treatment of glaucoma (1905). The first successful corneal transplantation was performed by the German surgeon Eduard Zirm (1863-1944) in 1906. In the following year, Sören Holth (1863-1937) reported on iridencleisis and Pierre Lagrange (1857-1928) of Bordeaux, France, was experimenting with sclerectomy, both for the treatment of glaucoma. In Madras, India, in 1909 Robert Elliot (1864-1936) was beginning to use his operation of sclerocorneal trephination for the treatment of glaucoma. Herbert Herbert (1865-1942) of England reported on small-flap sclerotomy in 1910. The American ophthalmologist Vard Hulen (1865-1939) devised a vacuum method of cataract extraction in 1911, and in 1915 one of his peers in New York City, Arnold Knapp (1869-1956), devised a method for the extraction of cataract with forceps. In Bucharest, Romania, Gheorghe Stanculeanu (1874-1944) reported a technique for cataract extraction in 1912. Ignacio Barraquer (1884-1965) of Madrid employed a special machine of his own invention to extract cataract by means of suction and aspiration (1917). The Japanese ophthalmologist Shinobu Ishihara (1879-1958) first introduced his tests for color blindness in 1917. Five years later Marius Tscherning (1854-1939) of Brussels, Belgium, described a photometric spectacle lens. Alan Woods (1889-1963) of Baltimore described an intradermal pigment test for sympathetic ophthalmitis in 1925. In Paris, Jules Gonin (1870-1935) reported on his operation of ignipuncture for treatment of detachment of the retina (1927). At the same time, Frederick Verhoeff (1874-1968) of the United States described a "buttonhole" iridectomy. Anton Elschnig (1863-1939) of Prague developed the method of corneal grafting (1930) which had previously been introduced by Arthur von Hippel (1841-1917). The work of Heine during the 1920s and 1930s provided the basis for the eventual manufacture of contact lenses. In 1930, Robert Moore (1878-1963) introduced a technique for the radiation treatment of choroidal neoplasms, and James Thomas (1893-1976) of England prepared a preliminary report on corneal transplantation. Alfred Vogt (1879-1943) of Germany described cyclodiathermy for the treatment of glaucoma in 1937. Retrolental fibroplasia was first reported by Theodore Terry (1899-1946) in 1942. The history of ophthalmology has been well described by Julius Hirschberg (1843-1925) in his 10-part *Geschichte Der Augenheilkunde* (1899-1918), Emil Bock (1857-1916) in *Die Brille Und Ihre Geschichte* (1903), Carl Greeff (1862-1938) in *Die Erfindung Der Augenglaser* (1921), Burton Chance (1868-1965) in *Ophthalmology* (1939), and Arnold Sorsby (1900-1980) in *A Short History of Ophthalmology* (1948).

ORTHOPEDIC SURGERY

Of all the surgical specialties orthopedic surgery has extended its territory most broadly. When first perceived as a true specialty at the turn of the twentieth century, orthopedics was primarily concerned with congenital bone deformities. Since then, especially in the United States, orthopedic surgery has absorbed from general surgery the management of fractures and dislocations. In addition, orthopedic surgeons have begun to dominate the practice of surgery of the hand, which includes extremity infections and tendon injuries.

As with many other surgical specialties, the push toward a formally recognized specialty of orthopedic surgery came much earlier in American than in Europe. Strong orthopedic groups had developed by the mid-nineteenth century, and specialized orthopedic institutions had been created in Boston and New York. American orthopedic surgery as a special discipline was less bound to general surgery than other specialties by years of tradition and was quite free to develop independently. Competition rather than dominance contributed to its evolution.

The American Orthopedic Association was founded in 1887 and became the first nationally affiliated group of orthopedic surgeons in the world. Within 2 years the *Transactions of the Association* were being published and disseminated throughout the world. The German Orthopedic Society began in 1902 as a splinter group from the Deutsche Gesellschaft für Chirurgie. In Great Britain the British Orthopaedic Society was founded in 1894 but lasted only a few years because organizational strength was lacking. The presently functioning British Orthopaedic Association was not begun until shortly after World War I.

The war brought great impetus to orthopedic surgery and helped forge its foundation as an accepted surgical specialty, especially after the American Board of Orthopaedic Surgery was established in 1934 and became the first such examining body for the specialty worldwide. In 1989, the board also began to give certificates of added qualification in hand surgery. Before 1980, 11,970 general certificates in orthopedic surgery had been awarded by the board, and during the 1980s an additional 5047 were given.

Like so many other surgical specialties, orthopedic surgery has been greatly refined during the twentieth century. Heinrich Albers-Schönberg (1865-1921) of Hamburg described osteosclerosis fragilis, or "marble bones," in 1903. In that same year Robert Osgood (1873-1956) of Boston and Carl Schlatter (1864-1934) of Zurich independently reported on lesions of the tibial tubercle that occur during adolescence. The first attempt at surgical lengthening of limbs was conducted by Alessandro Codivilla (1861-1912) of Bologna in 1905. Antonio Ceci (1852-1920) was the first to operate with the intent of using the musculature remaining above the amputation stump to form a motor unit for artificial limbs (1906). Fritz Steinmann (1872-1932) of Bern described a pin that was used to transfix bone for traction of fixation in 1907, and in that same year Albin Lambotte (1866-1956) developed an external fracture fixation device in which pins were used on either side of the fracture and were connected by a solid rod. Martin Kirschner (1879-1942) then wrote a paper on an apparatus for skeletal traction in long-bone fracture (1909). In 1910 Arthur Legg (1874-1939) of Boston, Jacques Calvé (1875-1954) of France, and Georg Perthes (1869-1927) of Leipzig described juvenile osteochondritis deformans. In 1911, Joel Goldthwait (1866-1961) of Harvard suggested that lumbago and sciatica might be due to intervertebral disk injury and Russell Hibbs (1869-1932) of New York City first reported on spinal fusion as a treatment of scoliosis. Albers-Schönberg provided a definitive description of osteopoikilosis in 1915. Fred Albee (1876-1945), a prominent American surgeon, was the first to employ living bone grafts as internal splints. His cutting machines and surgical saws were fully described in the classic treatise, *Bone-Graft Surgery* (1915). Vittorio Putti (1880-1940) greatly improved existing techniques in kineplastic surgery (1918). In 1923 Arthur Blundell Bankart (1879-1951) of England reported on an operative cure for chronic dislocation of the shoulder joint. Six years later Lorenz Bohler (1885-1973) of Vienna introduced several new methods and described a new apparatus for the treatment of fractures in *Technik Der Knochenbruchbehandlung*. A treatment developed by Hiram Orr (1877-1956) of Nebraska for open fractures was described in *Osteomyelitis and Compound Fractures and other Infected Wounds: Treatment by the Method of Drainage and Rest* (1929). Marius Smith-Petersen (1886-1953) described a flanged nail used for pinning a fracture of the neck of the femur in 1931 and introduced vitallium cup arthroplasty 8 years later. The demonstration of the causal role of intervertebral disk herniation in sciatica was initially described by William Mixter (1880-1958) and Joseph Seaton (1901-1963) of the United States in 1934. Gordon Gordon-Taylor (1878-1960) performed the first one-stage interinnominoabdominal, or hindquarter, amputation in 1935. Pins made of specially hardened stainless steel for use in the treatment of long-bone fractures were reported by H. Lowry Rush (1897-1965) in 1949. John Charnley (1911-1982) of England wrote a classic exposition of the nonoperative approach to fractures, *The Closed Treatment of Common Fractures* (1950), and a decade later described a type of arthroplasty. The history of orthopedic surgery has been aptly described by Arthur Keith (1866-1955) in *Menders of the Maimed* (1919), Osgood in *The Evolution of Orthopaedic Surgery* (1925), Edgar Bick (1902-1978) in *Source Book of Orthopaedics* (1948), and Bruno Valentin (1885-1969) in *Geschichte Der Orthopadie* (1961).

OTORHINOLARYNGOLOGICAL SURGERY

Laryngology and otology existed as separate specialties in Europe during much of the twentieth century. Conversely, in American university clinics the specialties of ophthalmology, otology, laryngology, and rhinology were commonly listed as a unified department. Nonetheless, otological and laryngological societies were founded in America before any such societies had appeared in England or continental Europe. Members of the American Ophthalmological and Otological Society, begun in 1864, were chiefly specialists from Boston, New York, and Philadelphia. The American Otological Society and the American Laryngological Society were founded in 1868 and 1879, respectively. These two organizations were elitist; the American Laryngological, Rhinological and Otological Society was established in 1895 to reach a larger and more egalitarian group of specialists. Among the earliest journals devoted to the specialty were the *Archives of Ophthalmology and Oto-Laryngology,* founded in 1869 by Knapp of New York City, and the *Journal of Laryngology and Otology,* edited by Mackenzie of England (1887).

In the United States the American Board of Otolaryngology, the second American certifying board, was incorporated in 1924. Among its current sponsoring organizations are the American Academy of Facial Plastic and Reconstructive Surgery, the American Academy of Otolaryngic Allergy, and the American Society for Head and Neck Surgery. These three organizations demonstrate the expansion of otorhinolaryngological surgery, which now includes such diverse surgical and medical disciplines as plastic and reconstructive surgery, head and neck surgery, and allergy treatment. By 1980 the American Board of Otolaryngology had awarded 9635 general certificates, and during the 1980s an additional 2585 were obtained.

Among the advances in laryngology during the twentieth century was Otto Freer's (1857-1932) report on an operation to correct deflection of the nasal septum (1902). Gustav Killian's (1860-1921) contributions were many and included a technique for the treatment of pathological conditions in the nasal sinuses (1903) and the introduction of suspension larngoscopy (1912). In 1907 Chevalier Jackson (1865-1958) of Philadelphia authored the first textbook on endoscopy, *Tracheo-Bronchoscopy, Esophagoscopy and Gastroscopy.* Two years later George Waugh (1875-1940) of England introduced blunt dissection tonsillectomy, and in the following year Samuel Whillis (1870-1953) described reverse "guillotine" tonsillectomy. Walter Howarth (1879-1962) of the United States authored an important account of the conservative treatment of sinusitis (1921). Independent of Howart, Robert Lynch (1880-1957) of New Orleans devised a different operation for the conservative treatment of sinusitis (1924). The St. Louis otorhinolaryngologist Arthur Proetz (1888-1966) described the displacement method of treatment for nasal sinusitis in 1926. St. Clair Thomson's (1859-1943) technique in the laryngofissure procedure for intrinsic cancer of the larynx was fully described in *Cancer of the Larynx* (1930).

In otology some of the most influential work was produced by Robert Bárány (1876-1936), including his caloric test for labyrinthine function and a pointing test for the localization of circumscribed cerebellar lesions (1906). George Jenkins (?-1939) of England suggested a type of fenestration operation for otosclerosis in 1913, which was improved by Gunnar Holmgren (1875-1954) of Sweden in 1923. Charles Ballance (1856-1926), an English surgeon, authored the important two-volume *Essays on the Surgery of the Temporal Bones* (1919). Dandy of Baltimore described an operation for the relief of an affliction characterized by vertigo, nausea, vomiting, tinnitus, and progressive deafness (1928). The first successful attempt to restore hearing in otosclerosis by means of fenestration was accomplished by Maurice Sourdille (1885-1961), a French otologist, in 1937. Samuel Kopetzky (1876-1950) of the United States improved the technique for the fenestration operation in 1941. Tympanoplasty was fully described by William Daggett (1900-1980) in 1949. The history of otorhinolaryngology has been written by Adam Politzer (1835-1920) in his two-volume *Geschichte Der Ohrenheilkunde* (1907-1913), Jonathan Wright (1860-1928) in *A History of Laryngology and Rhinology* (1914), and Robert Stevenson (1889-1967) and Douglas Guthrie (1885-1975) in *A History of Oto-Laryngology* (1949).

PLASTIC SURGERY

In virtually every surgical specialty some form of plastic and reconstructive surgery is involved. Consequently the plastic surgery specialists remained an abstract, disorganized group until well into the twentieth century. The successes in military surgery during World War I provided the greatest impetus for the eventual organization and economic viability of plastic surgery as a recognized surgical specialty. Nonetheless, not a single London Hospital had a designated plastic surgeon officially appointed to its staff until the 1930s.

In 1937 the American Board of Plastic Surgery received recognition as a subsidiary of the American Board of Surgery. Four years later the status of a major specialty board with the function of examining and awarding certificates was conferred on the American Board of Plastic Surgery. In 1990 the board began to award certificates of added qualifications in hand surgery. From its inception through 1979 the American Board of Plastic Surgery presented 2202 general certificates, and during the 1980s an additional 1576 were awarded.

Many of the currently used techniques of plastic and reconstructive surgery were first devised during the twentieth century. Hippolyte Morestin (1869-1919) initially described a method of mammaplasty in 1902. The first book on cosmetic surgery, *The Correction of Featural Imperfections* (1907), was privately published by a little-known physician from Chicago, Charles Miller (1880-1950). He was regarded as a surgical quack but was actually a surgical visionary, years ahead of his elitist and less creative academic colleagues. Vilray Blair (1871-1955) of St. Louis described a closed ramisection of the mandible for micrognathia or prognathism in 1909. In that same year, John Staige Davis (1872-1946) of Baltimore popularized a method of splinting skin grafts and later wrote the first comprehensive textbook on the specialty, *Plastic Surgery: Its Principles and Practice* (1919). In 1910 William Luckett (1872-1929) of New York City developed an operation for the correction of protruding ears (1910). The first complete work on cosmetic surgery, *Plastic and Cosmetic Surgery* (1911), was authored by Frederick Kolle (1872-1929) of the United States. Blair wrote the earliest textbook on maxillofacial surgery, *Surgery and Diseases of the Mouth and*

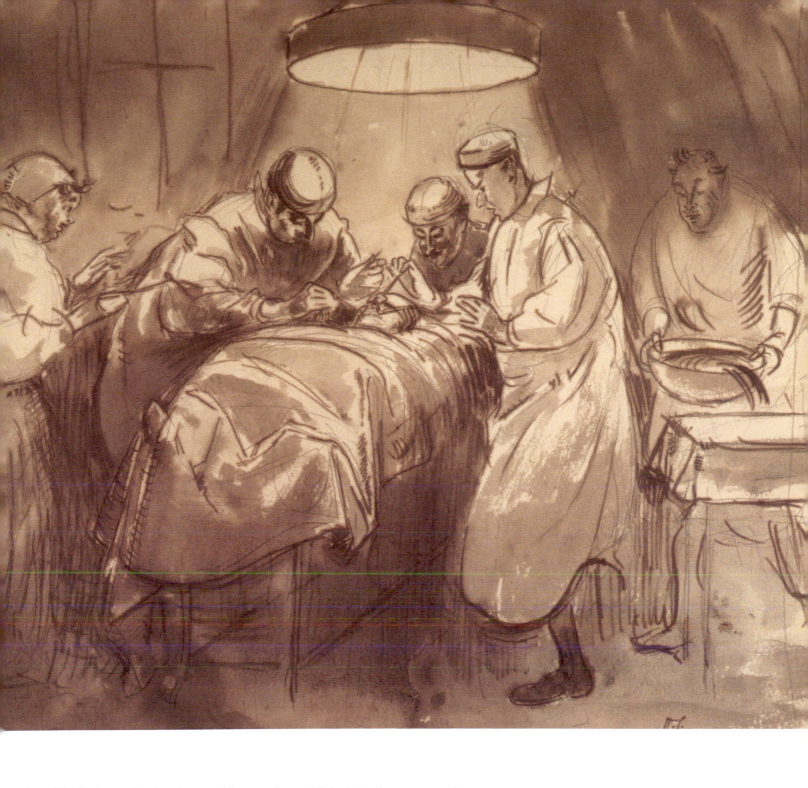

Jaws (1912). Immediately after World War I he established the first separate plastic surgery service in the United States at Barnes Hospital in St. Louis. Vladimir Filatov (1875-1956) of Odessa, Russia, used a tubed pedicle flap in 1916, and in the following year Harold Gillies (1882-1960) of London introduced a similar technique. John Roberts (1852-1924) of Philadelphia described the push-back procedure, or the backward displacement of the velum to ensure adequate speech (1918). Along with William Fry (1889-1963), Gillies authored a classic report on cleft palate repair in 1921. Seven years later William Wardill (1894-1960) of England also described an operation for cleft palate. Both Blair and James Brown (1899-1971) were instrumental in popularizing the use of split-skin grafts to cover large areas of granulating surfaces (1929) and to refine cleft lip repair (1930). Victor Veau (1871-1949) of Paris wrote a classic treatise on cleft palate repair, *Division Palatine,* in 1931. A masterpiece of twentieth-century plastic surgery was Jacques Joseph's (1865-1934) *Nasenplastik Und Sonitige Gesichtsplastik Nebst Einem Anhang Uber Mammaplastik* (1931). Earl Padgett (1893-1946) devised a dermatome, which allowed calibration of the thickness of skin grafts, in 1939.

342. Sir Harold Gillies operating during World War I. Gillies introduced the pedicle flap in 1917. His pioneering work, published in the classic *Plastic Surgery of the Face* (1920), evolved from his efforts in the First World War. Watercolor by Henry Tonks. Trained in surgery, Tonks eventually became director of the Slade School of Art in London. *(Reproduced by kind permission of the President and Council of the Royal College of Surgeons of England.)*

THORACIC SURGERY

Through the last decades of the nineteenth century, operative intervention in the heart, lungs, and other organs in the mediastinum and thoracic cage usually had fatal results. Accordingly, little interest was expressed in the establishment of such surgery as a specialty. As more and more papers on thoracic surgery were being presented during the first 20 years of the twentieth century, however, this attitude changed.

In 1898 John Murphy presented a lengthy oration on thoracic surgery at the annual meeting of the American Medical Association. This lecture, later published in the *Journal of the American Medical Association* as a four-part article, was one of the more important contributions to pulmonary surgery in the United States. It provided the impetus for the eventual establishment of various thoracic surgical societies and for the acceptance of thoracic surgery as a true surgical specialty.

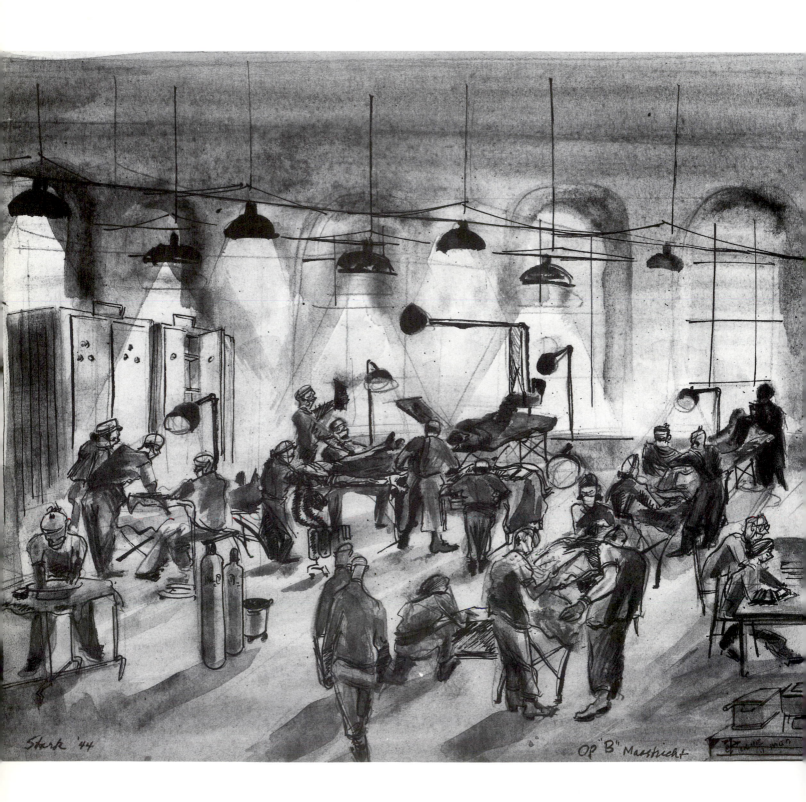

In 1917 the New York Thoracic Surgical Society, the first such organization worldwide, was founded. The founding of the American Association for Thoracic Surgery followed in the same year. Because of the exigencies of war, no other national societies were established until 1933, when the Society of Thoracic Surgeons of Great Britain and Ireland was begun.

The first journal devoted to the specialty, the *Journal of Thoracic Surgery* (1931) was published by the C. V. Mosby Company; the name was later changed to *The Journal of Thoracic and Cardiovascular Surgery*. The name change reflected the growth of cardiac surgery and the significant role it would assume in the evolution of the specialty, especially after World War II.

The certification of thoracic surgeons in the United States was first discussed by the American Association for Thoracic Surgery in 1936. At that time the consensus was that no need for certification existed. Ten years later, after the growth of thoracic surgery as a result of wartime injuries, a recommendation was made for the formation of a board of thoracic surgery in affiliation with the American Board of Surgery. The organization of the Board of Thoracic Surgery was quickly implemented, and its first meeting was held in 1948. In 1971 the Board of Thoracic Surgery became a primary board no longer affiliated with the American Board of Surgery and changed its name to the American Board of Thoracic Surgery. Before 1980, 3540 general certificates in thoracic surgery had been awarded, and during the 1980s an additional 1374 were presented.

The clinical advances in thoracic surgery during the twentieth century have been legendary. In 1902 Ludolph Brauer (1865-1951) first suggested the operation of cardiolysis. John Munro (1858-1910) of Boston was among the earliest to describe the feasibility of ligation of a patent arterial duct (1907). In 1913 Eugene Doyen (1859-1916) of France performed an experimental valvotomy. The first pericardiectomy for constrictive pericarditis was completed by Paul Hallopeau (1876-1924) of Paris in 1921, and two years later Elliott Cutler (1888-1947) of the United States performed a successful section of the mitral valve for relief of mitral stensosis. Also in 1923 Franz Volhard (1872-1950) and Viktor Schmieden (1874-1945) of Germany reported on a complete pericardiectomy for constrictive pericarditis. Henry Souttar (1875-1964) of England completed a successful mitral valvotomy in 1925. Wayne Babcock proposed an operation for thoracic aneurysm in 1926. Claude Beck (1894-1971) implanted pectoral muscle into the pericardium (1935) and attached a pedicled omental graft to the surface of the heart (cardioomentopexy) in 1935, thus providing collateral circulation to that organ. This feat was duplicated by Laurence O'Shaughnessy (1900-1940) in the following year. Ernst Sauerbruch (1875-1951) performed the first successful surgical intervention for cardiac aneurysm in 1931. In 1939 John Gibbon (1903-1973) constructed a prototypical heart-lung machine that was used successfully in an animal, and 15 years later he devised a pump oxygenator. Robert Gross (1905-1988) reported the first successful ligation of a patent arterial duct in 1939 and a resection for coarctation of the aorta with direct anastomosis of the remaining ends in 1945. John Alexander (1891-1954) resected a saccular aneurysm of the thoracic aorta in 1944. Alfred Blalock devised an operation for the relief of congenital defects of the pulmonary artery in 1945. Clarence Crafoord (1899-1984) of Stockholm wrote an important article on congenital coarctation of the aorta and its surgical treatment (1945). Willis Potts (1895-1968) of the United States anastomosed the aorta to a pulmonary artery (1946) for treatment of certain types of congenital heart disease. In 1948 Russell Brock (1903-1980) of England performed a pulmonary valvotomy for the relief of congenital pulmonary stenosis. Thomas Sellors (1902-1987) of England successfully divided the pulmonary valve for treatment of pulmonary stenosis in 1947. The first successful aortic valve homograft was performed by Gordon Murray (1894-1976) in 1956.

343. *Facing page,* Pen-and-ink wash by the American surgeon Richard B. Stark, who provided surgical care throughout the European theater during World War II. Stark has provided the following commentary for his painting, made in Maastricht, Holland, in 1944:

Our operating room occupied two areas. O.R. "A" had two tables for head and abdominal injuries. O.R. "B" resembled an assembly line of a well-lighted factory. Patients were being brought in or taken out incessantly by masked litter bearers, other patients were being "prepped" (area adjacent to the wound shaved or washed). Still others were undergoing major surgery, while the plaster casts of other patients were drying. Each operating table received a basic set of instruments for debridement (removing devitalized tissue, dirt, metal from the wound) which could be added to upon demand from the "master table." This table was presided over by a technician in cap, mask, gown and gloves.

A surgical team consisted of two surgeons, two nurses (one of whom was the anesthetist) and two enlisted corpsmen. The arrangement was flexible and depended upon the casualties presenting. The two surgeons could operate a case while the next patient was on their second table being prepped by the corpsmen. Alternately, the two surgeons could work independently upon a different case, each assisted by a corpsman. A table was provided so that the records (EMT, emergency medical tag) could be written up. In Maastricht we performed 96 operations in O.R. "B" in a 24-hour period.
(Courtesy Richard Boies Stark.)

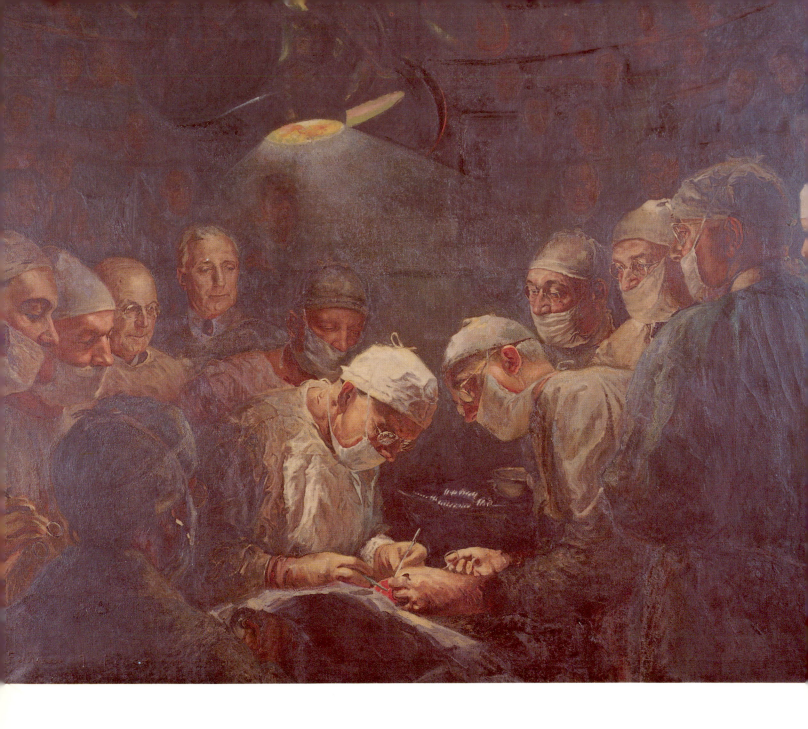

344. *The Babcock Surgical Clinic,* 1944–1945, by Furman Joseph Finck. In the tradition of Thomas Eakins's *The Gross Clinic* (1875) and *The Agnew Clinic* (1889) but with a twist. Finck's painting is a commemorative group portrait rather than a tribute to one great surgeon. Grouped around Babcock, who is shown watching the operation, are past and present deans, chairmen, and professors at Temple University. *(Temple University School of Medicine, Philadelphia.)*

UROLOGICAL SURGERY

Through the beginning of the twentieth century the urologist remained more a diagnostician of urological disorders than a clinical surgeon. When an operation was necessary, the patient was usually turned over to a general surgeon. Organization within the specialty was limited, and few urological hospitals or specific wards existed.

The first specialty organization devoted to urologic surgery, the American Association for Genito-Urinary Surgeons, was founded in 1886. It was soon joined by the American Urological Association, which commenced activities in 1902. The only periodical that published papers exclusively on urological topics in nineteenth-century America was the *Journal of Cutaneous and Genito-Urinary Diseases* (1887), which published the papers presented before the American Association for Genito-Urinary Surgeons. Early in the twentieth century the *American Journal of Urology* came into existence under the leadership of Hugh Young. In 1920, its name was changed to the *Journal of Urology* and it became the property of the American Urological Association.

Countries other than the United States soon had their own urological societies, including Europe's earliest, the Association Française d'Urologie in Paris, organized in 1896. Activities in the United States ultimately helped form the specialty and establish its present course. In 1935 the American Board of Urology was incorporated as an outgrowth of activities of the American Association of Genito-Urinary Surgeons, the American Urological Association, and the Section of Urology of the American Medical Association. From the founding of the board in 1935 through 1980, 7059 general certificates in urology were awarded, and during the 1980s an additional 2637 were obtained.

Like other surgical specialties, urological surgery grew out of general surgery and became a respected discipline largely on the merit of clinical advances that were made in the twentieth century. Among these were Peter Freyer's (1851–1921) popularization of the rectovesical method of prostatectomy (1901). Emerich Ullmann (1861-1937) successfully completed an autotransplantation of kidneys in dogs in 1902, and in the following year Fedor Krause (1856-1937) performed a total cystectomy and bilateral ureterosigmoidostomy. Hugh Young (1870-1945) reported on perineal prostatectomy (1903), radical prostatectomy for carcinoma (1905), and punch prostatectomy (1913) and first demonstrated vesiculography (1920). George Goodfellow (1856-1910) of the United States completed a perineal prostatectomy in 1891 but did not report it until 1904. Francis Watson (1853-1942) of Boston first performed a median perineal prostatectomy in 1889, although his definitive report on the subject was not written until 1905. In that same year a distensible bag for controlling hemorrhage after suprapubic prostatectomy was introduced by James Briggs (1869-1942). Friedrich Voelcker (1872-1955) and Alexander von Lichtenberg (1880-1949) of Germany authored a paper on cystograms in 1906. Francis Hagner (1873-1940) of New York City devised the open operation for relief of acute epididymitis (1906). Alexis Carrel transplanted a kidney from one animal to another in 1908. Among the most prominent early twentieth-century urologic textbooks was Joaquin Albarran's (1860-1912) *Médicine Operatoire Des Voies Urinaires,* published in 1909. In that same year Leo Buerger (1879-1943) of New York City reported on a direct irrigating observation and double catheterizing cystoscope. Franz Torek's (1861-1938) operation for undescended testicle was first described in 1909. A method for transurethral fulguration of bladder tumors, which led to the operation of transurethral prostatectomy, was introduced by Edwin Beer (1876-1938) in 1910. Urethrography was first described by John Cunningham (1877-?) of the United States (1910). John Squier (1873-1948) of Boston popularized suprapubic intraurethral enucleation of the prostate (1911). The modern method of ureterointestinal anastomosis followed the experimental research of Robert Coffey (1869-1933) of the United States (1911). Frank Hinman's (1880-1961) classic work on operative treatment of hydronephrosis was first introduced in 1918. John Caulk (1881-1938) introduced a cautery punch (1920). In 1922 John Geraghty (1876-1924) of the United States modified the perineal prostatectomy of Hugh Young, and in the following year a Foroblique panendoscope was devised by Joseph McCarthy (1874-1965). Maximilian Stern (1877-1946) reported on a cystoscope with a cutting current capable of operating in a water medium in 1926. Moses Swick (1900-1985) introduced Uroselectan for use in excretion urography in 1929, and 4 years later he described Hippuran. In the 1930s the most prominent textbook on prostate surgery was Alexander Randall's (1883-1951) *Surgical Pathology of Prostatic Obstructions* (1931). Samuel Harris (1880-1936) of Australia first described his suprapubic prostatectomy in 1927 and wrote a definitive paper on it in 1934. Frederic Foley (1891-1966) of the United States reported an operation for hydronephrosis in 1937. He remains eponymically linked with a retention bladder catheter that contains a device for inflating a retaining balloon. Jacob Fine (1900-1979) of Harvard first treated acute renal failure by means of peritoneal irrigation in 1946. The report of the first human to survive a kidney transplantation was authored by Richard Lawler (1895-1982) in 1950. Five years later David Hume (1917-1973) of Boston reported on nine cases of renal homotransplantation in humans. The history of urology, especially in the United States, has been exhaustively reviewed by Edgar Ballenger (1877-1945) in the two-volume *History of Urology,* prepared under the auspices of the American Urological Association (1933).

SUMMARY

The years after World War II have been highlighted by some of the most far-reaching changes ever to encompass the scientific discipline of surgery. Unlike in prior eras, however, most of the evolutionary shifts in modern times have been dictated more by socioeconomic pressures and technological breakthroughs than by individual clinical achievements. Surgery has undergone a social transformation in which research and technical advances have accelerated specialization, which in turn has contributed to the fragmentation of surgery as a unified profession.

In many respects the surgeon's greatest current challenges are to understand the socioeconomic forces that affect the practice of surgery and to learn how to effectively manage them. Many splendid schools of surgery now exist in virtually every major industrialized city, but none can lay claim to dominance in all the disciplines that make up surgery. Likewise, the presence of dominant individual personalities who help guide surgery is more unusual today than in previous times. National aims and socioeconomic status have become the overwhelming factors in securing and shepherding the future growth of surgery worldwide.

In the light of an understanding of the intricacies of surgical history, it seems an unenviable and obviously impossible task to predict what will happen in the future. In 1874 Erichsen wrote that:

> . . . the abdomen, chest, and brain will forever be closed to operations by a wise and humane surgeon.

A few years later Billroth remarked:

> A surgeon who tries to suture a heart wound deserves to lose the esteem of his colleagues.

Surgery, which began as a manual, magical art, has evolved into an integral aspect of science and technology. What the future will be for surgeons remains unknown. However, certain overriding concerns must be addressed.

The transformation of surgical care in the industrialized world from a "cottage industry" to a mammoth governmental-industrial-medical complex is undeniable. The central question for the surgical profession must now be: How does the profession view itself in relation to this cultural change and where does surgery fit into a rapidly altering system? The growth and consequent influence of large institutions such as government, major employers, and insurers on both surgeon and patient present previously unimagined perplexities today.

The economic and technological lessons of the nearly 50 years after World War II reveal the continuing importance of research in the advance of surgery. For centuries, surgery depended largely on discoveries and important advances in other medical disciplines for its own progress. In most respects this interdependence continues, and surgeons cannot define surgical research as experimental investigation completed strictly by surgeons. The interdisciplinary facets of biochemistry, biophysics, bioradiology, biomechanical engineering, and the like will be increasingly incorporated into the world of the surgeon.

Most important to the future conduct of surgery, surgeons must participate in the planning of health services research. Although surgeons who participate in basic biomedical research will always be needed, a similar need now exists for surgeons who can conceive original investigations into the socioeconomics of each country's health care delivery system.

Few surgeons have additional training in such fields as biostatistics, business administration, economics, epidemiology, government affairs, health services administration, public health, policy formation, and sociology. Until a "critical mass" of surgeons adopt an interdisciplinary approach to surgical health care, the crucial and often difficult process of making appropriate surgical policy decisions will be left to those outside the surgical profession.

Any surgeon who wishes to positively affect the health care delivery system of the future will need additional education in the social sciences. The future leaders of world surgery must be more than excellent clinicians who also investigate the basic sciences. They will be increasingly asked to make critical public policy decisions, and without proper education and experience they will be more likely to make ill-informed and potentially damaging ones.

The surgical community must accept the changes that are taking place in the health care delivery system. Power has shifted: the once dominant role of the surgeon has declined. Surgeons are no longer the heroes they were in the past, and the many dramatic alterations in surgical health care must be acknowledged with a sanguine outlook. The surgical profession has an absolute responsibility to be forthright with information about surgical care. Appropriate studies of the effectiveness of surgical treatment should be carried out for selected conditions, particularly when uncertainty leads to professional disagreement. Surgeons must foster the dissemination of reliable, scientifically based data to the public.

Surgeons must clarify their newfound role. They must realize that the practice of surgery can be conducted in a businesslike manner. This does not mean that the humanitarian aspects of medicine must be forgotten. The commitment to act on behalf of a sick patient and to be compassionate should always be preserved. Surgical health care is a right, not a privilege. The question that remains to be answered is: To what dollar amount does that right extend? Should all individuals be guaranteed an inguinal herniorrhaphy? a portosystemic shunt for esophageal varices? a heart transplantation?

Surgeons must provide effective leadership in determining the economic constraints that must be imposed to control expenditures and make services available to the poor and the uninsured. The surgical interests of the economically and socially disadvantaged and those who have limited access to health care must be ensured. Surgeons who are interested solely in patients who can pay for their care cannot consider themselves among the heirs of Hippocrates.

The most important issue that surgeons now face is not how to perform a better pancreaticoduodenectomy, for example, but how to determine the financial ramifications of performing such an operation when the patient's life expectancy is known to be less than a year. Should surgical care be rationed? From the present perspective it would appear that some rationing will be inevitable. If so, upon whom will the responsibility for making this surgical judgment fall?

Throughout the narrative of this illustrated history of surgery, the practice of surgery—the art, craft, and more recently the science, of working with the hands—has always been defined by its tools. From the crude flint instruments of stone age trephiners, to the bronze instruments of Egyptian and Roman surgeons, to the increasingly complex surgical instruments developed in the latter half of the nineteenth century, a better instrument usually lead to a better surgical result. Progress in surgical instrumentation and surgical technique went hand in hand.

During the last decades of the twentieth century there has been unprecedented progress in the development of new surgical tools, drugs, and imaging techniques, many of which have been offshoots of computer technology. These revolutionary enhancements to our craft, which have allowed for new life-saving surgical specialties like organ transplantation to arise, have not come without great social and economic cost.

It cannot be assumed that improvement in surgical technology must continue forever at its present pace; however, it should be expected that advancement will continue. If the study of surgical history offers any lesson, it is that progress can always be expected, at least in technology. There will be new surgical operations with better results. Although automation may ultimately robotize the surgeon's hand for some procedures, the practice of surgery will retain its historical roots as both a manual art and a science.

To study the fascinating history of our profession, with its many magnificent personalities and outstanding scientific and social achievements, may not necessarily help us predict the future of surgery. However, it does shed much light on the clinical practices of our own time. Although the future of the art, craft, and science of surgery remains unknown, it assuredly rests on a glorious past.

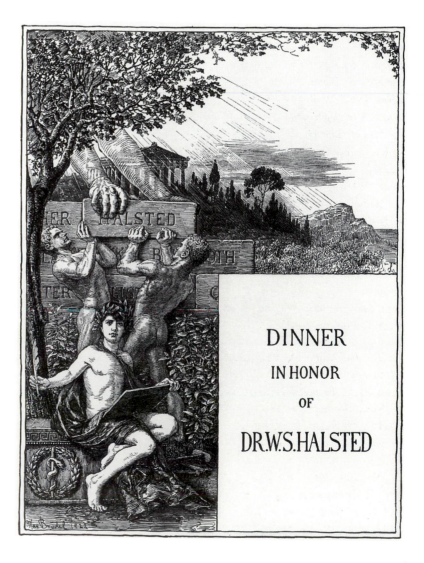

345. Invitation to a dinner during which a gold medal was presented to William S. Halsted by the National Dental Association, Baltimore, April 1, 1922. For this occasion the anatomical artist Max Brödel created an eloquent emblematic drawing symbolizing Halsted's achievements as a building block in the progress of surgery. In the lower left corner, a figure symbolizing the artist or a historian of surgery is dressed in the style of ancient Greece. Behind him, two muscle men place the building blocks of the temple of surgery, guided by what appear to be godlike hands. The building blocks bear various surnames; those of John Hunter, Joseph Lister, Bernhard von Langenbeck, Theodor Kocher, William Stewart Halsted, and Theodor Billroth may be deduced. In the distance is a Greek temple of Aesculapius. *(From the author's collection.)*

534

BIBLIOGRAPHY

ACKERKNECHT EH: *Medicine at the Paris Hospital, 1794-1848,* Baltimore, 1967, The Johns Hopkins Press.

ALLBUTT TC: *The historical relations of medicine and surgery to the end of the sixteenth century,* London, 1905, Macmillan.

ANONYMOUS: *Bibliography of the history of medicine, 1964-1969,* Bethesda, Md, 1970, National Library of Medicine.

ANONYMOUS: *Bibliography of the history of medicine, 1970-1974,* Bethesda, Md, 1975, National Library of Medicine.

ANONYMOUS: *Bibliography of the history of medicine, 1975-1979,* Bethesda, Md, 1980, National Library of Medicine.

ANONYMOUS: *Bibliography of the history of medicine, 1980-1984,* Bethesda, Md, 1986, National Library of Medicine.

ANONYMOUS: *Bibliography of the history of medicine, 1985-1989,* Bethesda, Md, 1990, National Library of Medicine.

ANONYMOUS: *A catalogue of printed books in the Wellcome Historical Medical Library.* I. Books printed before 1641, London, 1962, Wellcome Historical Medical Library.

ANONYMOUS: *A catalogue of printed books in the Wellcome Historical Medical Library.* II. Books printed from 1641 to 1850 (A-E), London, 1966, Wellcome Historical Medical Library.

ANONYMOUS: *A catalogue of printed books in the Wellcome Historical Medical Library.* III. Books printed from 1641 to 1850 (F-L), London, 1976, Wellcome Historical Medical Library.

ANONYMOUS: *Lister and the ligature, a landmark in the history of modern surgery,* New Brunswick, NJ, 1925, Johnson & Johnson.

ARRINGTON GE: *A history of ophthalmology,* New York, 1959, MD Publications.

BAILEY JB: *The diary of a resurrectionist 1811-1812, to which are added an account of the resurrection men in London and a short history of the passing of the Anatomy Act,* London, 1896, Swan Sonnenschein.

BAKAY L: *An early history of craniotomy: from antiquity to the Napoleonic era,* Springfield, Ill, 1985, Charles C Thomas.

BAKAY L: *Neurosurgeons of the past,* Springfield, Ill, 1987, Charles C Thomas.

BALLANCE CA: *A glimpse into the history of the surgery of the brain,* London, 1922, MacMillan.

BALLENGER EG: *History of urology* (2 vols), Baltimore, 1933, Williams & Wilkins.

BANKOFF G: *The story of surgery,* London, 1947, Arthur Barker.

BANKOFF G: *The story of plastic surgery,* London, 1952, Faber & Faber.

BARKER W: *The arteries: readings in the history of surgery,* Austin, Tex, 1988, Silvergirl.

BECK RT: *The cutting edge: early history of the surgeons of London,* London, 1974, Lund Humphries.

BENNION E: *Antique medical instruments,* Berkeley, 1979, University of California Press.

BICK EM: *Source book of orthopaedics,* Baltimore, 1948, Williams & Wilkins.

BICK EM: *Classics of orthopaedics,* Philadelphia, 1976, JB Lippincott.

BIGELOW HJ: *Ether and chloroform: a compendium of their history and discovery,* Boston, 1848, D Clapp.

BIGELOW HJ: A history of the discovery of modern anaesthesia. In *A century of American medicine, 1776-1876,* Philadelphia, 1876, Henry C Lea.

BILLINGS JS: Literature and institutions. In *A century of American medicine, 1776-1876.* Philadelphia, 1876, Henry C Lea.

BILLINGS JS: The history and literature of surgery. In Dennis FS: *System of surgery* (4 vols), Philadelphia, 1895, Lea Brothers.

BILLROTH CAT: *The medical sciences in the German universities,* New York, 1924, Macmillan.

BISHOP WJ: *A history of surgical dressings,* Chesterfield, 1959, Robinson & Sons.

BISHOP WJ: *The early history of surgery,* London, 1960, Robert Hale.

BLANCHARD CE: *The romance of proctology, which is the story of the history and development of this much neglected branch of surgery,* Youngstown, Ohio, 1938, Medical Success Press.

BLEKER J: *Die Geschichte Der Nierenkrankheiten,* Mannheim, 1972, Boehringer.

BODENHEIMER FS: *The history of biology,* London, 1958, Dawsons.

BOYES JH: *On the shoulders of giants, notable names in hand surgery,* Philadelphia, 1976, JB Lippincott.

BRADBURY S: *The evolution of the microscope,* Oxford, NY, 1967, Pergamon Press.

BRIEGER GH: *Medical America in the nineteenth century, readings from the literature,* Baltimore, 1972, The Johns Hopkins Press.

BROOKS S: *McBurney's point, the story of appendicitis*, New York, 1969, AS Barnes.

BROTHWELL D, SANDISON AT: *Diseases in antiquity: a survey of the diseases, injuries, and surgery of early populations*, Springfield, Ill, 1967, Charles C Thomas.

BROWN A: *Old masterpieces in surgery*, Omaha, 1928, private printing.

BUCK AH: *The growth of medicine from the earliest times to about 1800*, New Haven, 1917, Yale University Press.

BUCK AH: *The dawn of modern medicine*, New Haven, 1920, Yale University Press.

BUCY PC: *Neurosurgical giants: feet of clay and iron*, New York, 1985, Elsevier.

BURKE ME: *The Royal College of San Carlos, surgery and Spanish medical reform in the late eighteenth century*, Durham, NC, 1977, Duke University.

BUSCHAN GHT: *Chirurgisches Aus Der Volkerkunde*, Leipzig, 1902, B Konegen.

CABANES A: *Chirurgiens Et Blesses A Travers l'Histoire*, Paris, 1918, A Michel.

CAMERON CA: *History of the Royal College of Surgeons in Ireland*, Dublin, 1916, Fannin & Co.

CARTWRIGHT FF: *The development of modern surgery*, London, 1967, Arthur Barker.

CHANCE B: *Ophthalmology*, New York, 1939, PB Hoeber.

CHAUVEAU C: *Histoire Des Maladies Du Pharynx* (5 vols), Paris, 1901-1906, JB Baillière.

CIANFRANI T: *A short history of obstetrics and gynecology*, Springfield, Ill, 1960, Charles C Thomas.

CLAY RS: *The history of the microscope*, London, 1932, Griffin.

CLENDENING L: *Source book of medical history*, New York, 1942, PB Hoeber.

COLE F: *Milestones in anesthesia*, Lincoln, 1965, University of Nebraska Press.

COPE Z: *Pioneers in acute abdominal surgery*, London, 1939, Oxford University Press.

COPE Z: *The Royal College of Surgeons of England, a history*, London, 1959, Anthony Blond.

COPE Z: *A history of the acute abdomen*, London, 1965, Oxford University Press.

CORNER GW: *Anatomical texts of the earlier Middle Ages*, Washington, DC, 1927, Carnegie Institute.

COWEN DL, HELFAND WH: *Pharmacy: an illustrated history*, New York, 1990, Harry N Abrams.

CRESWELL CH: *The Royal College of Surgeons of Edinburgh, historical notes from 1505 to 1904*, Edinburgh, 1926, Oliver & Boyd.

DALLY AD: *Women under the knife: a history of surgery*, London, 1991, Hutchinson Radius.

DAVIS L: *Fellowship of surgery: a history of the American College of Surgeons*, Springfield, Ill, 1960, Charles C Thomas.

DENNIS FS: *The history and development of surgery during the past century*, New York, 1928, Private printing.

DEVECCHI P: *Modern Italian surgery and old universities of Italy*, New York, 1921, PB Hoeber.

DOBSON J: *Anatomical eponyms*, Edinburgh, 1962, Livingstone.

DOBSON J, MILNE R: *Barbers and barber-surgeons of London*, Oxford, 1979, Blackwell Scientific Publications.

DONAHUE MP: *Nursing, the finest art: an illustrated history*, St Louis, 1985, Mosby.

DORRANCE GM: *The operative story of cleft palate*, Philadelphia, 1933, WB Saunders.

DUNCUM BM: *The development of inhalation anaesthesia, with special reference to the years 1846-1900*, London, 1947, Oxford University Press.

EARLE AS: *Surgery in America*, New York, 1983, Praeger.

ELLIOTT IMZ: *A short history of surgical dressings*, London, 1964, Pharmaceutical Press.

ELLIS H: *A history of bladder stone*, Oxford, 1970, Blackwell.

ELLIS H: *Famous operations*, Media, Pa, 1984, Harwal Publishing.

ELLIS H: *The spleen: readings in the history of surgery*, Austin, Tex, 1988, Silvergirl.

FAULCONER A, KEYS TE: *Foundations of anesthesiology* (2 vols), Springfield, Ill, 1965, Charles C Thomas.

FERGUSSON W: *Lectures on the progress of anatomy and surgery during the present century*, London, 1867, J Churchill & Sons.

FISCHER G: *Chirurgie Vor 100 Jahren; Historische Studie*, Leipzig, 1876, FCW Vogel.

FISHBEIN M: *A history of the American Medical Association, 1847 to 1947*, Philadelphia, 1947, WB Saunders.

FISHER GJ: A history of surgery. In Ashhurst J: *The international encyclopedia of surgery* (6 vols), New York, 1881-1886, William Wood.

FISHMAN AP, RICHARDS DW: *Circulation of the blood: men and ideas*, New York, 1964, Oxford University Press.

FORT GF: *Medical economy during the Middle Ages*, New York, 1883, JW Bouton.

FOURMESTRAUX J: *Histoire De La Chirurgie Francaise (1790-1920)*, Paris, 1934, Masson.

FRANKLIN KJ: *A short history of physiology*, London, 1949, Staples Press.

FRIEDMAN SG: *A history of vascular surgery*, Mount Kisco, NY, 1989, Futura.

FULOP-MILLER R: *Triumph over pain*, New York, 1938, Literary Guild of America.

FULTON JF: *The great medical bibliographers, a study in humanism*, Philadelphia, 1951, University of Pennsylvania Press.

FULTON JF: *Selected readings in the history of physiology*, Springfield, Ill, 1966, Charles C Thomas.

FULTON JF, STANTON ME: *The centennial of surgical anesthesia*, New York, 1946, Henry Schuman.

GABKA J, VAUBEL E: *Plastic surgery past and present*, Basel, 1983, S Karger.

GARRISON FH: *An introduction to the history of medicine*, Philadelphia, 1929, WB Saunders.

GELFAND T: *Professionalizing modern medicine: Paris surgeons and medical science and institutions in the 18th century*, Westport, Ct, 1980, Greenwood Press.

GLASER H: *The road to modern surgery*, London, 1960, Lutterworth Press.

GLASER H: *The miracle of heart surgery,* London, 1961, Lutterworth Press.

GOLDSCHMID E: *Entwicklung Und Bibliographie Der Pathologisch-Anatomischen Abbildung,* Leipzig, 1925, KW Hiersemann.

GRAHAM H: *The story of surgery,* New York, 1939, Doubleday & Doran.

GRAHAM H: *Eternal Eve: the history of gynaecology and obstetrics,* Garden City, NY, 1951, Doubleday.

GRUN B: *The timetables of history, a horizontal linkage of people and events,* New York, 1982, Touchstone.

GRUNDER JWL: *Geschichte Der Chirurgie Von Den Urzeiten Bis Zu Anfang Des Achtzehnten Jahrhunderts,* Breslau, 1859, Trewendt & Granier.

GROSS SD: Surgery. In *A century of American medicine, 1776-1876,* Philadelphia, 1876, Henry C Lea.

GURLT EJ: *Geschichte Der Chirurgie Und Ihrer Ausubung* (3 vols), Berlin, 1898, A Hirschwald.

HAEGER K: *The illustrated history of surgery,* New York, 1988, Bell.

HALLER A: *Bibliotheca Chirurgica* (2 vols), Bern and Basel, 1774-1775, Haller & Schweighauser.

HARVEY SC: *The history of hemostasis,* New York, 1924, PB Hoeber.

HAU T: *Renal transplantation: readings in the history of surgery,* Austin, Tex, 1987, Silvergirl.

HELFREICH F: Geschichte Der Chirurgie. In Puschmann T: *Handbuch Der Geschichte Der Medizin* (3 vols), Jena, 1905, Gustav Fischer.

HERMAN J: *Urology, a view through the retrospectroscope,* Hagerstown, 1973, Harper & Row.

HILLER L: *Surgery through the ages; a pictorial chronical,* New York, 1944, Books, Inc.

HINMAN F: *American pediatric urology,* San Francisco, 1991, Norman Publishing.

HIRSCHBERG J: *Geschichte Der Augenheilkunde,* Leipzig, 1899-1918, W Engelmann.

HOCHBERG LA: *Thoracic surgery before the 20th century,* New York, 1960, Vantage Press.

HOOK DH, NORMAN JM: *The Haskell F. Norman library of science and medicine* (2 vols), San Francisco, 1991, Norman Publishing.

HORRAX G: *Neurosurgery: an historical sketch,* Springfield, Ill, 1952, Charles C Thomas.

HUARD PA, GRMEK MD: *Mille Ans De Chirurgie En Occident: Ve-XVe Siecles,* Paris, 1966, Roger Dacosta.

HUARD PA, GRMEK MD: *La Chirurgie Moderne: Ses Debuts En Occident: XVIe-XVIIe-XVIIIe Siecles,* Paris, 1968, Editions Dacosta.

HUBBELL AA: *The development of ophthalmology in America, 1800 to 1870,* Chicago, 1908, WT Keener.

HURWITZ A, DEGENSHEIN GA: *Milestones in modern surgery,* New York, 1958, Hoeber-Harper.

JAMESON EM: *Gynecology and obstetrics,* New York, 1936, PB Hoeber.

JOHNSON SL: *The history of cardiac surgery,* Baltimore, 1970, The Johns Hopkins University Press.

KEEN WW: *A sketch of the early history of practical anatomy,* Philadelphia, 1874, JB Lippincott.

KEITH A: *Menders of the maimed,* London, 1919, H Frowde.

KELLY EC: *Encyclopedia of medical sources,* Baltimore, 1948, Williams & Wilkins.

KEYS TE: *The history of surgical anesthesia,* New York, 1945, Schuman's.

KILLIAN H: *Meister Der Chirurgie Und Die Chirurgenschulen Im Deutschen Raum,* Stuttgart, 1951, G Thieme.

KLASEN HJ: *History of free skin grafting,* Berlin, 1981, Springer-Verlag.

LANDOR J: *The stomach: readings in the history of surgery,* Austin, Tex, 1985, Silvergirl.

LAUFMAN H: *The veins: readings in the history of surgery,* Austin, Tex, 1986, Silvergirl.

LEARMONTH J: *The contributions of surgery to preventive medicine,* London, 1951, Oxford.

LEONARDO RA: *History of surgery,* New York, 1943, Froben Press.

LEONARDO RA: *History of gynecology,* New York, 1944, Froben Press.

LEONARDO RA: *Lives of master surgeons,* New York, 1948, Frober Press.

LEVAY D: *The history of orthopaedics,* Park Ridge, 1990, Parthenon.

LONG ER: *A history of pathology,* Baltimore, 1928, Williams & Wilkins.

LUDMERER KM: *Learning to heal: the development of American medical education,* New York, 1985, Basic Books.

LUDOVICI LJ: *The discovery of anaesthesia,* New York, 1961, TY Crowell.

LYONS A, PETRUCELLI RJ: *Medicine, an illustrated history,* New York, 1978, Harry N Abrams.

MAGNUS HF: *Die Augenheilkunde Der Alten,* Breslau, 1901, JV Kern.

MALGAIGNE JF: *Histoire De La Chirurgie En Occident Depuis De VIe Jusqu' Au XVIe Siecle, Et Histoire De La Vie Et Des Travaux d'Ambroise Pare,* Paris, 1840, JB Baillière.

MALTZ M: *Evolution of plastic surgery,* New York, 1946, Froben Press.

MANJO G: *The healing hand: man and wound in the ancient world,* Cambridge, 1975, Harvard University Press.

MAULITZ RC: *Morbid appearances, the anatomy of pathology in the early nineteenth century,* Cambridge, 1987, Cambridge University Press.

McDOWELL F: *The source book of plastic surgery,* Baltimore, 1977, Williams & Wilkins.

McDOWELL F: *Plastic surgery: readings in the history of surgery,* Austin, Tex, 1987, Silvergirl.

McGREGOR DK: *Sexual surgery and the origins of gynecology,* New York, 1989, Garland Publishing.

McKAY WJS: *The history of ancient gynaecology,* London, 1901, Baillière, Tindall & Cox.

MEADE RH: *A history of thoracic surgery,* Springfield, Ill, 1961, CC Thomas.

MEADE RH: *An introduction to the history of general surgery,* Philadelphia, 1968, WB Saunders.

MILES A: *The Edinburgh school of surgery before Lister*, London, 1918, A & C Black.

MILLARD DR: *Cleft palate: the evolution of its surgery* (3 vols), Boston, 1976-1980, Little, Brown.

MILLER G: *Bibliography of the history of medicine of the United States and Canada, 1939-1960*, Baltimore, 1964, Johns Hopkins University Press.

MILNE JS: *Surgical instruments in Greek and Roman times*, Oxford, 1907, Clarendon Press.

MITCHELL-HEGGS F, RADCLIFFE HG: *The instruments of surgery*, Springfield, Ill, 1963, Charles C Thomas.

MOORE FD: American surgery, progress over two centuries. In Bower JZ, Purcell EF: *Advances in American medicine: essays at the bicentennial* (2 vols), New York, 1976, Josiah Macy.

MUKHOPADHYAYA G: *The surgical instruments of the Hindus*, Calcutta, 1914, Calcutta University Press.

MUMFORD JG: Narrative of surgery: a historical sketch. In Keen WW: *Surgery, its principles and practice* (8 vols), Philadelphia, 1906, WB Saunders.

MURPHY LJT: *The history of urology*, Springfield, Ill, 1971, Charles C Thomas.

NAEF AP: *The story of thoracic surgery*, Toronto, 1990, Hogrefe & Huber.

NISSEN R, WILSON R: *Pages in the history of chest surgery*, Springfield, Ill, 1960, Charles C Thomas.

NORMAN J: *Morton's medical bibliography, an annotated check-list of texts illustrating the history of medicine*, London, 1991, Scholar Press.

ORGAN CH, KOSIBA MM: *A century of black surgeons: the U.S.A. experience* (2 vols), Norman, Okla, 1987, Transcript Press.

ORR HW: *On the contributions of Hugh Owen Thomas of Liverpool, Sir Robert Jones of Liverpool and London, John Ridlon, M.D., of New York and Chicago, to modern orthopedic surgery*, Springfield, Ill, 1949, Charles C Thomas.

OSGOOD RB: *The evolution of orthopaedic surgery*, St Louis, 1925, Mosby.

OSLER W: *Incunabula Medica: a study of the earliest printed medical books, 1467-1480*, Oxford, 1923, Oxford University Press.

OSLER W: *Bibliotheca Osleriana*, Oxford, 1929, Oxford University Press.

PACKARD FR: *History of medicine in the United States* (2 vols), New York, 1931, PB Hoeber.

PANSIER P: *Histoire Des Lunettes*, Paris, 1901, A Maloine.

PARK R: *An epitome of the history of medicine*, Philadelphia, 1898, FA Davis.

PARKER G: *The early history of surgery in Great Britain: its organization and development*, London, 1920, A & C Black.

PELTIER LF: *Orthopedics: a history and iconography*, San Francisco, 1993, Norman Publishing.

PELTIER LF: *Fractures, a history and iconography of their treatment*, San Francisco, 1990, Norman Publishing.

PERSAUD TVN: *Early history of human anatomy, from antiquity to the beginning of the modern era*, Springfield, Ill, 1984, Charles C Thomas.

POLITZER A: *Geschichte Der Ohrenheilkunde* (2 vols), Stuttgart, 1907-1913, F Enke.

PORTAL A: *Histoire De l'Anatomie Et De La Chirurgie* (6 vols in 7), Paris, 1770-1773, P F Didot Le Jeune.

POUCHELLE M: *The body and surgery in the Middle Ages*, New Brunswick, 1990, Rutgers University Press.

POWER D: *A short history of surgery*, London, 1933, John Hale.

POWER D: *A mirror for surgeons; selected readings in surgery*, Boston, 1939, Little, Brown.

RANDERS-PHERSON J: *The surgeon's glove*, Springfield, Ill, 1960, Charles C Thomas.

RANG MC: *Anthology of orthopaedics*, Edinburgh, 1966, Livingstone.

RANSON FT: *Men and events in surgery*, Private printing.

RAVITCH MM: *A century of surgery, the history of the American Surgical Association* (2 vols), Philadelphia, 1981, JB Lippincott.

RICCI JV: *The genealogy of gynaecology; history of the development of gynaecology throughout the ages 2000 B.C.-A.D. 1800*, Philadelphia, 1943, Blakiston.

RICCI JV: *One hundred years of gynaecology, 1800-1900*, Philadelphia, 1945, Blakiston.

RICCI JV: *The development of gynaecological surgery and instruments from the hippocratic age to the antiseptic period*, Philadelphia, 1949, Blakiston.

RICHARDSON RG: *Surgery: old and new frontiers*, New York, 1968, Charles Scribner's Sons.

RICHARDSON RG: *The scalpel and the heart*, New York, 1970, Charles Scribner's Sons.

RING ME: *Dentistry: an illustrated history*, New York, 1985, Harry N Abrams and Mosby.

RIVINGTON W: *The medical profession*, Dublin, 1879, Fannin & Co.

ROBBINS G: *The breast: readings in the history of surgery*, Austin, Tex, 1984, Silvergirl.

ROBINSON J: *Biliary tract: readings in the history of surgery*, Austin, Tex, 1985, Silvergirl.

RODMAN JS: *History of the American Board of Surgery, 1937-1952*, Philadelphia, 1956, JB Lippincott.

ROGERS SL: *Primitive surgery: skills before science*, Springfield, Ill, 1985, Charles C Thomas.

ROHLFS H: *Die Chirurgischen Classiker Deutschlands* (2 vols), Leipzig, 1883-85, CL Hirschfeld.

ROSENBERG CE: *The care of strangers: the rise of America's hospital system*, New York, 1987, Basic Books.

ROSS JA: *The Edinburgh school of surgery after Lister*, Edinburgh, 1978, Churchill Livingstone.

RUCKER CW: *A history of the ophthalmoscope*, Rochester, Mn, 1971, private printing.

RUTKOW IM: History of surgery in the United States, *Surg Clin North Am* (special issue), Philadelphia, 1987, WB Saunders.

RUTKOW IM: *The history of surgery in the United States, 1775-1900*, I. Textbooks, monographs, and treatises, San Francisco, 1988, Norman Publishing.

RUTKOW IM: *Socioeconomics of surgery*, St Louis, 1989, Mosby.

RUTKOW IM: *The value of surgical history,* Arch Surg 126:953-956, 1991.

RUTKOW IM: *The history of surgery in the United States, 1775-1900.* II. Periodical and pamphlets, San Francisco, 1992, Norman Publishing.

SACHS E: *The history and development of neurological surgery,* New York, 1952, PB Hoeber.

SALEEBY CW: *Modern surgery and its making; a tribute to Lister-ism,* London, 1912, Herbert & Daniel.

SHAFER HB: *The American medical profession, 1783 to 1850,* New York, 1936, Columbia University Press.

SHANDS AR: *The early orthopaedic surgeons of America,* St Louis, 1970, Mosby.

SINGER CJ: *The evolution of anatomy,* London, 1925, Kegan Paul.

SINGER CJ: *A history of biology to about the year 1900,* London, 1959, Aberlard-Schuman.

SKINNER HA: *The origin of medical terms,* Baltimore, 1949, Williams & Wilkins.

SMITH E: *The Edwin Smith surgical papyrus* (2 vols), Chicago, 1930, University of Chicago Press.

SMITH S: The evolution of American surgery. In Bryant JD, Buck AH: *American practice of surgery* (8 vols), New York, 1906–1911, William Wood.

SORSBY A: *A short history of ophthalmology,* London, 1948, Staples Press.

SOUTH JF: *Memorials of the craft of surgery in England,* London, 1886, Cassel, (Edited by D Power).

SPARKMAN RS: *The Southern Surgical Association, the first 100 years, 1887-1987,* Philadelphia, 1989, JB Lippincott.

SPEERT H: *Obstetric and gynecologic milestones: essays in eponymy,* New York, 1958, Macmillan.

SPEERT H: *Iconographia gyniatrica: a pictorial history of gynecology and obstetrics,* Philadelphia, 1973, FA Davis.

SPEERT H: *Obstetrics and gynecology in America: a history,* Chicago, 1980, American College of Obstetricians and Gynecologists.

STARR P: *The social transformation of American medicine,* New York, 1982, Basic Books.

STARZL T: *Liver transplantation: readings in the history of surgery,* Austin, Tex, 1988, Silvergirl.

STEVENS A: *American pioneers in abdominal surgery,* Melrose, Mass, 1968, American Society of Abdominal Surgeons.

STEVENSON RS, GUTHRIE DJ: *A history of oto-laryngology,* Edinburgh, 1949, Livingstone.

STEWART FC: *The hospitals and surgeons of Paris,* New York, 1843, J & HG Langley.

THOMAS KB: *The development of anaesthetic apparatus,* Oxford, 1975, Blackwell.

THOMAS TG: Obstetrics and gynaecology. In *A century of American medicine, 1776-1876,* Philadelphia, 1876, Henry C Lea.

THOMPSON CJS: *The history and evolution of surgical instruments,* New York, 1942, Schuman.

THOMS H: *Classical contributions to obstetrics and gynecology,* Springfield, Ill, 1935, Charles C Thomas.

THORWALD J: *The century of the surgeon,* New York, 1957, Pantheon Books.

THORWALD J: *The triumph of surgery,* New York, 1960, Pantheon Books.

THORWALD J: *The patients,* New York, 1972, Harcourt, Brace, Jovanovich.

TIEMANN G: *American armamentarium chirurgicum,* New York, 1889, Private printing.

TILANUS CB: *Surgery: a hundred years ago,* London, 1925, Geoffrey Bles.

TRENDELENBERG F: *De Veterum Indorum Chirurgia,* Berolini, 1866, G Schade.

TRENDELENBERG F: *Die Ersten 25 Jahre Der Deutschen Gesellschaft Fur Chirurgie,* Berlin, 1923, J Springer.

TRUAX C: *The mechanics of surgery,* Chicago, 1899, Charles Truax.

VALENTIN B: *Geschichte Der Orthopadie,* Stuttgart, 1961, Georg Thieme.

WALKER AE: *A history of neurological surgery,* Baltimore, 1951, Williams & Wilkins.

WALL C: *The history of the Surgeons' Company, 1745-1800,* London, 1937, Hutchinson's.

WALLACE A: *The progress of plastic surgery: an introductory history,* Oxford, 1982, Oxford University Press.

WANGENSTEEN OH, WANGENSTEEN SD: *The rise of surgery from empiric craft to scientific discipline,* Minneapolis, 1978, University of Minnesota Press.

WELBOURN RB: *The history of endocrine surgery,* New York, 1990, Praeger.

WERSHUR LP: *Urology, from antiquity to the 20th century,* St Louis, 1970, Warren H Green.

WHIPPLE AO: *The evolution of surgery in the United States,* Springfield, Ill, 1963, Charles C Thomas.

WHIPPLE AO: *The story of wound healing and wound repair,* Springfield, Ill, 1963, Charles C Thomas.

WIDDESS JDH: *An account of the schools of surgery, Royal College of Surgeons, Dublin, 1789-1948,* Edinburgh, 1949, Livingstone.

WILKINS RH: *Neurosurgical classics,* New York, 1965, Johnson Reprint.

WRIGHT J: *A history of laryngology and rhinology,* Philadelphia, 1914, Lea & Febiger.

YOUNG A: *Scalpel, men who made surgery,* New York, 1956, Random House.

YOUNG JH: *Caesarean section, the history and development of the operation from earliest times,* London, 1944, HK Lewis.

YOUNG S: *The annals of the barber-surgeons of London, compiled from their records and other sources,* London, 1890, Blades, East & Blades.

ZEIS E: *Die Literatur Und Geschichte Der Plastischen Chirurgie,* Leipzig, 1863, W Engelmann.

ZIMMERMAN LM, VEITH I: *Great ideas in the history of surgery,* Baltimore, 1961, Williams & Wilkins.

539

INDEX

❧

A

Abbe, Robert, **492**
Abernethy, John, 277, **282**
Acrel, Olof, **298**
Acton, William, 348
Acupuncture chart, 70
Adair, Frank, 515
Adams, Robert, **377**
Addison, Thomas, **325**
Aesculapius, staff of, 38, 38
Aetius of Amida, 42, **47-48,**
    Tetrabiblion, 47-48, 47
Agnew, Cornelius Rea, **482**
Agnew, David Hayes, 453, **476**
Alanson, Edward, 277
Albarran, Joaquin, **427**, 531
Albee, Fred, 524
Albers-Schonberg, Heinrich, 524
Albert, Eduard, 397
Albinus, Bernard, 234
Albucasis, **57-59**
    Altasrif, 57-59, 58, 59
Alexander of Tralles, 42, **48-49**
Alexander, John, 529
Alexandrian surgery, 28-30
Allen, B B, 449
Allis, Oscar, **484**
Alt, Adolf, 522
American Academy of Facial, Plastic and Reconstructive Surgery, 525
American Association of Genito-Urinary Surgeons, 452
American Association of Obstetricians and Gynecologists, 518
American Association for Thoracic Surgery, 528
American Board of Colon and Rectal Surgery, 517
American Board of Neurological Surgery, 521
American Board of Obstetrics and Gynecology, 518
American Board of Ophthalmology, 522
American Board of Orthopaedic Surgery, 524
American Board of Otolaryngology, 525
American Board of Plastic Surgery, 526
American Board of Surgery, 513
American Board of Thoracic Surgery, 529
American Board of Urology, 531
American College of Obstetricians and Gynecologists, 518
American College of Surgeons, 508-509
American Gynecological Society, 452
American Journal of Ophthalmology, 555
American Journal of Urology, 531
American Ophthalmological Society, 452
American Orthopedic Association, 452
American Otological Society, 452
American Society for Head and Neck Surgery, 525
American Surgical Association, 452
American Urological Association, 531
Ammon, Freidrich von, **392**
Ammussat, Jean, **417**
Amputation, 146, 147, 169, 202-203, 289, 365, 375, 395, 435, 439
Amyand, Claudius, **278**
Anal abscess and fistula, 111-112, 112, 225, 517

Anatomical amphitheater, 159
Anatomy, 23-24, 41, 90, 107, 112-115, 127-140, 169, 188, 191, 235-238, 263, 268-270, 252-253, 287, 322-323
Andouille, Antoine, 243
Andrews, Edmund, 338, **480**
Andry, Nicholas, 232, **248**
Anel, Dominique, **247**, 256
Anesthesia, 94-95, 331-339, 332, 333, 442, 438, 445,
Aneurysm, 43, 276, 280
Angell, Henry, 450
Annals of Surgery, 452
Antisepsis and asepsis, 339-349, 345, 347, 491
Antyllus, **42-43**
Apothecaries, 358-359
Appendicitis, 489
Apprentice, surgical, 240-241
Aranzio, Guilio, 136, 161
Arceo, Francisco, 162
Archagathos of Sparta, 32
Archiv Fur Klinische Chirurgie, 393
Archiv Fur Ophthalmologie, 396, 522
Archiv Fur Pathologische Anatomie, 326
Aretaeus the Cappadocian, **37-38**
Arnald of Villanova, **105**
    Parabole, 105, 105
Arteriovenous aneurysm, 280
Asclepiades of Bithynia, **34**
Asclepiads, 21-22
Ashhurst, John, **486**
Atlee, John, **465**
Atlee, Washington, **471**
Auenbrugger, Leopold, 232
Autopsy, in nineteenth century, 324
Avenzoar, 60
Averroes, 60
Avicenna, **55-57**
    Canon, 56, 57, 83
Ayres, Daniel, **479**
Ayurvedic medicine, 66

B

Babcock, Wayne, 517, 529, 530
Bacteriology, 339-349
Baer, Benjamin, **490**
Baillie, Matthew, 232, 235-236, 325
Baker, George, 238-239
Baldwin, James, 519
Baldy, John, **499**
Balfour, Donald, 514
Ballance, Charles, 520, 521, 526
Ballenger, Edgar, 532
Ballingall, George, **375**
Bamberg Surgery, 92
Banister, John, **177-180**, 177
Bankart, Arthur Blundell, 524
Banting, Frederick, 506
Barany, Robert, 506, 526
Baraquer, Ignacio, 523
Barber-surgeon, 82, 85, 88, 91, 92, 101-102, 110-111, 122, 164-166, 169, 174-175, 180-181, 195, 208, 218, 220-221, 244, 261-262, 302,

---

Italic numbers indicate illustrations.
Boldface numbers indicate biographies.

541